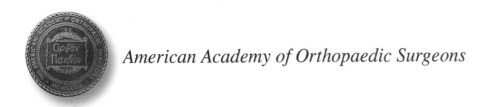

American Academy of Orthopaedic Surgeons

OKU
Orthopaedic Knowledge Update:

Sports Medicine

3

D1305045

American Academy of Orthopaedic Surgeons

OKU

Orthopaedic Knowledge Update:

Sports Medicine

3

Edited by
James G. Garrick, MD

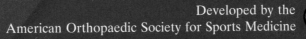
Developed by the
American Orthopaedic Society for Sports Medicine

Published 2004
by the American Academy of Orthopaedic Surgeons
6300 North River Road
Rosemont, IL 60018
1-800-626-6726

The material presented in Orthopaedic Knowledge Update Sports Medicine 3 has been made available by the American Academy of Orthopaedic Surgeons for educational purposes only. This material is not intended to present the only, or necessarily best, methods or procedures for the medical situations discussed, but rather is intended to represent an approach, view, statement, or opinion of the author(s) or producer(s), which may be helpful to others who face similar situations.

Some drugs or medical devices demonstrated in Academy courses or described in Academy print or electronic publications have not been cleared by the Food and Drug Administration (FDA) or have been cleared for specific uses only. The FDA has stated that it is the responsibility of the physician to determine the FDA clearance status of each drug or device he or she wishes to use in clinical practice.

Furthermore, any statements about commercial products are solely the opinion(s) of the author(s) and do not represent an Academy endorsement or evaluation of these products. These statements may not be used in advertising or for any commercial purpose.

Third Edition
Copyright © 2004 by the
American Academy of Orthopaedic Surgeons

ISBN 0-89203-332-0

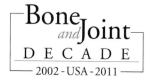

Acknowledgments

**Editorial Board,
OKU: Sports Medicine 3**

James G. Garrick, MD
Director, Center for Sports Medicine
Saint Francis Memorial Hospital
San Francisco, California

Thomas M. Best, MD, PhD, FACSM
Associate Professor of Orthopedics and Rehabilitation
 and Family Medicine
University of Wisconsin Medical School
Madison, Wisconsin

Marlene DeMaio, MD, CAPT, MC, USN
Department Head, Orthopaedics, Sports Medicine, and Podiatry
Assistant Professor, Department of Surgery
Uniformed Services University for the Health Sciences
Naval Medical Clinic
Annapolis, Maryland

Ben K. Graf, MD
Associate Professor, Department of Orthopaedics and Rehabilitation
University of Wisconsin Hospital
Madison, Wisconsin

W. Ben Kibler, MD
Medical Director, Sports Medicine Center
Lexington Clinic
Lexington, Kentucky

American Orthopaedic Society for Sports Medicine
Board of Directors, 2003-2004

William E. Garrett Jr, MD, PhD
 President
Thomas L. Wickiewicz, MD
 President-Elect
William A. Grana, MD, MPH
 Vice President
James R. Andrews
 Secretary
Bernard R. Bach Jr, MD
 Treasurer
Timothy N. Taft, MD
 Council of Delegates Chairman
Freddie H. Fu, MD
 Member At Large
Clarence L. Shields Jr, MD
 Past President
Claude T. Moorman, III, MD
 Member At Large
Peter J. Fowler, MD, FRCS
 Past President
Dean C. Taylor, MD
 Member At Large

American Academy of Orthopaedic Surgeons
Board of Directors, 2004

Robert W. Bucholz, MD
 President
Stuart L. Weinstein, MD
 First Vice-President
Richard F. Kyle, MD
 Second Vice-President
Edward A. Toriello, MD
 Treasurer
James H. Herndon, MD
 Past President
Vernon T. Tolo, MD
 Past President
Frederick M. Azar, MD
 Member-at-Large
Frances A. Farley, MD
 Member-at-Large
Laura L. Tosi, MD
 Member-at-Large
Oheneba Boachie-Adjei, MD
 Member-at-Large
Peter J. Mandell, MD
 Chair, Board of Councilors
Frank B. Kelly, MD
 Chair-Elect, Board of Councilors
Dwight W. Burney, III, MD
 Secretary, Board of Councilors
Glenn B. Pfeffer, MD
 Chair, Council of Musculoskeletal Specialty Societies
Mark C. Gebhardt, MD
 Chair-Elect, Council of Musculoskeletal Specialty Societies
Andrew N. Pollak, MD
 Secretary, Council of Musculoskeletal Specialty Societies
Leslie L. Altick
 Lay Member
Karen L. Hackett, FACHE, CAE
 (Ex Officio)

Staff

Mark Wieting
 Chief Education Officer
Marilyn L. Fox, PhD
 *Director, Department
 of Publications*
Lisa Claxton Moore
 Managing Editor
Keith Huff
 Senior Editor
Kathleen Anderson
 Medical Editor
Mary Steermann
 *Manager, Production and
 Archives*
David Stanley
 *Assistant Production
 Manager*

Sophie Tosta
 *Assistant Production
 Manager*
Mike Bujewski
 Database Coordinator
Susan Morritz Baim
 Production Coordinator
Dena M.Lozano
 *Desktop Publishing
 Assistant*
Courtney Astle
 Production Assistant
Karen Danca
 Production Assistant

Contributors

Christopher S. Ahmad, MD
Assistant Professor of Orthopaedic Surgery
College of Physicians and Surgeons
Columbia University
New York, New York

Annunziato Amendola, MD, FRCSC
Associate Professor, Orthopaedic Surgery
Department of Orthopaedic Surgery
University of Iowa
Iowa City, Iowa

Robert B. Anderson, MD
Chief, Foot and Ankle Service
Carolina's Medical Center
Miller Orthopaedic Clinic
Charlotte, North Carolina

Susanne L. Bathgate, MD
Assistant Professor, Division of Maternal
  Fetal Medicine
George Washington University
Washington, DC

Seth Baublitz, DO
Chief Resident, Orthopaedic Surgery
Department of Orthopaedic Surgery
Memorial Hospital
York, Pennsylvania

John S. Baxter, MD, JD
Director, Pentagon Flight Medicine Clinic
Arlington, Virginia

David T. Bernhardt, MD
Associate Professor
Department of Pediatrics
University of Wisconsin
Madison, Wisconsin

Thomas M. Best, MD, PhD, FACSM
Associate Professor of Orthopedics and
  Rehabilitation and Family Medicine
University of Wisconsin Medical School
Madison, Wisconsin

Anthony I. Beutler, MD
Director of Sports Medicine
Department of Family Practice
Malcolm Grow Medical Center
Andrews Air Force Base, Maryland

Robert T. Burks, MD
Professor of Orthopedic Surgery
Department of Orthopaedics
University of Utah
Salt Lake City, Utah

J.W. Thomas Byrd, MD
Nashville Sports Medicine &
  Orthopaedic Center
Nashville, Tennessee

R. Dana Carpenter, MS
Mechanical Engineering Department
Stanford University
Stanford, California

Dennis R. Carter, PhD
Professor and Biomedical Engineer
Rehabilitation R & D Center
VA Palo Alto Health Care Center
Palo Alto, California

E. Britton Chahine, MD
Assistant Professor, Obstetrics
  and Gynecology
George Washington University
Washington, DC

Brian J. Cole, MD, MBA
Midwest Orthopaedics
Rush-Presbyterian-St. Luke's
  Medical Center
Chicago, Illinois

George A. Corbett, MD
Fellow, Cincinnati Sportsmedicine and
Orthopaedic Center
Cincinnati, Ohio

Andrew J. Cosgarea, MD
Associate Professor of Orthopaedic Surgery
Director, Sports Medicine and
  Shoulder Surgery
Johns Hopkins University
Baltimore, Maryland

Marlene DeMaio, MD, CAPT, MC, USN
Department Head, Orthopaedics, Sports
  Medicine, and Podiatry
Assistant Professor, Department of Surgery
Uniformed Services University for
  the Health Sciences
Naval Medical Clinic
Annapolis, Maryland

Rebecca A. Demorest, MD
Pediatrics/Sports Medicine Fellow
Department of Pediatrics
University of Wisconsin-Madison
Madison, Wisconsin

William W. Dexter, MD, FACSM
Director, Sports Medicine
Department of Family Practice
Maine Medical Center
Portland, Maine

Pierre d'Hemecourt, MD
Children's Hospital
Division of Sports Medicine
Boston, Massachusetts

David C. Dome, MD
Lexington Sports Medicine Center
Lexington Clinic
Lexington, Kentucky

Laurie D. Donaldson, MD
Sports Medicine Fellow
Department of Family Practice
Maine Medical Center
Portland, Maine

Neal S. ElAttrache, MD
Associate and Fellowship Director
Sports Medicine
Kerlan-Jobe Orthopaedic Clinic
Los Angeles, California

Stephen Fealy, MD
Assistant Attending Orthopaedic Surgeon
Department of Sports Medicine
Hospital for Special Surgery
New York, New York

Jeff A. Fox, MD
Central States Orthopedic Specialists
Tulsa Sports Medicine and Wellness Center
Tulsa, Oklahoma

Matthew G. Friederichs, MD
Department of Orthopedics
University of Utah
Salt Lake City, Utah

Marc T. Galloway, MD
Cincinnati Sportsmedicine and
  Orthopaedic Center
Cincinnati, Ohio

Eugene G. Galvin, MD
San Francisco, California

Michael D. Gordon, MD
Clinical Institute in Orthopaedic Surgery
Tufts University School of Medicine
Department of Orthopaedic Surgery
New England Baptist Hospital
Boston, Massachusetts

Albert C. Hergenroeder, MD
Professor of Pediatrics
Chief, Section of Adolescent Medicine
  and Sports Medicine
Department of Pediatrics
Baylor College of Medicine
Houston, Texas

Michael H. Huo, MD
University of Texas SW
Dallas, Texas

William C. James III, MD
Midlands Orthopaedics
Columbia, South Carolina

Timothy S. Johnson, MD
Instructor
Department of Orthopaedic Surgery
Johns Hopkins School of Medicine
Baltimore, Maryland

W. Ben Kibler, MD
Medical Director
Sports Medicine Center
Lexington Clinic
Lexington, Kentucky

Marc R. Labbé, MD
Fellow
Mississippi Sports Medicine and
  Orthopaedic Center
Jackson, Mississippi

Gregory L. Landry, MD
Professor of Pediatrics
Head Medical Team Physician
University of Wisconsin Medical School
Madison, Wisconsin

John W. Larsen, MD
Oscar I. and Mildred S. Dodek Professor
Interim Chair, Department of Obstetrics and
  Gynecology
George Washington University
Washington, DC

Simon Lee, MD
Assistant Professor, Orthopaedic Surgery
Rush University Medical College
Chicago, Illinois

Susan L. Lewis, MD
Orthopedic Surgeon
Center for Sports Medicine
Saint Francis Memorial Hospital
San Francisco, California

Timothy A. Luke, MD
Clinical/Research Fellow
Department of Orthopaedics
Plancher Orthopaedics and Sports Medicine
New York, New York

C. Benjamin Ma, MD
Assistant Professor in Residence
Department of Orthopaedic Surgery
University of California-San Francisco
  Medical Center
San Francisco, California

Charles J. Macri, MD
Obstetrics and Gynecology
George Washington University
Washington, DC

Bert R. Mandelbaum, MD
Santa Monica, California

Stephen W. Marshall, PhD
Assistant Professor, Departments of Epi-
demiology
  and Orthopaedics
University of North Carolina
Chapel Hill, North Carolina

Gordon O. Matheson, MD, PhD
Professor and Chief
Division of Sports Medicine
Department of Orthopedic Surgery
Stanford University
Stanford, California

Edward R. McDevitt, MD
Chief of Surgical Services
Anne Arundel Medical Center
Annapolis, Maryland

Kathleen McHale, MD, FACS, COL, MC,
USA
Professor of Surgery
Chief, Orthopaedic Surgery
Department of Surgery
Uniformed Services University for the
  Health Sciences
Bethesda, Maryland

John McMullen, MS, ATC
Manager
Lexington Clinic Sports Medicine Center
Lexington Clinic
Lexington, Kentucky

Lyle J. Micheli, MD
Children's Hospital
Division of Sports Medicine
Boston, Massachusetts

Brett Miller, MD
Chief Resident, Orthopaedic Surgery
Department of Orthopaedics
University of Kansas
Kansas City, Kansas

Steve A. Mora, MD
Orange, California

Soheil Najibi, MD, PhD
Sports Medicine Fellow
Department of Orthopaedic Surgery
University of Iowa
Iowa City, Iowa

Kevin D. Plancher, MD, MS
Associate Clinical Professor
Department of Orthopaedics
Albert Einstein College of Medicine
New York, New York

Margot Putukian, MD, FACSM
Director of Athletic Medicine
Princeton University McCosh Health Center
Princeton, New Jersey

Scott A. Rodeo, MD
Associate Professor
Hospital for Special Surgery
New York, New York
Robert Sallis, MD, FACSM
Kaiser Permanente
Family Medicine and Sports Medicine
Rancho Cucamonga, California

Felix H. Savoie III, MD
Co-Director, Upper Extremity Service
Mississippi Sports Medicine and
  Orthopaedic Center
Jackson, Mississippi

Benjamin Shaffer, MD
Director, DC Sports Medicine Institute
Washington, DC

Mark E. Steiner, MD
Team Physician, Harvard University
Sports Medicine Section
New England Baptist Hospital
Boston, Massachusetts

Dean C. Taylor, MD, COL, MC, USA
Director, United States Army Joint and
  Soft Tissue Trauma (Sports Medicine)
  Fellowship
Keller Army Community Hospital
West Point, New York

Darryl B. Thomas, MD, MAJ, MC, USA
Orthopaedic Surgeon, Sports Medicine
  Fellow
Orthopaedic Surgery
Keller Army Community Hospital
West Point, New York

Joseph S. Torg, MD
Professor
Department of Orthopedics
Temple University School of Medicine
Philadelphia, Pennsylvania

Hechmi Toumi, PhD
Research Associate
Department of Orthopaedics and
  Rehabilitation
Department of Family Medicine
University of Wisconsin Medical School
Madison, Wisconsin

Lisa Wasserman, MD, FRCSC
Sports Medicine and Foot and Ankle Fellow
Department of Orthopaedics
University of Iowa
Iowa City, Iowa

Serena J. Young, MD
Fellow of Sports Medicine
Department of (Pediatric) Sports Medicine
Children's Hospital
Boston, Massachusetts

Preface

For more than 30 years, sports medicine has undergone gradual, evolutionary changes. Arthroscopy, imaging techniques, accelerated and aggressive rehabilitation, and finally, a review of long-term results of treatments have substantially changed the way we practice. Recently, however, changes of a more revolutionary nature are occurring. With the creation of an "official" curriculum for orthopaedic sports medicine fellowships (available for download at http://www.aossm.org) and the examination for Certificate of Special Qualification, the scope of "sports medicine" has been officially broadened. (The Orthopaedic Sports Medicine Curriculum for American Orthopaedic Society for Sports Medicine members appears in the Appendix.)

The goal of Orthopaedic Knowledge Update is to provide a useful, comprehensive, and accessible synthesis of the latest information and knowledge available. In addition to addressing this charge, we have attempted to broaden the base of "sports medicine" substantially beyond musculoskeletal problems. Issues such as eating disorders, osteoporosis, and the use of performance-enhancing substances are all topics about which we are assumed to be knowledgeable; thus, the expansion beyond musculoskeletal issues. Nonetheless, we have striven to present the salient advances in the more traditional aspects of orthopaedic sports medicine as well.

Our goal was to produce a volume dealing with sports medicine much as the *Journal of the American Academy of Orthopaedic Surgeons* does with the broader topic of orthopaedic surgery. Added to reviews of salient advances in traditional topics, we have attempted to temper enthusiasm with the writing and editing of mature, experienced practitioners who are acknowledged experts in the field.

Producing material for this volume is an onerous task. For the most part, the various chapter authors and section editors already had more than enough on their plates. For the section editors, Drs. Best, Kibler, Graf, and DeMaio, creation of this volume is especially prodigious. They recruited chapter authors, provided outlines, and reviewed and edited—sometimes on multiple occasions—every manuscript, in addition to producing their own chapters. Although we as orthopaedic surgeons are expected to give back something to our specialty, those from other disciplines had no such obligation, yet nearly one quarter of the chapter authors and one of the section editors (Dr. Best), all from other disciplines, rose to the occasion. I am eternally grateful for the time and expertise provided by all of the authors as well as the time, effort, and dogged determination of the Academy staff.

James G. Garrick, MD
Editor

Table of Contents

Section 1: Injuries of the Head and Spine

Section Editors: James G. Garrick, MD
Thomas M. Best, MD, PhD, FACSM

Section 2: Injuries of the Upper Extremity

Section Editor: W. Ben Kibler, MD

Section 3: Injuries of the Lower Extremity

Section Editor: Ben K. Graf, MD

Section 4: Systemic Injuries

Section Editors: James G. Garrick, MD
Thomas M. Best, MD, PhD, FACSM

Section 5: Medical Disorders in Athletes

Section Editor: Thomas M. Best, MD, PhD, FACSM

Section 6: Selected Sports-Related Issues
Section Editors: Marlene DeMaio, MD, CAPT, MC, USN
Thomas M. Best, MD, PhD, FACSM

Section 1

Injuries of the Head and Spine

Section Editors:
James G. Garrick, MD
Thomas M. Best, MD, PhD, FACSM

Chapter 1

Cervical Spine Injuries

Joseph S. Torg, MD

Introduction

Although all injuries require careful attention, the evaluation and management of cervical spine injuries require particular caution. The actual or potential involvement of the nervous system creates a high-risk situation in which the margin for error is low. An accurate diagnosis is imperative because the clinical picture does not always represent the seriousness of the injury at hand. A patient with an intracranial hemorrhage may initially have minimal symptoms yet can follow a precipitous downhill course, whereas a less severe injury, such as neurapraxia of the cervical spinal cord that is associated with alarming paresthesias and paralysis, will resolve swiftly and allow a return to activity. Although severe injuries are rare, the low incidence coincidentally results in little, if any, treatment experience for medical staff. Therefore, it is helpful to be familiar with guidelines for the prevention, classification, evaluation, management, and rehabilitation of injuries that occur to the cervical spine and related neural structures as a result of participation in competitive and recreational activities.

Diagnosis and Treatment

Cervical spine injuries can involve the bony vertebrae; intervertebral disks; ligamentous supporting structures; spinal cord, roots, and peripheral nerves; or any combination of these structures. Cervical spine injuries range from the cervical sprain syndrome to fracture-dislocation with permanent quadriplegia. Although severe injuries with neural involvement occur infrequently, those responsible for the emergency and subsequent care of patients with cervical spine injuries should possess a basic understanding of the variety of problems that can occur. A list of the various injuries that can occur to the cervical spine and related structures appears in Table 1.

Nerve Root and Brachial Plexus Injuries

Pinch-stretch neurapraxia of the cervical nerve roots or brachial plexus (also known as the burner syndrome) are the most common cervical injuries and the most poorly understood. After experiencing blunt force to the head, neck, or shoulder, patients typically report a sharp burning pain on the involved side that may radiate into the shoulder and down the arm to the hand. Weakness and paresthesia in the involved extremity lasting from several seconds to several minutes may accompany the injury. Characteristically, there is weakness of shoulder abduction (deltoid), elbow flexion (biceps), and external humeral rotation (spinati). The key to the nature of this lesion is its short duration and the presence of a full, pain-free range of neck motion. Although the majority of these injuries are short lived, they are worrisome because plexus axonotmesis occasionally occurs. Nonetheless, young patients may resume activity if the paresthesia completely abates, if full muscle strength in the intrinsic muscles of the shoulder and upper extremities is present, and most importantly, if full, pain-free range of cervical motion is maintained.

The etiology of burner syndrome has been attributed to two basic mechanisms: brachial plexus stretch and nerve root compression. Electrodiagnostic evidence indicates that stretch injuries to the brachial plexus typically involve only the upper trunk. Classification of these injuries is based on the staging system of Seddon. Neurapraxia, the mildest form of injury, represents a reversible aberration in axonal function. Focal demyelinization can occur, producing an electrophysiologic conduction block or conduction slowing. Complete recovery usually occurs immediately or within 2 weeks. Axonotmesis is an injury in which the axon and myelin sheath are disrupted, but the epineurium remains intact. Wallerian degeneration occurs distal to the point of injury; functional recovery may occur, but it can be incomplete and unpredictable. The most severe injury, neurotmesis, is rarely seen in athletes and results in complete disruption of the nerve. The prognosis for patients with neurotmesis is poor and recovery generally does not occur. Many of these injuries are mixed lesions, and classification using Seddon's system serves mainly to aid in describing a potential recovery course and prognosis.

Brachial plexus injuries are more likely to occur in younger patients with poorly developed neck muscula-

TABLE 1 | Injuries of the Cervical Spine and Related Structures

Nerve root brachial plexus injury

Stable cervical sprain

Muscular strain

Nerve root brachial plexus axonotmesis

Intervertebral disk injury (narrowing herniation) without neurologic deficit

Stable cervical fractures without neurologic deficit

Subluxations without neurologic deficit

Unstable fractures without neurologic deficit

Dislocations without neurologic deficit

Intervertebral disk herniation with neurologic deficit

Unstable fracture with neurologic deficit

Dislocation with neurologic deficit

ture. These are usually traction injuries resulting from lateral neck flexion away from the involved area and shoulder depression to the side of involvement. The point of brachial plexus injury is most likely to be a stretch injury occurring at Erb's point. Neck pain can be present but is usually not a prominent feature. When present, however, cervical spine radiographs are necessary. Pain and paresthesias involving the arm and shoulder are typically transient. On clinical examination, the result of Spurling's test (passive extension and lateral flexion of the head and neck) is negative. Weakness typically involves the deltoid, spinati, and biceps; if not evident on initial clinical examination, a follow-up examination is necessary.

Root lesions result from compression of the nerve root or dorsal root ganglion in the intervertebral foramen, and they are generally associated with radiologic evidence of cervical disk disease and/or developmental stenosis. In football players, these injuries usually occur when the player reaches the college or professional level. Hyperextension with lateral neck flexion is the common mechanism of injury. Neck pain and a decreased cervical range of motion may be present. On clinical examination, the result of Spurling's test is positive. Plain radiographs may be normal or demonstrate loss of normal cervical lordosis and changes consistent with degenerative disk disease. MRI is indicated for patients with a persistent neurologic deficit and prolonged or recurrent symptoms and will demonstrate either acute disk herniation or degenerative disk disease with asymmetric disk bulging. Patients often have developmental spinal stenosis, degenerative disk disease, and asymmetric disk bulging that result in root irritation with cervical hyperextension.

One study investigated the relationship between burner syndrome and cervical stenosis in patients age 15 to 18 years. A review of 69 cervical spine radiographs demonstrated a significant decrease in the Pavlov ratio

(the ratio of the AP diameter of the spinal cord to the AP diameter of the vertebral body) when compared with the control group. The authors hypothesized that developmental cervical stenosis predisposes an athlete to experience burner syndrome because of concomitant foraminal narrowing with nerve root compression.

Persistence of either paresthesia, weakness, limitation of cervical motion, or recurrent episodes requires that patients be protected from further exposure and undergo neurologic, electromyographic, and radiographic evaluation. A complete electromyographic examination, including both nerve conduction studies and a needle electrode examination, may be helpful. These studies should be delayed for 3 to 4 weeks from the time of the initial injury. Nerve conduction studies should include routine conduction and sensory nerve action potential evaluations. Electrode evaluation of the cervical spine musculature will help differentiate between preganglionic root injuries and plexus pathologies.

The signs and symptoms of the burner syndrome are transient and resolve within minutes. In patients whose pain and paresthesias abate, a normal neurologic examination and, most important, a full, pain-free range of cervical motion are required before returning to activity. Patients also must demonstrate normal strength on clinical examination before they can return to activity. Those patients who have recurrent symptoms without weakness require careful follow-up; continued symptoms associated with weakness preclude further participation in athletic activity.

In brachial plexus injuries, prevention is based on an aggressive neck and shoulder strengthening program. Neck rolls, the use of devices such as the cowboy collar, and high-profile shoulder pads also help prevent injuries, the latter by limiting the extent of lateral flexion and extension.

Electrodiagnostic studies may be helpful but are not mandatory in the management of burner syndrome resulting from a brachial plexus injury. It has been demonstrated that although there is no correlation between initial physical findings and the results of electrodiagnostic testing, evidence of muscular weakness at 72 hours after the injury does correlate with a positive electromyogram. Importantly, it has been reported that electromyography findings continue to appear long after weakness seems to have resolved in clinical examinations; therefore, abnormal electromyography findings should not be used as a criterion for exclusion from participation in athletic activity.

Acute Cervical Sprain Syndrome

An acute cervical sprain is a collision injury that occurs frequently in contact sports. Patients with acute cervical sprain syndrome report "jamming" the neck with subsequent pain localized to the cervical area. These patients typically have limited cervical spine motion without radiation of pain or paresthesias. Neurologic examination is negative, and radiographs are normal.

Stable cervical sprains and strains eventually resolve with or without treatment. The presence of a serious injury initially should be ruled out by determining the range of cervical motion and performing a thorough neurologic examination. Range of motion is evaluated by having the patient actively nod the head, touch the chin to the chest, extend the neck maximally, touch the chin to the left shoulder, touch the chin to the right shoulder, touch the left ear to the left shoulder, and touch the right ear to the right shoulder. If the patient is unwilling or unable to perform these maneuvers actively while standing erect, the evaluation of the range of motion should proceed no further. Patients with persistent paresthesia, weakness, or less than a full, pain-free range of cervical motion should wear a protective soft collar and cease participation in the inciting activity. The subsequent evaluation should include appropriate radiographic studies, including flexion and extension views to demonstrate fractures or instability.

In general, the treatment of athletes with acute cervical sprain syndrome should be tailored to the degree of severity of the injury. Immobilization of the neck using a soft collar and use of analgesics and anti-inflammatory agents until a full, spasm-free range of neck motion is regained is usually appropriate. Patients with a history of a collision injury, pain, and limited cervical motion should have routine cervical spine radiographs. In addition, lateral flexion and extension radiographs are indicated after the acute symptoms subside. Marked limitation of cervical motion, persistent pain, or radicular symptoms or findings may require MRI to rule out an intervertebral disk injury.

Intervertebral Disk Injuries

The acute herniation of a cervical intervertebral disk associated with neurologic findings rarely occurs as an isolated entity in athletes. However, an acute onset of transient quadriplegia in athletes who have experienced head impact but have no evidence of injury on cervical spine radiographs should prompt consideration of an acute rupture of a cervical intervertebral disk. Acute anterior spinal cord injury syndrome, as described by Schneider, may be observed in patients with instability associated with acute disk herniation. The author reports that acute anterior cervical spinal cord injury syndrome can be characterized as an immediate acute paralysis of all four extremities with a loss of pain and temperature to the level of the lesion; posterior column sensation of motion, position, vibration, and part of touch are preserved. The pressure of the disk is exerted on the anterior and lateral columns, whereas the posterior columns are protected by the denticulate ligaments. MRI or a CT

myelogram should be performed to substantiate the diagnosis. Anterior diskectomy and interbody fusion for patients with neurologic involvement or persistent disability because of pain should be considered.

Chronic cervical intervertebral disk injury without frank herniation or neurologic findings occurs with considerable frequency in athletes. Neck pain and limited cervical spine motion are associated with a history of injury. Radiographs may demonstrate disk space narrowing and marginal osteophytes. MRI frequently demonstrates evidence of disk bulge without herniation. In general, management is conservative and includes withholding permission to engage in athletic activity until the patient is asymptomatic and has regained a full range of cervical spine motion.

Cervical Vertebral Subluxation Without Fracture

Axial compression-flexion injuries incurred by striking an object with the top of the head can result in disruption of the posterior soft-tissue supporting elements, with angulation and anterior translation of the superior cervical vertebrae. Fractures of the bony elements do not appear on diagnostic radiographs, and the patient has no neurologic deficit. Flexion-extension radiographs demonstrate instability of the cervical spine at the involved level, which is manifested by motion, anterior intervertebral disk space narrowing, anterior angulation and displacement of the vertebral body, and fanning of the spinous processes. Demonstrable instability on lateral flexion-extension radiographs in young, vigorous patients requires aggressive treatment. When soft-tissue disruption occurs without an associated fracture, instability will likely result despite conservative treatment. When anterior subluxation greater than 20% of the vertebral body is caused by disruption of the posterior supporting structures, a posterior cervical fusion is recommended.

Cervical Fractures or Dislocations

Fractures or dislocations of the cervical spine may be stable or unstable and may or may not be associated with neurologic deficit. When fracture or disruption of the soft-tissue supporting structure violates or threatens to violate the integrity of the spinal cord, it is imperative to implement the following management and treatment principles: (1) protection of the spinal cord from further injury, (2) expeditious reduction, (3) attainment of rapid and secure stability, and (4) early initiation of a rehabilitation program.

Neurologic deficits commonly occur after initial injury when a patient with an unstable lesion is carelessly manipulated during transportation to a medical facility or subsequently managed inappropriately in a way that results in further encroachment on the spinal cord. Therefore, the first goal of treatment should be protection of the spinal cord and nerve roots from further injury.

TABLE 2 | Treatment Indications for Achieving Stability in Cervical Spine Fractures and Dislocations

Injury	Treatment
Stable compression fractures of the vertebral body Undisplaced fractures of the lamina or lateral masses Soft-tissue injuries without detectable neurologic deficit	Traction and subsequent protection with a cervical brace until healing occurs
Stable, reduced facet dislocations without neurologic deficit	Conservative treatment in a halo jacket brace until healing has been demonstrated by negative lateral flexion-extension radiographs
Unstable cervical spine fractures or fracture-dislocations without neurologic deficit	Either surgical or nonsurgical treatment to ensure stability
Unstable injuries without neurologic deficits and late instability following closed treatment and flexion-rotation injuries with unreduced locked facets	Surgical stabilization absolutely indicated
Unstable injuries without neurologic deficit and anterior subluxation >20%, certain atlantoaxial fractures or dislocations, and unreduced vertical compression injuries with neck flexion	Surgical stabilization relatively indicated
Cervical spine fractures with complete cord lesions	Reduction followed by stabilization by closed or open means, as indicated
Cervical spine fractures with incomplete cord lesions	Reduction followed by careful evaluation for surgical intervention

Once appropriate radiographs have been obtained and qualified orthopaedic and neurosurgical personnel are available, the malalignment of the cervical spine should be reduced as quickly and gently as possible. This will effectively decompress the spinal cord. A bulbocavernosus reflex, produced by pulling on the urethral catheter, indicates that spinal shock has worn off. Triggering this reflex stimulates the trigone of the bladder and produces a reflex contraction of the anal sphincter around the examiner's gloved finger. Although a bulbocavernosus reflex is generally a sign that no further neurologic recovery will occur below the level of injury, this is not always true and does not give license for the examination to proceed in an expectant manner. If maximum recovery is to be achieved, malalignment or dislocation of the cervical spine associated with quadriparesis should be reduced as quickly as possible by whatever means necessary.

The use of parenteral corticosteroids to decrease the inflammatory reactions of the injured spinal cord and surrounding soft-tissue structures is indicated in the management of acute cervical spinal cord injuries. The efficacy of methylprednisolone in improving neurologic recovery when given within the first 8 hours has been recently demonstrated. The recommended dose is a 30-mg/kg bolus of methylprednisolone administered intravenously followed by an infusion of 5.4 mg/kg/h for 23 hours.

The third goal of managing fractures and dislocations of the cervical spine is to ensure rapid and secure stability to prevent residual deformity and instability with associated pain and the possibility of further trauma to the neural elements. The method of immobilization depends on the postreduction status of the injury. The indications for nonsurgical and surgical methods for achieving stability in the management of cervical spine fractures and dislocations are summarized in Table 2. A more specific categorization of injuries to the cervical spine has recently been developed that divides injuries into those that occur in the upper cervical spine (C1-C2), middle cervical spine (C3-C4), or lower cervical spine (C5-C7). The differentiation is based on characteristic injury patterns observed at each level.

Upper Cervical Spine Fractures and Dislocations

Upper cervical spine fractures and dislocations involve C1 through C3. Although they rarely occur in sports, several specific injuries that do occur to the upper cervical vertebrae deserve mention. The transverse and alar ligaments are responsible for atlantoaxial stability. If these structures are ruptured from a flexion injury with translation of C1 anteriorly, the spinal cord can be impinged between a posterior aspect of the odontoid process and the posterior rim of C1. Patients with this type of injury report head trauma and neck pain (particularly with nodding) and may or may not have spinal cord symptoms. Lateral radiographs of the C1-2 articulation show increase of the atlanto-dens interval (ADI), which is normally 3 mm in adults. With transverse ligament rupture, the ADI may increase up to 10 to 12 mm depending on the status of the alar and accessory ligaments. The increase in the ADI, however, may only be seen when the neck is flexed. Atlantoaxial fusion may be the "conservative" treatment for this lesion.

Fractures of the atlas, first described by Jefferson, may be either posterior arch fractures or burst fractures. Posterior arch fractures are the more common of these two types, and satisfactory fibrous or bony union can be achieved with a brace support. Burst fractures result from an axial load transmitted to the occipital condyles, which then disrupt the integrity of both the anterior and posterior arches of the atlas. Radiographs demonstrate bilateral symmetric overhang of the lateral masses of the atlas in relation to the axis, with an increase in the paradontoid space on the open mouth view. Clinically, patients with burst fractures characteristically experience pain when nodding the head. Burst fractures are considered stable when the combined lateral overhang of the atlas measures less than 7 mm. When the transverse diameter of the atlas is 7 mm or greater than that of the axis, a transverse ligament rupture should be suspected.

Fractures of the odontoid are typically classified into three types. Type I, rare and stable lesions, are avulsions of the tip of the odontoid at the site of the attachment of the alar ligament. Type II are fractures through the base at or just below the level of the superior articular processes. Type III are fractures of the body of the axis. When the odontoid is not displaced, planograms may be required to identify the fracture. Although the mechanism of odontoid fractures has not been clearly delineated, they appear to be caused by head impact. Routine cervical spine radiographic studies for patients with odontoid fractures should include the open mouth view to identify lesions involving the odontoid as well as the atlas. If there is no radiographic evidence of injury and a fracture in this area is suspected, a CT scan or bending films may further delineate pathologic changes in this area.

Managing type II fractures is challenging. It has been reported that 36% to 50% of these fractures treated initially with a cervical brace fail to unite. Current management involves more aggressive surgical treatment with early stabilization. Fibrous unions or nonunited fractures of the odontoid must be stabilized surgically when they are noted to be unstable on flexion and extension views. Stabilization may be achieved either through posterior C1-2 wire fixation and fusion or anterior odontoid screw fixation.

Fractures through the arch of the axis, which are relatively rare, are also known as traumatic spondylolisthesis of C2 or hangman's fractures. The mechanism of injury for this type of fracture is generally recognized to be hyperextension. Fractures through the arch of the axis are inherently unstable, but they have been shown to heal with predictable regularity without surgical intervention.

Middle Cervical Spine Fractures and Dislocations
Although rare and generally not associated with fractures, acute traumatic lesions of the cervical spine at the C3-4 level have been reported to occur in football players who experience axial loading of the cervical spine. These lesions are classified as follows: (1) acute rupture of the C3-4 intervertebral disk, (2) anterior subluxation of C3 on C4, (3) unilateral dislocation of the joint between the articular processes, and (4) bilateral dislocation of the joint between the articular processes.

An episode of transient quadriplegia in an athlete who has experienced head impact but has no radiographic evidence of injury suggests acute rupture of the C3-4 intervertebral disk. The syndrome of acute anterior spinal cord injury may be observed. A cervical myelogram or MRI will substantiate the diagnosis. Anterior diskectomy and interbody fusion may be the most effective treatment of this lesion.

Anterior subluxation of C3 on C4 is caused by a shearing force through the intervertebral disk space that disrupts the interspinous ligament and the posterior supporting structure. Radiographs of patients with this type of injury demonstrate narrowing of the intervertebral disk space, anterior angulation and translation of C3 on C4, an increase in the distance between the spinous processes of the two vertebrae, and instability without fracture of the bony elements. Spinal fusion may be necessary for adequate stabilization in these patients; this is in contrast to cervical spine instability caused by a fracture in which adequate reduction and subsequent bony healing result in adequate stabilization. When patients have posterior instability, posterior fusion is preferable to anterior interbody fusion.

Unilateral facet dislocation at C3-4 may result in immediate quadriparesis. This injury involves the intervertebral disk space, the interspinous ligament, the posterior ligamentous supporting structures, and the one facet with resulting rotatory dislocation of C3 on C4 without fracture. In patients with unilateral facet dislocation at C3-4, strong skeletal traction does not usually yield a successful reduction, and closed manipulation under general anesthesia or open reduction is necessary to disengage the locked joint between the articular processes. Bilateral facet dislocation at the C3-4 level is a grave injury. Skeletal traction may not reduce the lesion, and the prognosis for this injury is poor.

Lower Cervical Spine Fractures and Dislocations
Lower cervical spine fractures or dislocations are those involving C4 through C7. The majority of fractures or dislocations of the cervical spine resulting from various athletic endeavors, with or without neurologic involvement, involve this segment. Although unilateral and bilateral facet dislocations occur, they are relatively rare. The vast majority of severe, athletically incurred cervical spine injuries are fractures of the vertebral body with varying degrees of compression or comminution.

Unilateral Facet Dislocations
Unilateral facet dislocations are caused by axial loading and flexion-rotation. The dislocation may be truly ligamentous without any associated vertebral fracture. In such instances, the facet dislocation is stable and is usually associated with neurologic involvement. Radiographs of patients with unilateral facet dislocations demonstrate less

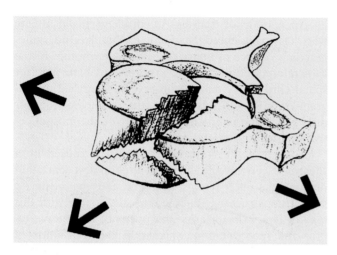

Figure 1 The axial load teardrop fracture is characterized by an anteroinferior corner teardrop fracture, a sagittal vertebral body fracture, and a fracture through the posterior arch. *(Reproduced with permission from Torg JS, Pavlov H, O'Neill MJ, Nichols CE Jr, Sennett B: The axial load teardrop fracture: A biomechanical, clinical and roentgenographic analysis. Am J Sports Med 1991;19:355-364.)*

than a 50% anterior shift of the superior vertebra on the inferior vertebra. Attempts should be made to reduce the facet dislocation by skeletal traction; however, as with similar lesions of the C3-4 level, it may not be possible to achieve a closed reduction with these types of injuries, in which instance open reduction under direct vision through a posterior approach with supplemental posterior element bone grafting should be done.

Bilateral Facet Dislocations

Bilateral facet dislocations are almost always associated with neurologic involvement and a high incidence of permanent quadriplegia. Lateral radiographs of patients with bilateral facet dislocations demonstrate greater than a 50% anterior displacement of the superior vertebral body on the inferior vertebral body. Immediate treatment, as previously described, consists of closed reduction with skeletal traction. Bilateral facet dislocations are generally reducible by skeletal traction and are stabilized with a halo brace and posterior fusion. Instability is directly related to the ease with which the lesion is reduced: the easier it is to reduce, the easier it is to redislocate. If skeletal traction is unsuccessful, either manipulative reduction under sedation or general anesthesia or open reduction under direct vision is recommended. When the dislocation is reduced in a closed procedure and the reduction is maintained, a halo brace should be used for 8 to 12 weeks to achieve immobilization. Corrective bracing should then continue for an additional 4 weeks.

Vertebral Body Compression Fractures

Compression fractures of the vertebral body are a result of axial loading and can be classified into five types.

Type I vertebral body compression fractures are simple wedge or vertebral end-plate compression fractures of the cervical vertebrae. These are common injuries that respond well to conservative management and rarely if ever are associated with neurologic involvement. It is important to differentiate these type I vertebral body compression fractures from compression fractures that are associated with disruption of the posterior element soft-tissue supporting structures. The latter type are unstable and are frequently associated with neurologic involvement, including quadriplegia.

Type II vertebral body compression fractures are isolated anterior-inferior vertebral body or axial load teardrop fractures with intact posterior elements, no displacement, and no neurologic involvement. Type II vertebral body compression fractures are relatively stable and may be treated conservatively.

Type III vertebral body compression fractures are comminuted burst vertebral body fractures with intact posterior elements and displacement of bony fragments into the vertebral canal that may put the spinal cord at risk. Late settling of type III vertebral body compression fractures with deformity can occur. Surgical stabilization is usually recommended.

Type IV vertebral body compression fractures are axial-load, three-part, two-plane vertebral body fractures that have three fracture parts: (1) anterior-inferior vertebral body teardrop fracture, (2) sagittal vertebral body fracture, and (3) disruption of the posterior neural arch (Figure 1). This lesion is unstable and is almost always associated with quadriplegia. Careful evaluation of routine AP radiographs or CT scans in patients with this type of injury is necessary to appreciate the sagittal vertebral body fracture, a finding with a grave prognosis.

Type V vertebral body compression fractures are three-part, two-plane compression fractures that are associated with disruption of posterior elements of an adjacent vertebra. Type V vertebral body compression fractures are extremely unstable.

Cervical Spinal Cord Neurapraxia and Transient Quadriplegia

The typical clinical scenario of cervical spinal cord neurapraxia with transient quadriplegia involves an athlete who experiences an acute transient neurologic episode of cervical spinal cord origin with sensory changes that may be associated with motor paresis involving both arms, both legs, or all four extremities after forced hyperextension, hyperflexion, or axial loading of the cervical spine. Sensory changes include burning pain, numbness, tingling, or loss of sensation; motor changes consist of weakness or complete paralysis. The episodes are transient, and complete recovery usually occurs in 10 to 15 minutes, although in some cases gradual resolution does not occur for 36 to 48 hours. Except for burning paresthesia, neck pain is not present at the time of injury, and patients typically experience complete return of motor function and full pain-free range of cervical motion. Routine radiographs of the cervical spine show no evidence of fracture or dislocation; however, a demonstrable degree of cervical spinal stenosis is usually present.

The most commonly used methods of determining the sagittal diameter of the spinal canal involve measuring the distance between the middle of the posterior surface of the vertebral body and the nearest point on the spinolaminar line. Using this technique, the average sagittal diameter of the spinal canal from the fourth to the sixth cervical vertebra is 18.5 mm (range, 14.2 to 23 mm) at a target distance of 1.4 meters. Values of less than 14 mm are uncommon and fall below the standard deviation for any cervical segment. Other measurements reported in the literature vary greatly. Variations in the landmarks and methods used to determine the sagittal distance as well as different target distances for radiography have resulted in inconsistencies in normal values. Therefore, the standard method of measurement for spinal stenosis is questionable.

The ratio method is an alternative method for determining the sagittal diameter of the spinal canal. Devised by Pavlov and associates, it compares the standard method of measurement of the spinal canal with the AP width of the vertebral body at the midpoint of the corresponding vertebral body (Figure 2). The ratio method compensates for variations in radiographic technique (the sagittal diameter of both the canal and the vertebral body are affected similarly by magnification factors, and the results are statistically significant). In one large study using the ratio method of determining the dimension of the spinal canal, a ratio of the spinal canal to the vertebral body of less than 0.80 was indicative of spinal canal narrowing. The ratio of the AP diameter of the spinal canal to that of the vertebral body is a consistent and reliable way to determine cervical stenosis in patients who have experienced an episode of cervical cord neurapraxia. However, the ratio has a very low predictive value and should not be used as a screening tool. Also, it has been observed that in patients with large vertebral bodies a ratio of 0.8 or less may occur in the presence of a normal size canal.

Cervical spinal cord neurapraxia is caused by diminution of the AP diameter of the spinal canal, either alone or in association with intervertebral disk herniation, degenerative changes, posttraumatic instability, or congenital anomalies. In patients with developmental cervical stenosis, forced hyperflexion or hyperextension of the cervical spine further decreases the caliber of an already narrow canal, which is explained by the pincer mechanism as described by Penning (Figure 3). In patients whose stenosis is associated with osteophytes or a herniated disk, direct pressure can occur, again when

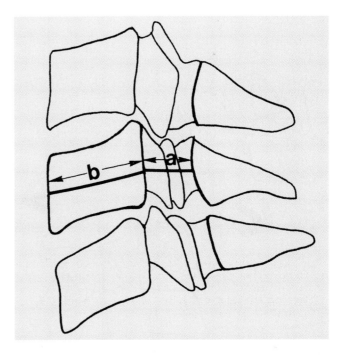

Figure 2 The ratio of the spinal canal to the vertebral body is the distance from the midpoint of the posterior aspect of the vertebral body to the nearest point on the corresponding spinolaminar line (a) divided by the anteroposterior width of the vertebral body (b). *(Reproduced with permission from Torg JS, Pavlov H, Genuario SE, et al: Neurapraxia of the cervical spinal cord with transient quadriplegia. J Bone Joint Surg Am 1986;68:1354-1370.)*

the spine is forced into extremes of flexion and extension. With an abrupt but brief decrease in the AP diameter of the spinal canal, the cervical cord is mechanically compressed, causing transient interruption of either motor or sensory function or both distal to the lesion. The neurologic aberration that results is transient and completely reversible.

The magnitude of the problem is greater than may be expected. Specifically, the reported incidence of transient paresthesia in all four extremities was 6 per 10,000 patients, whereas the reported incidence of paresthesia associated with transient quadriplegia was 1.3 per 10,000 in the one football season surveyed. From these data, it may be concluded that the prevalence of this problem is relatively high and that an awareness of the etiology, manifestations, and appropriate principles of management is warranted.

After an episode of cervical spinal cord neurapraxia with or without transient quadriplegia, the first issue raised usually involves the advisability of restricting activity. To address this issue, interviews were conducted of a cohort of 117 athletes who had cervical spine injuries associated with complete permanent quadriplegia when playing football. None of these patients recalled a prodromal experience of transient motor paresis. Conversely, none of the patients in this series who had experienced transient neurologic episodes subsequently sustained an injury that resulted in permanent neurologic

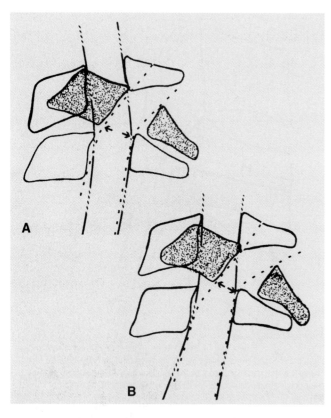

Figure 3 The pincer mechanism, as described by Penning, occurs when the distance between the posteroinferior margins of the superior vertebral body and the anterosuperior aspect of the spinolaminar line of the subjacent vertebra decrease with hyperextension; compression of the spinal cord occurs. With hyperflexion, the anterosuperior aspect of the spinolaminar line of the superior vertebra and the posterosuperior margin of the inferior vertebra would be the pincers. *(Reproduced with permission from Penning L: Some aspects of plain radiography of the cervical spine in chronic myelopathy. Neurology 1962;12:513-519.)*

injury. On the basis of these data, it was concluded that young patients who experienced an episode of cervical spinal cord neurapraxia with or without an episode of transient quadriplegia are not predisposed to permanent neurologic injury. Although this conclusion takes sides in a controversy about which many spine surgeons disagree, the data clearly support the position that cervical cord neurapraxia should not preclude an athlete from further participation in contact activities. The problem that needs to be addressed is the subsequent recurrent episodes of transient quadriplegia. The rate of recurrence for patients who returned to participation in tackle football was 56%; the risk of recurrence is correlated with the pathoanatomy (ie, the smaller the canal, the greater the risk) and is predictable (Figure 4).

Prevention

Although athletic injuries to the cervical spine that result in injury to the spinal cord occur infrequently, they are nevertheless catastrophic events. Accurate descriptions of the mechanism or mechanisms of injury transcend mere academic interest. Before preventive measures can be developed and implemented, the mechanism or mechanisms of injury must be accurately identified. Because the nervous system is unable to recover significant function after severe trauma, prevention assumes an important role.

Injuries resulting in spinal cord damage have been associated with football, water sports, wrestling, rugby, trampolining, and ice hockey. The use of epidemiologic data, biomechanical evidence, and cinematographic analysis has defined and supported the involvement of

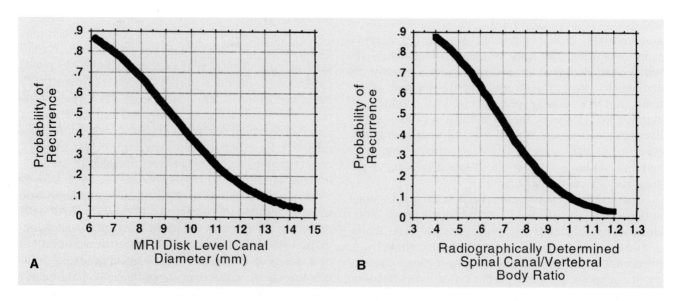

Figure 4 Graphs developed using logistic regression analysis in which the risk of recurrence can be plotted as a function of the disk level diameter measured on MRI (**A**) and the ratio of the spinal canal to the vertebral body calculated on the basis of a radiograph (**B**). The construction of these plots is based on the result that increased risk of recurrence is inversely correlated with canal diameter. Future cervical cord neurapraxia patients can be counseled regarding risk of recurrence based on the particular size of the spinal canal. *(Reproduced with permission from Torg JS, Corcoran TA, Thibault LE, et al: Cervical cord neurapraxia: Classification, pathomechanics, morbidity, and management guidelines. J Neurosurgery 1997;87:843-850.)*

axial load forces in cervical spine injuries occurring in football, demonstrated the success of appropriate rule changes in the prevention of these injuries, and emphasized the need for using epidemiologic methods to prevent cervical spine and similar severe injuries in other high-risk athletic activities.

To identify the causes of cervical quadriplegia and prevent cervical quadriplegia associated with participation in football consideration must be given to the role of the helmet–face mask protective system, the concept of the axial loading mechanism of injury, and the effect of rule changes banning spearing and the use of the top of the helmet as the initial point of contact in tackling.

The protective capacity of the modern football helmet has resulted in playing techniques that place the cervical spine at risk of injury with associated catastrophic neurologic sequelae. Cinematographic and epidemiologic data clearly indicate that cervical spine injuries associated with quadriplegia occurring as a result of participation in football are not hyperflexion accidents. Instead, they are caused by purposeful axial loading of the cervical spine as a result of spearing and head-first playing techniques (Figure 5). As an etiologic factor, the modern helmet–face mask system is secondary, contributing to these injuries because its protective capacity has permitted the head to be used as a battering ram, thus exposing the cervical spine to injury.

The role of hyperflexion has been classically emphasized in cervical spine trauma whether the injury was caused by a diving accident or participation in trampolining, rugby, or American football. Epidemiologic and cinematographic analyses have established that most instances of cervical spine quadriplegia that occur in football have resulted from axial loading. Far from being an accident or an untoward event, techniques are deliberately used that place the cervical spine at risk of catastrophic injury. Laboratory observations also indicate that athletically induced cervical spine trauma results from axial loading. Axial energy inputs applied to helmeted cadaver head-spine-trunk specimens produced fractures of the lower cervical spine when the impulse was applied to the crown of the helmet. Direct vertex impact imparted a larger force to the cervical vertebrae than forces applied further forward on the skull. Researchers investigating three different injury modes found that hyperflexion, hyperextension, and axial compression in anesthetized monkeys and axial compression produced cervical spine fractures and dislocations. Others have demonstrated that vertebral body fractures in the lower cervical spine are caused by the axial loading of isolated spinal units.

One study analyzed the relationships among head motion, local deformations of the cervical spine, and injury mechanisms using a cadaver head and neck model impacted in an anatomically neutral position. It was observed that the classic concepts of flexion and extension

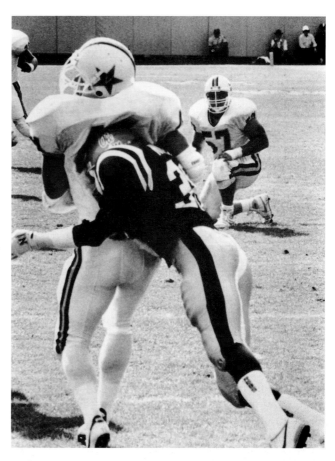

Figure 5 A college defensive back (dark jersey) is shown ramming an opposing ball carrier with his head, resulting in severe axial loading of the cervical spine. The defensive player suffered fractures of C4, C5, and C6 and was rendered quadriplegic. *(Reproduced with permission from Torg JS, Sennett B, Pavlov H, Leventhal MR, Glasgow SG: Spear tackler's spine: An entity precluding participation in tackle football and collision activities that expose the cervical spine to axial energy inputs. Am J Sports Med 1993;21:640-649.)*

of the cervical spine do not apply as a mechanism of injury to a vertically impacted head. They authors concluded that straightening of the cervical spine before injury may be a necessary element of the compressive-flexion mechanism.

In the course of a collision activity, such as tackle football, most energy inputs to the cervical spine are effectively dissipated by the energy-absorbing capacity of the cervical musculature via controlled lateral bending, flexion, or extension motion. However, the bones, disks, and ligamentous structures can be injured when contact occurs on the top of the helmet when the head, neck, and trunk are positioned in such a way that forces are transmitted along the longitudinal axis of the cervical spine.

When the neck is in the anatomic position, the cervical spine is extended as a result of normal cervical lordosis. When the neck is flexed to 30°, the cervical spine straightens. In axial loading injuries, the neck is slightly flexed, and normal cervical lordosis is eliminated, thereby converting the spine into a straight segmented

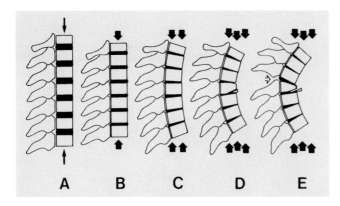

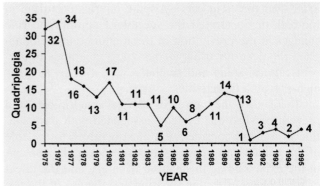

Figure 6 Biomechanically, the straightened cervical spine responds to axial loading forces like a segmented column. **A** and **B**, Axial loading of the cervical spine first results in compressive deformation of the intervertebral disks. **C**, As the energy input continues and maximum compressive deformation is reached, angular deformation and buckling occur. **D** and **E**, The spine fails in a flexion mode, with resulting fracture, subluxation, or dislocation. Compressive deformation leading to failure, with a resultant fracture, dislocation, or subluxation occurs in as little as 8.4 ms. *(Reproduced with permission from Torg JS, Vegso JJ, O'Neill MJ, Sennett B: The epidemiologic, pathologic, biomechanical, and cinematographic analysis of football-induced cervical spine trauma. Am J Sports Med 1990;18:50-57.)*

Figure 7 The effect of the 1976 rule changes banning spearing and head impact playing techniques was dramatic, and a sustained decrease in the occurrence of permanent cervical quadriplegia has occurred over a 20-year period. *(Reproduced with permission from Torg JS, Guille JT, Jaffe S: Injuries to the cervical spine in American football players. J Bone Joint Surg Am 2002;84:112-122.)*

column. Assuming the head, neck, and trunk components to be in motion, rapid deceleration of the head occurs when it strikes another object, such as another player, trampoline bed, or lake bottom. This results in the cervical spine being compressed between the rapidly decelerated head and the force of the oncoming trunk. When the maximum amount of vertical compression is reached, the straightened cervical spine fails in a flexion mode, and fracture, subluxation, or unilateral or bilateral facet dislocation can occur (Figure 6).

Refutation of the "freak accident" concept with the more logical principle of cause and effect has been most rewarding in dealing with problems of football-induced cervical quadriplegia. Definition of the axial loading mechanism in which a football player, usually a defensive back, makes a tackle by striking an opponent with the top of his helmet has been a key element in this process. Implementation of rule changes and the development of coaching technique that eliminate the use of the head as a battering ram have resulted in a dramatic reduction in the incidence of quadriplegia since 1976. Data on cervical spine injuries resulting from participation in football have been compiled by a national registry since 1971. Analysis of the epidemiologic data and cinematographic documentation clearly demonstrates that the majority of cervical fractures and dislocations were caused by axial loading. On the basis of these observations, rule changes banning both deliberate spearing and the use of the top of the helmet as the initial point of contact when tackling were implemented at the high school and college levels. A marked decrease in cervical spine injury rates subsequently occurred. The incidence of permanent cervical quadriplegia decreased from 34 in 1976 to 1 in the 1991 season (Figure 7).

One study evaluated 38 acute spinal cord injuries caused by diving accidents and observed that in most patients the cervical spine was fractured, the spinal cord was crushed as a result of the top of the head striking the bottom of a lake or pool. Another study, reporting on vertex impact and cervical dislocation in rugby players, observed that the spine is straight when the neck is slightly flexed and that significant force applied to the vertex when the spine is straight is transmitted down the long axis of the spine. Cervical spine flexion and dislocation result when the force exceeds the energy-absorbing capacity of the structures involved. Another study reported on the results of a national questionnaire survey by the Canadian Committee on the Prevention of Spinal Injuries due to Hockey that examined 28 injuries involving the spinal cord, 17 of which resulted in complete paralysis. They noted that the most common mechanism was a check in which the injured players struck the boards with the top of their heads, while their necks were slightly flexed. Reports in the recent literature that deal with the mechanism of injury of cervical spine injuries resulting from water sports (diving), rugby, and ice hockey support this thesis.

Guidelines for Return to Athletic Activities

Injuries to the cervical spine and associated structures as a result of participation in competitive athletic and recreational activities are common, and the frequency of injuries is inversely proportional to their severity. As indicated, the variety of possible injuries is considerable and the severity variable. The literature dealing with the diagnosis and treatment of these problems is also considerable. However, conspicuously absent is a comprehensive set of standards or guidelines for establishing criteria for permitting or prohibiting return to contact sports, boxing, football, ice hockey, lacrosse, rugby, and wrestling after injury to the cervical spinal structures. The explanation for

TABLE 3 | Guidelines for Return to Athletic Activities in Patients With Cervical Spine Abnormalities and Injuries

	Contraindication to Return to Athletic Activity		
	None	Relative	Absolute
Congenital Conditions			
Odontoid agenesis			X
Odontoid hypoplasia			X
Os odontoideum			X
Spina bifida occulta	X		
Atlanto-occipital fusion			X
Klippel-Feil anomaly			
Mass fusion of the cervical and upper thoracic vertebrae			X
Fusion of only one or two interspaces			
with associated limited motion, occipitocervical anomalies, or C2 involvement			X
with full cervical range of motion and no occipitocervical abnormalities, instability, disk disease, or degenerative changes	X		
Developmental Conditions			
Stenosis of the cervical spinal canal (ie, one or more vertebrae with canal-vertebral body ratio ≤ 0.8)			
and no other symptoms	X		
and motor or sensory manifestations of cervical cord neurapraxia		X	
and documented episode of cervical cord neurapraxia associated with ligamentous instability, MRI evidence of spinal cord defects, or swelling, symptoms or evidence of neurologic damage lasting longer than 36 hours, or multiple recurrences of cervical cord neurapraxia			X
Traumatic Injuries			
Upper cervical spine			
Almost all injuries of C1-C2 that involve fracture or ligamentous laxity			X
Healed nondisplaced Jefferson fractures in patients who are also pain free, have full range of cervical motion, and no evidence of neurologic injury		X	
Healed type I and type II odontoid fractures in patients who are also pain free, have full range of cervical motion, and no evidence of neurologic injury		X	
Healed lateral mass fractures of C2 in patients who are also pain free, have full range of cervical motion, and no evidence of neurologic injury		X	
Middle and lower cervical spine			
Ligamentous injuries			
> 3.5 mm of horizontal displacement of either vertebra in relation to the other			X
≤ 3.5 mm of horizontal displacement of either vertebra in relation to the other and depending on the patient's level of performance, physical habits, and position played		X	
> 11° of rotation of either adjacent vertebra			X
$\leq 11°$ of rotation of either adjacent vertebra and depending on the patient's level of performance, physical habits, and position played		X	

this void appears to be twofold. First, the combination of a litigious society and the potential for great harm should things go wrong makes doing nothing the easiest and perhaps most reasonable course of action. Second and perhaps most important, with the exception of transient quadriplegia, there is a lack of credible data pertaining to postinjury risk factors. Despite a lack of credible data, the guidelines presented in Table 3 are provided to assist physicians and patients and their families in deciding whether to permit or prohibit return to athletic activity after a cervical spine injury.

To develop these guidelines, four categories of cervical spine conditions have been identified for which a decision must be made whether a return to athletic activities is advisable and safe: congenital conditions, developmental conditions, traumatic injuries, and status following cervical spine fusion. For all of the conditions and injuries listed, return to athletic activity is not contraindicated (no recognized risk factors documented in the literature or known on the basis of anecdotal experiences), relatively contraindicated (permitting return to play predicated on less than unequivocal substantiated

TABLE 3 | Guidelines for Return to Athletic Activities in Patients With Cervical Spine Abnormalities and Injuries, continued			
	Contraindication to Return to Athletic Activity		
	None	**Relative**	**Absolute**
Fractures			
Healed stable compression fractures of the vertebral body without evidence of a sagittal component on AP radiographs and without involvement of either the ligamentous or posterior bony structures in asymptomatic patients with no evidence of neurologic injury and full pain-free range of cervical motion	X		
Healed stable end-plate fractures without evidence of a sagittal component on AP radiographs and without involvement of either the ligamentous or posterior bony structures in asymptomatic patients with no evidence of neurologic injury and full pain-free range of cervical motion	X		
Healed stable spinous process "clay shoveler" fractures in asymptomatic patients with no evidence of neurologic injury and full pain-free range of cervical motion	X		
Healed stable nondisplaced vertebral body compression fractures without evidence of a sagittal component on AP radiographs in asymptomatic patients with no evidence of neurologic injury and full pain-free range of cervical motion (Because these fractures can settle and cause increased deformity, patients with this type of fracture should be carefully observed.)		X	
Healed stable fractures involving the elements of the posterior neural ring in asymptomatic patients with no evidence of neurologic injury and full pain-free range of cervical motion (Because a rigid ring cannot break in one location, healing of paired fractures of the ring must be evident on radiographic and imaging studies.)		X	
Acute fractures of either the vertebral body or posterior bony structures with or without associated ligamentous laxity			X
Vertebral body fractures with evidence of a sagittal component on AP radiographs			X
Vertebral body fractures with or without displacement with associated posterior arch factures or ligamentous laxity			X
Comminuted vertebral body fractures with displacement into the spinal canal			X
Any healed fracture of either the vertebral body or the posterior bony structures in patients with associated pain, evidence of neurologic injury, and limitation of cervical motion			X
Healed displaced fractures involving the lateral masses with resulting facet incongruity			X
Spear tackler's spine (ie, developmental stenosis of the cervical canal, evidence of persistent straightening or reversal of the normal cervical lordotic curve on a standing lateral radiograph obtained with the patient in the neutral position, concomitant preexisting posttraumatic radiographic abnormalities of the cervical spine, and documentation of the patient using the spear tackling technique)			X
Intervertebral Disk Injuries			
Healed anterior or lateral disk herniation that is treated conservatively in patients who are asymptomatic, have no evidence of neurologic injury, and have full pain-free range of cervical motion	X		
Lateral or central disk herniation that has been treated with intervertebral diskectomy and interbody fusion in patients who have a solid fusion, are asymptomatic, have no evidence of neurologic injury, and have full pain-free range of cervical motion	X		
Acute or chronic (hard disk) herniation in patients with associated neurologic findings, pain, or significant limitation of cervical motion			X
Status Following Cervical Spine Fusion			
Stable single-level anterior or posterior fusion in patients who are asymptomatic, have no evidence of neurologic injury, and have full pain-free range of cervical motion	X		
Stable two- or three-level fusion in patients who are asymptomatic, have no evidence of neurologic injury, and have full pain-free range of cervical motion (*Because of the presumed increased stresses at the articulations of the adjacent uninvolved vertebrae and the propensity for the development of degenerative changes at these levels, these patients, with only rare exceptions, should not be permitted to return to athletic activity.)		X*	
Anterior or posterior fusion of four or more levels			X
Any fusion for instability of C1 regardless of radiographic evidence of successful fusion (An absolute contraindication exists because of the uncertainty of results of cervical fusion, the gracile configuration of C1, and the importance of the alar and transverse odontoid ligaments.)			X

data regarding risk as documented in the literature or by anecdotal experience), or absolutely contraindicated (significant risk factors documented in the literature or known on the basis of anecdotal experience) on the basis of a variety of parameters. Information compiled from over 1,200 cervical spine injuries documented by the National Football Head and Neck Injury Registry has provided insight into whether various conditions may predispose patients to more serious injury. A review of the literature provides significant data for a limited number of specific conditions. The analysis of many cervical spine conditions is predicated on an understanding of recognized mechanisms of injury and has permitted categorization on the basis of "educated" conjecture. Finally, in the development of the guidelines in Table 3, much reliance has been placed on personal experience that must be regarded as anecdotal; therefore, the criteria listed are intended only as guidelines. Each patient must be evaluated on an individual basis by assessing particular factors such as the level of athletic participation, position played, motivation, and risk assumption. Critical to the application of these guidelines is the implementation of coaching and playing techniques that preclude the use of the head as the initial point of contact in a collision situation. Exposure of the cervical spine to axial loading is an invitation to disaster and makes all safety standards meaningless.

Spinal Cord Resuscitation

The pathophysiology of lesions resulting in irreversible neurologic sequelae after injury to the cervical cord is similar to that for closed head injuries. Specifically, it is not the primary brain injury but the secondary injury phenomena (cerebral hypoxia and ischemia resulting from brain swelling) that cause the most damage. It has been well established in the literature that the release of excitotoxic substances, cell membrane depolarization, a rise in intracellular calcium concentration, and increased intracellular hydrostatic pressure result in increased neuronal pressure and rupture. It has been proposed that, with regard to permanent neurologic sequelae, the same phenomena occur in patients with acute spinal cord trauma. The secondary injury to the spinal cord caused by edema, hypoxia, and aberration of cell membrane potential is largely responsible for the neurologic deficit. The concept of spinal cord resuscitation, based in part on clinical observations lacking scientific format, has been proposed as an attempt to reverse the secondary injury phenomena and obtain maximum neurologic recovery. Such measures include support of both respiratory and hemodynamic function to facilitate spinal cord perfusion, prompt relief of cord deformation through realignment, intravenous administration of corticosteroids, and early spinal stabilization.

Prehospital Care

Medical team members who are responsible for the care of athletes who may sustain injuries to the cervical spine should consider several principles. The team physician or trainer should be designated as the person responsible for supervising on-the-field management of a potentially serious injury. Other principles require advance planning. All necessary emergency equipment must be available at the site of potential injury. At a minimum, this should include a spine board, stretcher, and equipment necessary for helmet removal and the initiation and maintenance of cardiopulmonary resuscitation. A properly equipped ambulance must be available as well as an accessible hospital equipped and staffed to handle emergency neurologic problems. A telephone must be available for communicating with emergency department staff, ambulance personnel, and other responsible individuals in case of an emergency. An unconscious athlete or an athlete with a spinal injury should not be treated hastily or haphazardly. Being prepared to handle this situation is the best way to prevent actions that could convert a repairable injury into a catastrophe.

Prevention of further injury is the single most important treatment objective. The first step should be to immobilize the patient's head and neck by supporting them in a stable position. Then, in the following order, breathing, pulse, and level of consciousness should be assessed. If the patient is breathing, the mouth guard, if present, should be removed, and the airway should be maintained. It may also be necessary to remove the face mask when the respiratory situation is threatened or unstable, when the athlete remains unconscious for a prolonged period, or when a cervical spine injury is suspected. The chin strap should be left on. Once it is established that the athlete is breathing and has a pulse, the neurologic status should be evaluated, noting the level of consciousness, response to pain, pupillary response, and any unusual posturing, flaccidity, rigidity, or weakness.

Next, the airway should be maintained and the patient should remain immobilized until emergency transportation is available or consciousness is regained. If the patient is face down when emergency transportation arrives, he or she should be logrolled onto a spine board. Gentle longitudinal traction should be exerted to support the head without attempting to correct alignment. No attempt should be made to move the patient except for transportation or cardiopulmonary resuscitation if necessary.

If the patient is not breathing or stops breathing, the airway must be established. If face down, the patient must be turned to a face-up position. The safest and easiest way to accomplish this is to logroll the patient into a face-up position. Ideally, the medical support team is made up of five members: the leader, who controls the head and gives the commands only; three members to roll; and a fifth member to help lift and carry when necessary. If time permits and a spine board is available, the athlete should be rolled directly onto it. However, breathing and circulation are much more important at this point. With all medical support team members in position, the athlete is rolled toward the assistants—one at the shoulders, one at the hips, and one at the knees. The leader maintains immobilization of the head by applying slight traction and must keep the head and spine in line with the body during the roll.

Heavy patients, including many athletes, can be lifted and carried more efficiently with a medical support team of six or more; a medical support team of this size is also preferred for patients with suspected spinal injuries. The Inter-Association Task Force recommends that a medical support team of six or more be used to lift and carry patients and that a scoop stretcher be used whenever possible. In the athletic arena, a sufficient number of certified athletic trainers, physicians, and emergency medical service personnel are usually on hand to effectively lift and carry patients in this manner. With a medical support team of six or more, one member immobilizes the neck by placing hands on the patient's shoulders (under the shoulder pads, if present) with the thumbs pointed away from the patient's face. The athlete's head will then be resting between the forearms of this member of the medical support team. The other six members position themselves alongside the patient—one on each side of the chest, pelvis, and legs. Hands are slid under the patient and any athletic equipment to provide a firm, coordinated lift. To lift, the team member immobilizing the neck gives the command to prepare to lift and lift. The other medical support team members lift the patient 4 to 6 inches off the ground, maintaining a coordinated lift to prevent any movement of the spine. One of the medical support team members at the thigh level must control the legs with his or her arms toward the feet so the splint can be slid into place from the foot end. After the splint is in place, with positions maintained, the team member immobilizing the neck gives the command to prepare to lower and lower, and the patient is lowered onto the splint.

In the case of larger patients, as many as 10 medical support team members should participate in the lift, with one on each side of the chest and pelvis, two at the legs, one at the head, and one with the splint. The Inter-Association Task Force does not recommend the use of a medical support team with fewer than four members to lift and carry patients with suspected spinal injuries, even smaller athletes and children, in part because of the weight of the athlete when wearing protective equipment.

The face mask should be removed as quickly as possible any time an athlete wearing a helmet is suspected of having a spinal injury, even if the patient is still con-

scious and regardless of respiratory status. The type of mask that is attached to the helmet determines the method of removal. Bolt cutters are used with the older single- and double-bar football helmet masks. The newer football helmet masks are attached with plastic loops and should be removed by cutting the loops with Dura Shears (EMT scissors) (Diversified Biotech, Boston, MA) or a Trainer's Angel (Trainer's Angel, Riverside, CA). The entire mask should be removed so that it does not interfere with further rescue efforts. Once the mask has been removed, rescue breathing should be initiated following the current standards of the American Heart Association.

Controversy currently exists among emergency medicine physicians and technicians on the one hand and team physicians and athletic trainers on the other regarding helmet removal. Existing emergency medical services guidelines mandate removal of protective headgear before the transport of a patient suspected of having a cervical spine injury to a fixed medical facility. These guidelines were implemented with motorcycle helmets in mind to facilitate both airway accessibility and the application of devices for immobilizing the cervical spine. This procedure clearly contradicts the long-standing principle adhered to by team physicians and athletic trainers that recommends leaving the helmet in place on the patient suspected of having a cervical spine injury until the patient is transported to a fixed medical facility.

This controversy is of more than academic interest because there have been instances in which emergency medical technicians under the directives of emergency department physicians who are unfamiliar with the nuances of the relationship between protective football gear (helmet and shoulder pads) and the injured cervical spine have refused to move the injured player before helmet removal. These instances represent more than an honest difference of opinion because they are clearly detrimental to the health and well-being of the patient. Removal of the football helmet and shoulder pads on site exposes a potentially injured spine to both unnecessary and awkward manipulation and disruption of the immobilizing capacity of the helmet and shoulder pads. In addition, removal of the helmet alone can subject a potentially unstable spine to hyperlordotic deformity.

According to the National Intercollegiate Athletic Association Guidelines for helmet removal, provided there are no special circumstances such as respiratory distress coupled with an inability to access the airway, the helmet should never be removed during the prehospital care of a patient with a potential head and neck injury unless the helmet does not hold the head securely such that immobilization of the helmet does not immobilize the head; the design of the helmet is such that even after removal of the face mask the airway cannot be controlled or ventilation provided; after a reasonable period, the face mask cannot be removed; and the helmet prevents immobilization for transportation in an appropriate position.

When such helmet removal is necessary in any setting, it should be done only by personnel trained in this procedure. If removal of the helmet is needed to initiate treatment or to obtain special radiographs, a specific protocol should be followed. With the head, neck, and helmet manually stabilized, the chin strap can be cut. While maintaining stability, the cheek pads can be removed by inserting the flat blade of a screwdriver or bandage scissor under the pad snaps and above the inner surface of the shell. While another member of the medical staff provides manual stability of the chin and neck, the medical staff members stabilizing the head place their thumbs or index fingers into the ear holes on both sides. By pulling both laterally and longitudinally, the helmet shell can be spread and eased off. If a rocking motion is necessary to loosen the helmet, the head-neck unit must not be allowed to move. The medical staff members participating in this important maneuver must proceed with caution and coordinate every move.

The initial diagnostic assessment of a patient with suspected or actual cervical spine trauma should include a routine radiographic examination. With the head, neck, and trunk still immobilized, the preliminary study includes an AP and lateral examination of vertebrae C1-C7. If a major fracture, subluxation, dislocation, or evidence of instability is not evident, open mouth and oblique views should be obtained. Depending on the neurologic and comfort status of the patient, lateral flexion and extension views should be obtained at some point. Although CT and MRI may provide more detailed information, horizontally oriented fractures and subtle subluxations are best identified on the routine radiographs. The choice of imaging technique will depend on the results of the routine examination, the neurologic status of the patient, physician preference, and the availability of the imaging modalities.

Summary

It is important to be familiar with the guidelines for the prevention, classification, evaluation, management, and return to play for injuries that occur to the cervical spine and related neural structures as a result of participation in competitive and recreational activities. Axial loading of the cervical spine has been clearly established as the primary injury mechanism, an observation with profound implications regarding implementation of preventive measures. Clinical entities peculiar to axial loading of the cervical spine and associated with irreversible cervical cord lesions have been described. In addition, more recently identified injury patterns have been emphasized. Specifically, those involving the middle cervical segment (C3-C4) and the more favorable response

of prompt reduction of these injuries have been delineated. The marked instability and grave prognosis of the axial load teardrop fracture are attributed to the associated sagittal vertebral body and posterior arch fractures. Spear tackler's spine has been described and classified as an absolute contraindication to participation in collision sports. Cervical cord neurapraxia with and without transient quadriplegia is neither associated with nor presages permanent neurologic sequelae; however, there is considerable risk of recurrence, which can be predicted on the basis of canal diameter data.

Return to activity guidelines have been proposed and relative risk assigned as follows: (1) no contraindication when no recognized risk factors documented in the literature are known on the basis of anecdotal experience; (2) relative contraindication when permitting return to play is predicated on less than unequivocal substantiated data regarding risk as documented in the literature or by anecdotal experience; and (3) absolute contraindication when significant risk factors are documented in the literature or known on the basis of anecdotal experience. The concept of spinal cord resuscitation is proposed as a means of obtaining maximum neurologic recovery by reversing the secondary injury phenomenon associated with acute spinal cord trauma.

Annotated Bibliography

Diagnosis and Treatment
Kelly JD IV, Aliquo D, Sitler MR, Odgers C, Moyer RA: Association of burners with cervical canal and foraminal stenosis. *Am J Sports Med* 2000;28:214-217.
    This article provides a comprehensive review of cervical root, brachial plexus, and peripheral nerve neurapraxias.

Thomas BE, McCullen GM, Yuan HA: Cervical spine injuries in football players. *J Am Acad Orthop Surg* 1999;7:333-347.
    The authors of this article report that avoiding spear tackling and wearing properly fitted equipment can markedly reduce the risk of serious injury in football players.

Torg JS, Guille JT, Jaffe S: Injuries to the cervical spine in American football players. *J Bone Joint Surg Am* 2002;84:112-122.
    This article attempts to answer basic questions dealing with epidemiology, prevention, pathomechanics, pathophysiology, and the histochemical responses of reversible and irreversible cervical cord injuries.

Prehospital Care
Kleiner DM, Almquist JL, Bailes J, et al: *Prehospital Care of the Spine-injured Athlete: A Document from the Inter-Association Task force for Appropriate Care of the Spine-Injured Athlete.* Dallas, Texas, National Athletic Trainers' Association, 2001.

This is a multiauthored, complete set of guidelines for on-the-field management of athletes with suspected spinal injuries.

Classic Bibliography

Bergfeld JA: Brachial plexus injury in sports: A five-year followup. *Orthop Clin North Am* 1988;23:743-744.

Bolhman HH: Anterior decompression and arthrodesis of the cervical spine: Long-term motor improvement. *J Bone Joint Surg Am* 1992;74:671-682.

Bracken MD, Shepard MJ, Collins WF, et al: A randomized, controlled trial of methylprednisolone or naloxone in the treatment of acute spinal-cord injury: Results of the Second National Acute Spinal Cord Injury Study. *N Engl J Med* 1990;322:1405-1411.

Chiles BW: Acute spinal injury. *N Engl J Med* 1996;334: 514-520.

Clancy WG Jr, Brand RL, Bergfield JA: Upper trunk brachial plexus injuries in contact sports. *Am J Sports Med* 1977;5:209-216.

Delamarter RB, Sherman J, Carr JB: Pathophysiology of spinal cord injury: Recovery after immediate and delayed decompression. *J Bone Joint Surg Am* 1995;77: 1042-1049.

Jefferson G: Fractures of the atlas vertebra. *Br J Surg* 1920;7:407.

Meyer SA: Cervical spinal stenosis and stingers in collegiate football players. *Am J Sports Med* 1994;22:158-166.

Nightingale RW, McElhaney JH, Richardson WJ, Best TM, Myers BS: Experimental impact injury to the cervical spine: Relating motion of the head and the mechanism of injury. *J Bone Joint Surg Am* 1996;78:412-421.

Pavlov H, Torg JS, Robie B, Jahre CL: Cervical spine stenosis: Determination with vertebral body ratio method. *Radiology* 1987;164:771-775.

Penning L: Some aspects of plain radiography of the cervical spine in chronic myelopathy. *Neurology* 1962;12: 513-519.

Scher AT: Vertex impact and cervical dislocation in rugby players. *S Afr Med J* 1981;59:227-228.

Schneider RC: The syndrome of acute anterior spinal cord injury. *J Neurosurg* 1955;12:95-123.

Seddon H: *Surgical Disorders of the Peripheral Nerves.* Edinburgh, Scotland, Churchill-Livingstone, 1972.

Tator CH, Edmonds VE, New ML: Diving: A frequent and potentially preventable cause of spinal cord injury. *Can Med Assoc J* 1981;124:1323-1324.

Tator CH, Edmonds VE: National survey of spinal injuries in hockey players. *Can Med Assoc J* 1984;130: 875-880.

Torg JS: Spinal cord resuscitation: A concept for today, in Delee JC, Drez D (eds): *Orthopaedic Sports Medicine: Principles and Practice.* Philadelphia, PA, WB Saunders, 1993, pp 183-186.

Torg JS, Corcoran TA, Thibault LE, et al: Cervical cord neurapraxia: Classification, pathomechanics, morbidity and management guidelines. *J Neurosurg* 1997;87:843-850.

Torg JS, Currier B, Douglas R, Hershman E, O'Leary PF: Spinal cord resuscitation. *Contemp Orthop* 1995;30: 495-509.

Torg JS, Pavlov H, Genuario SE, et al: Neurapraxia of the cervical spinal cord with transient quadriplegia. *J Bone Joint Surg Am* 1986;68:1354-1370.

Torg JS, Ramsey-Emrhein JA: Management guidelines for participation in collision activities with congenital, developmental, or postinjury lesions involving the cervical spine. *Clin J Sports Med* 1997;7:273-291.

Torg JS, Sennett B, Pavlov H, Leventhal MR, Glasgow SG: Spear tackler's spine: An entity precluding participation in tackle football and collision activities that expose the cervical spine to axial energy inputs. *Am J Sports Med* 1993;21:640-649.

Torg JS, Thibault L, Sennett B, Pavlov H: The Nicolas Andry Award: The pathomechanics and pathophysiology of cervical spinal cord injury. *Clin Orthop* 1995;321: 259-269.

Torg JS, Vegso JJ, O'Neill MJ, Sennett B: The epidemiologic, pathologic, biomechanical, and cinematographic analysis of football-induced cervical spine trauma. *Am J Sports Med* 1990;18:50-57.

Torg JS, Vegso JJ, Sennett B, Das M: The National Football Head and Neck Injury Registry: 14-year report on cervical quadriplegia, 1971 through 1984. *JAMA* 1985;254:3439-3443.

Chapter 2

Lumbar Spine Injuries

Lyle J. Micheli, MD

Serena J. Young, MD

Pierre d'Hemecourt, MD

Introduction

Back pain is common in the general population, with a lifetime prevalence approaching 85%. Ten percent to 15% of athletic injuries involve the spine. In the general population, these injuries are often self-limiting processes that respond well to conservative treatment. However, because the spines of athletes are exposed to a variety of repetitive forces that are sport-specific, back pain in athletes has been reported to be as high as 30% in some sports and often represents a continuum from childhood through adolescence and adulthood. Injury patterns will vary along this spectrum and overlap into the next age group. Rehabilitation depends on an accurate diagnosis. Athletic activities expose the young athlete to many cofactors, including anthropomorphic and sport-specific biomechanical factors. Growth cartilage, hormonal, and nutritional considerations create an interactive model for understanding injury and deformity of the athlete's spine.

Spine Anatomy and Biomechanics

The spine is divided into the anterior and posterior columns. The anterior column consists of the vertebral body, intervertebral disk, and attached anterior and posterior longitudinal ligaments. The posterior column consists of the neural arch, facet joints, spinal process, and the pars interarticularis. The triple joint complex of the intervertebral disk and bilateral facet joints forms a triangular base for support, force transfer, and synchronous motion.

In the anterior column, the vertebral body ends at the superior and inferior end plates. In children, there is an epiphyseal growth plate (epiphysis) and its contiguous ring apophysis. The vertebral end plate develops from the cartilaginous portion of the epiphysis and functions to nourish the disk through hydrostatic motion. The posterior arch also has primary growth centers in the pedicles bilaterally and one in the spinous process. The posterior arch closes during the first decade of life, whereas the vertebral body may continue growth late into the second decade of life. Exposure to asymmetric forces during this time may cause deformity.

The intervertebral disk is composed of an outer anulus fibrosus made of 10 to 20 layers of concentric lamellae. These organized collagen fibers, oriented 70° from vertical, are cross-hatched from layer to layer, surround the inner nucleus pulposus, and are enriched with glycoproteins to maintain hydration. The cartilaginous end plate separates the anulus fibrosus and nucleus pulposus from the vertebral body. The anulus fibrosus attaches to the ring apophysis and end plate in the periphery. Compressive forces increase intradiskal pressure and are transformed to tensile forces in the anulus fibrosus. Unlike in the adult, the cartilaginous end plate in the adolescent athlete is the first to fail with compressive loads. Except for its outer annular fibers, the intervertebral disk is primarily aneural and avascular.

The lower spine and pelvic ring are joined at the sacroiliac joint. Forces are transferred across the sacroiliac joint between the lower extremities to the trunk. With hip flexion, there is an ipsilateral posterior pelvic rotation and increased sacroiliac joint compression. Alternately, hip extension causes sacroiliac distraction. With increased extension, as occurs with sprinting, extension is transferred to the lumbar spine. The sacroiliac joint, which is flat until puberty, eventually develops corrugations that ultimately result in ankylosis late in life. The inferior sacroiliac articulation is a true synovial joint.

The spinal muscles can be divided functionally into the extensor-rotator and flexor-rotator muscles, which all insert into the thoracolumbar fascia. The extensor-rotator group of spinal muscles includes the latissimus dorsi, long spinal extensors, short spinal extensors (multifidi), and gluteus maximus. The flexor-rotator group of spinal muscles includes the rectus femoris, external oblique, internal oblique, and transverse abdominis.

The thoracolumbar fascia extends from the sacrum and iliac crest to the spinous processes and has a network of muscular attachments. It is important in the biomechanics of lumbar motion and stabilizes the spine in forward flexion. Furthermore, with its anterior attachments to the transversus abdominis and internal oblique

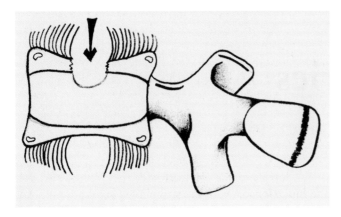

Figure 1 Schmorl's node.

muscles, it enhances coactivation with the posterior extensor group. This produces protective hydrostatic intraabdominal pressure that absorbs compressive forces.

The intraspinal ligaments provide stability and allow the transfer of tensile loads from one vertebra to another. The anterior longitudinal, posterior longitudinal, intraspinous, and supraspinous ligaments stabilize the vertebral bodies, whereas the iliolumbar, sacroiliac, sacrotuberous, and sacrospinous ligaments help anchor the lumbosacral spine to the pelvis. Most of the ligaments here are richly innervated and provide an important proprioceptive function.

Lumbar flexion and extension involve a constantly moving axis of rotation. In flexion, the axis of rotation is in the disk with a posterior distraction force. In extension, the compression is transferred to the posterior anulus fibrosus and facet joints. Axial rotation also involves a simultaneous compressive force at the facet, with a shear force at the posterolateral disk.

Risk Factors

Overuse Injuries
Repetitive microtrauma is often the key causative factor in spinal injuries of athletes. The cyclic loading of shear, tensile, and compressive forces often exceeds tissue elasticity and results in failure. This threshold may be surpassed in the total volume of hours per week or in excessive single-session drills of one motion.

Growth Process
In many sports, intense training begins at an early age. Growth cartilage is the weak link in the musculoskeletal system through adolescence. Repetitive or sudden overloading compressive forces may result in rupture of the end plate (Schmorl's node) or ring apophysis (limbus vertebrae) (Figure 1). Tensile forces may result in apophysitis or apophyseal avulsion. Sports in which athletes are exposed to repetitive asymmetric forces, as in rhyth-

mic gymnastics, may contribute to spinal curve deformity.

Incomplete ossification of the neural arch in the posterior arch may predispose athletes who participate in sports requiring hyperextension (for example, ballet and gymnastics) to stress fractures. This may result from abutment of the inferior articular process onto the inferior pars interarticularis or from repetitive traction or rotational activities.

Anthropomorphic Factors
Malalignment of the lower extremities may result in the improper transfer of ground forces to the lower trunk. One recent review of college athletes found that back pain was associated with lower extremity overuse injuries and laxity. In addition, weakness of the lower abdominal muscles and tight hip flexors can increase lumbar lordosis, which can result in a compressive load to the posterior elements and a shear force to the disk. Weakened lumbar extensor muscles have also been associated with chronic low back pain in the athlete.

Gender
Data regarding differences in risk of injury based on gender currently are derived primarily from observational studies. An increased incidence of spondylolysis has been noted in some female-dominated sports such as ballet, figure skating, and gymnastics. Additionally, sacral stress fractures have been noted to be predominant in female long-distance runners. The reasons for this are multifactorial. Bone homeostasis in the female athlete is regulated by multiple factors, including nutritional and hormonal balance. Physiologic training results in an anabolic response, whereas overtraining may result in a catabolic response. A negative caloric balance will diminish estrogen production, resulting in oligomenorrhea or amenorrhea, which may predispose the female athlete to lower bone density and subsequent stress fracture. The interrelatedness of disordered eating, oligomenorrhea/amenorrhea, and osteoporosis has been termed "the female athlete triad" (see chapter 28).

Sport-Specific Injuries
Sports injuries are either the result of acute macrotrauma or repetitive microtrauma. The forces applied across the spine are unique for each sport; for example, gymnastics involves repetitive flexion and extension of the lumbar spine, and disk degeneration has been strongly associated with this sport (11% in pre-elite athletes, 43% in elite athletes, and 63% in Olympic-level athletes). Training in excess of 15 hours per week has also been noted to be a risk factor. Herniation of the nucleus pulposus is seen with lumbar flexion, axial compression, and rotation, as occurs in weightlifting, rowing, collision sports, and bowling. Dance, figure skating, and

football (interior linesman position) involve repetitive hyperextension and are associated with posterior element overuse and spondylolysis.

Clinical Evaluation

The clinical history should include a review of the specific sports in which the patient participates and the patient's particular training volume. The mechanism of injury and nature and severity of the pain, including changes in its character, location, and radiation, should all be assessed. Pain aggravated by extension movements, such as those required during a tennis serve, suggest posterior element involvement, whereas pain aggravated by flexion movements or Valsalva maneuvers suggests discogenic involvement. Changes in neurologic symptoms, including bladder or bowel habits, should be determined. Response to medications, such as nonsteroidal anti-inflammatory drugs (NSAIDs), and any previous back injury should be noted. Lack of response to NSAIDs may indicate a primarily mechanical derangement such as spondylolysis or a neoplastic origin of the pain. Conversely, a patient with an osteoid osteotoma will present with pain that is temporarily resolved with NSAIDs.

"Red flag" symptoms identified when taking the medical history include night pain, immunosuppression (chronic corticosteroid or immunosuppressive medication use), history of a tumor, and systemic signs such as weight loss and fever. Peripheral joint involvement should be assessed for inflammatory conditions. Nutritional history, including eating disorders, and any previous stress fractures should be evaluated, and a menstrual history should be obtained in female athletes.

The physical examination of the athlete with a suspected lumbar spine injury should follow an orderly pattern, with attention paid to biomechanical analysis. The simple observation of gait may identify a lumbar shift, obvious motor weakness, and pain intensity. With the patient standing, forward spine flexion should be evaluated for pain reproduction, lumbar and hamstring tightness, and scoliosis. Examination in the standing position will also allow assessment of thoracolumbar fascia tightness, and spinal deformities such as thoracic kyphosis and flat back syndrome, which is a combination of hypokyphosis of the thoracic spine and hypolordosis of the lumbar spine.

This position will also expose thoracolumbar tightness as a flat back as well as thoracic kyphosis. Although back pain with extension may indicate posterior element pathology, greater sensitivity is gained with a single leg hyperextension test that reproduces unilateral pain. Conversely, pain with flexion or with both flexion and extension may indicate an injury with a discogenic origin. Toe walking and heel walking help assess gross motor strength of the S1 and L4 nerve roots. With the patient sitting, patellar tendon (L4) and Achilles tendon

(S1) reflexes can be tested. In this position, motor function of the extensor hallucis longus (L5), quadriceps (L3-4), and hip flexors (L2-3) can also be tested, and a sensory examination for the T12-S1 dermatomes can be done. With the patient in the supine position, the straight leg raise and Lasègue's sign test can be done to assess sciatic nerve root tension. The fabere test and Gaenslen's test can be done to check for sacroiliac joint inflammation. Peripelvic flexibility and biomechanics are also assessed in this position. The relative tightness of the hip flexors is assessed with the Thomas test and the hip extensors with the straight leg raise popliteal angle test, whereas tightness of the hip external rotators can be determined with rotation assessment.

Hip flexor tightness (Thomas test) and hamstring tightness (popliteal angle) should be noted. Piriformis tightness, limb length discrepancy, and pelvic obliquity are also assessed with the patient in the supine position. With the patient in the prone position, focal spinal tenderness and muscle tone should be assessed. Passive hip extension can be used to elicit a femoral nerve root tension sign. In a patient with perineal sensory changes, urinary retention, or bladder and bowel incontinence, perineal sensation should be assessed and rectal examination performed.

Acute Injuries

Fractures

Although uncommon in most athletes, acute thoracolumbar spine fractures as a result of severe trauma do occur in athletes who participate in contact sports. Bone failure occurs in combination with ligamentous and/or growth cartilage involvement. Falls during participation in equestrian sports, trampolining, skiing, snowboarding, hockey, and football have all been associated with thoracolumbar fractures as well as with cervical spine injuries. When such injuries occur, strict spinal precautions must be initiated and the patient assessed with full Advanced Trauma Life Support protocols, including the initial ABCDs (airway, breathing, circulation, neurologic disability) of trauma care. Proper immobilization with a spine board during transport is mandatory to prevent additional injury.

With traumatic injuries, spinal stability may be evaluated using Denis' three-column spinal stability assessment (Figure 2). The three columns are the anterior (containing the anterior longitudinal ligament, anterior half of the vertebral body, and anulus fibrosus), middle (containing the posterior half of the vertebral body and anulus fibrosus), and posterior columns (containing the bony neural arch with ligamentous structures). Spinal instability is defined when two columns are involved; it may be mechanical (progression of deformity) and/or neurologic.

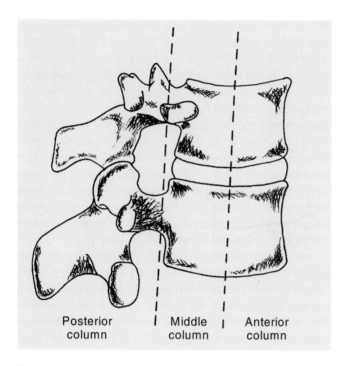

Figure 2 The three columns used to assess spinal stability (Denis) are the posterior column, the middle column, and the anterior column.

Evaluation should include obtaining a careful history of any weakness or paresthesias. A complete thoracic and abdominal examination should also be done for co-existing trauma, and AP and lateral radiographs should be obtained. When there is anterior compression approaching a 50% loss of height or involvement of two columns, a CT scan can help detect injury to the posterior arch. When neurologic involvement is suspected, MRI is essential. MRI using T1-weighted, T2-weighted, and fast spin echo and fast short tau inversion recovery methods provides greater detail for posttraumatic spinal cord injuries and soft-tissue impingement.

In pediatric patients, spinal cord injury without radiographic abnormality (SCIWORA) can occur. Although the etiology of this condition is unknown, SCIWORA may involve hyperlaxity of the spinal canal in relation to the relatively fixed spinal cord or a transient vascular compromise. SCIWORA most commonly occurs in the cervical region of young children; however, a thoracolumbar SCIWORA has been described in older children. Clinically, this condition may not demonstrate neurologic progression for several days.

The treatment of stable thoracic compression fractures involving less than a 50% loss of height includes the use of a thoracolumbosacral orthosis (TLSO) or Jewett extension brace for 6 to 12 weeks. Stable lumbar injuries should be treated with a TLSO for 4 to 6 weeks. Participation in athletic activites is prohibited during this period. Physical therapy and extensor strength exercises are started when the patient can tolerate them. In the child with suspected SCIWORA, bracing of the af-

fected cervical or thoracic area is appropriate for 3 months.

With minimal spine compression and no neurologic compromise, patients are allowed to return to participation in contact and noncontact sports when they are pain free and have attained full strength and flexibility. Conversely, more severe compression and/or neurologic deficit, particularly when occurring in the thoracic spine, may be a contraindication to participation in contact sports. For those patients requiring surgical stabilization with a single level fusion and no neurologic deficit, return to participation in contact sports is possible; however, these recommendations must be individualized. In general, if the patient remains asymptomatic during sports participation, single-level fusion of the thoracic or high lumbar spine is possible. However, patients and parents must understand the risks for disk degeneration of the levels adjacent to the fusion that may occur with athletic activities that require repetitive motion of the spine or contact sports. When instrumentation is used to treat the patient, contact sports are generally contraindicated. All patients must understand the risk for disk degeneration of the adjacent levels before returning to contact sports participation.

Acute Disk Herniation

Clinically significant herniated nucleus pulposus is estimated to occur in 2% of the general population at some point, usually in adults (mean age, 35 years). However, of young athletes who report back pain, 10% have a discogenic etiology, but not all of them experience pain as a result of acute disk herniations. Adults with acute disk herniations are more likely to report sciatica, whereas younger athletes will typically report back and buttock pain, often with dramatic postural deformity and lumbar tightness. Loading the spine in flexion and rotation, as occurs in weightlifting, contact sports, and possibly rowing, is thought to put athletes at great risk for this type of injury.

On physical examination, patients with acute disk herniation typically have decreased lumbar and peripelvic flexibility, varying amounts of leg or back pain, and possibly a sciatic shift. A detailed neurologic examination and neurotension tests (including straight leg raising and femoral nerve stretch testing) should be performed. If the history has indicated any question of bladder or bowel symptoms, a careful neurologic examination for sensation and motor function of the perineum including rectal examination must be done to rule out cauda equina syndrome. Although CT may help make a diagnosis, MRI best demonstrates acute disk herniation. An intravenous contrast agent used in conjunction with MRI will help differentiate the scar tissue of a previous disk surgical procedure from a recurrent herniation.

Treatment consists of initial rest for comfort and then activity within the limits of pain. About 90% of adult nucleus pulposus herniations resolve within 3 months without surgical excision. In younger athletes, even fewer require surgery. Nonsurgical interventions include minimal rest followed by activity modification. Activities such as prolonged sitting, jumping, and spine hyperflexion or extension and straining are prohibited. NSAIDs and occasionally oral corticosteroids are used. A rigid brace in 15° of lordosis can be quite helpful in the initial phase to unload the disk and allow more rapid mobilization. This minimizes the detrimental effects of bed rest.

The patient then begins a physical therapy program that includes aerobic exercise, peripelvic flexibility, core stabilization, and sport-specific conditioning. Early use of epidural corticosteroid injections has been shown to improve progress in rehabilitation. Some patients may require partial diskectomy. Indications for partial diskectomy, which are the same for athletes as nonathletes, include progressive neurologic deficit, cauda equina syndrome (emergent), or unresolved pain. Standard procedures include a microscopic diskectomy or microendoscopic diskectomy. In those treated nonsurgically, return to athletic activity is usually allowed in 3 to 6 months. After surgery, aggressive rehabilitation is necessary and return to athletic activity may be possible in 6 to 12 weeks.

Apophyseal Injuries

In the skeletally immature athlete, physeal and apophyseal cartilage is present at the vertebral end plates in the spine. Macrotrauma can result in apophyseal avulsion. The pathomechanics of this type of injury are thought to involve sudden traction or compression force on the cartilage. Spine extension can cause anterior vertebral endplate apophyseal avulsion, and spine flexion can cause posterior apophyseal avulsion (Figure 3). Acute compression in flexion may result in a limbus vertebra. Typical findings include increased paraspinal muscle tone. In patients with posterior avulsions, canal compromise can occur. Physical findings can mimic those of herniated nucleus pulposus or spinal stenosis. MRI can help assess whether herniated disk material is within the fracture. CT may be needed to help define a small fragment laterally.

Contusions, Strains, and Sprains

Contusions can result from a direct blow to the back and will often lead to hematoma formation, swelling, and pain. Muscle and tendon strains can occur with excessive stretching during a concentric or eccentric contraction. A sprain occurs when a ligament stretches beyond its elastic limit. Inadequate warm-up and stretching pose the greatest risk for strains and sprains.

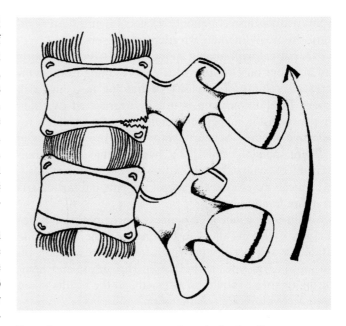

Figure 3 Apophyseal avulsion. The arrow indicates the direction of force.

Treatment for contusions, strains, and sprains usually consists of ice application, relative rest, and early mobilization.

Overuse Injuries
Spondylolysis
Isthmic spondylolysis is a stress fracture of the pars interarticularis, most often in the lower lumbar vertebrae. This injury usually occurs as a result of cyclic loading of the inferior articular facet onto the inferior lamina and pars interarticularis. It may also be caused by an acute macrotraumatic overload. This type of stress fracture occurs with higher and more repetitive forces and more pain in athletes than in nonathletes (nonathletes are predisposed to develop these fractures with minimal stresses and may be asymptomatic). Whether lumbar spondylolysis is congenital or acquired was once a matter of debate. Although the congenital hypothesis has been discounted, in addition to mechanical risk factors, there may be genetic risk factors for the development of lumbar spondylolysis. Family history of a first-degree relative with lumbar spondylolysis has been noted in patients with this type of fracture. In addition, there is an increased incidence of spina bifida occulta in patients with lumbar spondylolysis. In the general population, the incidence of lumbar spondylolysis is 4.4% at 6 years of age and 6% by adulthood. In the athletic population, however, this incidence may be exceeded depending on the sport. In one study, 47% of young athletes with low back pain were reported to have lumbar spondylolysis. This type of fracture has been identified in as many as 32% of gymnasts and 33% of ballet dancers. Lumbar

spondylolysis also commonly occurs in figure skaters, interior football linemen, wrestlers, and divers.

A patient with lumbar spondylolysis typically reports an insidious onset of low back pain resulting from an increased volume or intensity of training in a high-risk sport. In addition, pain is usually aggravated by spine hyperextension maneuvers required by the athlete's respective sport. Sciatic symptoms are occasionally present, possibly caused by hypertrophic ligamentum flavum or synovial proliferation at the pseudarthrosis, which can develop at the site of the pars interarticularis fracture nonunion.

Pain is reproduced in patients during physical examination by asking them to hyperextend the back while standing and performing single leg hyperextension on the ipsilateral side of the lesion. Hip flexor and hamstring tightness should be assessed and the results taken into account during rehabilitation.

In the patient with extension-based pain, plain radiographs of the lumbar spine should be obtained, including an AP view to look for evidence of scoliosis, spina bifida occulta, or transitional vertebrae and a lateral view to look for evidence of spondylolisthesis. Radiographic evidence of spina bifida occulta increases the suspicion for spondylolysis as a source of back pain because the association is very high between spina bifida occulta and spondylolysis. By contrast, the presence of transitional vertebrae may itself be an explanation for the pain originating from impingement of the transitional vertebrae on the pelvic rim. Although oblique views may provide evidence of more subtle unilateral spondylolysis, they lack sensitivity because only 32% of these fractures fall within the range of the oblique x-ray beam. A bone scan using single-photon emission computed tomography (SPECT) is required to identify evidence of subtle prespondylolytic stress reaction. A standard planar technetium Tc 99m bone scan is far less sensitive. If the SPECT bone scan shows a lesion, a 3-mm reverse gantry CT is done that is isolated to the level of increased bone scan activity. This better defines the lesion as early, intermediate, or terminal (sclerotic) and minimizes radiation exposure. CT can also be used to assess healing when needed. Recently, MRI has been shown to be useful in assessing pars interarticularis stress fractures. In addition, it does not expose patients to radiation and better defines other disk pathology. The MRI techniques that have shown promise in defining pars interarticularis defects include the reverse angle oblique axial T1-weighted images and duel echo at steady state. However, studies are needed to confirm that MRI has the sensitivity of SPECT. Furthermore, SPECT bone scans can show evidence of other pathology such as inflammation at a transitional vertebrae, pseudarthrosis, sacroiliac inflammation, and occult osteoid osteomas.

The risk of persistent pain and spondylolisthesis progression is a primary concern in patients with lumbar spondylolysis. Because it is a stress fracture of the pars interarticularis, the logical goal of treatment for young athletes with this type of injury would be osseous union. However, once a bone lysis occurs, distraction forces at the fracture site act in a manner that is similar to distraction forces in stress fractures of the lateral femoral neck, base of the fifth metatarsal, and anterior tibia. Therefore, attaining osseous union can be difficult, and pain-free function with a fibrous union or possibly a unilateral bony union is acceptable. It has been reported that 73% of early lesions unite, whereas lesions with established nonunions usually do not. Several studies have demonstrated that a good clinical outcome is not always related to osseous union. Furthermore, in patients with bilateral pars interarticularis defects and minor slippage, the risk of spondylolisthesis progression in athletes mirrors that in the general population, with only 10% to 12% demonstrating an increase of more than 10%. This increase in spondylolisthesis progression usually occurs during growth acceleration.

Treatment varies with regard to brace wear and participation in athletic activities. Brace types range from simple lumbar corsets to rigid thoracolumbar braces. Most treatment protocols that call for no brace or the use of corset braces also recommend prohibiting participation in athletic activities for 3 to 6 months. Retrospective analyses of these treatment protocols generally report good clinical outcomes in 78% to 82% of patients. One review, however, showed that early rigid antilordotic bracing might enhance spinal stability and be useful in safely returning the patient to participation in athletic activities in 4 to 6 weeks. The patients examined in this review were required to be pain free (no pain on hyperextension) before returning to participation in athletic activities. The treatment protocol included continuation of full-time bracing for 4 to 6 months. Lumbar flexion abdominal strengthening exercises as well as psoas and hamstring stretching were emphasized in the rehabilitation program. If the patient was pain free at 4 months, brace use was gradually discontinued. If the patient was still symptomatic at 4 months, other pathologies were considered. Case studies have shown that electromagnetic stimulation may be helpful in treating patients who experience nonunion of their fractures.

Surgical intervention, usually fusion, is reserved for the young athlete who has intractable pain with athletic activities and activities of daily living. Surgical intervention is also indicated in patients with spondylolisthesis exceeding a 50% slippage, progressive slippage, neurologic deficit, and intractable pain. In patients in whom the disk above is suspected in the pain etiology, a diskogram is indicated.

Degenerative Disk Disease

One or more degenerative disks can cause intermittent aching low back pain. One study reported that 48% of adult patients had discogenic pathology. The spectrum of disk pathologies includes disk overuse resulting in dehydration and desiccation, annular tears, protrusions or diffuse segmental spondylosis, and end plate fracturing in the immature spine. In addition, disk material or inflammation can cause nerve root encroachment. Although many disk changes are a normal part of the aging process, abnormal MRI findings of disk degeneration in completely asymptomatic adults have been reported to occur in 15% to 30% of patients. Nonetheless, participation in certain sports, such as gymnastics, poses an increased risk of disk injury. Other high-risk activities such as weightlifting, contact sports, and rowing involve repetitive axial loading with flexion of the spine, which increases stress on the anulus fibrosus from increased intradiskal pressures and torsional strain. In young athletes, these forces may produce end plate injuries at the thoracolumbar region, resulting in Schmorl's nodes and fragmented end plates (Figure 1). Similar end plate changes occur in the thoracic spine in patients with Scheuermann's disease. In the thoracolumbar region, these changes are referred to as atypical Scheuermann's or lumbar Scheuermann's disease.

Patients with degenerative disk disease may report axial and referred pain. Radicular pain indicates inflammation of the nerve root. Young athletes with lumbar Scheuermann's disease may report painful hypokyphosis and hypolordosis (flat back) with resultant flexion overload of the thoracolumbar juncture. In patients with thoracic Scheuermann's disease, however, hyperkyphotic vertebral injury and deformity are limited to the thoracic spine.

Physical examination should include a careful review of peripelvic and thoracolumbar flexibility. In patients with lumbar Scheuermann's disease, plain radiographs are often diagnostic. In patients with early adult disk disease, plain radiographs are normal. In patients with advanced degenerative disk disease, the disk space is usually narrowed with osteophyte formation and evidence of facet hypertrophy can be detected. MRI can help assess the extent of degenerative disk disease and stenosis. For some patients, a diskogram may be needed to assess whether fusion or intradiskal electrothermy is indicated.

The treatment of athletes with degenerative disk disease typically includes relative rest with cross training and physical therapy to address flexibility and core stabilization. Athletes with lumbar Scheuermann's disease may benefit from a temporary TLSO in 15° of extension, which may be advanced as needed. Anti-inflammatory medications are also useful. Sport-specific training is essential to return the athlete to participation and is directed by symptoms. For patients who do not respond to this treatment, such as those with anulus fibrosus shrinkage and neurolysis, intradiskal electrothermal therapy may be appropriate. Satisfactory results have been reported using this treatment in 53% to 73% of patients. Although intradiskal electrothermal therapy is less invasive than fusion, recovery time is still 4 to 6 months.

Lordotic Low Back Pain

During the adolescent growth spurt, the thoracolumbar fascia and peripelvic tendons may be unable to keep up with the growth acceleration of the spine. Consequently, a number of tissues are subjected to traction and compression with cyclic loading and injuries can result, including traction injury to the spinous process and iliac crest apophyses, impingement of the spinous process and facet joints, and potentially pseudarthrosis of transitional vertebrae (Bertolotti syndrome). Although the clinical presentation of this type of injury is variable, it usually mimics a spondylolytic process. Patients often manifest painful hyperextension but may also show pain on flexion from the traction component. This is usually a diagnosis of exclusion; however, careful review of a bone scan may show some increased uptake in the spinous process, iliac crest, or transitional pseudarthrosis (seen initially on plain radiographs).

Treatment involves exercises that address pelvic and thoracolumbar inflexibility as well as antilordotic strengthening. With the exception of injurious motions such as a back walkover in gymnastics, participation in athletic activities is usually permitted. The athlete gradually resumes all motion as the therapeutic exercises are performed. Patients who do not improve may benefit from bracing. In addition, a corticosteroid injection into an inflamed facet or transitional pseudarthrosis can be quite helpful in the rehabilitation process.

Sacroiliac Inflammation

Sacroiliac inflammation may occur as a result of trauma or with repetitive asymmetric loading of the pelvis, as occurs in patients with a limb-length discrepancy. Pain in the sacroiliac region is problematic because this is a watershed zone for pain referral, and physical examination techniques of this region are insensitive. Treatment regimens address core stabilization with attention to the oblique muscle groups. Rotary torso motion is also effective in gaining strength in the oblique muscle groups. Occasionally, corticosteroid and/or anesthetic injections are used for diagnostic and therapeutic purposes.

Spinal Curve Deformity: Scoliosis and Kyphosis

Adolescent idiopathic scoliosis has a prevalence of 2% to 3% in the general population, with a female to male ratio of 4:1 that includes significant curvature. The prevalence may be higher among participants in specific sports; for example, in ballet the incidence of adolescent idiopathic scoliosis has been noted to be as high as 24%. Adolescent idiopathic scoliosis has also been recognized to occur with a tenfold increase in incidence among rhythmic gymnasts. Increased spinal curvature has also been identified in swimmers, throwers, and rowers. The various mechanisms of injury that have been proposed include cyclic loading with asymmetric torques to the growing spine, delayed menarche, and ligamentous laxity. Painful scoliosis is uncommon and should initiate a search for other causes such as a tethered cord, syrinx, tumor, or herniated disk.

Sagittal curve deformity is seen with kyphosis in the midthoracic region. This deformity is seen predominantly in male athletes and is associated with repetitive loading in flexion in the immature spine. Sports in which the risk for sagittal curve deformity is greatest include gymnastics, wrestling, water skiing, and swimming.

The treatment of scoliosis and kyphosis deformities in athletes is similar to treatment for the nonathletic population. The decision whether to brace depends on the magnitude of the deformity and the Risser score. Commonly used braces include the Boston underarm TLSO brace and the Charleston brace. Many athletes may be permitted to fully participate in athletic activities (including contact sports) without a brace. Although exercise does not alter the scoliotic curve, it is encouraged to improve general stabilization and flexibility. With kyphosis, upper back strengthening and abdominal exercises are an integral part of treatment.

Rehabilitation

Rehabilitation for patients with spinal injuries progresses through three phases: acute care, recovery, and sport-specific (functional) care. Each phase is important in helping patients to safely return to participation in athletic activity without recurrence of injury.

In the acute care phase, a short period of rest lasting a few days is allowed. During the subsequent subacute phase, the patient is gradually mobilized, and analgesia and anti-inflammatory medications are used to treat pain. Aerobic conditioning, flexibility, and isometric strength are addressed with exercise. It is during this phase that additional rehabilitative modalities such as icing, ultrasound, or iontophoresis are most useful.

Recovery is the longest phase of rehabilitation. During recovery, an accurate diagnosis is important in the design of a rehabilitation program that will avoid further damage to injured tissue. An extension-based program is used for patients with disk involvement, and a flexion-based program is used for patients with posterior element injuries. However, each particular patient and pathology may define a different neutral zone. In recovery, inflexibilities must be addressed to allow fluid lumbopelvic motion. Core stabilization involves progressively strengthening isolated muscle groups and advancing to coactivation techniques, such as Swiss ball and Pilates exercises. Pilates, widely used by ballet dancers, is now becoming increasingly used for both fitness and rehabilitation of athletic injuries. This system of exercise was developed by Joseph Pilates and Clara Pilates in the early 20th century. Pilates can be done as either mat-based exercises or exercises using special pieces of equipment. The key components of this system include a series of exercises and physical movements including stretching, strengthening, and balancing of the body components that are often done in association with specific breathing patterns. Although Pilates has been of particular use for the prevention and treatment of injuries in dancers, it has now become widely used by the general public and, in some cases, for sports rehabilitation. It is essential to have an instructor who has been trained in the Pilates technique and programs in order to ensure proper use of the apparatus and proper sequence of exercises with appropriate resistance and safety measures, as well as to give attention to individual specific requirements and limitations in the performance of the total exercise program.

The entire closed chain must be addressed, including lower extremity and hip rotational muscles. Because each athletic activity has particular requirements, rehabilitative exercises must be tailored to the needs of each patient. For all athletes, aerobic conditioning is used throughout the entire recovery phase.

The functional phase in rehabilitation is reached once the athlete has gained full strength and endurance. Nonetheless, sport-specific training is crucial to avoid reinjury, which, for example, includes techniques to improve the golf swing of golfers or the pelvic tilt of a ballet dancer in extension. Sport-specific plyometric drills are used during the functional phase as well.

Summary

Because back pain in athletes is a relatively common complaint, it is essential to make a specific diagnosis and determination of the etiology of the pain; treatment, rehabilitation, and return to play determinations vary greatly depending on the diagnosis. Using a sport-specific history and careful and systematic physical examination, combined with additional imaging techniques as indicated, an appropriate plan of treatment and return to play can usually be developed for the young athlete with back pain. Most importantly, the complaint of back pain must not be simply ascribed to a muscle strain or sprain without careful assessment. In particular, certain infectious and neoplastic processes may become symptomatic in the course of athletic participation and be incorrectly ascribed to repetitive microtrauma or macrotrauma etiology.

Annotated Bibliography

Risk Factors

Soler T, Calderone C: The prevalence of spondylolysis in the Spanish elite athlete. *Am J Sports Med* 2000;28: 57-62.

This article documents the prevalence of spondylolysis in specific sports, which are then classified according to risk.

Trainor TJ, Wiesel SW: Epidemiology of back pain in the athlete. *Clin Sports Med* 2002;21:93-103.

This article overviews the epidemiology and risk factors for back pain in athletes, particularly the young athlete, with special emphasis on spondylolysis.

Tsirikos A, Papagelopoulos PJ, Giannakopoulos PN, et al: Degenerative spondyloarthropathy of the cervical and lumbar spine in jockeys. *Orthopedics* 2001;24:561-564.

This article provides a sport-specific review of back and neck injuries in jockeys.

Watson KD, Papageorgiou AC, Jones GT, et al: Low back pain in schoolchildren: The role of mechanical and psychosocial factors. *Arch Dis Child* 2003;88:12-17.

This is a cross-sectional study of nonspecific low back pain in British schoolchildren. The authors suggest that psychosocial factors rather than mechanical factors (such as bookbag weight) are more important etiologic factors of this type of low back pain.

Clinical Evaluation

d'Hemecourt PA, Gerbino PG II, Micheli LJ: Back injuries in the young athlete. *Clin Sports Med* 2000;19:663-679.

This article summarizes the most common etiology of back injuries (specifically in young athletes) and provides rationale for treatment.

McTimoney CA, Micheli LJ: Current evaluation and management of spondylolysis and spondylolisthesis. *Curr Sports Med Rep* 2003;2:41-46.

This article is the most recent overview of reports on the current evaluation and management of spondylolysis and spondylolisthesis in the adolescent.

Staendaert CJ, Herring SA: Spondylolysis: A critical review. *Br J Sports Med* 2000;34:415-422.

This is a literature review of the current diagnosis and treatment of spondylolysis.

Sys J, Michielsen J, Bracke P: Nonoperative treatment of active spondylolysis in elite athletes with normal x-ray findings: Literature review and results of conservative treatment. *Eur Spine J* 2001;10:498-504.

This article provides a review of both the English and non-English literature on the conservative management of spondylolysis in elite athletes.

Udeshi UL, Reeves D: Routine thin slice MRI effectively demonstrates the lumbar pars interarticularis. *Clin Radiol* 1999;54:615-619.

The authors of this article report that the pars interarticularis can be adequately imaged using smaller (3-mm) slices than previously used.

Watkins RG: Lumbar disc injury in the athlete. *Clin Sports Med* 2002;21:147-165.

This review article overviews the diagnosis, assessment, and treatment of discogenic pain specific to the athlete.

Spinal Curve Deformity: Scoliosis and Kyphosis

Omey ML, Micheli LJ, Gerbino PG II: Idiopathic scoliosis and spondylolysis in the female athlete: Tips for treatment. *Clin Orthop* 2000;372:74-84.

This article focuses on treatment techniques for athletes with both scoliosis and spondylolysis and, in particular, on the use of bracing and exercise.

Wood KB: Spinal deformity in the adolescent athlete. *Clin Sports Med* 2002;21:77-92.

This is a current overview of the athletic participation of children with spinal deformities, including those under treatment with bracing or those who have had surgical interventions.

Rehabilitation

d'Hemecourt PA, Zurakowski D, Krimeler S, Micheli LJ: Spondylolysis: Returning the athlete to sports participation with brace treatment. *Orthopedics* 2002;25:653-657.

This article establishes return to sport parameters for patients with spondylolysis who were conservatively managed with the Boston overlapping brace.

Fellander-Tsai L, Micheli LJ: Treatment of spondylolysis with external electrical stimulation and bracing in adolescent athletes: A report of two cases. *Clin J Sport Med* 1998;8:232-234.

Two patients were treated successfully with a bone growth stimulator. Both patients had previously failed conventional conservative brace treatment therapy.

Classic Bibliography

Fredrickson BE, Baker D, Mc Hollick WJ, et al: The natural history of spondylolysis and spondylolisthesis. *J Bone Joint Surg Am* 1984;66:699-707.

Goldstein JD, Berger PE, Windler GE, Jackson DW: Spine injuries in gymnasts and swimmers: An epidemiologic investigation. *Am J Sports Med* 1991;19:463-468.

Greene TL, Hensinger RN, Hunter LY: Back pain and vertebral changes simulating Scheuermann's disease. *J Pediatr Orthop* 1985;5:1-7.

Hellstrom M, Jacobson B, Sward L: Radiologic abnormalities of the thoracolumbar spine in athletes. *Acta Radiol* 1990;31:127-132.

Ikata T, Morita T, Katoh S, Tachibana K, Maoka H: Lesions of the lumbar posterior end plate in children and adolescents. *J Bone Joint Surg Br* 1995;77:951-955.

Micheli LJ, Wood R: Back pain in young athletes: Significant differences from adults in causes and patterns. *Arch Pediatr Adolesc Med* 1995;149:15-18.

Mundt DJ, Kelsey JL, Golden AL, et al: An epidemiologic study of sports and weightlifting as a possible risk factors for herniated lumbar and cervical discs: The Northeast Collaborative Group on Low Back Pain. *Am J Sports Med* 1993;21:854-860.

Rosen PR, Micheli LJ, Treves S: Early scintigraphic diagnosis of bone stress and fractures in athletic adolescents. *Pediatrics* 1982;70:11-15.

Chapter 3

Head Injuries in Athletics: Mechanisms and Management

Margot Putukian, MD, FACSM

Introduction

Head injury and concussion occur commonly in sports, and these injuries can pose significant risks for morbidity and mortality. Over the past several years, there have been tremendous developments in the assessment, treatment, and rehabilitation of athletic head injuries. In addition, although previous emphasis has been on the development of various classification systems and guidelines for return to play, what has evolved is a better understanding of the natural history of traumatic brain injury in the athlete. The development of new assessment tools, such as neuropsychologic testing, has questioned many assumptions and enhanced the knowledge base for the natural history of these injuries.

Epidemiology

Traumatic brain injuries are generally the result of motor vehicle accidents, falls, or violent acts and are twice as common in males than females. One million head injuries are treated in North American emergency departments annually. The incidence is estimated to be 100 injuries per 100,000 persons, and 52,000 deaths occur annually as a result of traumatic brain injuries. Individuals who are age 15 to 24 years as well as those older than 75 years account for the majority of patients with traumatic brain injuries, with accidents or trauma being the most likely cause in the youth population and falls being the most common mechanism in those older than 75 years. Alcohol is involved in 50% of traumatic brain injuries. An estimated 2.5 to 6.5 million people survive traumatic brain injuries, but some continue to experience posttraumatic symptoms and deficits. Athletic activities are the cause of traumatic brain injuries in only 3% of patients hospitalized for traumatic brain injuries, 90% of which are mild.

Head injuries comprise 4.5% of all sports-related injuries in high school athletes and 19% of all nonfatal high school football-related injuries. At the elementary, junior, and high school levels, football accounts for the highest incidence of head injuries in any sport. At the college level, concussions account for roughly 1.6% to 8.5% of all injuries, with an incidence of 0.06 to 0.55 injuries per 1,000 athlete exposures (Table 1). Although ice hockey and football tend to account for the highest incidence of injuries, several sports, including men's and women's soccer and lacrosse, have a similar incidence of injuries. Interestingly, sports activities that are performed with and without helmets appear to have similar incidence rates. The mechanism of injury tends to be player-to-player contact, with the exceptions being field hockey (in which the mechanism of injury tends to be contact with the stick) and women's lacrosse, women's softball, and baseball (in which the mechanism of injury tends to be contact with the ball).

Pathophysiology

Once the pathophysiology and mechanisms of head injuries are understood, the severity of and recovery from head injuries can be predicted, and head injuries can potentially be prevented as well. With the most severe brain injury (diffuse brain injury), anatomic changes can occur, including disruption of axonal and myelin sheath structures throughout the white matter of the hemispheres and brainstem, petechial hemorrhages in periventricular regions, and chromatolysis and cell loss throughout the cortical gray matter and brainstem nuclei. With cumulative and repetitive injury, cerebral hemispheric atrophy can occur. Much of the information known about the mechanisms of injury in sports-related or traumatic brain injuries is derived from animal research models.

Acceleration forces occur when a moving head strikes a nonmoving object, such as when an athlete falls and strikes the ground. Impact or compressive forces occur when a moving object strikes a stationary head, such as when an athlete's head is struck by a ball or other moving object. Rotational forces are associated with shearing stresses, and these are believed to be associated with more severe injuries and structural injuries. In sports, these forces often occur in combination, with the most severe injuries being a result of both rotational and acceleration forces.

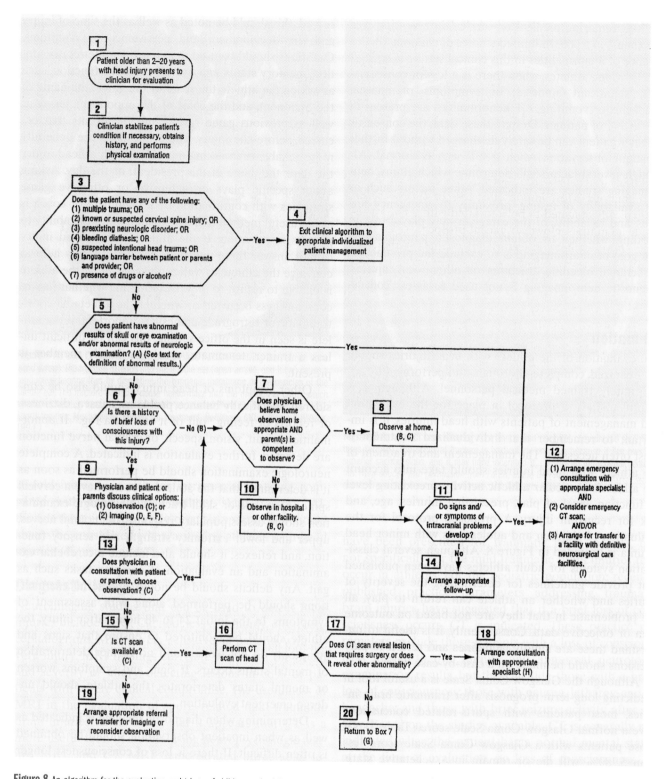

Figure 8 An algorithm for the evaluation and triage of children and adolescents with minor head trauma. *(Reproduced with permission from The management of minor closed head injury in children: Committee on Quality Improvement, American Academy of Pediatrics, Commission on Clinical Policies and Research, American Academy of Family Physicians. Pediatrics 1999;104:1407-1415.)*

Classification Systems

In 2002, a recognized group of medical personnel with expertise in sports-related mild traumatic brain injuries published their revised definition of concussion (as dis-

cussed previously) and developed a protocol for treating sports-related head injuries that included clinical history, evaluation, neuropsychologic testing, imaging procedures, research methods, management and rehabilita-

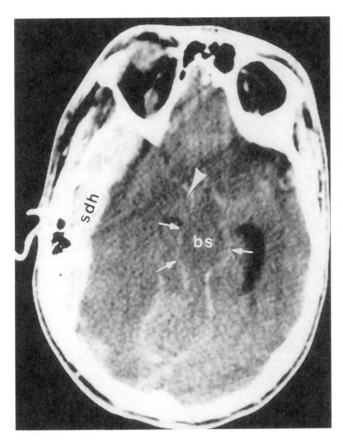

Figure 1 An axial CT scan demonstrating an acute subdural hematoma (sdh) on the right side, with herniation of the medial temporal lobe into the tentorial notch (*arrowhead*). The midbrain is outlined by subarachnoid hemorrhage in the perimesencephalic cistern (*arrows*). bs = brainstem. *(Reproduced with permission from Fu FH, Stone DA (eds): Sports Injuries: Mechanisms, Prevention, Treatment. Baltimore, MD, Williams & Wilkins, 1994.)*

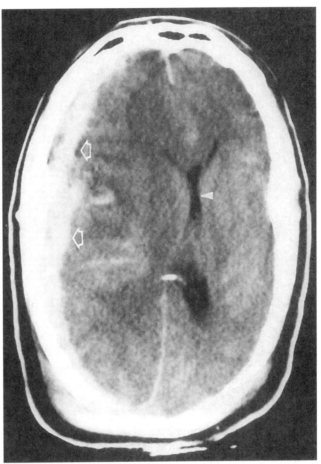

Figure 2 Typical appearance of an acute subdural hematoma (*open arrows*) on an axial CT scan. The degree of shift of the midline structures (*arrowhead*) is greater than the thickness of the subdural hematoma, suggesting significant parenchymal injury to the hemisphere in addition to the hematoma. *(Reproduced with permission from Fu FH, Stone DA (eds): Sports Injuries: Mechanisms, Prevention, Treatment. Baltimore, MD, Williams & Wilkins, 1994.)*

ing brain is compromised. The adolescent athlete, however, will have symptoms earlier and sooner after subdural injury. Symptoms in the adolescent athlete are more often the result of compression of normal brain substance, whereas the symptoms in the adult athlete are the result of a mass effect.

Epidural hematomas are less common than subdural hematomas and are caused by the disruption of the high-pressure meningeal arterial vasculature, most commonly the middle meningeal artery. Patients with epidural hematomas usually report an initial loss of consciousness followed by apparent recovery and a lucid interval. Minutes to hours later (rarely days), severe headache, deterioration in mental status, pupillary abnormalities (ipsilateral pupil dilates), loss of consciousness, and decerebrate posturing with weakness on the opposite side of the bleed will occur. Unfortunately, only one third of patients will have this classic presentation (Figure 3), underscoring the need to maintain a high index of suspicion for these vascular emergencies.

Cerebral contusions, intracerebral hemorrhages, and subarachnoid hemorrhages are other examples of focal brain injuries. (Subarachnoid hemorrhages occur rarely in sports and therefore are beyond the scope of this chapter.) Cerebral contusions generally are caused by impact injuries (either coup or contrecoup) and are a result of damaged parenchymal vessels on the surface of the brain. These injuries often occur on the inferior surface of the frontal or temporal lobes because of the presence of the bony ridges and prominences of the bone inside the skull. Patients with cerebral contusions often report a very brief loss of consciousness and prolonged posttraumatic confusion. In addition, they may have signs of increased intracranial pressure or focal neurologic deficits. Most isolated cerebral contusions have a good outcome, but if the contusions are large or are associated with increased intracranial pressure or posttraumatic seizures, the outcome can be poor. If cerebral contusions compress underlying brain tissue, ischemia and infarction of these areas can occur.

Intracerebral hemorrhages or hematomas occur when the small caliber arterioles within the brain paren-

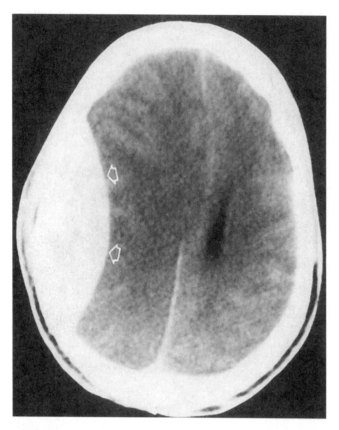

Figure 3 An axial CT scan showing the typical appearance of an epidural hematoma (arrows). *(Reproduced with permission from Fu FH, Stone DA (eds): Sports Injuries: Mechanisms, Prevention, Treatment. Baltimore, MD, Williams & Wilkins, 1994.)*

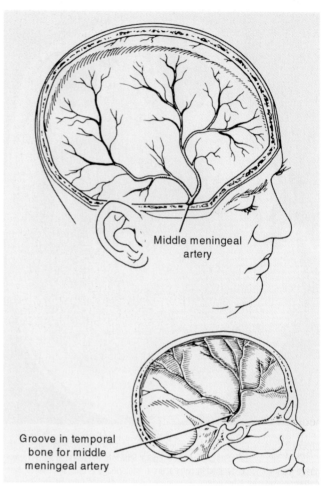

Figure 4 The middle meningeal artery is tethered in a groove in the temporal bone and is easily lacerated by fractures through this bone. Hemorrhage from the middle meningeal artery causes an epidural hematoma. *(Reproduced with permission from Fu FH, Stone DA (eds): Sports Injuries: Mechanisms, Prevention, Treatment. Baltimore, MD, Williams & Wilkins, 1994.)*

chyma bleed, which most commonly affects the frontal or temporal lobes. Tensile or shearing forces cause this bleeding, and the patient presentation will depend on the size and location of the lesion, as well as whether associated pathology, such as contusions or edema, is present. If the patient is conscious at presentation, the mortality rate is low; if the patient is unconscious at presentation, the mortality rate approaches 45%. Approximately 50% of patients with intracerebral hemorrhages or hematomas will have headaches; other symptoms include confusion, nausea, vomiting, and focal neurologic deficits, all of which can develop over hours to days. Cerebral contusions and hemorrhages both can occur in association with hydrocephalus and changes associated with a mass effect (Figures 4 and 5).

Diffuse Brain Injuries

Diffuse brain injury occurs when there is no identifiable lesion. These injuries are typically categorized on a spectrum of injury in which the degree of anatomic disruption correlates with the severity of brain dysfunction. Diffuse axonal injury represents the most severe injury along this spectrum, and cerebral concussion represents the most mild. Diffuse axonal injury is often associated with residual psychologic, personality, and neurologic

deficits. These injuries do not occur commonly in athletes.

Concussion was defined almost 40 years ago as a clinical syndrome characterized by immediate and transient impairment of neurologic function secondary to mechanical forces. More recently, this definition was modified to characterize concussion as a complex pathophysiologic process affecting the brain that is induced by traumatic biomechanical forces. Several common features of concussion have also been described, which help determine the nature of concussive injuries. Concussions can occur as the result of either a direct blow or an impulsive force transmitted from one part of the body; they typically result in short-lived impairment with rapid onset and spontaneous resolution; they cause symptoms that reflect functional disturbances more commonly than neuropathologic changes; they result in a graded set of syndromes that may or may not include loss of consciousness, and resolution generally follows a

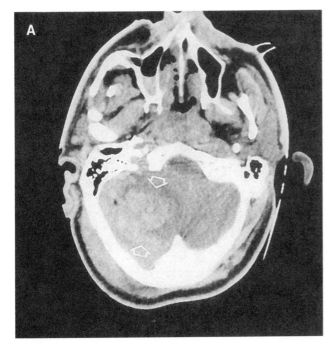
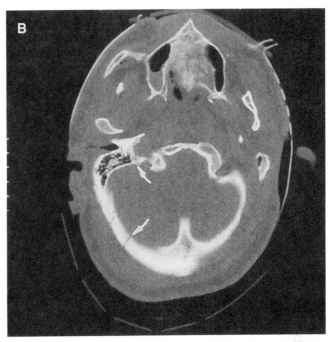

Figure 5 Axial CT scans demonstrate a hemorrhagic contusion to the right cerebellar hemisphere (*open arrows*) (**A**) associated with a fracture through the floor of the posterior fossa on the right side (*solid arrows*) (**B**). (*Reproduced with permission from Fu FH, Stone DA (eds): Sports Injuries: Mechanisms, Prevention, Treatment. Baltimore, MD, Williams & Wilkins, 1994.*)

sequential course; and they are generally associated with normal results on structural neuroimaging studies. This definition is very useful in assessing sports-related mild traumatic brain injuries.

The hallmark of concussion is confusion. Two types of memory dysfunction, posttraumatic amnesia and retrograde amnesia, are important symptoms that predict the severity of injury. The signs and symptoms of cerebral concussion are listed in Table 2. Several symptoms of head injury, including headache, fatigue, and nausea, are ubiquitous, occurring commonly in individuals who have not experienced head trauma. Therefore, distinguishing individuals with mild traumatic brain injuries from those with less significant injuries or those without injuries can be difficult. If an athlete experiences trauma to the head and headache is the only symptom, it is difficult to define this injury as a concussion unless transient confusion or disorientation or other symptoms are present. Therefore, the presence and persistence of retrograde amnesia and posttraumatic amnesia should be assessed and followed closely.

It is essential when evaluating the athlete with head injuries to also consider associated injuries such as scalp lacerations, skull fractures, and/or cervical spine injuries. Cervical spine injuries occur in 5% to 10% of patients with severe head injuries. If the athlete is unconscious, the spine should be considered unstable until proven otherwise. Skull fractures may be identified by palpable malalignment of the calvarium, cranial nerve injuries, rhinorrhea, otorrhea, "raccoon eyes," Battle's sign, or

TABLE 2	Signs and Symptoms of Cerebral Concussion
Loss of consciousness
Confusion
Posttraumatic amnesia
Retrograde amnesia
Disorientation
Delayed verbal and motor responses
Inability to focus
Headache
Nausea/vomiting
Visual disturbances (photophobia, blurry vision, double vision)
Disequilibrium
Feeling "in a fog" or "out of it"
Vacant stare
Emotional lability
Dizziness
Slurred/incoherent speech
Excessive drowsiness

(*Adapted with permission from Garrett WE Jr, Kirkendall DT, Squire DL (eds): Principles and Practice of Primary Care Sports Medicine. Philadelphia, PA, Lippincott Williams & Wilkins, 2001, p 337.*)

hemotympanum. If these signs and symptoms are evident, the athlete should be transported to a medical facility for additional imaging studies and a neurosurgical consultation if indicated. Skull fractures are associated with an increased risk for intracranial infection and a

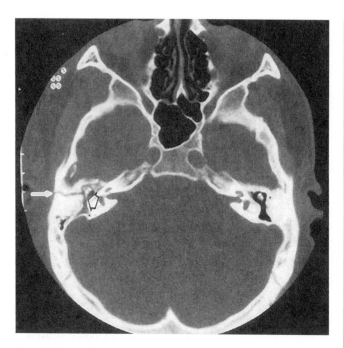

Figure 6 An axial CT scan showing a basilar skull fracture involving the petrous bone (*solid arrow*). The fracture extends into the middle ear (*open arrow*), and it can cause a conductive hearing loss by disrupting the tympanic membrane or the ossicles of the middle ear. The fracture also can cause hemorrhage into the middle ear cavity, which results in hearing loss. (*Reproduced with permission from Fu FH, Stone DA (eds): Sports Injuries: Mechanisms, Prevention, Treatment. Baltimore, MD, Williams & Wilkins, 1994.*)

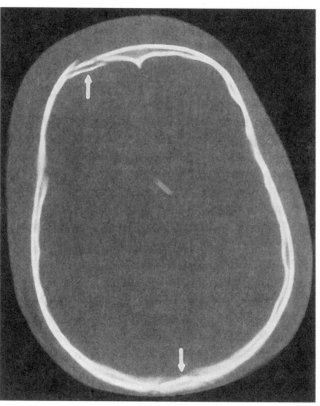

Figure 7 An axial CT scan showing right frontal and occipital comminuted skull fractures (*arrows*). The occipital fracture is particularly ominous because it lies over the superior sagittal sinus, and it may have lacerated it, causing an intracranial hematoma. (*Reproduced with permission from Fu FH, Stone DA (eds): Sports Injuries: Mechanisms, Prevention, Treatment. Baltimore, MD, Williams & Wilkins, 1994.*)

20-fold increase in risk for intracranial bleeding compared with head injuries without skull fracture. Although these injuries rarely occur in sports, they should always be considered when assessing athletes with head injuries (Figures 6 and 7).

Diagnostic Imaging

Neuroimaging studies that can be used to detect focal injuries include MRI, CT, and, less commonly, electroencephalograms. MRI is very sensitive; in patients with severe injury, MRI findings correlate with both the depth and severity of injury, detecting lesions in 88% of patients with severe clinical compromise. The usefulness of MRI in the evaluation of sports-related mild traumatic brain injuries is less clear, and it appears that CT is a more useful tool. In studies using neuropsychologic testing, MRI, and CT, MRI demonstrated intracranial lesions more often than CT, although both MRI and CT detected those lesions requiring surgical treatment. Given its superiority in detecting fractures, subarachnoid hemorrhages, and evidence of other bleeding, the initial diagnostic imaging modality of choice should almost always be CT, provided it is indicated and available.

Although it is difficult to determine when these diagnostic imaging tests should be ordered, guidelines

have been presented for traumatic brain injuries, but not specifically for the mild traumatic brain injuries that occur in athletes. For the pediatric population, recently published practice parameters addressing traumatic brain injuries have suggested that if a brief loss of consciousness occurs, CT is indicated. These practice parameters exclude those patients with a loss of consciousness longer than 1 minute and abnormal neurologic examination results, but they include those with a brief loss of consciousness; those with nausea, lethargy, and/or headache; and those with brief seizure activity after injury. Based on the studies available, CT is generally not indicated when the patient has a normal mental status at the time of evaluation, no loss of consciousness, no abnormalities on neurologic (including funduscopic) examination, and no evidence of skull fracture. In these patients, observation in the emergency department, clinic, or at home by a competent adult is believed to be safe and reasonable.

In both adults and children, the likelihood of intracranial abnormalities in the absence of loss of consciousness or focal neurologic deficits is quite low. In population-based studies, the incidence of CT abnormalities requiring medical or surgical intervention was less than 1 in 5,000. In limited studies of children, the incidence of abnormalities in this clinical setting is negligible. In young athletes, when there is a loss of consciousness, significant amnesia, or symptoms of nausea, headache, or vomiting, CT abnormalities are present in 0% to 7% of patients. Despite these data, the consensus is that a patient can be safely discharged without further inpatient observation when a CT scan is normal. Although several factors will determine which, if any, neuroimaging studies are indicated, other factors such as the availability of testing, proximity to emergency services, and reliability of the caregiver may play a role in deciding whether to obtain diagnostic neuroimaging. The goal of neuroimaging is to exclude the presence of intracranial bleeding, fractures, or other focal injuries; diagnostic neuroimaging is not used to assess concussions.

Evaluation

The evaluation of the athlete with head injuries should be organized, complete, thorough, and performed by appropriately trained medical personnel. Although it is helpful to have a protocol in place for the evaluation and management of patients with head injuries, it is important to remember that individualized treatment is most often necessary. The management and treatment of the athlete with head injuries should take into account the athlete's particular athletic activity, preexisting level of function, level of play, preexisting injuries, age, and risk for recurrent injury. A proposed protocol for the evaluation of children and adolescents with minor head trauma is provided in Figure 8. Although several classification systems for adult athletes have been published that provide guidelines for determining the severity of injuries and whether an athlete can return to play, all are problematic in that they are not based on outcome data or objective data. Consequently, it is useful to understand these are simply guidelines and return to play decisions should be made on a case-by-case basis.

Although the Glasgow Coma Scale is a useful tool in predicting long-term prognosis after traumatic brain injuries, most patients with sports-related concussions have a normal Glasgow Coma Scale score (Table 3). Of those patients with a Glasgow Coma Scale score less than 5, 80% will die or remain in a vegetative state, whereas of those with a Glasgow Coma Scale score greater than 11, more than 90% will have complete recovery. Increases in Glasgow Coma Scale scores are associated with improved prognosis; therefore, serial assessments are useful.

Because the medical history is critical in determining the extent of a head injury, when possible, it should be obtained directly from the injured athlete and be as complete as possible. If the mechanism of injury was observed, this should be noted as well as the time of injury and the development and persistence of symptoms. Questions should be used to assess the athlete's orientation, memory status, and overall cognitive function, such as asking the athlete the score of the game, the name of the opponent, and the color of the opponent's jersey as well as previous game results and the events that occurred before the injury. These questions are generally more reliable than asking an athlete with a head injury the date, the name of the president, or the day. Asking about specific plays or defensive or offensive game strategies with confirmation by a teammate or coach is also a useful method to assess memory and the ability to process information. If the athlete with a head injury cannot answer these questions correctly, it may help to convince the athlete as well as the coach that the athlete is unable to return to play. Determining whether loss of consciousness occurred or whether the athlete has post-traumatic or retrograde amnesia is important; if the athlete is seen in the office setting, this can be difficult unless a trainer, teammate, coach, or family member is present.

Other symptoms of head injury should also be considered, specifically balance problems, nausea, dizziness, or reports of feeling "out of it" or "in a fog." If abnormalities in gait, vision, speech, or cranial nerve function are detected, further evaluation is indicated. A complete neurologic examination should be performed as soon as it is determined that the athlete does not have a cervical spine injury and/or skull fracture. Neurologic examination should assess pupillary response, the cranial nerves, upper and lower extremity strength and sensory function, and reflexes; it should also include a cerebellar examination and an evaluation of complex tasks such as gait. Any deficits should be noted, and serial examinations should be performed along with assessment of symptoms. In the initial 24 to 48 hours after injury, the athlete should be monitored to ensure that signs and symptoms do not worsen and no further deterioration of mental status occurs. If signs and symptoms worsen or mental status deteriorates, the athlete should undergo emergent evaluation.

Determining when diagnostic imaging is indicated as well as when inpatient observation should be obtained is often difficult. If there is loss of consciousness longer than 5 seconds, concern that a skull fracture may be present, or any evidence of focal neurologic deficits, diagnostic imaging should be considered. If an athlete with a head injury has a lucid interval followed by a decline in mental status, or if symptoms worsen, diagnostic imaging should be done. If an athlete with a head injury cannot be observed closely in a safe environment by a responsible caregiver, then inpatient observation may be necessary.

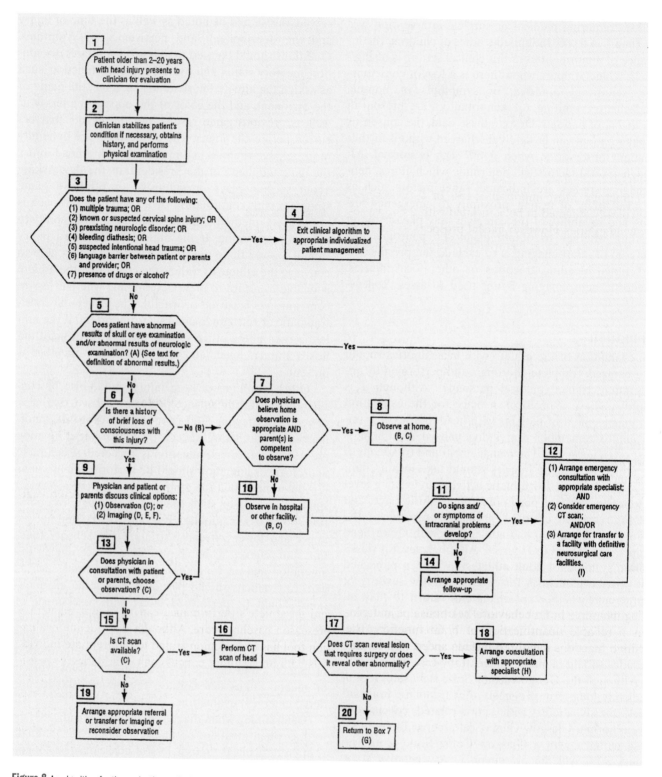

Figure 8 An algorithm for the evaluation and triage of children and adolescents with minor head trauma. *(Reproduced with permission from The management of minor closed head injury in children: Committee on Quality Improvement, American Academy of Pediatrics, Commission on Clinical Policies and Research, American Academy of Family Physicians. Pediatrics 1999;104:1407-1415.)*

Classification Systems

In 2002, a recognized group of medical personnel with expertise in sports-related mild traumatic brain injuries published their revised definition of concussion (as dis-

cussed previously) and developed a protocol for treating sports-related head injuries that included clinical history, evaluation, neuropsychologic testing, imaging procedures, research methods, management and rehabilitation, prevention, education, future directions, and medicolegal considerations. Although this protocol presented no new research information, it updated the current thinking regarding the treatment of athletes with head injuries, recognized the importance of using neuropsychologic testing as the cornerstone of evaluation, and recommended that a progression of activity be used to determine whether an athlete should return to play.

The weaknesses of using previously established classification systems to treat sports-related head injuries are numerous. Most importantly, loss of consciousness was typically assumed to be associated with the most severe head injuries. However, recent prospective research using neuropsychologic testing has confirmed that loss of consciousness does not predict severity of injury; instead, posttraumatic amnesia appears to be a more sensitive indicator. In addition, classification systems for head injuries, which usually assign a grade to injury types, do not describe the clinical course of recovery, do not relate specific symptoms, and often do not detail the extent of memory or cognitive dysfunction. For these reasons, no single classification system is appropriate for establishing a comprehensive treatment protocol for sports-related head injuries. To do so, more research is needed to clarify the factors that help assess severity of injury and when return to play is indicated. It may be appropriate to assess the number and severity of symptoms and to determine whether posttraumatic amnesia, retrograde amnesia, and/or loss of consciousness has occurred.

Neuropsychologic Testing

Neuropsychologic testing assesses cognitive function and is well established in its ability to assess acute and chronic mild traumatic brain injuries. Neuropsychologic testing measures brain behavioral relationships and provides a reliable quantification of brain function. The cognitive functions measured include speed of information processing, attention, concentration, reaction time, visual scanning, visual tracking, memory recall, and problem solving. Neuropsychologic testing is more sensitive than traditional medical testing and neuroimaging in assessing deficits after mild traumatic brain injuries. In studies of patients with severe head injuries, neuropsychologic testing results correlated with the location and size of lesions on initial MRI scans and at 1- and 3-month follow-up. Neuropsychologic testing has been used to successfully evaluate both acute and chronic sports-related mild traumatic brain injuries. Over the past 10 years, there has been an exponential increase in research using neuropsychologic tests to evaluate mild traumatic brain injuries, and it is becoming an increasingly important tool in preparticipation evaluations of athletes at risk for head injury.

TABLE 3 | Glasgow Coma Scale	
	Score*
Eye opening	
Eyes open spontaneously	4
Eyes open to verbal command	3
Eyes open only with painful stimuli	2
No eye opening	1
Verbal response	
Oriented and converses	5
Disoriented and converses	4
Inappropriate words	3
Incomprehensible sounds	2
No verbal response	1
Motor response	
Obeys verbal commands	6
Response to painful stimuli (upper extremities)	
Localizes pain	5
Withdraws from pain	4
Flexor posturing	3
Extensor posturing	2
No motor response	1

*Total score = eye opening + verbal response + motor response

(Adapted with permission from Garrett WE Jr, Kirkendall DT, Squire DL (eds): Principles and Practice of Primary Care Sports Medicine. Philadelphia, PA, Lippincott Williams & Wilkins, 2001, p 340.)

Sideline evaluations of athletes with suspected head injuries should include some sort of testing of cognitive function. The use of a standardized assessment tool (the standardized assessment for concussion or SAC) has been advocated by some. This includes tests assessing memory for recent events, digit recall, listing the months in reverse order, and list recall. A point system is used, and an athlete's performance can be compared with a preseason baseline score. Although this sideline evaluation tool has been demonstrated to differentiate individuals with and without concussions in athletics, its sensitivity has been questioned. One concern that has been raised is that athletes with normal scores are considered concussion free when, in fact, they may have concussions. This sideline assessment is not as sensitive as a full battery of neuropsychologic tests and misses several facets of cognitive function that these larger batteries entail. In addition, the use of these sideline assessments will no longer demonstrate deficits at 48 hours, when more sensitive testing demonstrates persistent deficits, underscoring their limited use for definitive treatment. In other words, there may be a high rate of false-negative results using limited sideline cognitive assessment. Although using these sideline assessment tests is better than using no sideline assessment tool at all, they should be used with caution, and should not take the place of clinical evaluations.

Ideally, a full, preseason neuropsychologic battery of tests should be performed on all athletes who participate in any contact sports in which a significant risk for mild traumatic brain injuries exists. The use of neuropsychologic testing as part of a preparticipation physical examination for athletes involved in sports with a significant risk for mild traumatic brain injuries can significantly improve the quality of care to these athletes. In addition, it can help assess the severity of injury and make determinations regarding whether an injured athlete may return to play. Neuropsychologic tests can demonstrate deficits when the physical examination and other diagnostic imaging test results are normal. Neuropsychologic tests often demonstrate to the athlete and coach that the athlete is not yet ready for participation and can provide the team physician with objective information to help make decisions regarding return to play.

There are several computerized versions of neuropsychologic testing batteries (for example, CogSport, CogState Ltd, Victoria, Australia; HeadMinder, HeadMinder Inc, New York, NY; and ImPACT, ImPACT, Pittsburgh, PA) that can help make these tests easy to administer in a group setting. The results, however, may very well be less sensitive than standard neuropsychologic batteries that involve more time and individualized test administration. Many of the computerized versions of neuropsychologic testing batteries also miss certain aspects of cognitive function, but they remain superior to classic medical testing in detecting injury and assessing recovery. In addition, many of these have now been validated with prospective research studies involving athletes.

With the tremendous popularity of neuropsychologic studies to assess mild traumatic brain injuries in athletes, several questions remain unanswered. How sensitive is neuropsychologic testing, and is it too sensitive? At what point is it safe for an injured athlete to return to play? Is there a point at which athletes can protect themselves and not be at undue risk for a second injury? In addition, with repetitive neuropsychologic testing, athletes tend to score better because of a practice effect on certain neuropsychologic tests. How much of a practice effect is there for different neuropsychologic tests, and how much should be expected? If athletes do not improve when retested, does this mean a deficit exists? Many of these questions should be answered as additional research is completed.

Return to Play Considerations

Making decisions regarding return to play remains the ultimate challenge to the physician treating the athlete with a head injury. There are several factors to consider when making these decisions; although guidelines are

useful, decisions should be individualized. For focal lesions, there is not much to guide the sports physician in terms of return to play. However, for mild traumatic brain injuries, certain standards should be met, including ensuring that the athlete is asymptomatic before returning to play and following a gradual progression from no activity to full activity. The goal is to return the athlete to play as soon as possible, without placing the athlete at an increased risk for additional injuries.

Any athlete with symptoms should not be allowed to return to play, even if the only symptom is a mild headache. In addition, if athletes have prolonged duration of symptoms or significant memory dysfunction, their return to play should be delayed. It is also imperative before return to play is considered that the results of the neurologic and cognitive examinations be normal. If available, neuropsychologic testing should be used to assess cognitive function; ideally, the results of neuropsychologic testing done after an injury should be compared with preinjury test results to ensure that function is normal.

Once the athlete is ready to consider returning to play, the first step should be a cardiovascular challenge. This should entail at least 15 to 20 minutes of cardiovascular activity only that raises the heart rate and allows athletes to break a sweat without putting them at risk for trauma. If exertion alone causes any symptoms to recur, then the athlete is not yet ready to return to play. If the athlete is able to participate in cardiovascular activity without any symptoms, then the next step is to allow the athlete to perform some sport-specific skills, again without risk of contact. For basketball players, this can include shooting baskets; for football players, this can include throwing passes. These activities allow the athlete to return to practice, remain part of the team, and gain confidence, while continuing to protect the athlete from recurrent injury. If the athlete remains symptom free, full practice without restrictions can be resumed. If the athlete does well in full practice without restrictions, full play can be instituted.

Certain guidelines suggest a slower progression to full play, including periods of no activity, light aerobic activity, sport-specific training (cardiovascular), noncontact training drills, full-contact practice after medical clearance, and return to play. These guidelines also suggest that each step take a minimum of 24 hours; if symptoms recur, the athlete should drop back to the previous stage of the progression. Although these guidelines are reasonable, in certain situations, advancing the athlete more slowly may be appropriate because individual circumstances differ.

Ideally, each of these steps should occur within a 24-hour period. Many team physicians will allow an athlete to return to play earlier by using a comparable progression that requires less than 24 hours for each step. Individualized decisions should be made based on the severity and duration of symptoms, the results of neurologic and cognitive examinations, and several other important athlete-specific factors, including age, level of play, sport, position played, and any previous history of mild traumatic brain injuries. The most important factor to consider is likely the athlete's readiness to return to play. The athlete with a head injury is commonly apprehensive about returning to full play, especially if the injury was associated with any loss of function. There may be concern that another injury may lead to permanent loss of function. Because physicians, parents, and coaches often assume the athlete wants to return to play, it is essential that the athlete is asked whether he/she is comfortable returning to play so that emotional readiness is assessed and no assumptions are made.

Ensuring a close follow-up is essential in the overall management of the athlete with head injuries. Depending on the severity of injury, follow-up can occur several hours later or within 24 to 48 hours. It is also important to provide the athlete and the athlete's caregiver with home instructions. Basic information should include instructions to refrain from any sports activities until follow-up evaluation, avoid alcohol and other sedative medications, and avoid aspirin and other medications that increase risk of bleeding; a list of the symptoms or signs that warrant emergent follow-up should also be provided. These instructions are very important for younger athletes for whom participation in gym class may need to be restricted.

Information regarding activity restrictions, observational needs, and ensuring that follow-up tests and evaluations are done must be clearly communicated to athletes, athletic trainers, coaches, administrators, parents, and caregivers (if applicable). Once follow-up is complete and the return to play progression is started, communication is again essential. This remains true even when full clearance is given to the athlete to participate. Although true for any injury, return to play after a head injury deserves special attention, given the potential risk for complications with mild traumatic brain injuries.

Making clearance decisions for sports participation after focal injuries is more difficult because there is little information to guide the physician. Reasonable guidelines have been published based on clinical judgment and experience. For example, guidelines recommend that any athlete with focal injuries (subdural, epidural, or intracerebral hematomas and subarachnoid hemorrhages) or diffuse axonal injuries should not participate in sports activities if persistent postconcussive symptoms, permanent central neurologic sequelae (organic dementia, hemiplegia, and homonymous hemianopsia), hydrocephalus, spontaneous subarachnoid hemorrhages from any cause, or symptomatic neurologic or pain-producing abnormalities about the foramen magnum are present. Additionally, any athlete who has undergone a surgical procedure should be discouraged from

continued participation in contact and collision sports. If an athlete has had a focal lesion with no underlying brain injury and no history of surgical intervention, it has been suggested that the athlete should not participate in contact or collision sports for at least 1 full year after complete recovery from injury.

Complications of Head Injury

In addition to skull fractures, intracranial bleeding, cervical spine injuries, and scalp lacerations, complications of head injury include seizures, postconcussive syndrome, second impact syndrome, and chronic traumatic encephalopathy, all of which should be considered when making return to play decisions and communicating with athletes, families, coaches, and administrators. It is important to understand that for the athlete with a mild traumatic brain injury, the risk for a second concussion is four to six times higher than for the athlete who has never had a concussion.

Seizures

Seizures complicate roughly 5% of traumatic brain injuries and most commonly occur within the first week after injury. Seizures often occur in association with skull fractures with undersurface brain contusion or irritation. They are more likely to occur in adults than children younger than 16 years. Other risk factors for seizure include seizures within 1 week of trauma, posttraumatic amnesia for longer than 12 hours, intracranial bleeding, or neurologic deficit after injury. Posttraumatic epilepsy can occur even when an electroencephalogram is normal. Seizures that occur after head trauma are treated similarly to those that occur without trauma.

Postconcussive Syndrome

Postconcussive syndrome and headache can also occur after mild traumatic brain injuries; symptoms include persistent headache, inability to concentrate, irritability, fatigue, vertigo, sleep and gait disturbances, visual complaints, and emotional lability (Table 4). The same biochemical changes appear to occur in patients with postconcussive syndrome that occur in those with mild traumatic brain injuries and posttraumatic migraines. All appear to have impaired glucose utilization and changes in the levels of excitatory amino acids, electrolytes, serotonin, catecholamines, endogenous opioids, and neuropeptides. Strict criteria are used to define postconcussive syndrome, and these are presented in Table 5. However, many physicians use postconcussive syndrome to describe the general condition of any athlete who has persistent symptomatology after mild traumatic brain injuries, even if the strict criteria are not met.

TABLE 4	Signs and Symptoms of Postconcussive Syndrome

Loss of intellectual capacity

Poor recent memory

Personality changes

Headaches

Dizziness

Lack of concentration

Poor attention

Fatigue

Irritability

Phonophobia/photophobia

Sleep disturbances

Depressed mood

Anxiety

(Adapted with permission from Garrett WE Jr, Kirkendall DT, Squire DL (eds): Principles and Practice of Primary Care Sports Medicine. Philadelphia, PA, Lippincott Williams & Wilkins, 2001, p 337.)

TABLE 5	Proposed Criteria For Postconcussive Syndrome

History of head injury that includes at least two of the following:

Loss of consciousness for 5 minutes or more

Posttraumatic amnesia of 12 hours or more

Onset of seizures (posttraumatic epilepsy) within 6 months of head injury

Current symptoms (either new symptoms or substantially worsening preexisting symptoms) to include:

At least the following two cognitive difficulties

Learning or memory (recall)

Concentration

At least three of the following affective or vegetative symptoms:

Easy fatigability

Insomnia or sleep/wake cycle disturbances

Headache (substantially worse than before injury)

Vertigo/dizziness

Irritability and/or aggression on little/no provocation

Anxiety, depression, or lability of affect

Personality change (eg, social or sexual inappropriateness and childlike behavior)

Aspontaneity/apathy

Symptoms associated with a significant difficulty in maintaining premorbid occupational or academic performance or with a decline in social, occupational, or academic performance

(Reproduced with permission from Brown SJ, Fann JR, Grant I: Postconcussional disorder: Time to acknowledge a common source of neurobehavioral morbidity. J Neuropsychiatry Clin Neurosci 1994;6:15-22.)

Variability exists in terms of the onset and persistence of postconcussive syndrome symptoms. In addition, little is known about what puts an athlete at risk for developing postconcussive syndrome. It is difficult to differentiate postconcussive syndrome from persistent symptoms, recurrent symptoms, unrelated symptoms, and/or trauma-induced migraines, which can make return to play decisions and other treatment decisions challenging. The treatment of postconcussive syndrome may include psychotherapy, behavioral modifications, medications, biofeedback, and physical therapy. Although tricyclic antidepressants and β-blockers have shown favorable results in the treatment of postconcussive syndrome and posttraumatic headaches, additional research is needed.

Second Impact Syndrome

Second impact syndrome was initially described in 1984 as the complication of sustaining a second impact before full recovery from a first trauma. In this situation, brain edema, persistent deficits, and ultimately death can occur. The force of either impact can be minimal, and the symptoms after the first impact can also be mild. Once the second impact occurs, deterioration occurs within seconds to minutes, with worsening mental status, dilated and fixed pupils, respiratory failure, and death. Although the etiology of second impact syndrome is unclear, it has been hypothesized to result from changes in cerebral blood flow that occur after trauma. With traumatic brain injuries, an increase in the sensitivity of the cerebral vasculature occurs; with a second impact, dysfunction in the vascular autoregulation occurs. An increase in vascular congestion also occurs as well as a resultant increase in intracranial pressure, which is believed to cause herniation of the brain, resultant compromise, and ultimately respiratory failure, coma, and death.

Despite this hypothesis, there is a lack of consensus about whether second impact syndrome exists. All of the reports of second impact syndrome have been in young children, and critical review of individual cases raises questions as to how common this entity is. Nonetheless, those who believe that second impact syndrome exists recommend that a patient with a traumatic brain injury be asymptomatic and fully recovered from the first insult before being put at risk for a second injury. Whether second impact syndrome exists or not, it is important to prohibit athletes with traumatic brain injuries from participating in athletic activities until they are completely asymptomatic; it is also important to continue to discern the parameters that define "normal" cognitive function.

Chronic Traumatic Encephalopathy

Chronic traumatic encephalopathy, first described in 1928 as the "punch drunk syndrome" in athletes, is a premature loss of normal central nervous system function resulting from a complication of recurrent head injury. Chronic traumatic encephalopathy is also known as dementia pugilista and is further characterized by cognitive and personality deficits and abnormalities in the cerebellar, pyramidal, and extrapyramidal systems. Although it is unclear why some individuals develop chronic traumatic encephalopathy, it is known that chronic traumatic encephalopathy can occur in the absence of injuries that cause associated loss of consciousness. Most of the information regarding chronic traumatic encephalopathy in athletics has come from the sport of boxing, where chronic traumatic encephalopathy occurs in 9% to 25% of professional boxers and appears to correlate to the number of fights and the length of a boxer's career. Neuropathologic changes as well as structural changes have been demonstrated in chronic traumatic encephalopathy. In one study of professional boxers, CT scans were obviously abnormal in 7% and borderline abnormal in 22%.

Attempts have been made to minimize the risks of developing chronic traumatic encephalopathy in boxing by changing some of the rules regarding mild traumatic brain injuries. Some states have mandated a time suspension for boxers who experience a mild traumatic brain injury to prevent them from returning to play too early. One state issues a 45-day suspension after a mild injury, a 60-day suspension after a moderate concussion, and a 90-day suspension and a normal CT and electroencephalogram after any severe concussion. These mandates, although conservative, were put in place to minimize the risk for complications after mild traumatic brain injuries in a sport in which the ultimate goal of each participant is to knock out the opponent.

There has been some recent concern that repetitive heading (striking the ball with the head) in soccer may lead to chronic traumatic encephalopathy. This concern has been fueled by cross-sectional data with poor methodology and lack of control subjects, retrospective studies evaluating former players, and the assumption that heading is the culprit. Concussion does occur in soccer players, and the mechanism of injury is usually related to contact of the head with the ground, goal post, or an opponent's head or body. In none of these studies, however, has the effect of concussion been separated from the effect of purposeful heading of the ball. There are no prospective data to support the contention that heading is dangerous, and it was concluded that most, but not all, of the studies presented suggest that heading a soccer ball does not cause cognitive deficits. Severe and cumulative concussions appear to be more of a concern for soccer players.

Future Research

There have been many advances in the evaluation and treatment of mild traumatic brain injuries over the past several years. Electrophysiologic recording, balance testing, and identifying biochemical markers (such as mye-

lin basic protein, S-100B, and neuron-specific enolase) appear to demonstrate deficits with concussive insult and may some day be useful in assessing injury. Advances in neuroimaging include the development of gradient echo MRI, perfusion MRI, and diffusion-weighted MRI that have greater sensitivity than traditional MRI in detecting structural abnormalities. Other imaging techniques that demonstrate promise in the evaluation of mild traumatic brain injuries include positron emission tomography, single-photon emission CT, and functional MRI. In addition, genetic research has demonstrated a potential hereditary predisposition that may put certain individuals at an increased risk for mild traumatic brain injuries. These apoE4 markers have also been associated with an increased incidence of Alzheimer's disease and chronic traumatic encephalopathy. It has been theorized that the presence of genetic markers may also place certain individuals at risk for second impact syndrome. It may be possible in the future to detect those at risk for injury and use this information in the rehabilitation of patients with mild traumatic brain injuries.

Summary

Mild traumatic brain injuries occur commonly in sports and can have significant short- and long-term consequences. Appropriate treatment entails a management protocol that is complete and thorough, with special attention to detecting vascular emergencies and associated cervical spine injuries and skull fractures. Neuropsychologic testing has become a useful tool in the assessment of mild traumatic brain injuries and recovery in athletes. The use of neuropsychologic testing as part of a preseason evaluation of athletes who are at risk for mild traumatic brain injuries should be considered when available. Athletes should be asymptomatic and have normal neurologic and cognitive examination results before returning to participation. Return to full athletic participation should progress in a gradual fashion, with an increase in both exertion and risk for contact. Decisions regarding return to play are challenging and should be made on an individualized basis. Future research will likely continue to change the way brain injuries are treated and improve the overall medical care of the athlete.

Annotated Bibliography

Epidemiology

National Center for Injury Prevention and Control: *Traumatic Brain Injury in the United States: A Report to Congress.* Atlanta, GA, Centers for Disease Control and Prevention, 1999, pp 1-28. Available at: http://www.cdc.gov/ncipc/pub-res/tbi_congress/tbi_congress.htm#html. Accessed November 13, 2003.

This is a report to Congress on the complexity of traumatic brain injury.

Rehabilitation of persons with traumatic brain injury. *NIH Consens Statement* 1998;16:1-41.

The statement provides state-of-the-art information regarding effective rehabilitation measures for persons who have suffered a traumatic brain injury and presents the conclusions and recommendations of the consensus panel regarding these issues.

Pathophysiology

Aubry M, Cantu R, Dvorak J, et al: Summary and agreement statement of the 1st International Symposium on Concussion in Sport, Vienna 2001. *Clin J Sport Med* 2002;12:6-11.

This article provides recommendations for the improvement of safety and health of athletes who may experience concussive injuries. The authors provide an excellent summary of the Vienna Conference, including a review of return to play guidelines and a consensus of sports medicine experts on concussion.

Diagnostic Imaging

Jagoda AS, Cantrill SV, Wears RL, et al: Clinical policy: Neuroimaging and decision making in adult mild traumatic brain injury in the acute setting. *Ann Emerg Med* 2002;40:231-249.

This is a review of emergency department imaging considerations for adult patients with brain trauma.

Johnston KM, Ptito A, Chankowsky J, Chen JK: New frontiers in diagnostic imaging in concussive head injury. *Clin J Sport Med* 2001;11:166-175.

This is a review of the diagnostic imaging tools used for evaluating patients with concussive brain injuries, with an emphasis on new techniques such as functional MRI.

The management of minor closed head injury in children: Committee on Quality Improvement, American Academy of Pediatrics, Commission on Clinical Policies and Research, American Academy of Family Physicians. *Pediatrics* 1998;104:1407-1415.

This article provides a recent review of head injury in the pediatric population.

Classification Systems

Cantu RC: Return to play guidelines after a head injury. *Clin Sports Med* 1998;17:45-60.

The author provides revised return to play guidelines for patients with head injuries.

Lovell MR, Iverson GL, Collins MW, McKeag D, Maroon JC: Does loss of consciousness predict neuropsychological decrements after concussion? *Clin J Sport Med* 1999;9:193-198.

In this sentinel article, the authors demonstrate that loss of consciousness does not correlate with severity of injury after concussion.

Neuropsychologic Testing

Collie A, Maruff P: Computerized neuropsychological testing. *Br J Sports Med* 2003;37:2-3.

The authors discuss various computerized versions of neuropsychologic tests in the athletic setting.

Collins MW, Grindel SH, Lovell MR, et al: Relationship between concussion and neuropsychological performance in college football players. *JAMA* 1999;282:964-970.

This article reports on the assessment of football players with concussions using neuropsychologic testing.

Echemendia RJ, Putukian M, Mackin RS, Julian L, Shoss N: Neuropsychological test performance prior to and following sports-related mild traumatic brain injury. *Clin J Sport Med* 2001;11:23-31.

This is a prospective evaluation of male and female college athletes (in various sports) with and without concussions using neuropsychologic testing.

Erlanger D, Feldman D, Kutner K, et al: Development and validation of a Web-based neuropsychological test protocol for sports-related return-to-play decision making. *Arch Clin Neuropsychol* 2003;18:293-316.

In this study, the authors validate a Web-based protocol using neuropsychologic testing in athletes with concussions.

Erlanger D, Saleba E, Barth J, Almquist J, Webright W, Freeman J: Monitoring resolution of concussions symptoms in athletes: Preliminary results of a Web-based neuropsychological test protocol. *J Athl Train* 2001;36:280-287.

In this article, the authors report on the use of a Web-based neuropsychologic test protocol for evaluating athletes with concussions.

Maroon JC, Lovell MR, Norwig J, Podell K, Powell JW, Hartl R: Cerebral concussion in athletics: Evaluation and neuropsychological testing. *Neurosurgery* 2000;47:659-672.

The authors provide a review of concussion in athletes with emphasis on the use of neuropsychologic testing.

McCrea M, Guskiewicz KM, Marshall SW, et al: Acute effects and recovery time following concussion in collegiate football players: The NCAA Concussion Study. *JAMA* 2003;290:2556-2563.

This prospective, multicenter study assesses the acute effects of concussion in college football players using balance testing and neuropsychologic testing.

McCrea M, Kelly JP, Randolph C, Cisler R, Berger L: Immediate neurocognitive effects of concussion. *Neurosurgery* 2002;50:1032-1042.

The authors review cognitive deficits that occur acutely after concussion.

Putukian M, Echemendia RJ, Mackin RS: The acute neuropsychologic effects of heading in soccer: A pilot study. *Clin J Sport Med* 2000;10:104-109.

The results of this prospective pilot study demonstrate no effect of heading on the cognitive function of male and female college soccer players as assessed using neuropsychologic testing.

Return to Play Considerations

Guskiewicz KM, McCrea M, Marshall SW, et al: Cumulative effects associated with recurrent concussion in collegiate football players: The NCAA Concussion Study. *JAMA* 2003;290:2549-2555.

This prospective, multicenter study assesses the occurrence of concussion and risk for recurrent injury in college football players.

Complications of Head Injury

Boden BP, Kirkendall DT, Garrett WE: Concussion incidence in elite college soccer players. *Am J Sports Med* 1998;26:238-241.

This prospective study assesses the mechanisms of concussion in male and female college soccer players within one conference. Results demonstrated that concussions in soccer occurred as a result of head-to-opponent, head-to-ground, or head-to-goalpost contact and not purposeful heading.

Cantu RC: Epilepsy and athletics. *Clin Sports Med* 1998; 17:61-69.

This is a review of epilepsy in athletics, with a discussion of return to play considerations.

Cantu RC: Second-impact syndrome. *Clin Sports Med* 1998;17:37-44.

The author provides a review of the literature on second-impact syndrome.

Kirkendall DT, Garrett WE Jr: Heading in soccer: Integral skill or grounds for cognitive dysfunction? *J Athl Train* 2001;36:328-333.

The authors of this study review the literature concerning heading in soccer as it relates to the possibility of brain injury. Their findings support the concept that if brain injury occurs as a result of long-term soccer play, then the most likely culprit is not heading the ball, but more likely concussive injury.

McCrory PR: Second impact syndrome. *Neurology* 1998; 50:677-683.

This article is a review of the literature regarding second-impact syndrome; the author questions whether second-impact syndrome exists.

Future Research

Kors EE, Terwindt GM, Vermeulen FL, et al: Delayed cerebral edema and fatal coma after minor head trauma: Role of the CACNA1A calcium channel subunit gene and relationship with familial hemiplegic migraine. *Ann Neurol* 2001;49:753-760.

The authors of this study address genetic markers that may predispose patients to brain injury.

Classic Bibliography

Barcellos S, Rizzo M: Posttraumatic headaches, in Rizzo M, Tranel D (eds): *Head Injury and Postconcussive Syndrome*. New York, NY, Churchill Livingstone, 1996, pp 1-18.

Bergsneider M, Hovda DA, Shalmon E, et al: Cerebral hyperglycolysis following severe traumatic brain injury in humans: A positron emission tomography study. *J Neurosurg* 1997;86:241-251.

Colorado Medical Society: *Guidelines for the Management of Concussion in Sports*. Denver, CO, Sports Medicine Committee, Colorado Medical Society, 1991.

Elson LM, Ward CC: Mechanisms and pathophysiology of mild head injury. *Semin Neurol* 1994;14:8-18.

Gentry LR, Godersky JC, Thompson B, Dunn VD: Prospective comparative study of intermediate-field MR and CT in the evaluation of closed head trauma. *AJR Am J Roentgenol* 1988;150:673-682.

Graham DI: Neuropathology of head injury, in Narayan RK, Wilberger JE Jr, Povlishock JT (eds): *Neurotrauma*. New York, NY, McGraw-Hill, 1996, pp 46-47.

Hovda DA, Lee SM, Smith ML, et al: The neurochemical and metabolic cascade following brain injury: Moving from animal models to man. *J Neurotrauma* 1995;12: 903-906.

Jordan B, Jahre C, Hauser A, et al: CT of 338 active professional boxers. *Radiology* 1992;185:509-512.

Jordan BD, Relkin NR, Ravdin LD, et al: Apolipoprotein E epislon4 associated with chronic traumatic brain injury in boxing. *JAMA* 1997;278:136-140.

Katayama Y, Becker DP, Tamura T, et al: Massive increases in extracellular potassium and the indiscriminate release of glutamate following concussive brain injury. *J Neurosurg* 1990;73:889-900.

Katayama Y, Cheung MK, Alves A, et al: Ion fluxes and cell swelling in experimental traumatic brain injury: The role of excitatory amino acids, in Hoff JT, Betz AL (eds): *Intracranial Pressure VII*. Berlin, Germany, Springer, 1989, pp 584-588.

Levin HS, Amparo E, Eisenberg JM, et al: Magnetic resonance imaging and computerized tomography in relation to the neurobehavioral sequelae of mild and moderate head injuries. *J Neurosurg* 1987;66:706-713.

Levin HS, Williams D, Crofford MJ, et al: Relationship of depth of brain lesions to consciousness and outcome after closed head injury. *J Neurosurg* 1988;69:861-866.

Martland HS: Punch drunk. *JAMA* 1928;91:1103-1107.

Mayeux R, Ottman R, Tang MX, et al: Genetic susceptibility and head injury as risk factors for Alzheimer's disease among community-dwelling elderly persons and their first-degree relatives. *Ann Neurol* 1993;33:494-501.

Mortimer JA: Epidemiology of post-traumatic encephalopathy in boxers. *Minn Med* 1985;68:299-300.

Packard RC, Ham LP: Pathogenesis of posttraumatic headache and migraine: A common headache pathway? *Headache* 1997;37:142-152.

Practice parameter: The management of concussion in sports (summary statement): Report of the Quality Standards Subcommittee. *Neurology* 1997;48:581-585.

Report of the Ad Hoc Committee to Study Head Injury Nomenclature: Proceedings of the Congress of Neurological Surgeons in 1964. *Clin Neurosurg* 1966;12:386-394.

Saunders RL, Harbaugh RE: The second impact in catastrophic contact-sports head trauma. *JAMA* 1984;252-538-539.

Teasdale GM, Nicoll JA, Murray G, et al: Association of apolipoprotein E polymorphism with out come after head injury. *Lancet* 1997;350:1069-1071.

Troncoso JC, Gordon B: Neuropathology of closed head injury, in Rizzo M, Tranel E (eds): *Head Injury and Postconcussive Syndrome*. New York, NY, Churchill Livingstone, 1996, pp 47-56.

Yamakami I, McIntosh TK: Alterations in regional cerebral blood flow following brain injury in the rat. *J Cereb Blood Flow Metab* 1991;11:655-660.

Section 2

Injuries of the Upper Extremity

Section Editor:
W. Ben Kibler, MD

Chapter 4

Integrated Biomechanics of the Shoulder and Elbow

W. Ben Kibler, MD

Introduction

The skillful, efficient, and safe function of the shoulder and elbow during overhead athletic activities requires balancing the generation of forces and motions necessary to move the shoulder and elbow to propel a ball or racquet, and control these forces and motions for precision of performance and protection of the joints from excessive loading. The body achieves this balance by integrating the physiologic muscle activations and the resulting biomechanical forces and motions throughout all the segments or links of the kinetic chain. As a result, no single segment or link is required to generate all of the required force or absorb all of the resulting loads in normal function. Dysfunction of this integrated mechanism can cause or result in local segment overload, which may be associated with overt injury, altered physiology and/or biomechanics, or decreased performance. To diagnose and effectively treat such dysfunction, it is important to understand the integrated physiology and biomechanics of force generation and force control and the clinical implications for evaluation and treatment.

Force Generation

The local and distant forces that are necessary to achieve skilled shoulder and elbow function have been explored in great detail in the literature. It has been shown that these forces and loads are high in magnitude and are repetitively applied. It has also been shown that most of the forces that are measured at the joints are not generated by anatomic or physiologic factors in close proximity to the joint. This is probably because of the relatively small cross-sectional area of the muscle around the joints, which results in limited force generation capability, and the mechanical disadvantage of the moment arms around the joint, which are too close to the center of motion. All recent studies have confirmed that the kinetic chain is the body's mechanism for optimum force generation.

This mechanism results from a coordinated sequenced pattern of muscle activations that produce sequenced biomechanical forces and motions that, in turn, create optimal positioning and motion of the terminal segment of the kinetic chain. The kinetic chain appears to generate 50% to 60% of the total force from the proximal segments of the chain, the legs, and trunk. This proximally generated force is then transmitted to the distal segments by sequenced, coupled motions of the intervening segments and results in interactive moments, forces generated at joints by the position and motion of distant segments that are similar to the motion of the butt of a whip creating large force and motion at the tip.

A key clinically observable manifestation of this integration of proximal force generation and distal movement is long axis rotation (Figure 1), a motion defined by coupled scapular stabilization, glenohumeral rotation, and forearm pronation. Long axis rotation has been termed the missing link in the kinetic chain because it explains how the segments are integrated in a multisegmental action, creating a composite motion. It creates a relatively stiff moment arm (the arm from the shoulder to the wrist) that maximizes centripetal action, transforms linear momentum to more efficient angular momentum, and occurs as the last joint action immediately before ball release or ball impact to maximize the force delivered to the hand or racquet. This motion is clinically observable and analyzable, and its components (trunk stability, scapular stability, shoulder internal rotation, and forearm rotation) are measurable. Assessing long axis rotation can be a key part of the evaluation of shoulder and elbow dysfunction.

Force Control

As with the generation of forces and motions, the control of all of the forces and loads at the shoulder and elbow is not totally dependent on local anatomic and physiologic factors. The medial collateral ligament of the elbow would have to be 2.5 times its normal thickness to be able to withstand the observed valgus loads in the baseball throw. The muscular activations required to maintain concavity and compression of the glenohumeral joint are 2.7 times higher when the gleno-

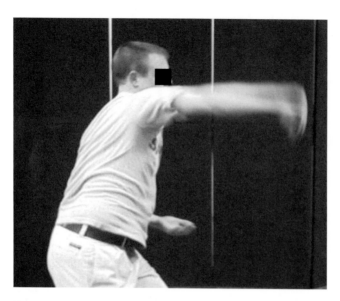

Figure 1 Long axis rotation. Note the coupling of shoulder internal rotation (on a stabilized scapula) with forearm rotation.

humeral angle is greater than 29.3°. In both instances, the kinetic chain produces interactive moments that increase control of the generated forces at the local joint. The major component of the varus acceleration at the elbow that protects against generated valgus load results from the interactive moment created by shoulder internal rotation. Trunk rotation and control of scapular protraction and retraction produce the coupled interactive moment of scapulohumeral rhythm to maximize glenohumeral concavity and compression.

The proximal kinetic chain activations that produce most of the forces and motions also produce a proximal stability that allows a distal mobility. The patterns of activation create anticipatory postural adjustments that stabilize the body as a counterforce to the forces produced by the rapid movements of the distal segments (which can be illustrated by attempting to throw a ball hard while standing on ice). Finally, because the muscles around the distal segments do not have to be primarily used in force generation or control, they may be activated for precision and control of performance.

Integrated Activity

Advantages
There are several advantages to this mechanism of integration of proximal and distal segments. It allows placement of larger, bulkier muscles in the central core, which creates a large moment of inertia against pertubation while still allowing a stable base for distal mobility. In addition, it places most of the "engine" of force development in the central core, allowing small changes in rotation around the central core to have large changes in rotation in the distal segments. Because of the relatively smaller mass in the distal segments, the moment

of inertia of the distal segment is less, allowing the summation of high peripheral velocities. Finally, by allowing joint force control to be influenced by preprogrammed joint positioning and interactive moments instead of local ligament size or feedback-based muscle activation, the ligaments can be smaller in size, and the smaller muscles can be activated for precision and control of performance variables.

Disadvantages
This integrated mechanism may break down at any segment in the linkage system, creating a domino effect in the rest of the kinetic chain. Kinetic chain breakage, which may occur from injury, acquired deficits in flexibility or strength, or muscle imbalances, can result in any or all of the following scenarios: decreased force to the terminal segment, resulting in decreased performance parameters (for example, velocity and power); "catch up" in the distal segments, with more force or energy development required from the smaller distal segments; and alterations in the interactive moments, which may change the loads at distal joints. These deficits are seen in association with shoulder or elbow injury in 67% to 100% of patients. The most common deficits are hip rotation inflexibility, trunk muscle weakness and/or inflexibility, scapular dyskinesis, and glenohumeral internal rotation deficit.

Decreased force or energy to the terminal segment of the kinetic chain will occur if the remaining segments are activated and positioned in the same manner as for a "normal" kinetic chain. The functional result will be altered force and energy to the ball or racquet. The other functional adaptation, which is commonly used by athletes, is to play "catch up," with distal segments increasing their contribution to the entire chain activation. "Catch up" is difficult to maintain over an extended period of activity because of the small margin of error in the kinetic chain. Mathematical analysis has shown that a 20% decrease in trunk kinetic chain energy to the shoulder requires a 34% increase in shoulder velocity or a 70% increase in shoulder mass to achieve the same energy in the terminal segment. This study was corroborated by a clinical study that showed kinetic chain breakage at the knee (less knee bend during the tennis serve) created 23% to 27% more load at the shoulder and elbow in athletes who played "catch up" and maintained the same service velocity. The absolute magnitude of the resulting forces was over 50 Nm, placing these athletes in a high-risk category for strain injury.

Alteration of interactive moments occurs because of alteration in the position and/or motion of the proximal segments. Alterations in scapular motion and position, collectively termed scapular dyskinesis, are associated with proximal biomechanical causes. Altered scapular

TABLE 1 | Terms Used to Describe Throwing Compensations

Term	Meaning	Possible Cause
Overstriding	Forward stride is too long	Weak back leg, not maintaining one leg stance position
Lateral lean	Body is tilted over hip	Weak plant leg hip muscles
Opening up	Plant leg is lateral to the line to home plate	Weak trunk and plant leg hip muscles
Slow arm	Excessive trunk extension and arm behind body	Weak trunk, upper body not pulled through
Short arming	Scapular elevation, arm is close to body, and lack of full elbow extension	Weak low trap, hyperactive upper trap, scapular dyskinesis, glenohumeral internal rotation deficit
Dropping down	Altered arm position relative to body	Loss of acromial tilt/elevation, weak rotator cuff, weak plant leg hip muscles
Unable to reach set point	Alteration in position of hand in cocking	Weak trunk muscles, lack of scapular retraction, glenohumeral internal rotation deficit
Dropped elbow	Elbow is below shoulder level in acceleration	Weak plant leg hip muscles, scapular dyskinesis, weak rotator cuff

TABLE 2 | Kinetic Chain Alterations Associated With Shoulder and Elbow Injuries

Alteration	Shoulder Injury	Reference
Hip internal rotation deficit, scapular dyskinesis, glenohumeral internal rotation deficit	Posterior glenoid labral tears	Burkhart et al, 2000
Scapular dyskinesis	Instability, impingement	Warner et al, 1992
Scapular dyskinesis	Impingement	McClure et al, 2001
Glenohumeral internal rotation deficit	Impingement	Tyler et al, 2000
Scapular dyskinesis	Rotator cuff tear	Paletta et al, 1997
Trunk weakness	Impingement	Young et al, 1996
Scapular muscle weakness	Impingement	Cools et al, 2003

protraction increases strain on the anterior band of the inferior glenohumeral ligament and decreased rotator cuff activation intensity. Altered scapular rotation and posterior tilt are associated with decreased subacromial space and impingement. Altered knee flexion alters long axis rotation by increasing elbow valgus loads and shoulder internal rotation, abduction, and distraction loads. Hip rotation inflexibility is seen in association with 50% of arthroscopically demonstrated posterior labral tears.

Clinical Implications

Alterations in the integrated biomechanical sequencing that may be associated with shoulder or elbow dysfunction in the symptomatic athlete may be observed by evaluating the throwing or serving motion and by a comprehensive clinical examination of all segments of the kinetic chain.

One of the first clinically observable effects of kinetic chain breakage may be alteration in a performance factor, such as decreased ball velocity, altered ball accuracy, or a breakdown in the athlete's normal throwing or serving mechanics. These alterations may be seen in the face of minimal clinical symptoms of pain or injury.

Many terms have been used by coaches, players, and physicians to describe the alterations in the observable mechanics. These terms usually relate to altered body posture or body segment motion, but they may also be related to kinetic chain compensations or "catch up" (Table 1). Physical examination should be done to evaluate possible anatomic or biomechanical causes in athletes in whom kinetic chain compensations or "catch up" are noted.

All throwing, serving, or overhead athletes who have shoulder or elbow dysfunction (altered performance, pain, or injury) from atraumatic or microtraumatic origin should be clinically evaluated from a kinetic chain perspective because of the high incidence of associated proximal alterations (Table 2). A large proportion of the examination can involve screening, with more inclusive evaluation conducted for areas of abnormality identified during examination or from observation. A minimal screening examination should include evaluation of one-leg stability (Figure 2), trunk posture, sit and reach flexibility, scapular position and motion, and true glenohumeral internal and external rotation with the scapula stabilized.

The goal of rehabilitation of shoulder and elbow injuries should be reestablishment of the integrated physiology and biomechanics, the specific principles and guidelines of which are discussed in detail in chapter 10.

Summary

Athletes integrate patterned coordination of muscle activations, coordinated generation and control of forces,

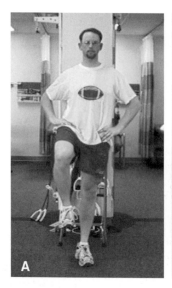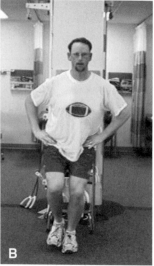

Figure 2 One-leg stability evaluation includes one-leg stance (**A**) and squat (**B**).

and sequencing of joint positions and motions to produce skillful athletic activities involving the shoulder and elbow. Alteration in this integrated mechanism is frequently associated with shoulder and elbow injury. Evaluation protocols can be devised to screen for proximal alterations; the results can then help direct treatment.

Annotated Bibliography

Force Generation
Marshall RN, Elliott BC: Long axis rotation: The missing link in proximal to distal segmental sequencing. *J Sports Sci* 2000;18:247-254.

This article provides the scientific basis for the concept of long axis rotation and demonstrates the mechanism of integrated coupling of biomechanical motions to produce power.

Force Control
Hirashima M, Kadota H, Sakurai S, et al: Sequential muscle activity and its functional role in the upper extremity and trunk during overarm throwing. *J Sports Sci* 2002;20:301-310.

The authors of this article used sophisticated electromyography and force analysis to demonstrate the proximal to distal muscle activation patterns and resulting forces at each body segment. They demonstrate that the activation pattern at the elbow is used primarily for precision control rather than force development.

Integrated Activity
Burkhart SS, Morgan CD, Kibler WB: Throwing injuries in the shoulder: The dead arm revisited. *Clin Sports Med* 2000;19:125-158.

This article describes findings associated with arm symptoms and demonstrates the common incidence of kinetic chain alterations in patients with arthroscopically proven labral injuries.

Cools AM, Witvrouw EE, Declercq GA, Danneels LA, Cambier DC: Scapular muscle recruitment patterns: Trapezius muscle latency with and without impingement symptoms. *Am J Sports Med* 2003;31:542-549.

The authors of this article are the first to document alterations in activation patterns in the muscles responsible for scapular stabilization in retraction and protraction in patients with shoulder symptoms.

Elliott B, Fleisig G, Nicholls R, Escamilia R: Technique effects on upper limb loading in the tennis serve. *J Sci Med Sport* 2003;6:76-87.

The authors of this article analyzed tournament play and found that significant increases in loads and forces in the shoulder and elbow resulted from a specific proximal kinetic chain defect: lack of effective knee flexion during cocking.

Kibler WB, McMullen J: Scapular dyskinesis and its relation to shoulder pain. *J Am Acad Orthop Surg* 2003; 11:142-152.

The authors of this article outline the roles of the scapula in function and discuss the effect of the alteration of scapular motion and position in shoulder function and dysfunction. The authors also describe methods of evaluation and treatment.

McClure PW, Michener L, Sennett BJ, Karduna AR: Direct 3-dimensional measurement of scapular kinematics during dynamic movements in vivo. *J Shoulder Elbow Surg* 2001;10:269-277.

This article describes the actual movements of the scapula during arm motions and documents the importance of tilt and external rotation as well as upward rotation.

Clinical Implications
Burkhart SS, Morgan CD, Kibler WB: The disabled throwing shoulder: Spectrum of pathology. Part I: Pathology and biomechanics. *Arthroscopy* 2003;19:404-420.

Burkhart SS, Morgan CD, Kibler WB: The disabled throwing shoulder: Spectrum of pathology. Part II: Evaluation and treatment of SLAP lesions in throwers. *Arthroscopy* 2003;19:531-539.

Burkhart SS, Morgan CD, Kibler WB: The disabled throwing shoulder: Spectrum of pathology. Part III: The SICK scapula, scapular dyskinesis, the kinetic chain, and rehabilitation. *Arthroscopy* 2003;19:641-661.

This three-part article places the disabled throwing shoulder (dead arm) in a context of adaptive changes in flexibility and strength that alter the ball and socket kinematics of the glenohumeral joint. A framework for understanding the pathoetiology of the combination of partial rotator cuff injury, glenoid labral injury, and glenohumeral instability that occur together in athletes is presented. The authors also discuss treatment of the anatomic injury and the associated local and distant adaptive changes. The causative factors that appear to be basic to the process include a tight posteroinferior capsule causing glenohumeral internal rotation deficit, peel-back forces causing superior labrum anterior and posterior lesions, hyperexternal rotation of the humerus, and scapular protraction resulting from loss of control of scapular retraction.

Tyler TF, Nicholas ST, Roy T, et al: Quantification of posterior capsular tightness and motion loss in patients with shoulder impingement. *Am J Sports Med* 2000;28: 668-674.

This article documents the effect of glenohumeral internal rotation deficit on shoulder motion and resulting impingement.

Classic Bibliography

Fleisig GS, Andrews JR, Dillman CJ: The kinetics of baseball pitching with implications about injury mechanisms. *Am J Sports Med* 1995;23:233-239.

Happee R, van der Helm FC: Control of shoulder muscles during goal directed movements. *J Biomech* 1995; 28:1179-1191.

Kibler WB: Biomechanical analysis of the shoulder during tennis activities. *Clin Sports Med* 1995;14:79-85.

Paletta GA Jr, Warner JJ, Warren RF, Deutsch A, Altchek DW: Shoulder kinematics with two-plane x-ray evaluation in patients with anterior instability or rotator cuff tearing. *J Shoulder Elbow Surg* 1997;6:516-527.

Putnam CA: Sequential motions of body segments in striking and throwing skills. *J Biomech* 1993;26:125-135.

Warner JJ, Micheli LJ, Arslanian LE, Kennedy J, Kennedy R: Scapulothoracic motion in normal shoulders and shoulders with glenohumeral instability and impingement syndrome: A study using Moire topographic analysis. *Clin Orthop* 1992;285:191-199.

Young JL, Herring SA, Press JM, Casazza BA: The influence of the spine on the shoulder in the throwing athlete. *J Back Musculoskeletal Rehabil* 1996;7:5-17.

Zattara M, Bouisset S: Posturo-kinetic organisation during the early phase of voluntary limb movement. *J Neurol Neurosurg Psychiatry* 1988;51:956-965.

stability episodes (25 patients). Tissue quality was superior in the group of first-time dislocators, including better soft-tissue vascularity, less retraction, and the perception of easier reparability. In contrast, tissue in recurrent dislocators was more pale, stiff and inelastic, and of poorer quality. Bony lesions were not seen in the acute first-time dislocator group. In the recurrent dislocation group, however, 40% had a nonengaging Hill-Sachs lesion, and 16% had a glenoid impact bony lesion. This nonrandomized trial documented a higher success rate with early treatment, with no recurrent dislocations and only one subluxation reported in the first-time dislocator group (recurrence rate, 4%). In comparison, those treated for recurrent instability had a failure rate of 16% (8% with recurrent dislocations and 8% with recurrent subluxations).

Not every first-time dislocator is an appropriate candidate for early surgical stabilization. Patient age, activity level, and desire to return to preinjury status are important factors that must be weighed on an individual basis. Dislocation itself is only one criterion influencing treatment decision making. Disadvantages of immediate surgical stabilization include the complications of surgery, cost, and inconvenience.

Recurrent Anterior Instability

Patients with recurrent shoulder instability are disabled in terms of both shoulder function and general health status. The spectrum of this disability ranges from pain and apprehension during specific activities to episodic subluxation and recurrent dislocation. A thorough medical history must include information about previous events and treatment. Arm position at the time of dislocation should be determined. The relationship of symptoms to activity, such as in which position symptoms are provoked, may suggest the predominant direction of instability.

Range of motion in patients with recurrent anterior instability is usually normal; however, range of motion in the throwing population has been shown to be greater in external rotation. Assessment of anterior instability involves both objective laxity translation testing and subjective instability tests. Anterior laxity tests include the anterior drawer test and the load and shift test. In each, the amount of translation and the quality of the end point are assessed under load. The presence of subjective symptoms (ie, reproducing the patients' sense of apprehension or pain) during translation may further corroborate the diagnosis. Inferior translation is assessed by the sulcus sign.

A recent study examined the intrareliability and interreliability of manual techniques in assessing anterior humeral head translation. The authors found intrareliability to be only 54% and interreliability to be only 37% and concluded that manual assessment of humeral head translation was unreliable. They further noted that use of an "end feel" component to the examination actually decreased the reliability of the examination.

In addition to standard radiographs, additional views that help assess recurrent instability include the West Point and the Stryker's notch views. CT has been shown to be valuable in quantifying the degree of glenoid bone loss. In a recent cadaveric study, glenoid osseous defects were created to simulate bony Bankart lesions. Both CT and the West Point view were found to provide precise measurements of the size of the glenoid defect. In another study, glenoid rim morphology was studied in 100 consecutive shoulders with recurrent anterior instability. Three-dimensional reconstructed CT images (with the humeral head digitally "eliminated") provided an accurate interpretation of glenoid rim morphology comparable to that obtained using arthroscopic assessment. MRI and magnetic resonance arthrography remain popular imaging tools despite their relative inaccuracy in interpreting labral pathology.

Nonsurgical treatment of recurrent instability includes activity modification to reduce risk and rehabilitation to improve functional strength. Patients who are unwilling to accept activity modification or those with athletic or functional impairment are candidates for surgical stabilization.

Examination Under Anesthesia

Examination under anesthesia (EUA) is an integral part of shoulder instability assessment, particularly in instances of diagnostic uncertainty. Recent studies have reinforced its value. In one study, 30 patients with documented unilateral posttraumatic recurrent anterior instability were assessed using EUA in multiple directions and rotations. The authors found testing helpful when performed at both 40° and 80° of external rotation and when assessing instability in the anteroinferior direction, with a reported sensitivity of 83% and a specificity of 100%. Another study assessed glenohumeral translation in 50 patients with surgically confirmed anterior instability while the patients were awake and under anesthesia. Examination of patients while they were awake was reported to be unproductive, but EUA proved helpful in confirming both the direction and degree of instability.

Open Versus Arthroscopic Repair

Open stabilization certainly is the historic standard for the treatment of anterior shoulder instability. Recurrence rates of 3% to 5% have been documented in several long-term studies. Arthroscopic techniques have made considerable inroads, however, with many studies demonstrating outcomes comparable to, and in some instances, better than those for open stabilization. Open repair involves anatomic restoration of the capsulola-

Chapter 5

Acute Shoulder Injuries

Benjamin Shaffer, MD

Seth Baublitz, DO

Introduction

The evaluation and treatment of acute shoulder injuries are areas of active inquiry. Advances in understanding the pathophysiology of instability, improvements in arthroscopic instrumentation and technique, and better clinical outcome reporting have advanced the optimal treatment of acute shoulder problems.

Anterior Instability

Acute Anterior Dislocation

Anterior dislocation is the most common instability pattern affecting the glenohumeral joint, constituting over 90% of reported instability events. More common in contact and collision sports such as football, rugby, and hockey, the instability event usually results from application of a violent external rotation or extension force to the vulnerably positioned (usually abducted and externally rotated) arm.

Normal Functional Anatomy and Shoulder Stability Mechanisms

Normal glenohumeral stability is rendered by a complex interaction among static (labrum and glenohumeral capsular ligaments) and dynamic (cuff, deltoid, biceps, and scapular rotator musculature) restraints. The most studied of the static restraints are the glenohumeral capsular ligaments, which have been anatomically and biomechanically characterized as distinct structures. The most important is the inferior glenohumeral ligament complex, consisting of an anterior band, axillary pouch, and posterior band (Figure 1). This complex acts as a sling to support the humeral head and resist anterior translation when the arm is abducted. The importance of dynamic stabilizers, including the rotator cuff and scapular rotators, has been emphasized in several recent studies. For example, one cadaveric study compared dynamic glenohumeral joint stability in the end-range of motion with that in the midrange by investigating the force component generated by the rotator cuff muscles. The rotator cuff was found to provide substantial anterior dynamic

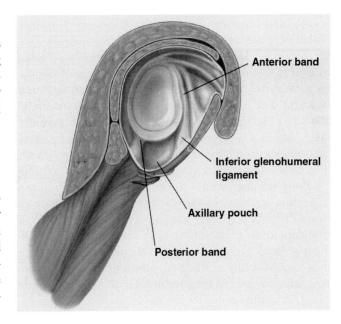

Figure 1 This cut-away cross section displays the inferior glenohumeral ligament, the most important static restraint to anterior translation. The inferior glenohumeral ligament is composed of the anterior band, axillary pouch, and posterior band. *(Reproduced with permission from Lashgari CJ, Leesa M, Yamaguchi K: Arthroscopic shoulder anatomy, in Tibone J, Shaffer BS, Savoie FH III, Davis CS (eds): Shoulder Arthroscopy. New York, NY, Springer Verlag, 2003.)*

stability to the glenohumeral joint in both mid- and end-ranges of motion. The authors postulated that enhancement of the internal and external rotators might dynamically stabilize a lax glenohumeral joint in the end-range of motion.

Pathophysiology of Instability

The Bankart lesion is the most common pathologic finding, seen in approximately 97% of initial traumatic anterior shoulder dislocations. Less commonly, the capsuloligamentous complex can avulse from the humeral rather than glenoid side, resulting in a humeral avulsion of the glenohumeral ligament (HAGL) lesion. In a recent retrospective series of 547 shoulders (529 patients), lateral capsule avulsion from the humeral neck was considered the cause of instability in 41 patients (7.5%). Thirty-five were detected at the time of the index instability procedure, whereas six of these were noted only at revision for a failed instability surgery. In analyzing their data, the authors noted that these lesions were generally found in older patients. The incidence of HAGL lesions was as high as 39% in a select group of patients in which the initial dislocation was caused by violent trauma, no Bankart lesion occurred, but multidirectional laxity was present.

Although historically considered the "essential" lesion, ongoing basic science and clinical studies suggest that factors other than the Bankart lesion are responsible for instability, including capsular patholaxity, bony injury, and rotator interval insufficiency. Capsular patholaxity has been the most widely implicated cofactor. Strain before capsular detachment has been shown to lead to permanent irrecoverable plastic deformation. In a recent cadaveric study, the inferior glenohumeral ligament was subjected to repetitive cyclic strains in 33 shoulders. Subfailure cyclic loading induced capsular laxity, which was largely unrecoverable. Clinically, these repetitive stresses may explain the acquired laxity seen in patients with recurrent instability.

Bony lesions include those of the glenoid rim and impaction fractures of the humeral head (Hill-Sachs lesions). Rim lesions that exceed approximately 25% of the glenoid articular surface may require grafting. Hill-Sachs lesions greater than 30% of the articular surface may require bone grafting or nonanatomic reconstruction. Insufficiency of the rotator interval has been implicated in contributing to instability, particularly in patients with posterior and/or multidirectional instability.

Presentation and Evaluation

The patient with an acute shoulder dislocation will be in considerable discomfort and will usually hold the arm at the side in slight abduction and external rotation. The deltoid loses its rounded contour and instead appears flat, with prominence anteriorly and loss of normal posterior fullness. A diligent prereduction neurologic examination must be done to rule out axillary nerve injury, which occurs in 9% to 18% of anterior shoulder dislocations.

At minimum, the initial radiographic evaluation should include a true AP view (perpendicular to the plane of the scapula rather than the thorax) and an axillary lateral view. Additional views may be helpful in delineating associated bony pathology (for example, the West Point view to help visualize bony avulsions of the glenoid rim and the Stryker's notch view to help visualize Hill-Sachs lesions). More sophisticated imaging studies, such as CT, are reserved for dislocations that are irreducible, chronic, or associated with fracture, including a large Hill-Sachs lesion component. Except for patients older than 40 years or those with relevant postreduction clinical findings suggestive of possible rotator cuff injury, MRI has little value in the evaluation of the acutely dislocated shoulder.

Treatment

Reduction of an acute anterior dislocation should be performed as early as possible and in some patients may be achieved without anesthesia. On-the-field reduction depends on clinical experience and specific circumstances. If there is any concern that on-the-field reduction cannot be done without causing further injury, radiographs should be obtained before manipulation. Careful neurologic assessment is important before any treatment to establish baseline status. Reduction is often fairly easy if undertaken promptly, whereas manipulation several hours later in the emergency department will usually require that the patient receive medication for pain relief and muscle relaxation. There is no consensus as to the best protocol for medication. Although narcotic and sedative medication administered intravenously have an established track record, an intraarticular injection can provide good pain relief, facilitate reduction, and obviate the potential complication of respiratory depression.

One recent prospective randomized study of 30 patients with acute anterior dislocations compared intraarticular lidocaine (IAL) to intravenous sedation in manipulative reduction. Pain relief, success of the Stimson technique, and time to achieve reduction were similar. Time spent in the emergency department, however, was considerably less for the IAL group (75 minutes compared with 185 minutes in the sedation group, $P < 0.01$). The cost of IAL was also less ($0.52 for IAL compared with $97.64 for intravenous sedation). The authors concluded that reduction with IAL required fewer resources in terms of cost, time, and personnel compared with traditional intravenous sedation. In another randomized study of 54 anterior dislocations, IAL was less effective than intravenous narcotics and sedation in relieving prereduction pain, although equally effective in overall pain relief.

Natural History of Anterior Dislocation

The natural history of primary anterior shoulder dislocations is well established. Nonsurgical treatment leads to recurrence rates varying from 17% to 96%. Most authors report recurrence directly related to age, with those younger than 20 years having the highest incidence. One recent study evaluated risk factors for recurrence. In a retrospective examination of 180 patients, the authors found age to be the most reliable predictor of recurrence, with the highest incidence occurring in patients between the ages of 21 and 30 years. Despite careful stratification of activities into three different levels of risk, however, the authors were unable to demonstrate any relationship between type of sports activity and recurrence.

A recent retrospective review of 253 consecutive anterior shoulder stabilizations examined prognostic variables influencing recurrence. Identified risk factors included the presence of a workers' compensation issue, a voluntary instability pattern, a previous instability surgery, shorter periods of postoperative immobilization, and age. Factors that were found to have no relationship to recurrent instability included gender, pattern of instability, presence of a labral tear, presence of a Hill-Sachs lesion, or experience of the surgeon.

Immobilization

The value of immobilization remains unclear, with most studies concluding that it offers little benefit against recurrence. Current guidelines suggest some minimal period of immobilization for comfort, followed by early isometric exercises and restoration of motion and strength. A shorter period of immobilization is probably warranted in older athletes because of their decreased recurrence risk and the increased likelihood of stiffness.

Two recent studies have questioned the traditional wisdom of sling immobilization in internal rotation and suggested immobilization in external rotation instead. In a cadaveric study, contact forces between the glenoid and labrum were measured after creating a Bankart lesion. Contact force between the detached labrum and glenoid was reported to be greatest at 45° of external rotation, with no contact force detectable with internal rotation. In a clinical study, two groups of first-time dislocators were treated with immobilization in either external or internal rotation for 3 weeks. At an average follow-up of 15.9 months for the internal rotation group, the recurrence rate was 30%. In comparison, at an average follow-up of 13.7 months for the external rotation group, the recurrence rate was 0%. The anterior apprehension sign in the two groups was not statistically different; it was positive in 2 of 14 patients (14%) in the internal rotation group without recurrence, and 1 of 20 patients (5%) in the external rotation group ($P = 0.35$). The authors concluded that immobilization in external rotation following shoulder dislocation probably improves tissue coaptation and may decrease recurrence.

Braces, which prevent the shoulder from being placed in a vulnerable position, play only a limited role in the treatment of instability. Their relevance is usually for the in-season athlete for whom expedient surgical intervention is not a realistic option. In addition, because they often compromise function in athletes playing skilled positions in which above-the-shoulder or overhead function is critical for effectiveness, braces are limited in their usefulness.

Treatment of the First-Time Dislocator

Because of the predictably high recurrence rate following a first-time dislocation, some authors have advocated primary stabilization in young athletes. Justifications for this approach include proven recurrence rates as high as 90% among young and/or high-demand athletes; consequences of recurrence on subsequent activities, including risk of lost playing time or subsequent second season injury; and evidence that intervention before the development of capsular laxity and bony pathology may yield better results than delayed surgical intervention. This suggests that additional joint damage to the capsule and articular structures accrue with recurrent instability episodes.

Several recent series have compared the effectiveness of immediate arthroscopic stabilization versus nonsurgical treatment of the first-time dislocator. One study examined 28 adolescents between 12 and 17 years of age who were followed for an average of 7.1 years following initial dislocation. All nonsurgically treated patients showed clinical evidence of instability, whereas those treated surgically had no recurrent dislocations. In a second series, 40 patients younger than 30 years were prospectively randomized to receive either 3 weeks of immobilization and rehabilitation or arthroscopic stabilization using a transglenoid technique. At an average follow-up of 32 months, the rate of recurrence was significantly different, with recurrence occurring in 47% of the nonsurgical group compared with only 15.9% of the surgically treated group. Disease-specific quality of life was significantly better in the surgically treated group. An interesting finding of this study was the presence of an average 15% deficit in disease-specific quality of life, even among nonsurgically treated patients who did not experience recurrence. Shoulder function following even a single dislocation did not return to normal. The results of longer-term 6-year follow-up on this group of patients were recently reported. At average follow-up of 75 months, recurrence in the nonsurgically treated group was 75% compared with 15.4% in the surgically treated group.

A prospective randomized study examined a group of young, active West Point cadets who were first-time dislocators. After either nonsurgical treatment consisting of 4 weeks of immobilization followed by rehabilitation (14 patients) or arthroscopic Bankart repair with a bioabsorbable tack (10 patients), 75% of nonsurgically treated patients experienced recurrence on return to their demanding activities. In comparison, those treated with arthroscopic stabilization had only an 11% recurrence rate at 2-year minimum follow-up.

Data comparing the results of immediate repair of the first-time dislocator versus delayed intervention of the recurrent instability patient are sparse. One study compared the arthroscopic findings in first-time dislocators (10 patients) to patients with multiple recurrent instability episodes (25 patients). Tissue quality was superior in the group of first-time dislocators, including better soft-tissue vascularity, less retraction, and the perception of easier reparability. In contrast, tissue in recurrent dislocators was more pale, stiff and inelastic, and of poorer quality. Bony lesions were not seen in the acute first-time dislocator group. In the recurrent dislocation group, however, 40% had a nonengaging Hill-Sachs lesion, and 16% had a glenoid impact bony lesion. This nonrandomized trial documented a higher success rate with early treatment, with no recurrent dislocations and only one subluxation reported in the first-time dislocator group (recurrence rate, 4%). In comparison, those treated for recurrent instability had a failure rate of 16% (8% with recurrent dislocations and 8% with recurrent subluxations).

Not every first-time dislocator is an appropriate candidate for early surgical stabilization. Patient age, activity level, and desire to return to preinjury status are important factors that must be weighed on an individual basis. Dislocation itself is only one criterion influencing treatment decision making. Disadvantages of immediate surgical stabilization include the complications of surgery, cost, and inconvenience.

Recurrent Anterior Instability

Patients with recurrent shoulder instability are disabled in terms of both shoulder function and general health status. The spectrum of this disability ranges from pain and apprehension during specific activities to episodic subluxation and recurrent dislocation. A thorough medical history must include information about previous events and treatment. Arm position at the time of dislocation should be determined. The relationship of symptoms to activity, such as in which position symptoms are provoked, may suggest the predominant direction of instability.

Range of motion in patients with recurrent anterior instability is usually normal; however, range of motion in the throwing population has been shown to be greater in external rotation. Assessment of anterior instability involves both objective laxity translation testing and subjective instability tests. Anterior laxity tests include the anterior drawer test and the load and shift test. In each, the amount of translation and the quality of the end point are assessed under load. The presence of subjective symptoms (ie, reproducing the patients' sense of apprehension or pain) during translation may further corroborate the diagnosis. Inferior translation is assessed by the sulcus sign.

A recent study examined the intrareliability and interreliability of manual techniques in assessing anterior humeral head translation. The authors found intrareliability to be only 54% and interreliability to be only 37% and concluded that manual assessment of humeral head translation was unreliable. They further noted that use of an "end feel" component to the examination actually decreased the reliability of the examination.

In addition to standard radiographs, additional views that help assess recurrent instability include the West Point and the Stryker's notch views. CT has been shown to be valuable in quantifying the degree of glenoid bone loss. In a recent cadaveric study, glenoid osseous defects were created to simulate bony Bankart lesions. Both CT and the West Point view were found to provide precise measurements of the size of the glenoid defect. In another study, glenoid rim morphology was studied in 100 consecutive shoulders with recurrent anterior instability. Three-dimensional reconstructed CT images (with the humeral head digitally "eliminated") provided an accurate interpretation of glenoid rim morphology comparable to that obtained using arthroscopic assessment. MRI and magnetic resonance arthrography remain popular imaging tools despite their relative inaccuracy in interpreting labral pathology.

Nonsurgical treatment of recurrent instability includes activity modification to reduce risk and rehabilitation to improve functional strength. Patients who are unwilling to accept activity modification or those with athletic or functional impairment are candidates for surgical stabilization.

Examination Under Anesthesia

Examination under anesthesia (EUA) is an integral part of shoulder instability assessment, particularly in instances of diagnostic uncertainty. Recent studies have reinforced its value. In one study, 30 patients with documented unilateral posttraumatic recurrent anterior instability were assessed using EUA in multiple directions and rotations. The authors found testing helpful when performed at both 40° and 80° of external rotation and when assessing instability in the anteroinferior direction, with a reported sensitivity of 83% and a specificity of 100%. Another study assessed glenohumeral translation in 50 patients with surgically confirmed anterior instability while the patients were awake and under anesthesia. Examination of patients while they were awake was reported to be unproductive, but EUA proved helpful in confirming both the direction and degree of instability.

Open Versus Arthroscopic Repair

Open stabilization certainly is the historic standard for the treatment of anterior shoulder instability. Recurrence rates of 3% to 5% have been documented in several long-term studies. Arthroscopic techniques have made considerable inroads, however, with many studies demonstrating outcomes comparable to, and in some instances, better than those for open stabilization. Open repair involves anatomic restoration of the capsulolabral complex. A recent study reported the outcome following open Bankart repair for recurrent anterior instability in 78 patients. At minimum 2-year follow-up, the recurrence rate (defined as symptomatic subluxation or dislocation) was 13%; patients who had a postoperative episode of trauma were excluded, however, which potentially resulted in an underestimation of the rate of true failure. Two other recent studies also suggest that recurrence rates following open repair may be higher than previously reported. In a retrospective follow-up of 54 patients following open Bankart repair with suture anchors, 17% experienced recurrent instability at 4- to 9-year follow-up. Another retrospective study evaluated 66 collision and contact athletes in a US military academy after open Bankart/capsulorrhaphy repair. At an average 47-month follow-up, 23% were noted to have recurrent instability, including 3% with recurrent dislocations and 20% with recurrent subluxations. These studies may help level the playing field of instability outcome studies, which under current scientific scrutiny may have been held to a higher standard for success than traditional open repair studies. Analyzing open repair outcomes with these newer tools may explain the discrepancy of arthroscopic and open repair results.

Alternative open repair techniques include the Putti-Platt, Magnuson-Stack, and Bristow-Laterjet procedures. These nonanatomic techniques do not address the underlying cause of instability and although still favored as primary procedures by some, are generally reserved for salvage or revision situations. In one recent follow-up study of Putti-Platt capsulorrhaphy procedures performed in 66 shoulders, redislocation occurred in only 3%. However, the authors of this study noted a definite increased rate of glenohumeral osteoarthritis, graded as moderate in 20% and severe in 6% of shoulders. A recent prospective study reported on 30 shoulders after the Bristow-Laterjet procedure. At an average 15.1-year follow-up, the recurrence rate was only 3.4%. Although a Bristow-Laterjet procedure may play a role in addressing glenoid bone deficiency, particularly when involving more than 25% of the glenoid fossa, this procedure was shown to compromise external rotation (average loss, 11°), and overhead athletes who undergo this procedure are typically unable to return to preinjury activity level. Other associated complications include articular cartilage damage, nonunion of the coracoid bone block, migration of hardware, and neurovascular injury.

Arthroscopic stabilization procedures have evolved considerably. Some outcomes continue to be published regarding transglenoid techniques, although current literature seems to be increasingly focused on the use of either bioabsorbable tacks or suture anchors. In a recent study following military cadets for an average of 37 months after arthroscopic stabilization using bioabsorbable tacks, the recurrence rate was 12%. Factors associated with recurrence included a history of bilateral shoulder instability, a 2+ sulcus sign, and poor quality capsulolabral tissue. In a recent study following 20 patients for an average of 3.4 years after arthroscopic stabilization with a bioabsorbable tack, a 30% recurrence rate was noted in patients with documented recurrent anterior dislocations. In light of these results, the authors recommended not using the technique for patients whose instability began with an initial dislocation.

Other bioabsorbable tack–related complications include reports of foreign-body reaction and synovitis. One recent report examined 52 patients undergoing arthroscopic stabilization using a poly-L-lactic acid tack. Nineteen percent developed delayed onset of symptoms of pain and/or progressive stiffness at an average 8 month follow-up (range, 3 to 19 months). Nine of the 10 patients who underwent arthroscopy demonstrated gross implant debris and considerable glenohumeral synovitis. Three of these patients exhibited significant full-thickness chondral injury to the humeral head, and arthroscopic débridement was effective in resolving pain and stiffness in seven patients.

The development of suture anchors has eliminated some of the problems related to earlier techniques. Arthroscopic Bankart repair using suture anchors replicates the open approach. Twin anterior portals permit mobilization of the labrum, glenoid preparation, anchor placement, suture passage, and labral fixation (Figure 2). Associated capsular patholaxity and rotator interval deficiency can be definitively addressed as needed (Figure 3). Recurrence rates after stabilization with suture anchors have generally been low. In one recent study, 30 patients, most of whom had sports-related recurrent anterior posttraumatic instability, underwent arthroscopic Bankart repair using suture anchors. At a minimum 2-year follow-up, none experienced recurrent dislocation, and only 2 (7%) demonstrated a positive relocation sign, which is indicative of possible subtle residual instability. Using multiple outcome criteria, including the grading scale of Rowe, the simple shoulder test, the American Shoulder and Elbow Surgeons system, and the Medical Outcomes Study 36-Item Short Form, overall good and excellent results were reported in 96% of patients.

Glenoid bone deficiency, an engaging Hill-Sachs lesion, the absence of a discrete Bankart lesion, and an attenuated capsuloligamentous complex have been associated with poor outcomes following arthroscopic surgery. In addition, some authors have reported an increased risk of recurrence in young, male athletes who participate in collision sports. Bony Bankart lesions have long been considered an indication for open surgical intervention. One recent report examined the outcome of 194 consecutive patients undergoing arthroscopic stabilization using suture anchors. At an average follow-up of 27 months, the 173 shoulders without significant bone defects had a 4% recurrence rate. In contrast, of the 21

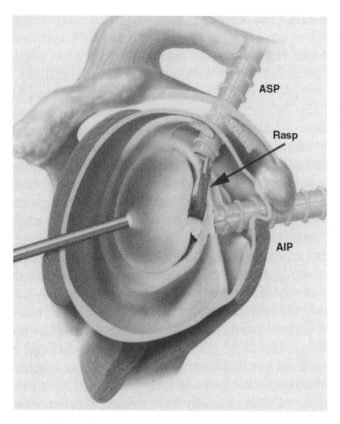

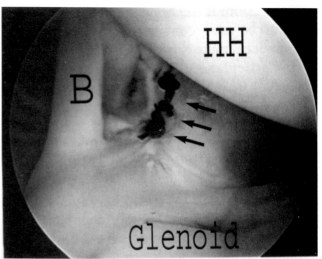

Figure 3 In this lateral decubitus arthroscopic view of a right shoulder, absorbable polydioxanone sutures (*arrows*) were used to achieve closure of the rotator interval in a patient with a significant sulcus sign and arthroscopic appearance of interval deficiency. B = Bankart lesion, HH = humeral head. *(Reproduced with permission from Abrams JS: Arthroscopic treatment of posterior instability, in Tibone J, Shaffer BS, Savoie FH III, Davis CS (eds): Shoulder Arthroscopy. New York, NY, Springer Verlag, 2003.)*

Figure 2 Twin anterior portals are seen in this cross-sectional illustration. Viewed from the posterior portal, the rasp (*arrow*) is introduced from the anterosuperior portal (ASP), mobilizing the labrum from the anterior glenoid. The anteroinferior portal (AIP) facilitates anchor insertion along the anteroinferior glenoid rim. *(Reproduced with permission from Levine RG, Iannotti SJ, Matthews LS: Arthroscopic anterior capsulolabral repair using suture anchor technique, in Tibone J, Shaffer BS, Savoie FH III, Davis CS (eds): Shoulder Arthroscopy. New York, NY, Springer Verlag, 2003.)*

ficient glenoid as the shape of an inverted pear in 18 of these patients, 11 (61%) of which had recurrent instability following Bankart repair. All of the patients with an engaging Hill-Sachs lesion (3 of 3) had recurrent instability. The authors concluded that the presence of an inverted pear-shaped glenoid (ie, the inferior glenoid is narrower than the superior glenoid) or an engaging Hill-Sachs lesion (ie, the lesion engages the anterior glenoid rim in the position of flexion abduction/external rotation) is a contraindication to arthroscopic repair (Figure 4).

Small bony lesions are probably less of a risk factor. A recent study of 25 shoulders in which a small (< 25% of the length of the anterior glenoid rim) bony Bankart lesion was present showed overall good results using suture anchors, with shoulder function and stability restored in 23 patients (92%). All were able to resume sports activities, with most returning to the same preinjury level of participation. The mean loss of external rotation was 9.7°, which the authors attributed to the medial capsulolabral anchor fixation site. Another recent study has described a method of assessing glenoid bone deficiency arthroscopically. In 56 patients and 10 cadavers, the bare spot was a reliable reference from which glenoid bone loss could be determined (Figure 5). This constant landmark was proposed to be a clinically useful tool to determine the necessity of possible bone grafting in cases of glenoid rim deficiency (Figure 6).

The importance of addressing associated capsular patholaxity has received considerable recent attention. Several studies have evaluated the efficacy of adjunctive measures to treat associated capsular patholaxity at the

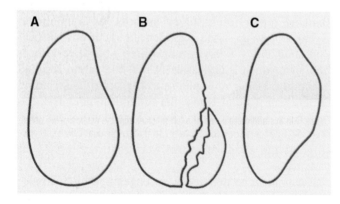

Figure 4 A, The normal shape of the glenoid is that of a pear (larger below than above). **B,** A bony Bankart lesion can create an inverted-pear configuration of the glenoid. **C,** A compression Bankart lesion can also create an inverted-pear configuration of the glenoid. *(Reproduced with permission from Burkhart SS, DeBeer JF: Traumatic glenohumeral bone defects and their relationship to failure of arthroscopic Bankart repairs: Significance of the inverted pear glenoid and the humeral engaging Hill-Sachs lesion. Arthroscopy 2000;16:677-694.)*

shoulders with significant osseous Bankart or Hill-Sachs lesions, 14 (67%) had recurrent instability. The authors further described the arthroscopic appearance of the de-

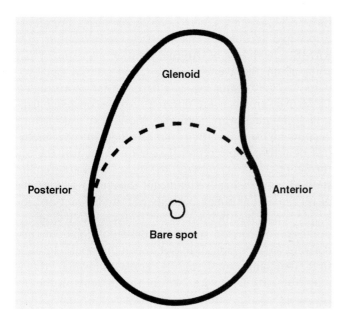

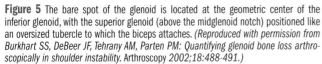

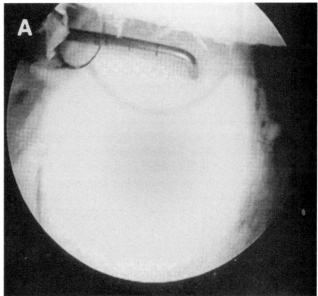

Figure 5 The bare spot of the glenoid is located at the geometric center of the inferior glenoid, with the superior glenoid (above the midglenoid notch) positioned like an oversized tubercle to which the biceps attaches. *(Reproduced with permission from Burkhart SS, DeBeer JF, Tehrany AM, Parten PM: Quantifying glenoid bone loss arthroscopically in shoulder instability.* Arthroscopy 2002;18:488-491.)

time of arthroscopic Bankart repair. In one such study, an arthroscopic inferior capsular split/shift procedure was done in addition to suture anchor Bankart repair in 29 patients. At 2- to 5-year follow-up, the recurrence rate was 6.9%. The results of electrothermal-assisted capsulorrhaphy used to supplement arthroscopic Bankart repair for recurrent anterior instability have also been recently reported. In one study, 42 patients with recurrent instability who were also involved in contact sports underwent arthroscopic capsulolabral repair with either a suture anchor and horizontal mattress suture or an absorbable tack, supplemented by thermal shrinkage (using a monopolar radiofrequency probe) of the middle, anteroinferior, and posteroinferior glenohumeral ligaments. At an average follow-up of 28 months, 7% experienced traumatic redislocation. Thirty-eight of 42 patients (90%) returned to participation in their previous sport.

In another study, 53 patients underwent arthroscopic Bankart repair with suture anchors along with interval plication in 26% and capsular soft-tissue tightening with laser capsulorrhaphy in 91%. At an average 33-month follow-up, the rate of recurrence was 10.5%. Eighty-nine percent of the patients were able to return to their desired level of activity. The success rate of each of these procedures has been credited to addressing associated pathology.

Literature regarding the results of arthroscopic versus open stabilization for the collision or contact athlete is confounding. In general, most arthroscopic studies have identified participation in contact or collision

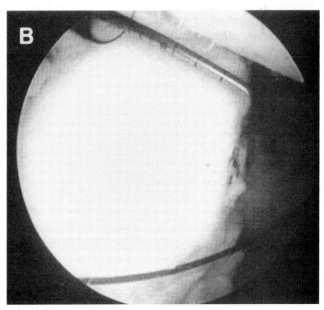

Figure 6 In this arthroscopic view of a left shoulder from the anterosuperior portal, the tip of the hook probe rests on the bare spot of the glenoid, and the 3-mm laser marks on the probe indicate a 12-mm distance (4 marks on the probe) from the bare spot to the posterior glenoid rim (**A**); the probe is placed just inferior to the bare spot (**B**), showing that the distance from the bare spot to the anterior glenoid rim is 6 mm (2 marks) and suggesting a 6-mm bone loss from compression of the anterior glenoid, which represents a 25% reduction in the diameter of the inferior glenoid. *(Reproduced with permission from Burkhart SS, DeBeer JF, Tehrany AM, Parten PM: Quantifying glenoid bone loss arthroscopically in shoulder instability.* Arthroscopy 2002;18:488-491.)

sports as a significant risk factor. Some authors have reexamined the results of both open and arthroscopic repairs in contact and collision sports populations. In a recent study of 58 American football players (43 high school, 11 college, and 4 professional athletes) at an average follow-up of 37 months after open Bankart repair, no postoperative dislocations and two subluxations were reported, a recurrence rate of 3%. Fifty-two of the 58 patients (90%) returned to playing football for at least 1 year. A recent survey of National Football League and National Hockey League team orthopaedists examined the role of arthroscopic management of anterior instability in professional contact sport athletes. Of 20 professional athletes (12 football players and 8 hockey players) who underwent arthroscopic stabilization, successful outcomes at a minimum 2-year follow-up were achieved in only 75%. This included 11 of 12 football players, but only 4 of 8 hockey players. Based on these data, the authors do not recommend arthroscopic stabilization for hockey players.

In another study, 14 collision and contact athletes younger than 20 years underwent arthroscopic stabilization using suture anchors. The authors drew a distinction between contact (in which athletes are at risk of contact but do not intentionally engage in collision) and collision (football, rugby, lacrosse, and hockey) sports. At an average 38.9-month follow-up, 14% (2 of 14) of the collision athletes experienced recurrence, but none (0 of 8) of the contact athletes experienced recurrence. Overall, 91% of the athletes returned to organized high school or college sports. The authors concluded that collision athletics, rather than all contact sports, are the more specific risk factor in athletes being considered for arthroscopic stabilization.

Fifty-six patients underwent one of three different stabilization procedures for recurrent instability experienced playing Australian Rules football. At a mean follow-up of 29.4 months, arthroscopic suture repair yielded a 70% recurrence rate, and repair with biodegradable tacks a 38% recurrence rate; 75% of the recurrences resulted from minimal trauma. Open capsular shift with Bankart repair also resulted in a high (30%) recurrence rate, although half of these injuries were caused by violent trauma. The authors advocated open surgery for athletes participating in Australian Rules football.

The authors of one arthroscopic study suggest that the high reported recurrence rates among contact and collision sport athletes may actually be attributable to bony deficiency in this population rather than their activities. In a review of 101 contact athletes (96 South African rugby players and 5 American football players), the rate of recurrence after arthroscopic Bankart repair using suture anchors was only 6.5% in the absence of glenoid deficiency or a Hill-Sachs lesion, but 89% in the presence of a significant bone defect.

Proponents of arthroscopic stabilization cite the reported advantages of decreased morbidity, preserved motion, improved cosmesis, shorter surgical time, and enhanced ability to visualize and completely address pathoanatomy. A recent meta-analysis compared arthroscopic and open techniques. Outcomes of 1,946 patients in 45 arthroscopic repair series were compared with

those of 724 patients in 14 open repair series. For all arthroscopic techniques, the average redislocation rate was 18%, with loss of external rotation averaging 5°. In comparison, the average redislocation rate for open repairs was 7.9%, with loss of external rotation averaging 11°. However, when the different arthroscopic stabilization techniques were analyzed, those that used suture anchors had significantly better results than other methods of arthroscopic repair. Comparison of just the arthroscopic anchor repairs to open Bankart repairs showed no statistically significant difference in the rate of recurrence, although patients who underwent arthroscopic repair had better external rotation. In a nonrandomized comparison study, 63 consecutive patients underwent arthroscopic Bankart repair or open capsular shift. Outcomes were slightly worse following arthroscopic stabilization, with 24% of the patients in the arthroscopy group reporting unsatisfactory results compared with 18% of the patients in the open repair group.

Patients with a discrete Bankart lesion, a robust inferior glenohumeral ligament, no significant capsular laxity, and absence of other concomitant intra-articular pathology are ideal candidates for arthroscopic repair, and there is a high likelihood of success when this procedure is properly performed by an experienced arthroscopist. If the surgeon adheres to rigid selection criteria, results can approach or equal those of open repair techniques; however, when arthroscopic repair is done in young, high-risk patients and those with excessive capsular laxity and/or significant bone defects, instability may recur. The disadvantages of arthroscopic repair include complications of the various techniques, the technically demanding nature of the procedure, generally higher failure rates, and difficulty in easily determining and addressing associated capsular patholaxity. The advantages of open repair techniques include providing surgeons with the ability to restore capsular tension more precisely and to access and definitively repair the rotator interval.

Postoperative Protocol

A period of postoperative immobilization has been advocated by most authors because of the higher reported failure rate with arthroscopic procedures. Recently, one study presented an accelerated rehabilitation program. Sixty-two patients were prospectively randomized to undergo either 3 weeks of immobilization and a conventional rehabilitation program or an accelerated rehabilitation program, consisting of staged range-of-motion and strengthening exercises beginning on the first postoperative day after arthroscopic Bankart repair. At an average 31-month follow-up, no differences were seen in the recurrence rate (no patients reported redislocation), but the accelerated rehabilitation group reported less pain, greater overall satisfaction, quicker resumption of functional range of motion, and earlier return to functional activities. However, these data may not be easily extrapolated to the general population because the patient population in this study was older (average age, 28 years), carefully selected, excluded athletes, and required that patients have a classic Bankart lesion and a robust labrum for inclusion.

Complications of Instability Surgery

Complications of surgery for anterior instability (both open and arthroscopic repair) include persistent or recurrent instability, loss of motion, weakness, and neurovascular injury. Subscapularis rupture following open anterior shoulder instability repair is a rare complication, but it must be considered in the patient with pain, instability, increased external rotation, and a positive lift-off test result. Complications related to implants include improper placement, suture breakage, anchor unloading or pullout, knot abrasion within the joint, and instrument failure. A recent report described eight patients with complications following shoulder surgery in which metal anchors had been used. Of these, five were the result of open reconstruction for anterior instability. Three of these five had extraosseous positioning of the anchor implant. Three patients developed severe articular damage.

Neurologic complications were the focus of one recent study that reported an 8.2% incidence of neurologic deficit after open anterior shoulder stabilization. Of 282 patients treated for recurrent anterior instability, 7 (2.5%) had sensory disturbances only, 16 (5.7%) had sensorimotor neuropathies, and 8 (2.8%) had a more defined deficit in one or two cords or peripheral nerves. Complete resolution occurred in most patients, but the deficit persisted in 4 (18% of those with neurologic complications).

Revision Shoulder Stabilization

Shoulder stability can usually be restored with a revision Bankart procedure; however, the results are less predictable than those of primary repair. Success depends on accurate recognition of the cause of the instability, which most commonly includes glenoid deficiency, anterior capsular and/or subscapularis tendon deficiency, and large Hill-Sachs lesions, and the ability to definitively address technical challenges. One study retrospectively reviewed the results of revising 50 failed anterior instability repairs. At an average follow-up of 4.7 years, the authors reported good and excellent results in 78% of patients. All 17 patients with significant postoperative trauma as the cause of their failed anterior stability repair had excellent results after revision surgery. However, only 22 of the 33 patients with atraumatic recurrent instability (67%) had satisfactory results

after revision surgery. Overall, the authors reported a high percentage of satisfactory results following revision surgery, but they concluded that patients with atraumatic recurrence, those with voluntary dislocations, and those who have undergone multiple prior stabilization attempts were at significantly greater risk for poor results with revision repair.

Posterior Instability

The diagnosis and treatment of posterior instability of the shoulder continues to pose a considerable clinical challenge. It may present as a frank dislocation or, more commonly, as recurrent posterior subluxation. Posterior dislocations, accounting for 4% of all glenohumeral joint dislocations, may present as acute (< 6 weeks from time of injury) or chronic. Approximately 50% to 80% of posterior dislocations are unrecognized at the time of initial presentation, underscoring the importance of thorough physical and radiographic examinations. In athletes, a direct blow to the anterior shoulder or, more commonly, a posteriorly directed force to a flexed, internally rotated, and adducted shoulder is the typical mechanism of injury. Posterior subluxation can be related to a specific traumatic event (in 50% of patients) or repetitive minor traumatic episodes. Athletes participating in swimming or overhead activities may be subject to tensile failure of the posterior capsule from repetitive microtrauma, thereby precipitating symptoms of posterior instability.

Traumatic posterior instability affects both the posterior labrum and the capsuloligamentous tissue. Convincing biomechanical evidence suggests that injury to the anterior capsular structures may also be necessary for a patient to develop posterior glenohumeral instability. Although reverse Bankart lesions were historically considered uncommon, recent clinical series suggest a much higher incidence of capsulolabral detachment in athletes with a traumatic posterior dislocation (Figure 7).

Presentation and Evaluation

Unlike anterior dislocations, most acute posterior dislocations reduce spontaneously. Patients with an acute posterior dislocation usually present with the arm in an adducted, internally rotated position. The coracoid is typically prominent, and the dislocated humeral head creates a posterior fullness. Although sometimes subtle, a lack of external rotation and inability to supinate the forearm are the hallmarks of diagnosis. Radiographic evaluation should consist of a three-view trauma series. The axillary view will reveal an empty glenoid with the humeral head displaced posteriorly. An apical oblique view may show an associated anteromedial humeral head impaction fracture (reverse Hill-Sachs lesion) and/or posterior glenoid rim fracture. As with anterior

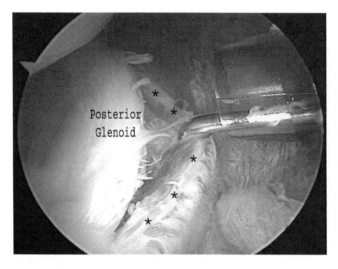

Figure 7 In this lateral decubitus arthroscopic view of a right shoulder from an anterosuperior portal, a probe displaces the posterior labral detachment (reverse Bankart lesion) seen here from the 10-o'clock position. * = labrum. *(Reproduced with permission from Abrams JS: Arthroscopic treatment of posterior instability, in Tibone J, Shaffer BS, Savoie FH III, Davis CS (eds): Shoulder Arthroscopy. New York, NY, Springer Verlag, 2003.)*

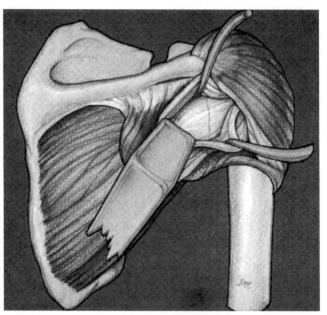

Figure 8 The posterior shoulder capsule is exposed during the open approach to posterior stabilization using the infraspinatus-splitting approach. The natural plane is developed by incising through the tendinous raphe between the two muscle bellies. This approach permits direct exposure over the midglenoid. To avoid injury to the suprascapular nerve, sharp dissection more than 15 mm medial to the glenoid rim should be avoided. *(Reproduced with permission from Shaffer BS, Conway J, Jobe FW, Kvitne RS, Tibone JE: Infraspinatus muscle-splitting incision in posterior shoulder surgery. Am J Sports Med 1994;22:113-120.)*

instability, CT may be useful for quantifying bone loss.

The more common presentation of posterior instability includes pain, instability, or both when the arm is placed in the provocative position of flexion, adduction, and internal rotation. Patients may describe crepitus or clicking in certain positions. Approximately 50% of patients with posterior instability will be able to voluntarily demonstrate their instability pattern by positioning and muscle activation. These patients must be distinguished from the habitual dislocator who willfully subluxates the shoulder for secondary gain.

Reproduction of the instability should be attempted during physical examination. Stability tests include the posterior drawer test, load and shift test, and jerk test. Instability testing more frequently elicits symptoms rather than discernable translation. The jerk test attempts to reproduce the clunk of reduction or a patient's sense of instability/reduction by manually attempting to replicate the voluntary instability maneuver. The arm is flexed to 90° and posteriorly loaded, followed by extension of the loaded arm, yielding a clunk and/or reproduction of the patient's sense of reduction from a dislocated position. Examination should also include assessment of laxity in anterior and inferior directions. A positive sulcus sign may indicate excessive inferior capsular laxity, suggesting that the posterior subluxation may be a component of a bidirectional or multidirectional instability pattern.

Treatment

When necessary, acute dislocations are treated with a traction-countertraction reduction technique facilitated by appropriate relaxation. The shoulder is immobilized in a neutral position for 4 to 6 weeks. Rehabilitation follows, with emphasis on parascapular and rotator cuff strengthening. The documented incidence of recurrence after posterior dislocation is lower than that after anterior instability. Chronic dislocations, large humeral head fractures, significant glenoid rim fractures, and displaced lesser tuberosity fractures may necessitate surgical management.

Many patients with recurrent posterior instability, particularly those whose onset is atraumatic, are effectively treated with a strengthening program. Surgical intervention is reserved for those who have symptomatic involuntary instability and for whom nonsurgical measures are not successful. Numerous surgical techniques have been described to treat symptomatic involuntary posterior instability. Results of bony procedures, such as glenoid osteotomy, bone blocks, and rotational osteotomy of the humerus, have been based on small series of patients and have shown inconsistent results. Soft-tissue surgical procedures include reverse Bankart repair, reverse Putti-Platt procedure, and posteroinferior capsular shift (Figure 8). Success rates of open posterior capsular repair range from 80% to 95%. In one recent series of 14 athletes with recurrent posterior instability treated via open posterior capsulorrhaphy, 13 patients reported good or excellent results according to a modified Rowe grading system. In another long-term follow-up study, 31 patients (33 shoulders) were treated with open posterior capsulorrhaphy with lateral advancement of the teres minor and infraspinatus insertions. A significant decrease in the mean subjective instability score was documented after surgery, and results were maintained over time. Complications were rare, and revision procedures were uncommon.

Recently, arthroscopy has played a major role in the identification and treatment of posterior instability pathology. One recent series evaluated 27 patients who underwent arthroscopic posterior capsular shift for recurrent instability. At an average 39-month follow-up, all but one patient had stable shoulders. In a study of 39 patients, arthroscopic stabilization with suture anchors and capsular plication when necessary demonstrated a success rate of 92% at a minimum 2-year follow-up. Finally, in a smaller recent follow-up of nine athletes with posterior labral detachment, arthroscopic stabilization using a bioabsorbable tack was effective in eliminating instability and returning all athletes to contact sports and weight lifting at a minimum 2-year follow-up.

Acromioclavicular Joint Dislocation

The acromioclavicular (AC) joint is one of the most vulnerable and commonly injured joints in athletics, particularly among those who participate in contact sports such as football, hockey, and rugby. Subluxations and dislocations result from direct force or indirect forces transmitted through the upper extremity. Most commonly, the athlete falls directly onto the acromion while the humerus in an adducted position. Injury to the capsular ligaments (AC ligaments), extracapsular ligaments (coracoclavicular ligaments), and supporting musculature (deltoid and trapezius) can result in instability of the AC joint.

Rockwood's modification of Allman and Tossy's original classification system for defining the extent of injury to the AC joint remains the standard; in this system, AC joint injuries are divided into six different types. Types I, II, and III involve progressive degrees of injury to the AC joint capsule and coracoclavicular ligaments. Type I involves isolated injury to the AC joint capsule. Type II involves a greater degree of injury, with disruption of the AC joint capsule in addition to some degree of incomplete tearing of the coracoclavicular ligaments. In a type III separation, both the AC joint capsule and coracoclavicular ligaments are completely disrupted, often with significant (superior) displacement of the clavicle relative to the acromion. Types IV and VI, in which the clavicle is displaced posteriorly and inferiorly, respectively, are extremely uncommon. Type V is an exaggerated type III injury, in which there is considerable additional injury to the envelope of surrounding soft tissue, the deltotrapezial fascia. The increased severity of this injury leads to a greater degree of displacement that

can be appreciated both clinically and radiographically with vertical joint displacement between 100% and 300%.

An alternative classification scheme has been recently proposed, based on recognizing previously unreported medial instability of the AC joint. In 36 patients with acute (n = 25) and chronic (n = 12) Rockwood grade II, III, and V injuries, medial instability was assessed by performing cross-body adduction AP radiographs, defined as displacement of the medial edge of the acromion under or medial to the lateral edge of the clavicle (which represents loss of the strut function of the clavicle to stabilize the scapula). Of the 25 acute injuries, 21, including all of the type II injuries, demonstrated medial subluxation. Of the 12 chronic injuries examined, 7 showed instability. The authors reported a direct relationship between the presence of instability and the association of symptoms. Based on the results of this study, the authors believed that this "functional" classification, in addition to routine radiographs, might have some predictive value in identifying patients who may benefit from surgical intervention.

Presentation and Evaluation

Physical examination of the injured AC joint depends on injury severity. Findings include swelling, ecchymoses, deformity, tenderness, and abnormal translation. Optimal radiographs for evaluating these injuries include an AP view of both AC joints on a single film (when possible), an axillary view to assess anteroposterior displacement and evaluate for intra-articular fracture, and the 10° to 15° cephalic tilt (Zanca) view. Stress views have been recommended to differentiate type II from type III injuries in some cases.

Treatment

Optimal treatment for AC joint injuries has varied little over the past decade. Nonsurgical treatment, using either a sling or figure-of-8 device, continues to be the preferred method of management for type I and type II AC joint separations. Although most patients are able to successfully return to participation in sports, a small percentage (9% to 23%) will experience chronic symptoms that may limit participation.

Complications of nonsurgical treatment include persistent symptoms of pain, fatigue, and posttraumatic arthritis. These symptoms can often be managed with a judicious corticosteroid injection, but they may require distal clavicle excision. Outcome studies have shown that surgical excision provides generally good results if the joint is stable. However, some studies have indicated that resection of the distal clavicle for some type II separations, particularly in athletes, may not be as innocuous as previously thought. Careful examination to exclude subtle AC joint instability may be necessary before resection of the chronically symptomatic grade II AC joint separation.

Most authors continue to recommend early surgical treatment of types IV, V, and VI AC joint injuries because of the morbidity associated with marked clavicle displacement in relation to the scapula. Several surgical options have been described, including AC ligament repair, coracoclavicular ligament repair, coracoacromial ligament transfer (the Weaver and Dunn procedure), dynamic muscle transfer, distal clavicle resection, and various combinations of these procedures. Complications of surgical management include loss of reduction, failure or migration of hardware, infection, coracoclavicular ossification, excessive shortening of the clavicle, and postoperative arthritis. One recent series suggested that the consequences after grade I and II AC sprains are underestimated. The authors clinically and radiographically evaluated 24 patients at a mean follow-up of 6.3 years after conservative treatment of grade I and II injuries. At latest follow-up, 7 patients reported activity-related pain, 8 presented with anteroposterior instability, and 12 exhibited AC joint tenderness and a positive result on the cross-body adduction test. Radiographic studies showed degenerative changes (13 patients), ossification of the coracoclavicular ligament (2 patients), degenerative changes and coracoclavicular ligament ossification (3 patients), and distal clavicle osteolysis (3 patients). Treatment of type III AC joint injuries remains controversial, although most continue to be treated nonsurgically.

Investigations comparing surgical to nonsurgical management have failed to show any difference in regard to overall outcome and pain relief. Evidence suggests that patients treated nonsurgically return to work and athletics earlier and are more likely to have normal range of motion and strength. Complication rates after surgery appear to be higher than those associated with conservative treatment. A recent meta-analysis of the literature was performed to determine which factors influenced surgical decision making regarding the treatment of young adults with a severely displaced AC joint dislocation. Of 24 articles found using a Medline search from 1966 through 1997, 14 reported surgical outcomes, 5 reported nonsurgical outcomes, and 5 reported both surgical and nonsurgical outcomes in the same series. Of these five, only two studies were prospective and randomized. There was no statistically significant difference between patients who underwent surgical (n = 833) and nonsurgical treatment (n = 439). The authors found that surgery led to a higher rate of complications, including further surgery (59% versus 6%), infection (6% versus 1%), restriction in range of motion (14% versus 5%), weakness (13% versus 8%), and pain (7% versus 4%). However, surgery was superior with respect to deformity (3% reported unsatisfactory outcomes in the surgical group versus 37% in the nonsurgical group). The au-

thors concluded that based on available evidence, there was not any apparent reason to recommend a surgical procedure for patients with grade III AC joint separations.

The complications of surgical treatment include loss of reduction, clavicle fracture, deltotrapezius detachment, infection, and hardware migration. Surgery for grade III AC joint separations seems to be appropriate in patients who perform repetitive lifting, overhead work, manual labor, or athletes participating in noncontact sports. The most recent reports in the literature support an individualized approach to these injuries, with nonsurgical management recommended for all but a select group of patients. Some authors advocate primary surgical repair in competitive overhead (throwing) athletes, manual laborers, and the occasional patient in whom cosmetic outcome poses an issue. Early anatomic surgical repair may permit better outcome than delayed reconstruction, but this remains unproven.

Recent evidence, however, suggests that conservative treatment may compromise function in some athletes. For example, in a group of 20 athletes evaluated at 1 year after grade III AC joint separation, 4 of 20 (20%) were found to have suboptimal results, although none reported outcomes that were poor enough to require surgery. Objective strength evaluation using a bench press revealed an average of 17% weakness, which corresponded to subjective reports of weakness and fatigue with maximal overhead effort.

Most surgical reconstructions for AC joint injuries are done in patients with chronic symptoms; the most commonly used procedure is the Weaver and Dunn procedure with coracoacromial ligament transfer. A small but growing body of evidence suggests that this procedure may be inadequate to restore normal stability. In one study, 21 cadaveric shoulders underwent Weaver and Dunn reconstruction and were biomechanically tested. The reconstructed AC joint showed considerably increased anteroposterior translation (41.9 mm in the Weaver and Dunn procedure group versus 9.1 mm in the intact joint group) and superoinferior AC joint motion (13.6 in the Weaver and Dunn procedure group versus 2.7 mm in the intact joint group). Another study found that neither the trapezoid nor conoid were able to effectively compensate for loss of AC joint capsular function during anteroposterior loading; the authors reported that the AC joint ligaments should be considered discrete biomechanical structures worthy of reconstruction. Finally, the coracoacromial ligament has been found to be weaker than the intact coracoclavicular ligaments. In load-to-failure testing, semitendinosus, gracilis, and long toe extensor tendon grafts were significantly (three to 10 times) stronger and stiffer than coracoacromial ligament transfer. On this basis, it has been suggested that tendon grafts may permit a better biologic reconstruction for chronic AC joint separations.

Sternoclavicular Joint Injuries

Sternoclavicular (SC) joint dislocations account for a very small percentage of shoulder injuries. The more common anterior dislocation is produced by posteriorly directed forces applied to the anterolateral shoulder, resulting in reciprocal anterior displacement of the medial clavicle. Posterior dislocations may result from a direct blow to the anteromedial clavicle or an anteriorly directed force applied to the posterolateral aspect of the shoulder. Recent experimental selective cutting studies have demonstrated the relative importance of the SC ligaments. In 24 unpaired cadaver specimens, the posterior capsule was found to be the most important restraint to anterior and posterior translation. The costoclavicular and interclavicular ligaments were found to have little biomechanical resistance.

Presentation and Evaluation

Patients with an anterior dislocation may present with a visible, prominent, and easily palpable medial clavicle. Physical findings of a posterior dislocation may be more subtle. A sulcus sign at the SC joint or prominence of the lateral manubrium can be masked by significant swelling. Inquiries should be made about associated dyspnea, dysphagia, and throat tightness. Compression of nearby vascular or visceral structures can cause signs of venous congestion or abnormal pulses.

Asymmetry of the SC joint may be seen on a routine chest radiograph. The 40° cephalic tilt or "serendipity" view is the best plain radiograph for patients with SC joint asymmetry, and it may permit identification of the direction of dislocation. The direction and degree of instability can be better delineated with axial CT. MRI is rarely necessary to assess SC joint injury, but it can help assess associated soft-tissue injury.

Treatment

Mild (no ligamentous disruption) and moderate (incomplete ligamentous disruption) sprains of the SC joint are treated symptomatically, with short-term immobilization and pain control. Good long-term outcomes have been documented following the nonsurgical management of complete anterior SC joint dislocations. Closed reduction of acute anterior dislocations can be attempted with general anesthesia or narcotic medications and/or muscle relaxants. Reduction is obtained with traction to the abducted, slightly externally rotated arm, while applying gentle pressure over the medial clavicle. Temporary sling immobilization provides definitive treatment, even if closed reduction fails or immediate redislocation occurs.

Open reduction is rarely indicated and is associated with high redisplacement rates and life-threatening complications, usually the result of the migration of pins. A recent study found that of three reconstructive methods performed in 36 cadaver specimens with simulated SC joint instability, a figure-of-8 semitendinosus reconstruction had superior biomechanical properties compared with either intramedullary ligament or subclavius tendon reconstruction techniques.

Management of posterior SC joint injuries should involve consultation with a vascular or trauma surgeon because of the proximity of vital underlying structures. Closed reduction, using a technique similar to that used for anterior dislocations, is recommended for patients older than 25 years who present within 7 days of the injury. A percutaneous towel clip applied under general anesthesia may help facilitate reduction. Once the reduction is stable, immobilization for approximately 6 weeks allows for soft-tissue healing.

Open reduction of a posterior SC joint dislocation is indicated in patients with unsuccessful or unstable closed reductions. The SC joint is usually stable after repair, and soft-tissue reconstruction is rarely necessary. In patients younger than 25 years, medial clavicular physeal injury can mimic anterior SC joint dislocation. CT is particularly helpful in delineating this entity. Closed reduction should be performed for patients with posterior physeal injuries who present within 10 days of injury. Open reduction is reserved for patients with signs of thoracic outlet obstruction.

Fractures

Proximal Humerus Fractures

Proximal humerus fractures in the athlete are uncommon and usually result from high-energy trauma. These injuries occur more frequently in the skeletally immature and older osteoporotic athlete. Management strategies are similar to those instituted for the nonathletic patient. Stable, nondisplaced fractures are treated nonsurgically with early range-of-motion exercises. Displaced fractures require closed reduction and, if unstable, fixation (Figure 9). Percutaneous pinning is an attractive option for treating two-part neck fractures and valgus impacted fractures with minimal comminution. Indications for open reduction and internal fixation of displaced fractures include unstable, comminuted two- and three-part fractures and displaced tuberosity fractures.

Fractures of the greater tuberosity are commonly associated with anterior glenohumeral dislocation (7% to 15% of all greater tuberosity fractures). The greater tuberosity usually reduces into its bed after reduction of the glenohumeral dislocation. Currently, most authors believe that 5 mm or more of displacement is the threshold for considering surgery. Some authors have advocated open reduction and internal fixation for as little as 3 mm of displacement in athletes and laborers who participate in overhead activities. Open reduction is usually performed through a superior deltoid-splitting

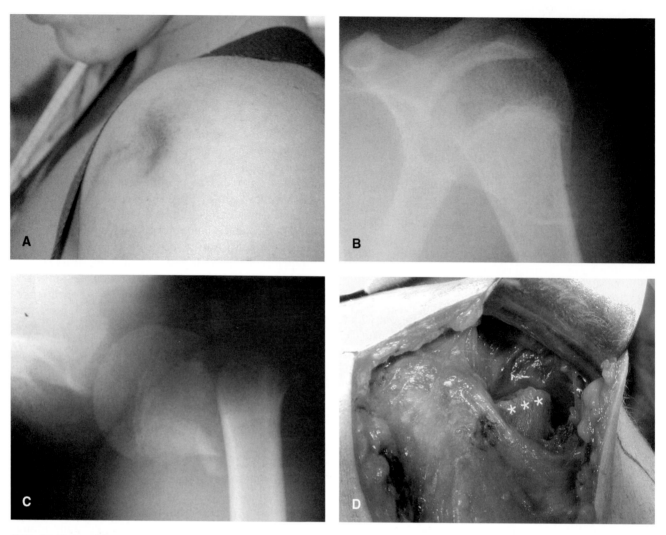

Figure 9 A, Photograph demonstrating a "dimple" at the site of a proximal humerus fracture that occurred when this 16-year-old patient fell while skateboarding. AP radiograph (**B**) demonstrates the two-part proximal humerus fracture, whereas an axillary view (**C**) more graphically shows the degree of displacement. **D,** Photograph showing penetration of the deltoid by fracture fragment (*asterisks*).

approach, followed by screw fixation or fixation with nonabsorbable suture. Three-part fractures are treated with a tension band technique. Four-part fractures and fracture-dislocations are uncommon among athletes, and open reduction and internal fixation may be needed to treat these injuries in younger patients. In most cases, four-part fractures and fracture-dislocations require treatment with prosthetic replacement because of humeral head vascular compromise and the risk of osteonecrosis.

Clavicle Fractures

Most clavicle fractures are caused by direct trauma, such as a fall onto the shoulder. Uncommon associated injuries include ipsilateral scapula and rib fractures, pneumothorax, and neurovascular injury. AP and apical oblique radiographs are used to confirm the diagnosis. CT may be valuable for better defining comminuted or intra-articular fractures.

Medial third clavicle fractures can be successfully managed with nonsurgical treatment, with the exception of posteriorly displaced fractures that threaten underlying neurovascular structures. In skeletally immature athletes, medial-third clavicle fractures may represent a fracture through the medial clavicular physis near the SC joint (Figure 10). The middle third clavicle is the most common site of fracture. Most midshaft fractures will go on to achieve union and most patients will have excellent functional results when treated nonsurgically. Treatment involves use of supportive measures such as a sling and use of analgesics rather than attempts at reduction. However, there are some recent reports suggesting that significantly displaced midclavicular fractures may have a higher than previously appreciated rate of nonunion. In a prospective randomized clinical trial of 100 patients with 100% displaced midshaft clavicle fractures, patients were treated nonsurgically with either a figure-of-8 clavicle brace or sling, or surgically with open reduction and internal fixation using a low-profile compression plate. At an average 12-month follow-up, all fractures treated surgically had united compared with 24% nonunions in the nonsurgical treatment group. Thirty percent of patients in the nonsurgical treatment group developed neurologic complaints with overhead use compared with only 6% in the surgical treatment group. Forty-four percent of patients in the nonsurgical treatment group reported being displeased with the cosmetic appearance of their shoulders, one third of which would have preferred surgery to their final nonsurgical treatment result. One caveat to the apparent advantages of surgery is that 30% of patients in the surgical treatment group requested removal of hardware after fracture union. Also, 4% of the patients in the surgical treatment group had adhesive capsulitis requiring surgical intervention.

Lateral clavicle fractures have been classified into three types based on the fracture's relationship to the coracoclavicular ligaments. Type I lateral clavicle fractures occur lateral to the coracoclavicular ligaments, have a very high union rate, and require no special treatment. Type II lateral clavicle fractures occur in the vicinity of the coracoclavicular ligaments and are further subdivided into two types: type IIA fractures, which occur medial to both coracoclavicular ligaments and remain attached to the lateral fragment; and type IIB fractures, in which the conoid ligament is torn but the trapezoid ligament remains attached to the lateral fragment. Type II lateral clavicle fractures have been shown to have a higher rate of nonunion compared with other clavicle fractures because the forces across the fracture site are similar to those seen in grade III AC joint separations. Type III lateral clavicle fractures have intra-articular extension into the AC joint, potentially predisposing a patient to posttraumatic degenerative arthritis. A type IV lateral clavicle fracture is a physeal fracture of the lateral clavicle, which can occur in skeletally immature athletes. Displacement of the lateral clavicle occurs superiorly through a tear in the thick periosteal tube surrounding the distal clavicle. Because the lateral clavicular physis, along with the AC and coracoclavicular ligaments, usually remains intact, these fractures are stable and respond favorably to closed treatment.

Type I, type III, and type IV clavicle fractures heal readily with nonsurgical treatment. Type II injuries, however, may be unstable secondary to the weight of the arm and displacing muscular forces and have a higher incidence of nonunion than other clavicle fractures. A recent retrospective review examined the outcome of 30 patients with type II distal clavicle fractures treated either surgically or nonsurgically. In this nonrandomized study, at an average follow-up of 53.5 months, all 14 patients treated with surgical coracoclavicular stabilization achieved union compared with only 9 of 16 patients (56%) who were treated nonsurgically. Of the seven pa-

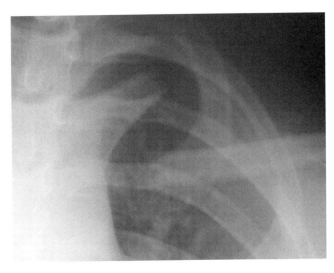

Figure 10 This AP "serendipity" radiograph demonstrates a fracture through the physis of the medial clavicle in a 14-year-old football player who experienced blunt trauma when hit directly by an opposing player's helmet. The patient underwent open reduction and internal fixation with suture fixation and healed uneventfully.

tients who were treated nonsurgically and did not achieve unions, five were asymptomatic and exhibited no difference in functional outcome compared with patients whose fractures united.

Factors implicated in contributing to the risk of clavicle nonunion include initial severity of trauma and the degree of fracture shortening (> 20 mm). These fractures may be better treated with open reduction and internal fixation using plate and screws or an intramedullary device. In a recent Swedish analysis of 245 patients with clavicle fractures, 46% continued to have sequelae, including nonunions, pain during activity, pain at rest, and cosmetic defect. The authors emphasized that treatment and follow-up of clavicle fractures should not be focused exclusively on radiographic evidence of nonunion. Other less common indications for primary surgical management include open fractures, neurovascular or skin compromise, the presence of concomitant displaced scapular neck fractures, and patients with multiple trauma who require upper extremity use for transfers and ambulation.

Scapula Fractures

Fractures of the scapula account for only 3% to 5% of all shoulder girdle injuries. They generally result from high-energy trauma and are likely associated with other osseous and soft-tissue injuries. The most common scapula fractures include ipsilateral rib fractures, clavicle fractures, shoulder dislocations, pulmonary injuries, and brachial plexus injuries.

The majority of scapula fractures are extra-articular, involving the body, spine, glenoid neck, acromion, and/or coracoid. Most scapula fractures can be adequately evaluated using multiple plain radiographs.

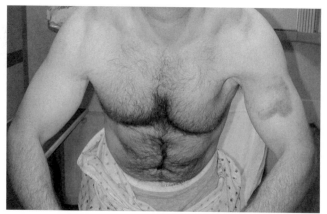

Figure 11 This 32-year-old man experienced an acute injury during a "decline" bench press. With his shoulders slightly flexed, he adducts both shoulders isometrically. The defect in the left anterior axillary crease shows the visible defect of his pectoralis major muscle tear.

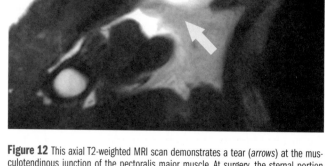

Figure 12 This axial T2-weighted MRI scan demonstrates a tear (*arrows*) at the musculotendinous junction of the pectoralis major muscle. At surgery, the sternal portion of the pectoralis major tendon was torn in an oblique plane approximately 1 cm from the humeral insertion.

Nonsurgical treatment, consisting of immobilization and early range of motion, is preferred for most fractures and results in satisfactory outcomes. Fractures that may require surgical consideration include displaced acromion fractures (with compromise of the subacromial space), markedly displaced coracoid fractures associated with neurovascular compression or coracoclavicular rupture, coracoid tip avulsion, and glenoid neck fractures with either 1 cm of medial translation of the glenoid fossa or more than 40° of angulation.

Approximately 10% of all scapula fractures are intra-articular. Of the six described types of glenoid cavity fractures, the most common is an anterior glenoid avulsion fracture, which usually occurs during anterior glenohumeral dislocation or subluxation. Its counterpart is the posterior lip fracture, which occurs in association with a posterior dislocation. The other varieties of glenoid cavity fractures typically have a transverse or oblique fracture pattern through the glenoid fossa. Radiographic evaluation of these fractures consists of plain radiographs and CT, which allows for assessment of articular incongruity as well as displacement. Arthroscopic examination may also play a role in assessing articular step-off.

Open reduction and internal fixation is indicated for glenoid fossa fractures with more than 5 mm of articular step-off and significant peripheral rim fractures associated with recurrent instability. The largest single-center series of patients treated surgically for displaced intra-articular fractures included 22 patients for whom the surgical approach was determined based on the Ideberg classification; the fractures of 16 patients were approached posteriorly and 6 were approached anteriorly. At an average 10-year follow-up, surgery was successful in 17 (77%). Results were good in the absence of associated complete brachial plexus injury and when postop-

erative complications (deep infection and hardware failure) were avoided.

Muscle and Tendon Injuries

Ruptures of the pectoralis major muscle are uncommon, although the incidence of this injury may be underreported. All documented cases of rupture of the pectoralis major muscle in athletes have occurred in men. A recent meta-analysis of 112 cases of pectoralis major muscle rupture found that the injury occurs most commonly in sports during weight training or wrestling. Most ruptures are complete and involve the sternal head at or near the humeral insertion site. The mechanism of injury usually involves eccentric contraction of the muscle against extreme loads with the arm in a position of abduction, extension, and external rotation.

Diagnosis of the injury may be difficult until initial swelling and ecchymoses resolve. The anterior axillary fold may have an abnormal contour and appear webbed when the arm is in 90° of abduction. Medial retraction of the pectoralis major muscle may create abnormal bulging of the anterior chest wall. Physical examination is the mainstay of diagnosis (Figure 11); however, plain radiographs can help exclude uncommon concomitant bony injury, such as avulsed bone fragments. MRI can aid in earlier detection of the injury when physical examination findings are inconclusive; it may also aid in the identification of partial tears. Several recent studies have confirmed that MRI allows accurate evaluation of injuries to the pectoralis major muscle and aids in determining indications for surgical intervention (Figure 12).

Nonsurgical treatment is appropriate for incomplete tears or the rare muscle belly injury. Surgical treatment is advocated for athletes or active patients who wish to return to their preinjury level of participation in sports. The benefits of surgical intervention include fewer symptoms, improved cosmesis, and restoration of strength. In a recent study of 21 patients (22 pectoralis tendon tears), surgical treatment outcomes of 10 tears were compared with nonsurgical treatment outcomes of 12 tears. In the surgical treatment group, peak torque returned to 99% of the uninjured side, and work performed returned to 97% of the opposite side. In distinction, peak torque and work performed returned to only 56% that of the injured side in the nonsurgical treatment group. Although treatment groups were not randomized, this study suggests that the surgical treatment of pectoralis tendon tears is superior to nonsurgical treatment. In another smaller study, 13 patients were treated surgically and four patients were treated nonsurgically for distal pectoralis major rupture; subjective results were considerably better in the surgical treatment group (96%) than the nonsurgical treatment group (51%). Isokinetic strength testing showed higher adduction strength in the surgical treatment group (102% of the opposite side) than the nonsurgical treatment group (71% of the opposite side).

Previous studies have suggested that repair of chronic pectoralis major muscle tears may not be possible after 6 months. Repair in the acute setting is technically easier because dissection is not complicated by scar tissue and adhesions; therefore, surgical repair should be done within the first 8 weeks. Isolated reports suggest, however, that results may not necessarily be compromised by the late repair of chronic pectoralis major muscle tears. In a recent retrospective study of 17 acute and chronic tears in which the results of early repair were compared with those of late repair (average, 7 months; range, 10 weeks to 14 months), no significant subjective or objective differences in outcome were seen. At odds with this conclusion was a study comparing the outcomes of 32 patients who were treated for acute tears and 8 patients who were treated for chronic tears (average time from injury to repair, 22.6 months). Two chronic tears (25%) and one acute tear (3%) were found to be irreparable. Although all patients were able to resume normal unrestricted activities by 3 months postoperatively, with no significant difference in the range of motion between the two groups reported, there was a significant difference in return to activities. In the acute treatment group, all patients were able to return to their preinjury level of training. Most of the patients who were treated for chronic tears were unable to return to their preinjury level of weight training.

Neurologic Injuries
Brachial Plexus Injuries
Neurologic injuries in athletics are relatively uncommon and easily overlooked. Most of these injuries are associated with contact or collision sports such as football, rugby, hockey, and wrestling. The most common problem is a burner or stinger. This injury is thought to be a transient neurapraxia caused by injury to the brachial plexus or a cervical root as a result of traction, compression, or a direct blow. The athlete typically reports radiating pain, numbness, or tingling down one limb that is usually transient (lasting less than 1 minute). Although weakness of the deltoid or rotator cuff can occur, it may not appear until several hours or days after the injury. Initial diagnosis is based on physical examination. Formal workup is required when neurologic findings are present, symptoms persist, or the patient has a history of previous brachial plexus injury. When necessary, diagnostic testing includes plain radiographs, MRI, and electrodiagnostic testing to ascertain the level and severity of the lesion. Several authors have documented an association between cervical canal and foraminal stenosis and the increased risk of burners caused by extension and compression. Cervical stenosis or degenerative disk disease should be considered in the athlete experiencing recurrent or chronic burners.

Athletes can generally return to participation in athletic activities after resolution of symptoms and restoration of normal strength. Permanent sequelae, such as proximal arm weakness or chronic dysesthetic pain, are rare. Preventive strategies include initiation of a neck strengthening program, use of cervical orthosis, and correcting errors in sport-specific practices (for example, teaching football players proper tackling techniques). Patients with confirmed cervical pathology may require counseling with respect to possible discontinuation of contact and other high risk sports. Because patients with burners have unilateral symptoms exclusive to the upper extremity, any evidence of bilateral upper extremity or lower extremity symptoms warrants evaluation for spinal cord injury.

Axillary Nerve Injuries
The axillary nerve is the most commonly injured peripheral nerve in the athlete participating in contact sports. Axillary nerve injury may result from stretching during glenohumeral dislocation or a direct blow to the anterolateral deltoid. The clinical presentation is variable, ranging from mild sensory loss over the lateral deltoid to overt weakness of shoulder abduction and extension. A careful neurologic examination is required to make the diagnosis, particularly when concomitant soft-tissue or bony trauma is present. Electromyography and nerve conduction velocity studies help confirm the diagnosis, and in the absence of clinical improvement, these studies should be repeated 3 months after injury.

Prognosis after axillary nerve injury appears to be related to the mechanism of injury. Patients with axillary nerve palsy caused by glenohumeral dislocation generally do well with a rehabilitation program emphasizing range of motion and muscle strengthening during neurologic recovery. Surgical exploration is indicated when no sign of nerve recovery occurs within 3 to 6 months. Prognosis for recovery in athletes who injure the axillary nerve as the result of a direct blow, however, is guarded. In one series of 11 contact athletes with direct trauma to the axillary nerve, although none had complete recovery, 10 returned to preinjury levels of activity. Because surgical intervention did not positively influence outcome, it is not indicated in this group of patients. Despite variability in recovery, prognosis for return to function is typically good. Athletes who sustain axillary nerve injury are permitted to return to participation in contact sports as soon as they achieve full active range of motion and when manual muscle strength is good to excellent.

Summary

Acute shoulder injuries continue to receive considerable clinical and basic science attention. Improved understanding of the pathophysiology of instability, combined with advances in arthroscopic techniques, have led to improved outcomes in the treatment of anterior, posterior, and multidirectional instability. The importance of careful patient selection for arthroscopic stabilization continues to receive emphasis. Most injuries to the AC joint continue to be treated nonsurgically, with little evidence-based outcome data to justify surgical intervention. However, recent investigations recommend anatomic reconstruction of the coracoclavicular ligaments rather than using the less anatomic coracoacromial ligament transfer (Weaver and Dunn procedure). Most fractures about the proximal humerus, clavicle, and scapula can be successfully treated without surgery. Tears of the pectoralis major can usually be successfully repaired even when treatment is delayed. Neurologic injuries about the shoulder are relatively uncommon and usually recover spontaneously.

Annotated Bibliography

Anterior Instability

Allegra F, Vincenzo C, Lodispoto F: Abstract: Anatomic lesion differences in first time dislocators compared with multiple dislocators: Prospective study on arthroscopic Bankart repair. *Arthroscopy* 2003;19(suppl 2):28.

At the time of arthroscopy, the authors observed better soft-tissue quality and less joint damage in first-time dislocators compared with patients with multiple recurrent instability episodes. After arthroscopic stabilization, recurrence rates were lower in the primary shoulder dislocation group.

Apreleva M, Hasselman CT, Debski RE, Fu FH, Woo SL, Warner JJ: A dynamic analysis of the glenohumeral motion after simulated capsulolabral injury: A cadaver model. *J Bone Joint Surg Am* 1998;80:474-480.

This cadaveric study evaluated the effects of varying degrees of capsulolabral injury on the kinematics of the gleno-humeral joint in abduction and external rotation. The simulation of a large Bankart lesion or sectioning of the anterior joint capsule did not cause dislocation. Division of the entire joint capsule resulted in a significant increase in posterior translation during abduction.

Bokor DJ, Conboy VB, Olson C: Anterior instability of the glenohumeral joint with humeral avulsion of the glenohumeral ligament: Review of 41 cases. *J Bone Joint Surg Br* 1999;81:93-96.

The authors retrospectively reviewed a consecutive series of 547 shoulders in 529 patients undergoing surgery for anterior instability of the glenohumeral joint. A lateral capsule avulsion from the humeral neck was identified as the cause of instability in 41 patients (7.5%).

Bottoni CR, Wilckens JH, DeBerardino TM, et al: A prospective randomized evaluation of arthroscopic stabilization versus non-operative treatment in patients with acute, traumatic, first-time shoulder dislocations. *Am J Sports Med* 2002;30:576-580.

This article compares nonsurgical treatment with arthroscopic Bankart repair for acute, traumatic shoulder dislocations in young athletes. A 75% recurrence rate was observed in the group managed with immobilization and rehabilitation. Only 11% developed recurrent instability after arthroscopic stabilization with a bioabsorbable tack.

Burkhart SS, DeBeer JF: Traumatic glenohumeral bone defects and their relationship to failure of arthroscopic Bankart repairs: Significance of the inverted pear glenoid and the humeral engaging Hill-Sachs lesion. *Arthroscopy* 2000;16:677-694.

This article identifies specific bone defects (the inverted-pear glenoid and the humeral engaging Hill-Sachs lesion) related to the recurrence of instability after arthroscopic Bankart repair. A 4% recurrence rate was observed in patients without bone defects, whereas a 67% recurrence rate was seen in patients with significant bone defects. The findings support the use of open reconstruction for patients with significant glenoid bone loss, particularly contact athletes.

Burkart SS, Debeer JF, Tehrany AM, Parten PM: Quantifying glenoid bone loss arthroscopically in shoulder instability. *Arthroscopy* 2002;18:488-491.

The authors describe a method for arthroscopically quantifying the percentage of inferior glenoid bone loss using the glenoid bare spot as a central reference point.

Cohen NP, Timothy T, Montgomery KD, Hershman EB, Nisonson B: Abstract: Arthroscopic shoulder stabilization in professional contact athletes. *Arthoscopy* 2002; 18(suppl 2):SS-43.

At minimum 2-year follow-up, arthroscopic Bankart repair yielded a successful outcome in 92% of National Football League football players compared with 50% of National

Hockey League hockey players undergoing arthroscopic shoulder stabilization.

Cole BJ, L'Insalata J, Irrgang J, Warner JJ: Comparison of arthroscopic and open anterior stabilization: A two to six-year follow-up study. *J Bone Joint Surg Am* 2000;82: 1108-1114.

Thirty-nine patients with discrete Bankart lesions underwent arthroscopic stabilization with an absorbable tack device. Twenty-four patients with combined anterior and inferior translation and arthroscopically observed capsular laxity underwent an open capsular shift. No significant differences were found between these two groups in respect to prevalence of failure or other outcome measures. This article emphasizes the importance of refining selection criteria based on findings at the time of surgery.

Dora C, Gerber C: Shoulder function after arthroscopic anterior stabilization of the glenohumeral joint using an absorbable tack. *J Shoulder Elbow Surg* 2000;9:294-298.

The authors report a high rate of residual instability and incomplete functional recovery in shoulders stabilized with a bioabsorbable tack. Based on their results, the authors discontinued the use of bioabsorbable tacks for the treatment of recurrent dislocators.

Ellenbecker TS, Bailie DS, Mattalino AJ, et al: Intrarater and interrater reliability of a manual technique to assess anterior humeral head translation of the glenohumeral joint. *J Shoulder Elbow Surg* 2002;11:470-475.

This clinical evaluation of the manual anterior humeral head translation test revealed poor overall interrater reliability and only fair intrarater reliability.

Faber KJ, Homa K, Hawkins RJ: Translation of the glenohumeral joint in patients with anterior instability: Awake examination versus examination with the patient under anesthesia. *J Shoulder Elbow Surg* 1999;8:320-333.

In 50 patients with traumatic anterior shoulder instability, examination under anesthesia was found to be more effective than awake examination in confirming the direction and degree of instability.

Freehill MQ, Harms DJ, Huber SM, Atlihan D, Buss DD: Poly-L-lactic acid tack synovitis after arthroscopic stabilization of the shoulder. *Am J Sports Med* 2003;31: 643-647.

This study reports on complications after arthroscopic stabilization with a poly-L-lactic acid tack. Nineteen percent of 52 patients developed pain or stiffness at an average 8-month follow-up. Glenohumeral synovitis was present in all patients and was effectively treated with arthroscopic débridement.

Gartsman GM, Roddey TS, Hammerman SM: Arthroscopic treatment of anterior-inferior glenohumeral instability: Two to five-year follow-up. *J Bone Joint Surg Am* 2000;82:991-1003.

The investigators reported persistent instability in only 4 of 53 patients after arthroscopic Bankart repair with suture anchors. The investigators concluded that the success rate was the result of addressing associated pathology, particularly with laser thermal capsulorrhaphy.

Gill TJ, Zarins B: Open repairs for the treatment of anterior shoulder instability. *Am J Sports Med* 2003;31:142-153.

An excellent review of both the current and historical open techniques used for the treatment of anterior shoulder instability. Indications for surgery, surgical technique, and postoperative rehabilitation are thoroughly discussed.

Hatrick C, O'Leary S, Miller B, Goldberg J, Sonnabend D, Walsh W: Abstract: Should acute anterior dislocation of the shoulder be treated in external rotation? 48th Annual Meeting of the Orthopaedic Research Society, Dallas, Texas, February, 2002. Available at: http://www.ors.org/Transactions/48/0830.PDF. Accessed March 29, 2004.

After the creation of a Bankart lesion in a cadaveric shoulder, contact forces between the glenoid labrum and the glenoid were measured with a force sensor. Maximum contact force between the glenoid and labrum was reported to be greatest at 45° of external rotation.

Hattrup SJ, Cofield RH, Weaver AL: Anterior shoulder reconstruction: Prognostic variables. *J Shoulder Elbow Surg* 2001;10:508-513.

In this retrospective review of 253 serial anterior shoulder stabilization procedures, the presence of a workers compensation issue, voluntary instability pattern, shorter periods of immobilization, and patient age were found to have a negative influence of the result of surgery.

Ho E, Cofield RH, Balm MR, Hattrup SJ, Rowland CM: Neurologic complications of surgery for anterior shoulder instability. *J Shoulder Elbow Surg* 1999;8:266-270.

Neurologic deficit was reported in 8.2% of patients after open anterior shoulder stabilization. Neurologic injury did not interfere with the outcome of the stabilization procedure.

Hovelius L, Sandstrom BC, Rosmark DL, Saeboe M, Sundgren KH, Malmqvist BG: Long-term results with the Bankart and Bristow-Laterjet procedures: Recurrent shoulder instability and arthropathy. *J Shoulder Elbow Surg* 2001;10:445-452.

This study documents long-term results after Bristow-Laterjet repair in 30 shoulders. At an average of 15-year follow-up, the authors report a patient satisfaction rate of 98% and a recurrence rate of only 3.4%.

Itoi E, Hatakeyama Y, Kido T, et al: A new method of immobilization after traumatic anterior dislocation of the shoulder: A preliminary study. *J Shoulder Elbow Surg* 2003;12:413-415.

The authors reported a 0% recurrence rate after initial traumatic anterior shoulder dislocation in patients immobilized in a position of external rotation for 3 weeks.

Itoi E, Lee SB, Amrami KK, Wenger DE, An KN: Quantitative assessment of classic anteroinferior bony Bankart lesions by radiography and computed tomography. *Am J Sports Med* 2003;31:112-118.

Using a cadaveric model, the authors demonstrated that CT and the West Point radiographic view provide accurate size estimation of glenoid osseous defects.

Kaar TK, Schenck RC Jr, Wirth MA, Rockwood CA Jr: Complications of metallic suture anchors in shoulder surgery: A report of 8 cases. *Arthroscopy* 2001;17:31-37.

The authors reported complications associated with metallic suture anchors, including extraosseous positioning, migration, and severe articular damage.

Kim SH, Ha KI, Jung MW, Lim MS, Kim YM, Park JH: Accelerated rehabilitation after arthroscopic Bankart repair: A prospective randomized clinical study. *Arthroscopy* 2003;19:722-731.

The investigators documented a quicker resumption of functional range of motion, earlier return to function, and less postoperative pain with an accelerated rehabilitation program after arthroscopic Bankart repair.

Kirkley A, Griffen S, Richards C, Miniaci A, Mohtadi N: Prospective randomized clinical trial comparing the effectiveness of immediate arthroscopic stabilization versus immobilization and rehabilitation in first traumatic dislocations of the shoulder. *Arthroscopy* 1999;15:507-514.

This prospective randomized study evaluated the effectiveness of immobilization and rehabilitation versus arthroscopic transglenoid suture stabilization in young patients with first-time traumatic dislocations. The authors document a significant reduction in redislocation and improvement in disease-specific quality of life with early arthroscopic stabilization.

Kraplinger FS, Gosler K, Wischatta R, Wambacher M, Sperner G: Predicting recurrence after primary anterior traumatic shoulder dislocation. *Am J Sports Med* 2002; 30:116-120.

This retrospective study evaluated factors influencing recurrence rates after primary anterior traumatic shoulder dislocation. Patients between the ages of 21 and 30 years were found to the have the highest risk of recurrence. Statistical analysis revealed no correlation between sports participation and recurrence rates.

Lee SB, Kim KJ, O'Driscoll SW, Morrey BF, An KN: Dynamic glenohumeral stability provided by the rotator cuff muscles in the mid-range and end-range of motion: A study in cadavera. *J Bone Joint Surg Am* 2000;82:849-857.

Using cadaveric testing, the authors of this study concluded that the rotator cuff provides substantial anterior dynamic stability to the glenohumeral joint in both the midrange and end range of motion. Their findings suggest that despite lax capsuloligamentous restraints, dynamic stabilizers may effectively stabilize the glenohumeral joint in the end range of motion.

Levine WN, Arroyo JS, Pollock RG, Flatow EL, Bigliani JU: Open revision stabilization surgery for recurrent anterior glenohumeral instability. *Am J Sports Med* 2000; 28:156-160.

This is a retrospective review of 50 patients who underwent revision anterior stabilization surgery for failed anterior glenohumeral instability procedures. Factors associated with poor results of revision repair included atraumatic cause of failure, voluntary dislocations, and multiple prior stabilization attempts.

Magnusson L, Kartus J, Ejerhed L, Hultenheim I, Sernert N, Karlsson J: Revisiting the open Bankart experience: A four- to nine-year follow-up. *Am J Sports Med* 2002;30:778-782.

This article reports a 17% recurrent instability rate after open Bankart repair with suture anchors at 4- to 9-year follow-up. The authors emphasize the importance of long-term follow-up when assessing stability after surgical reconstruction.

Mazzocca AD, Brown FM, Carreira DS, Hayden J, Romeo AA: Abstract: Arthroscopic stabilization of collision athletes. American Orthopaedic Society for Sports Medicine Web site. Available at: http://www.aossm.org/Downloads/pdf/2002%20AOSSM%2028%20AM%20abstracts.pdf. Accessed March 31, 2004.

The authors identified 14 collision and contact athletes younger than 20 years who underwent arthroscopic stabilization with suture anchors. Ninety-one percent of collision and contact athletes returned to organized sports and did not experience redislocation at latest follow-up.

Metcalf MH, Savoie FH, Smith KL, Matsen FA III: Abstract: Meta-analysis of surgical reconstruction for anterior shoulder instability: A comparison of arthroscopic and open techniques. *Arthroscopy* 2002;18(suppl 2): SS-47.

This meta-analysis found that recurrence rates after arthroscopic suture anchor stabilization were equivalent to those for open Bankart reconstruction. Less loss of external rotation was observed in patients who underwent suture anchor repair.

Miller SL, Cleeman E, Auerbach J: Flatow El: Comparison of intra-articular lidocaine and intravenous sedation for reduction of shoulder dislocations: A randomized, prospective study. *J Bone Joint Surg Am* 2002;84:2135-2139.

The authors evaluated the value of intra-articular lidocaine injection versus intravenous sedation in manipulative reduction of acute anterior shoulder dislocations. Intra-articular lidocaine injection was found to be less expensive and require less time in the emergency department and fewer nursing resources than intravenous sedation.

Mishra DK, Fanton GS: Two-year outcome of arthroscopic Bankart repair and electrothermal-assisted capsulorrhaphy for recurrent traumatic anterior shoulder instability. *Arthroscopy* 2001;17:844-849.

Forty-two patients underwent capsulolabral repair and treatment of associated capsular laxity with electrothermal-assisted capsulorrhaphy. At average follow-up of 28 months, 90% of patients returned to their previous sport. Seven percent experienced a traumatic redislocation.

Oliashirazi A, Mansat P, Cofield RH, Rowland CM: Examination under anesthesia for evaluation of anterior shoulder instability. *Am J Sports Med* 1999;27:464-468.

The authors assessed unilateral posttraumatic recurrent anterior instability using examination under anesthesia. They concluded that examination under anesthesia was a useful adjunct in diagnosing shoulder instability and recommended testing in the anteroinferior direction and varying degrees of external rotation.

Pollack RG, Wang VM, Bucchieri JS, et al: Effects of repetitive subfailure strains on the mechanical behavior of the inferior glenohumeral ligament. *J Shoulder Elbow Surg* 2000;9:427-435.

In this cadaveric study, the IGHL was subjected to repetitive cyclic strains in 33 shoulders. Repetitively applied subfailure strain resulted in increased ligament length that appeared to be largely unrecoverable.

Porcellini G, Campi F, Paladini P: Arthroscopic approach to acute bony Bankart lesion. *Arthroscopy* 2002; 18:764-769.

The authors addressed bony Bankart lesions less than 3 months old and involving less than 25% of the glenoid with an arthroscopic modified Bankart technique. At two-year follow-up, all 25 patients resumed athletic activity, and no recurrence of instability was reported.

Postacchini F, Gumina S, Cinotti G: Anterior shoulder dislocation in adolescents. *J Shoulder Elbow Surg* 2000; 9:470-474.

At a mean of 7.1 years after an initial anterior dislocation, the authors documented an 86% recurrence rate in 28 patients age 12 to 17 years. During the follow-up period, all nonsurgically treated patients showed clinical signs of instability, whereas surgically treated patients experienced no recurrent instability.

Roberts SN, Taylor DE, Brown JN, Hayes MG, Saies A: Open and arthroscopic techniques for the treatment of traumatic anterior shoulder instability in Australian Rules football players. *J Shoulder Elbow Surg* 1999;8: 403-409.

Results of three different stabilization procedures for recurrent instability in Australian Rules football players are reported. The authors suggest that open surgery in Australian Rules football players provides the most secure repair and reduces the risk of recurrence.

Romeo AA, Carreira D: Abstract: Outcome analysis of arthroscopic Bankart repair: Minimum two year follow-up, in *Program and Abstracts of the American Shoulder and Elbow Surgeons 16th Open Meeting*, March 18, 2000, Orlando, FL. Paper #36.

Thirty patients underwent arthroscopic Bankart repair using suture anchors. At a minimum two-year follow-up, the authors reported no recurrent dislocations and 96% good or excellent clinical results.

Stein DA, Jazrawi L, Bartolozzi AR: Arthroscopic stabilization of anterior shoulder instability: A review of the literature. *Arthroscopy* 2002;18:912-924.

This article reviews the technical reasons for improved arthroscopic results and describes technical aspects of suture anchor and bioabsorbable tack stabilization. The authors summarize the results of previous and current reports on arthroscopic management of anterior shoulder instability.

Sugaya H, Moriishi J, Kon DM, Tsuchiya A: Glenoid rim morphology in recurrent anterior glenohumeral instability. *J Bone Joint Surg Am* 2003;85:878-884.

Three-dimensional reconstructed CT with elimination of the humeral head was found to be comparable to arthroscopic assessment in evaluating glenoid morphology.

Tauro JC: Arthroscopic inferior capsular split and advancement for anterior and inferior shoulder instability: Technique and results at 2-5 year follow-up. *Arthroscopy* 2000;16:451-456.

This study reports on a modification of Bankart repair. In conjunction with suture anchor repair, the author successfully used an inferior capsular split and advancement to address inferior capsular laxity.

Uhorchak JM, Arciero RA, Huggard D, Taylor DC: Recurrent shoulder instability after open reconstruction in athletes involved in collision sports. *Am J Sports Med* 2000;28:794-799.

At an average of 47 month follow-up, 23% of 66 collision and contact athletes were found to have recurrent instability following open Bankart/capsulorrhaphy repair.

van der Zwaag HM, Brand R, Obermann WR, Rozing PM: Glenohumeral osteoarthritis after Putti-Platt repair. *J Shoulder Elbow Surg* 1999;8:252-258.

The authors report long-term results of Putti-Platt capsulorrhaphy for recurrent anterior dislocation. Although the re-dislocation rate was 3%, glenohumeral arthrosis was noted in 61% of shoulders.

Posterior Instability

Abrams J: Abstract: Arthroscopic stabilization of recurrent posterior subluxation, in *Program and Abstracts of the American Shoulder and Elbow Surgeons 18th Annual Meeting*, October 24-27, 2001, Napa, CA. Paper #26.

The author addressed recurrent posterior subluxation in 39 patients with arthroscopic suture anchor repair and capsular plication when necessary. Pain and instability were corrected in 92% at minimum 2-year follow-up.

Antoniou J, Harryman DT: Posterior instability. *Orthop Clin North Am* 2001;32:463-473.

In this review of the pathophysiology, evaluation, and treatment of posterior instability, the authors discuss their preferred method of treatment and report on their experience in treating 41 patients with primary posteroinferior instability.

Kim SH, Ha KI, Park JH, et al: Arthroscopic posterior capsular shift for the traumatic recurrent unidirectional posterior subluxation of the shoulder. *J Bone Joint Surg Am* 2003;85:1479-1487.

At an average of 39-month follow-up, arthroscopic posterior capsular shift resulted in stable shoulders in all but one patient. The procedure also reliably relieved pain and restored function.

Mair SD, Zarzour R, Speer KP: Posterior labral injury in contact athletes. *Am J Sports Med* 1998;26:753-758.

Nine athletes were found to have posterior labral detachment at the time of arthroscopy. All athletes returned to at least one full season of sports competition after posterior labral reattachment.

Misamore GW, Facibene WA: Posterior capsulorrhaphy for treatment of traumatic recurrent posterior subluxation of the shoulder in athletes. *J Shoulder Elbow Surg* 2000;9:403-408.

Fourteen athletes with traumatic posterior instability of the shoulder were treated surgically with an open posterior capsulorrhaphy procedure. At a mean 45-month follow-up, 13 of 14 patients returned to unrestricted sports without recurrence of pain or instability.

Richards RR, Harniman E, Beaton DE: Abstract: A long term follow-up of posterior shoulder stabilization for recurrent posterior glenohumeral instability, in *Program and Abstracts of the American Shoulder and Elbow Surgeons 18th Annual Meeting*, October 24-27, 2001, Napa, CA. Paper #28.

The results of posterior capsulorrhaphy combined with lateral advancement of the teres minor and infraspinatus insertions were associated with a good level of function and maintained over time.

Acromioclavicular Joint Dislocation

Basamania CJ, Higgins LD, Witkowski EG: Abstract: Medial instability of the shoulder: A new concept of the pathomechanics of acromioclavicular separations, in *Program and Abstracts of the American Shoulder and Elbow Surgeons 18th Annual Meeting*, October 24-27, 2001, Napa, CA. Paper #49.

The authors assessed medial instability of the scapula using cross-body adduction AP radiographs. A classification was proposed based on the degree of medial subluxation, defined as displacement of the medial edge of the acromion under or medial to the lateral edge of the clavicle. A direct relationship was noted between instability and association of symptoms.

Clarke HD, McDann PD: Acromioclavicular joint injuries. *Orthop Clin North Am* 2000;31:177-186.

This article summarizes the surgical and nonsurgical indications for treating the complete spectrum of AC joint pathology. The most current literature regarding the controversial treatment of grade III injuries is reviewed.

Jones HP, Lemos MJ, Schepsis AA: Salvage of failed acromioclavicular joint reconstruction using autogenous semitendinosus tendon from the knee: Surgical technique and case report. *Am J Sports Med* 2001;29:234-237.

This article describes the surgical technique for the revision of a failed Weaver and Dunn/Gortex augmentation procedure using semitendinosus tendon.

Lee SJ, Nicholas SJ, Akizuki KH, McHugh MP, Kremenic IJ, Ben-Avi S: Reconstruction of the coracoclavicular ligaments using tendon grafts: A comparative biomechanical study. *Am J Sports Med* 2003;31:648-655.

In load to failure testing, tendon graft reconstructions were found to be significantly stronger and stiffer than coracoacromial ligament transfers. The authors concluded that early motion, accelerated rehabilitation, and decreased failure rates can be anticipated after tendon graft reconstruction.

Mouhsine E, Garofalo R, Crevoisier X, Farron A: Grade I and II acromioclavicular dislocations: Results of conservative treatment. *J Shoulder Elbow Surg* 2003;12:599-602.

Only 52% of patients remained asymptomatic at an average of 6.3 years after conservative treatment of grade I and II

AC joint injuries. Radiographic abnormalities were observed in all but 4 of 24 patients.

Perlmutter GS, Deshmukh A, Wilson DR, Zilberfarb J: Abstract: Effect of subacromial decompression on the stability of the acromioclavicular joint: Biomechanical testing in a cadaveric model, in *Program and Abstracts of the American Shoulder and Elbow Surgeons 16th Open Meeting*, March 18, 2000, Orlando, FL. Paper #3.

The authors concluded that Weaver and Dunn reconstruction did not restore the stability provided by the native ligaments in vitro. They recommended using supplemental fixation when performing Weaver and Dunn reconstruction.

Phillips AM, Smart C, Groom AF: Acromioclavicular dislocation: Conservative or surgical therapy. *Clin Orthop* 1998;353:10-17.

This article provides a definitive meta-analysis of the literature regarding the treatment of grade III AC joint separations. Based on this review, the authors conclude that surgery appears to have no value in comparison with nonsurgical treatment. Specific outcomes and complications are discussed, along with analysis of problems associated with proper study design and required power analysis that preclude easy conclusions.

Schlegel TF, Burks RT, Marcus RL, Dunn HK: A prospective evaluation of untreated acute grade III acromioclavicular separation. *Am J Sports Med* 2001;29:699-703.

The objective of this study was to document the natural history of untreated grade III AC joint injuries and provide a baseline by which to judge other proposed methods of treatment. Twenty patients underwent a nonsurgical protocol for treatment of a grade III AC joint injury. At 1-year follow-up, patients reported no limitation of shoulder motion in the injured extremity and no difference between sides in rotational shoulder muscle strength.

Sternoclavicular Joint Injuries
Medvecky MJ, Zuckerman JD: Sternoclavicular joint injuries and disorders. *Instr Course Lect* 2000;49:397-406.

This is a comprehensive review of the anatomy, mechanism of injury, clinical presentation, and evaluation of both anterior and posterior SC joint injuries. The authors provide accepted individual treatment strategies based on the current literature. Medial clavicular physeal injuries are also discussed.

Spencer EE Jr, Kuhn JE: Biomechanical analysis of reconstructions for sternoclavicular joint instability. *J Bone Joint Surg Am* 2004;86:98-105.

The authors compared methods of reconstruction in 36 cadavers with simulated sternoclavicular joint instability. A figure-of-8 semitendinosus technique was found to have superior biomechanical properties.

Spencer EE, Kuhn JE, Huston LJ, Carpenter JE, Hughes RE: Ligamentous restraints to anterior and posterior translation of the sternoclavicular joint. *J Shoulder Elbow Surg* 2002;11:43-47.

The authors of this cadaveric study determined that the posterior capsule of the sternoclavicular joint is the most important restraint to anterior and posterior translation.

Fractures
Naranja RJ Jr, Iannotti JP: Displaced three- and four-part proximal humerus fractures: Evaluation and management. *J Am Acad Orthop Surg* 2000;8:373-382.

This article presents an overview of the classification, evaluation, treatment principles, and specific surgical approach for three- and four-part proximal humerus fractures.

Nowak J, Holgersson M, Larsson S: Abstract: Can we predict sequelae following fractures of the clavicle based on initial findings? A prospective study with 9-10 years follow-up, in *Program and Abstracts of the American Shoulder and Elbow Surgeons 18th Open Meeting*, February 16, 2002, Dallax, TX. Paper #1

Two-hundred eight patients with clavicle fractures were evaluated at 9- to 10-year follow-up. Forty-six percent continued to have sequelae, including nonunion, pain during activity, pain during rest, and cosmetic defect.

Rokito AS, Zuckerman JD, Shaari JM, Eisenberg DP, Cuomo F, Gallagher MA: A comparison of nonoperative and operative treatment of type II distal clavicle fractures. *Bull Hosp Jt Dis* 2002-2003;61:32-39.

In this nonrandomized study, at an average follow-up of 53.5 months, all patients treated with coracoclavicular stabilization achieved union compared with only 56% of patients who were treated nonsurgically.

Schandelmaier P, Blauth M, Schneider C, Krettek C: Fractures of the glenoid treated by operation: A 5- to 23-year follow-up of 22 cases. *J Bone Joint Surg Br* 2002; 84:173-177.

The authors reported 10-year results after open reduction and internal fixation of 22 consecutive displaced fractures of the glenoid. Surgery was successful in 77% of patients, and the best results were obtained when infection and brachial plexus palsy were avoided.

Smith CA, Rudd J, Crosby LA: Abstract: Results of operative versus non-operative treatment for 100% displaced mid-shaft clavicle fractures: A prospective randomized clinical trial, in *Program and Abstracts of the American Shoulder and Elbow Surgeons 16th Open Meeting*, March 18, 2000, Orlando, FL. Paper #31.

The authors randomly compared surgical versus nonsurgical treatment of 100% displaced midshaft clavicle fractures and reported no nonunions, decreased neurologic symptoms, and no failures of hardware in the surgical group; however, 30 patients requested hardware removal.

Muscle and Tendon Injuries

Bak K, Cameron EA, Henderson IJ: Rupture of the pectoralis major: A meta-analysis of 112 cases. *Knee Surg Sports Traumatol Arthrosc* 2000;8:113-119.

The authors of this meta-analysis found that pectoralis major rupture occurs most commonly during weight training or wrestling. Most reported ruptures were complete and located at the insertion to the humerus.

Basamania CJ: Abstract: Pectoralis major ruptures: A comparison of repair of acute and chronic injuries, in *Program and Abstracts of the American Shoulder and Elbow Surgeons 15th Open Meeting*, February 7, 1999, Anaheim, CA. Paper #8.

Patients undergoing acute and chronic repair of pectoralis major ruptures all returned to normal unrestricted activity by 3 months; however, patients treated for chronic tears were unable to return to their preinjury level of weight training.

Connell DA, Potter HG, Sherman MF, Wickiewicz TL: Injuries of the pectoralis major muscle: Evaluation with MR imaging. *Radiology* 1999;210:785-791.

In this study of 15 pectoralis major injuries, the authors concluded that MRI enables the identification of partial versus complete tears and acute versus chronic tears.

Hanna CM, Glenny AB, Stanley SN, Caughey MA: Pectoralis major tears: Comparison of surgical and conservative treatment. *Br J Sports Med* 2001;35:202-206.

In this study of 22 complete distal pectoralis major muscle ruptures, the authors found that surgical repair resulted in a greater recovery of peak torque and work preformed than conservative management. Surgical repair also resulted in better subjective functional outcomes.

Schepsis AA, Grafe MW, Jones HP, Lemos MJ: Rupture of the pectoralis major muscle: Outcome after repair of acute and chronic injuries. *Am J Sports Med* 2000;28:9-15.

This study reviews the subjective and objective outcomes of 17 cases of distal pectoralis major tendon ruptures, comparing the results of primary repair in the acute setting with delayed repair in the chronic setting. No difference in outcome was seen, although surgical intervention was reported to be superior to nonsurgical treatment. The literature is comprehensively reviewed.

Neurologic Injuries

Koffler KM, Kelly JD: Neurovascular trauma in athletes. *Orthop Clin North Am* 2002;33:523-534.

This is a thorough review of the diagnosis and management of neurovascular injuries in athletes. Although particular focus is given to brachial plexus injuries, axillary nerve injuries and other less common injuries are also discussed.

Perlmutter GS: Axillary nerve injury. *Clin Orthop* 1999;368:28-36.

This is a review of the epidemiology, presentation, and evaluation of axillary nerve injuries. The author also discusses alternative treatment strategies and results.

Classic Bibliography

Bannister GC, Wallace WA, Stableforth PG, Hutson MA: The management of acute acromioclavicular dislocation: A randomised prospective controlled trial. *J Bone Joint Surg Br* 1989;71:848-850.

Bergfeld JA, Andrish JT, Clancy WG: Evaluation of the acromioclavicular joint following first- and second-degree sprains. *Am J Sports Med* 1978;6:153-159.

Bigliani LU, Pollock RG, McIlveen SJ, Endrizzi DP, Flatow EL: Shift of the posteroinferior aspect of the capsule for recurrent posterior glenohumeral instability. *J Bone Joint Surg Am* 1995;77:1011-1020.

de Jong KP, Sukul DM: Anterior sternoclavicular dislocation: A long-term follow-up study. *J Orthop Trauma* 1990;4:420-423.

Deutsch A, Altchek DW, Veltri DM, Potter HG, Warren RF: Traumatic tears of the subscapularis tendon: Clinical diagnosis, magnetic resonance imaging findings, and operative treatment. *Am J Sports Med* 1997;25:13-22.

Galpin RD, Hawkins RJ, Grainger RW: A comparative analysis of operative versus nonoperative treatment of grade III acromioclavicular separations. *Clin Orthop* 1985;193:150-155.

Hershman EB, Wilburn AJ, Bergfeld JA: Acute brachial neuropathy in athletes. *Am J Sports Med* 1989;17:655-659.

Larsen E, Bjerg-Nielsen A, Christensen P: Conservative or surgical treatment of acromioclavicular dislocation: A prospective, controlled, randomized study. *J Bone Joint Surg Am* 1986;68:552-555.

Lazarus MD, Sidles JA, Harryman DT II, Matsen FA III: Effect of a chondral-labral defect on glenoid concavity and glenohumeral stability: A cadaveric model. *J Bone Joint Surg Am* 1996;78:94-102.

Miller MD, Johnson DL, Fu FH, et al: Rupture of the pectoralis major muscle in a collegiate football player: Use of magnetic resonance imaging in early diagnosis. *Am J Sports Med* 1993;21:475-477.

O'Brien SJ, Neves MC, Arnoczkmy SP, et al: The anatomy and histology of the inferior glenohumeral ligament complex of the shoulder. *Am J Sports Med* 1990; 18:449-456.

Perlmutter GS, Apruzzese W: Axillary nerve injuries in contact sports: Recommendations for treatment and rehabilitation. *Sports Med* 1998;26:351-361.

Press J: Zuckerman JD, Gallagher M, Cuomo F: Treatment of grade III acromioclavicular separations: Operative versus nonoperative management. *Bull Hosp Joint Dis* 1997;56:77-83.

Rockwood CJ, Williams G, Young D: Disorders of the acromioclavicular joint, in Rockwood CJ, Matsen F (eds): *The Shoulder*. Philadelphia, PA, WB Saunders, 1998, pp 483-553.

Weinstein DM, McCann PD, McIlveen SJ, Flatow EL, Bigliani LU: Surgical treatment of complete acromioclavicular dislocations. *Am J Sports Med* 1995;23:324-331.

Wolfe SW, Wickiewicz TL, Cavanaugh JT: Ruptures of the pectoralis major muscle: An anatomic and clinical analysis. *Am J Sports Med* 1992;20:587-593.

Chapter 6

Chronic Shoulder Injuries

W. Ben Kibler, MD

David C. Dome, MD

Introduction

Many concepts regarding rotator cuff injury, labral tears, and impingement are evolving because several studies have been completed that shed light on the normal function, pathoetiology, and clinical presentation of chronic shoulder injuries. This chapter focuses on presenting new principles to guide the evolving understanding and proper evaluation and treatment of these conditions.

Rotator Cuff Function Relating To Normal Shoulder Biomechanics

The rotator cuff, either as a whole or in part, plays a secondary role in initiating and controlling active rotation of the humerus in the glenoid of the arm. The total cross-sectional area of the rotator cuff muscles is not large enough to create the measured forces or speeds required in throwing, and the tendons are at a biomechanical disadvantage for initiating rotation because of their close insertion to the axis of rotation and the resulting shorter lever arms. The rotator cuff muscles provide only 18% of the total force to move the arm forward. The individual portions of the rotator cuff may exhibit high levels of muscle activation during rotation, but these levels are most commonly associated with high activation levels in the deltoid and parascapular muscles.

The rotator cuff must create efficient rotation via its most important biomechanical function as a compressor cuff. The points of insertion and the lines of muscle pull create a biomechanical disadvantage for rotation and a mechanical advantage for compression (Figure 1). When the glenohumeral angle is between –30° and 30°, the muscles can act efficiently by pulling in a relatively straight line, thereby pulling the humerus into the glenoid socket and increasing the concavity and compression of the shoulder joint. This allows the large primary motors (the deltoid, latissimus dorsi, and pectoralis major) to rotate and elevate the arm around a stable base, with minimal joint shearing or translation. This effect is more pronounced at lower angles of arm elevation and helps the muscles to initiate elevation.

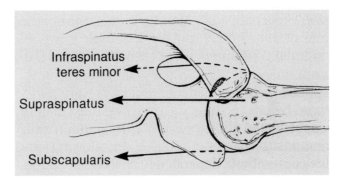

Figure 1 The line of optimum pull of the rotator cuff muscle works to compress the humeral ball into the glenoid socket. *(Reproduced with permission from Kelley MJ, Clark WA: Orthopaedic Therapy of the Shoulder. Philadelphia, PA, Lippincott Williams & Wilkins, 1994, p 85.)*

Recent electromyographic studies on the timing of rotator cuff muscle activation confirm these biomechanical principles. They show that efficient rotator cuff activation is preceded by parascapular muscle (upper and lower trapezius and serratus anterior) and deltoid activation. Conversely, alterations in the timing and intensity of rotator cuff activation have been demonstrated in patients with shoulder injuries.

The compressor cuff function is the primary source of dynamic glenohumeral joint stability in the midranges of joint motion because all of the passive capsular constraints and ligaments should be physiologically lax in this range. Their coordinated action keeps the humeral head centered in the glenoid, allowing true ball-and-socket kinematics. These muscles work in co-contraction force couples, using reciprocal inhibition muscle patterns to balance the intensity of activation.

The rotator cuff also has a variable effect as a humeral head depressor. This effect is thought to be integrated with but occasionally separate from the compressor function. The depressor effect is more effective at arm elevation angles greater than 90°. The subscapularis and infraspinatus/teres minor act as a force couple to depress the humeral head in the glenoid socket and decrease humeral head impingement.

Clinical Application

Rotator cuff function is best restored in rehabilitation by integration of rotator cuff activation with other muscles that control shoulder rotation, emphasizing exercises that use cocontraction/stabilization force couples and emphasizing humeral head depression. Conditioning of rotator cuff function for maximum performance must also include exercises that use co-contraction force couples and are coordinated with exercises that develop maximum strength of the surrounding musculature.

Etiologic Factors for Rotator Cuff Tendinopathy

Terminology

Most recent studies have established that rotator cuff "tendinitis" is not the correct term to clinically or pathologically describe the histologic changes observed via imaging or biopsy in patients with rotator cuff symptoms. There are no inflammatory findings (for example, edema or invasion by macrophages). "Tendinosis" is the correct pathologic term because ample evidence of the degenerative nature of the changes is provided using imaging or biopsy. However, this term does not suggest how the degenerative changes are initiated. From a clinical point of view, the term "tendinopathy" is the best general descriptor of the clinical presentation of tendon injuries. It encompasses the combination of tendon injury, pain, swelling, and impaired performance, without creating a bias for certain types of treatment ("itis"), and it signals a need for a comprehensive evaluation of the intrinsic and extrinsic etiologic factors that create the tendinosis.

Intrinsic Factors

There is little evidence for a "smoking gun" (that is, one specific etiologic factor) that is responsible for rotator cuff injury and tears. It appears that a variable mixture of intrinsic and extrinsic factors create the lesion.

Intrinsic factors can include inferior tissue mechanical properties, poor microvascular blood supply, aging tissues, and internal overload. The presence and relative effect of each is controversial. There is evidence that the hypovascular zone in the distal end of the tendon is actually hypervascular in patients with impingement. Although younger tissues have a better healing capability, there appear to be no studies that specifically correlate age with increased tearing at a specific strain. Aging probably decreases the quality of the tendon internal structures, making them more susceptible to the internal effects of tissue overload or the external effects of compression or shear.

Tension overload has been studied extensively as a causative factor. Several studies have demonstrated high levels of tension in the critical zone, as well as a possible differential strain pattern, with more strain being developed on the articular surface in shoulders that are put through arcs of abduction motion. It also appears that there is less tolerance for excessive strain on the articular surface of the tendon. These strain patterns may cause injury by direct mechanical disruption of the cells, but they may also exert an effect by influencing the control of apoptosis (programmed cell death).

Apoptosis

Apoptosis is a physiologic process that is essential to maintain the constancy of tissue mass. However, abnormal regulation of apoptosis has been implicated in the onset and progression of many disease processes. Apoptotic cells die from the inside—they shrink, condense their nuclear material, lose their intercellular contacts, and are phagocytosed by their cellular neighbors. Apoptosis is a process of degenerative change, the complete results of which become fully expressed over time. Because the cell membranes are not disrupted, no intracellular contents are released, with minimal resulting reactive inflammation. During the apoptotic degenerative process, the production of normal extracellular matrix is altered, making it weaker and disorganized. Apoptosis can be initiated by a wide variety of stimuli, including cyclic strain. Cyclic strain at a high level of intensity and duration triggers stress-activated protein kinases, which influence the regulation of apoptosis. Studies of ruptured supraspinatus tendons have demonstrated the presence of twice as many apoptotic cells compared with the normal subscapularis tendon from the same patient.

The implication of apoptosis as an etiologic factor may help unify some of the diverse findings in rotator cuff or other tendinopathies. It does explain the lack of an inflammatory response and the findings of tendinosis. It also provides a clue regarding the role of tension overload in tendinopathy. The load may be an absolute overload (normal tissues, supraphysiologic load) or a relative overload (normal load, weakened tissues). In either instance, the strain or load seen by the tendon, cell, and/or the intracellular contents may trigger the release of stress-activated protein kinases and start the pathologic sequence.

Extrinsic Factors

Extrinsic factors usually are the result of subacromial impingement lesions. No known studies have demonstrated that external compression is the primary factor in producing rotator cuff tendinopathy. Many factors such as acromioclavicular joint arthritis, acromial morphology, intra-articular injury, scapular dyskinesis, and muscle weakness and/or imbalance can alter the geometry of the subacromial space and create the external compression. In a rat model of the creation of rotator cuff disease, extrinsic compression did not cause injury until overuse activity was added.

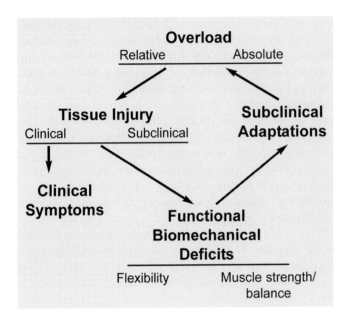

Figure 2 The negative feedback vicious cycle represents the process of alteration in mechanics and physiology that may precede the actual anatomic injury.

TABLE 1 | Classification of Causative Factors in Impingement
Primary
Subacromial
Bone spurs
Hypertrophic synovitis
Secondary
Intra-articular
Anterior instability
Superior labral tears
Biceps injury
Extra-articular
Nonsubacromial
Muscle weakness/imbalance
Muscle inflexibility
Scapular dyskinesis

Negative Feedback Vicious Cycle

The process of extrinsic and intrinsic tendon damage is thought to produce a compromised tendon, either by altering the intracellular or the mechanical environment. These relative or absolute loads create physiologic and biomechanical alterations. Continued use may increase the strains to the point at which apoptosis and tendinosis are created. This process can be described as a negative feedback vicious cycle (Figure 2), with the eventual production of an anatomic alteration (a complete or a partial tendon tear or tendinopathy with impaired performance). Much more research needs to be done regarding the role of each of these factors.

Clinical Implications

The clinical presentation of rotator cuff tendinopathy should trigger an examination of possible extrinsic factors (acromioclavicular joint injury, acromial spurs, intra-articular injury, and scapular dyskinesis) and intrinsic factors (rotator cuff strength and/or imbalance, muscle inflexibility, and activities of overload or overuse). In addition to eliminating the extrinsic factors, treatment should modify the intrinsic factors (via cocontraction and eccentric muscle strengthening and modification of load and use).

External Impingement in Throwing Athletes

The shoulder dysfunction that is characterized by symptoms of impingement has been subclassified into two or three categories. External impingement denotes the classic impingement of the rotator cuff under the acromial arch that was first described by Neer. External impingement in throwing athletes appears to have a generally different pathoetiology than in the more common scenario described in older patients by Neer. The major causative factor advocated by Neer was alteration in the subacromial space, usually from encroachment by bone spurs. These alterations were assumed to be the primary causative factors producing pathology and symptoms.

In throwing athletes, the presenting symptom complex may be similar, but impingement is more frequently a secondary phenomenon. Throwers and other overhead athletes are generally younger than patients with primary impingement. Throwing athletes exhibit fewer radiographic findings associated with classic impingement (ie, fewer bone spurs and a lower incidence of type III acromions). Conversely, throwing athletes have a higher incidence of clinically significant intra-articular problems such as labral lesions and instabilities.

The causes of secondary external impingement may be subclassified as intra-articular or nonsubacromial extra-articular (Table 1). Intra-articular causes include anterior instability (the instability/impingement complex described by Jobe), superior labral tears, or biceps injury. All of these causes decrease the concavity/compression effect of the humerus on the glenoid and allow superior humeral translation with impingement.

Nonsubacromial extra-articular causes primarily involve muscle weakness and/or inflexibility. Muscle weakness may involve the parascapular or the rotator cuff muscles. Alterations in scapular stabilizer activation sequencing (the lower trapezius being activated later than in control subjects), fatigue and decreased muscle activation in protraction in serratus anterior, and decreased lower trapezius muscle strength have been found in young patients with external impingement.

These same muscle alterations along with tightness of the pectoralis minor muscle have been associated with alteration in scapular kinematics (decreased posterior tilt and external rotation, leading to lack of acromial elevation) in patients with impingement.

Clinical Implications

The variety of underlying causes that produce the symptoms and signs of external impingement demonstrates that this is a syndrome. Rigorous evaluation of the various intra-articular, subacromial, and nonsubacromial extra-articular causes should be undertaken in the history, physical examination, and diagnostic imaging. It is not uncommon to find multiple alterations (labral injury and scapular dyskinesis or rotator cuff weakness and glenohumeral instability) associated with external impingement symptoms. A complete and accurate diagnosis of all alterations is required to initiate effective treatment.

Internal Impingement in Throwing Athletes

The term "internal impingement" was first used to describe the posterior-based symptoms and anatomic lesions that occur in throwing athletes. The anatomic injuries most commonly found in patients with internal impingement were superior glenoid labral tears and articular-sided partial-thickness rotator cuff tears. As originally described, the lesions found at surgery were caused by primary impingement of the undersurface of the posterior supraspinatus against the superior glenoid as the arm was brought into horizontal abduction and external rotation in throwing. However, several studies now document that this impingement position is achieved in normal external rotation. Therefore, just as in external impingement in throwers, internal impingement is now being regarded as a secondary phenomenon, producing symptoms as a result of altered mechanics in the scapuloglenohumeral articulation.

One proposed causative mechanism of the altered mechanics is acquired anterior microinstability caused by stretching of the anterior capsule. This capsular stretch would allow the glenohumeral articulation to move into a hyperangulation position of increased external rotation and horizontal abduction and thereby create the rotator cuff and labral lesions associated with mechanical wear. There have been no biomechanical studies to date that show that this mechanism works as proposed.

A second proposed causative mechanism of the altered mechanics is acquired glenohumeral internal rotation deficit (GIRD). This deficit is created by progressive contracture of the posterior glenohumeral capsule and decreased static and dynamic flexibility of the posterior shoulder muscles. This tight capsule has been demonstrated on biomechanical testing to create a supe-

rior shift in the glenohumeral contact point (posterosuperiorly in cocking and anterosuperiorly in follow-through) so that the instant center of rotation of the humerus is not centered in the glenoid and true ball-and-socket kinematics do not occur in the midranges of shoulder rotation. This initiates a pathologic cascade that climaxes in the cocking phase of throwing. As the shoulder horizontally abducts and excessively externally rotates around the new contact point, shear forces at the biceps anchor and posterosuperior labrum increase through an excessive peel-back action of the biceps on the labrum, producing a posterior glenoid labral lesion. Additionally, the anterior capsule becomes apparently lax as a result of the altered posterosuperior contact point and loss of tension in the capsule, and there are increased shear and torsional forces on the rotator cuff as the other joint constraints fail. These forces create a hypertwist load mechanism on the rotator cuff, increasing the load on the vulnerable articular side of the cuff. The anterior capsule may also eventually fail in tension, thereby creating a true stretch. All of these consequences are worsened by scapular dyskinesis, producing an excessive protraction that creates an antetilted glenoid (more posterior contact), increases anterior capsular tensile loads, and magnifies the peel-back effect.

Clinical Implications

Labral lesions and partial rotator cuff tears represent pathoanatomy (anatomic alteration). In most patients, these injuries are the result of a process of injury that started with altered mechanics (pathomechanics) and altered muscle strength, balance, and/or inflexibility (pathophysiology). These factors must be taken into account when evaluating and treating these athletes.

Superior Glenoid Labral Tears

Superior glenoid labral tears have been described as superior labrum anterior and posterior (SLAP) tears, identifying the superior labrum as the affected structure and the tear location as being anterior and posterior to the biceps root. They may be seen as isolated injuries but are most frequently seen in association with other problems, such as partial-thickness or full-thickness rotator cuff tears, microtrauma or macrotrauma instability, and external impingement. Proposed mechanisms of injury all involve the biceps—repetitive overhead arm motions with tensile or more likely peel-back forces applied to the labrum, a fall or sudden load on the outstretched arm and tensed biceps, or occasionally a fall and a direct blow on the lateral aspect of the humerus.

SLAP injuries are most commonly associated with articular-sided rotator cuff injuries. This is not surprising given the way these two structures interact to maintain static and dynamic stability (ball-and-socket kinematics) of the glenohumeral joint. This association is also demonstrated by the fact that the rotator cuff injuries may be lesion specific. Anterior rotator cuff lesions are frequently associated with predominantly anterior SLAP lesions (giving rise to the acronym SLAC, which stands for superior labrum anterior cuff), and the posterior cuff injuries may be associated with predominantly posterior labral lesions.

The clinical presentation of superior glenoid labral tears may be subtle and difficult to appreciate. In many cases, there may be a lag between the time of acute trauma and the onset of symptoms. When the injury is the result of repetitive throwing, there may be no specific trauma—only a gradual increase in symptoms. The symptoms may be similar to those for rotator cuff tendinopathy (pain, painful arc, weakness, and easy fatigue), or they may be related to decreased performance. Internal derangement symptoms (popping, clicking, sliding, and dead arm) may also be present. Careful attention to the history can frequently alert the examiner to include labral tear as part of the differential diagnosis.

Clinical Examination for Patients With Rotator Cuff Tendinopathy, Impingement, and Labral Injury

The clinical examination should be viewed as making a significant contribution to the total understanding of the shoulder problem, along with the history, imaging, and findings at surgery. Clinical examination is one of the keys to understanding the anatomic alterations that underlie the presentation of shoulder dysfunction. However, because of the interaction of the bony alignment, ligamentous and labral functions, individual and coupled muscle activations, and kinetic chain input, multiple sources of possible alteration exist. Also, frequently there may be multiple anatomic alterations present that result in symptoms. Therefore, the examiner must approach the shoulder examination from a broad-based "victims and culprits" approach, realizing that the source of symptoms (impingement and labral tear) may not always be the sole source of the problem (GIRD, altered mechanics, and rotator cuff weakness). Also, the examiner must have a variety of clinical tests to use when assessing the shoulder. Currently, none of the clinical tests for labral injury have been shown to be reliable and accurate enough to be diagnostic in themselves. Clinical examination is a skill, similar to arthroscopic labral repair, and just as with surgical skills, it will improve with practice. As the examination becomes more reproducible, its effectiveness will increase. Comprehensive reviews of all of the published clinical tests for the shoulder exist and can be a major aid in improving the depth of testing and the information yield of the clinical examination.

The anatomic alterations in the shoulder have been the primary focus of the clinical examination in the past.

The clinical examination should evaluate the physiologic and biomechanical alterations as well. A good screening examination for these types of alterations includes hip rotation and flexion/extension flexibility, hip/trunk stability on a planted leg, lumbar flexibility, assessment of scapular control, and scapular stabilized assessment of glenohumeral rotation.

Nonsurgical Treatment

Most of the physiologic and biomechanical alterations that are associated with the anatomic alterations in patients with shoulder injuries are best addressed by nonsurgical means. These include GIRD, pectoralis minor and hip-related inflexibility, scapular stabilizer and rotator cuff weakness and imbalance, and poor stroke or throwing mechanics. They are present from 49% to 94% of the time.

Restoration of muscle strength, balance, flexibility, and proper kinetic chain function may improve the dynamic stability of the shoulder joint to allow asymptomatic function. Even if this goal is not achievable, restoration of kinetic chain function and scapular stabilization provides a biomechanical and physiologic base for postoperative rehabilitation.

Nonsurgical treatment should be based on the complete and accurate diagnosis of all of the alterations found on history and physical examination. The goals of the program should include proximal segment control (core stability), scapular stabilization, shoulder muscle flexibility, rotator cuff balance, and power production. Rehabilitation should be considered as a flow of activity rather than as a specific time-based protocol. The pace and direction of the flow should be individualized and is based on achievement of each successive goal.

If patients fail to progress at a reasonable pace through the flow of rehabilitation, if their levels of function remain poor after achieving kinetic chain and scapular control, or if their anatomic alterations preclude any significant participation in rehabilitation, surgical treatment should be instituted.

Surgical Treatment

The principles underlying the surgical repair of superior labral lesions are becoming more unified. Arthroscopic treatment is capable of addressing all of these lesions. Most treatment protocols recommend using suture anchors and suture tying over tack stabilization. The major issue in the surgical repair of labral lesions involves proper identification of the lesion and criteria for determining satisfactory stabilization of the lesion. Identification of the lesion solely by arthroscopic visualization can be difficult because of the variable anatomy of the superior labrum. Identification of anatomically or functionally significant lesions can be enhanced by a good preoperative history; a clinical examination with positive results on labral tests, such as the anterior slide, O'Brien's active compression, biceps stress, and Mayo shear tests; imaging using either CT or MRI with contrast; arthroscopic demonstration of anatomic fraying, tears, or separation of the labrum from the glenoid with glenoid roughness or yellowish degenerative tissue; and a positive peel-back of the labrum and biceps root with humeral abduction/external rotation. Treatment goals should include débridement of frayed or torn tissue, glenoid rim abrasion, and sufficient fixation points to securely reattach the labrum to the prepared glenoid rim and eliminate the biceps peel-back. Elimination of the peel-back is thought to be most important in restoring the function of the biceps/labral complex.

Arthroscopic labral repair should be combined with arthroscopic or open repair of all of the associated intra-articular or extra-articular injuries that are identified by the examination, imaging, or arthroscopy.

Indications and principles for external impingement surgery are also becoming clearer, and the key point is establishing the exact causative factors before undertaking surgery. Many instances of nonsubacromial extra-articular external impingement are secondary to physiologic and biomechanical causes and are largely treated by nonsurgical rehabilitation. The impingement symptoms created by secondary intra-articular causes are treated by surgical correction of those lesions with subacromial treatment only if lesions are demonstrated at arthroscopy. Impingement that are the result of primary subacromial causes may be treated with surgical acromioplasty if nonsurgical treatment is not successful. Arthroscopic treatment in this select group of athletes appears to yield reliable results, with relief of symptoms and decreased morbidity being reported when the results of arthroscopic treatment are compared with those of open procedures. Treatment goals for surgical acromioplasty include proper visualization of the entire subacromial space, removal of bursal and other soft tissue, determining the anatomic integrity of the rotator cuff, adequate removal of anterior and lateral acromial bone to create a type I acromion, coplaning the distal clavicle, and complete elimination of the compression by viewing dynamic arm motion.

Indications and principles for surgical treatment of partial and complete rotator cuff tears continue to evolve. This is mainly because of the lack of precise knowledge of the pathoetiology and natural history of rotator cuff injuries. There are imprecise indications for surgery even in the face of documented rotator cuff tears. It is a well-established fact that a relatively high percentage of rotator cuff tears are functionally asymptomatic. Even in the presence of symptoms, prospective studies have shown that pain relief and increased range of motion can be achieved in up to 50% of patients with nonsurgical treatment. Strength is not significantly changed, however, and improvement in total functional capability is variable. Poor prognostic factors for pain relief or predictable functional improvement include pain interrupting sleep, tears greater than 1 cm, symptoms present for more than 1 year, and severe weakness of abduction or external rotation on initial examination.

At this time, both arthroscopic and mini-open surgical techniques have been demonstrated to be effective in relieving symptoms of pain, improving strength, and increasing function in terms of functional outcome measures in all types of tears from partial-thickness to moderate-sized complete tears. There continues to be much debate and a lack of consensus on many other aspects of rotator cuff surgery, including whether to take down a partial rotator cuff tear entirely or repair it through the cuff; the role of anterior and posterior releases in mobilizing for repair; optimum suture configuration—simple, mattress, or Mason-Allen type; and fixation geometry—single-row or double-row anchors, bone tunnels, or a combination of both.

The literature does suggest several techniques that can help in surgical decision making and surgical treatment. Complete probing and evaluation from intra-articular and bursal sides will help determine the size, depth, and location of partial-thickness tears. Most recommendations continue to emphasize that symptomatic partial tears that involve more than 50% of the width of the tendon should be treated with repair techniques. Evaluation of the width of the rotator cuff footprint can give an estimation of the degree of articular-sided partial tearing. More than 6 mm of footprint exposure suggests a 50% full-thickness loss. Reconstitution of the total footprint contact area is thought to be optimal. In partial-thickness tears, this appears to be best accomplished by complete tear takedown and suture anchor repair.

There is a small subset of articular-sided partial rotator cuff tears in which the injury is in the substance of the tendon with a flap configuration and an intact footprint. These can be repaired by arthroscopic through-and-through suture repairs, with the passing instruments (usually spinal needles) being introduced from the subacromial space through the tear and the stitches being passed from an anterior intra-articular portal through the needles and tied in the subacromial space. Bursal-sided partial tears have less healing capability and require treatment similar to that for complete tears for relief of symptoms. These tears are more frequently associated with subacromial impingement.

Efficacious surgical treatment of complete rotator cuff tears is based on the following three principles: tear pattern recognition, secure fixation, and restoration of the footprint. Proper tear pattern recognition is crucial. Many repairs fail because of lack of proper tear pattern recognition, resulting in increased tension and poor restoration of anatomy when nonanatomic repair is attempted.

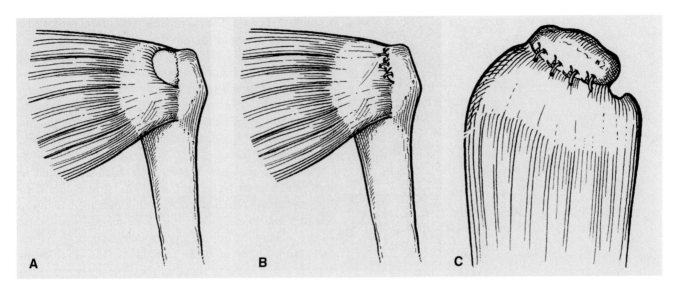

Figure 3 **A** through **C,** Crescent-shaped tears have their greatest extent transverse to the tendon and may be reattached by mobilization and repair in a transverse fashion. *(Reproduced with permission from Burkhart SS: A stepwise approach to arthroscopic rotator cuff repair based on biomechanical principles. Arthroscopy 2000;16:82-90.)*

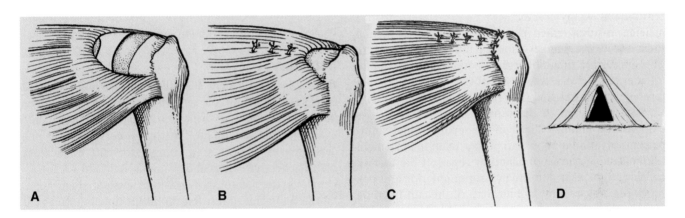

Figure 4 Suture repair. **A** through **D,** U-shaped tears have their greatest extent longitudinal to the tendon and may be reattached by margin convergence and then transverse repair. *(Reproduced with permission from Burkhart SS: A stepwise approach to arthroscopic rotator cuff repair based on biomechanical principles. Arthroscopy 2000;16:82-90.)*

Complete tear patterns can be broadly divided into two types: crescent-shaped or U-shaped (with several variations). Crescent-shaped tears do not usually retract far from the greater tuberosity and can usually be directly repaired back to the greater tuberosity (Figure 3). Their greatest extent is most frequently in a transverse direction to the longitudinal axis of the tendon. The surgeon should always check the anterior and posterior attachments of the crescent-shaped tear because these tissues are usually plastically deformed and are not normal. They must be débrided to allow high-quality tissue attachment. There is usually adhesion formation on both surfaces that needs to be removed to allow complete mobilization to decrease tension on the repair.

U-shaped tears frequently have their greatest extent in a longitudinal direction to the tendon (Figure 4). The medial point of the tear does not represent retraction but represents the shape that an L-shaped or T-shaped tear assumes with muscle contraction. Mobilization of the two leaves of the tendon by release of the subacromial and intra-articular adhesions will allow better recognition of the tear pattern. The longitudinal component can be repaired by margin convergence, and the transverse component, now a crescent-shaped tear, can then be repaired to the bone. This can be conceptualized as a "U to T" or a "U to L" repair.

Margin convergence by longitudinal side-to-side closure of the leaves of the tear progressively decreases the strain on the lateral margins of the tear so that the resulting strain on the lateral transverse margin is within the tolerance for repair. It is usually easiest to place the transverse fixation anchors in the bone and the stitches in the lateral part of the tendon first without tying them and use them as traction sutures to place the longitudi-

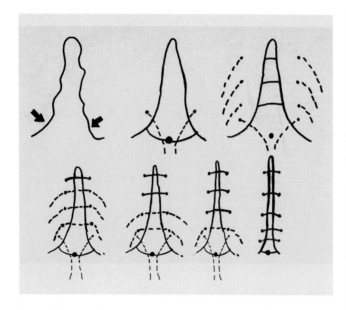

Figure 5 The stitches should be placed from lateral to medial using each successive stitch as a traction stitch, then tied from medial to lateral, zipping up the repair.

nal side-to-side stitches in order from lateral to medial. Each successive suture becomes the next stay suture. The sutures are then tied from medial to lateral, zipping up the repair. The transverse sutures reattaching the tendon to bone are tied last (Figure 5).

Secure fixation of the repair can be optimized by emphasizing minimal shear on the repair, proper suture placement in the tendon, and proper fixation placement. Minimal shear can be obtained by repair of the tear according to the tear pattern, by proper anterior and posterior releases, and by mobilization of the cuff from the subacromial and intra-articular adhesions. If these adhesions are not removed, they may act as proximal tethers, increasing shear at the distal repair site as motion is regained and muscle activation force is applied.

Suture placement in the tendon is the subject of much study. The types of suture placement may be categorized as simple, mattress, or combination (modified Mason-Allen). Although there is literature favoring each type of suture placement, it is probably more important how securely the sutures are tied (proper loop security of tendon to bone and knot security within the throws of the knot) and how much load is carried across each suture. Cyclic biomechanical testing has demonstrated that knot security is enhanced by using braided suture, alternating post limbs of the sutures, and past pointing to minimize slack within the stitch. Double loading each suture anchor increases the number of fixation points, thus decreasing the load on each individual suture.

Fixation placement should result in proper position of the cuff to bone and optimum pullout strength of the fixation device or construct. Suture anchors should be placed at a 45° angle to increase the anchor's resistance

to pullout. For single-row repairs, they are placed 4 to 5 mm off the articular margin. Biomechanical testing under cyclic loading indicates that these constructs are stronger than fixation by transosseous tunnels. However, in osteopenic bone, tunnels may be the fixation type of choice. The entrance to the tunnels should also be close to the articular margin, and the exits on the humerus should be placed far enough apart to allow a good bony buttress.

Lately, double-row repairs have been advocated to maximize suture placement, load per suture, and fixation placement. The rows consist of either medial suture anchors and lateral bone tunnels or medial and lateral suture anchors. Clinical reports demonstrate good results from either of these techniques. The double-row repairs also appear to result in the closest reapproximation of the total geometry of the rotator cuff footprint. Most repairs replicate the width but not the size of the original insertion. By allowing a larger, more physiologic area of contact, these double-row repairs have a theoretical ability to increase healing potential and ultimate tensile strength of the repair construct.

Summary

Athletes with chronic shoulder injuries often present with an unclear mix of symptoms, signs, and alterations in performance, and several principles can help guide evaluation and treatment. The rotator cuff functions in a closed-chain manner as a compressor cuff to increase concavity/compression and maintain ball-and-socket kinematics. The rotator cuff should be evaluated and rehabilitated to achieve restoration of this function. Both extrinsic and intrinsic factors play a role in producing rotator cuff tendinopathy. The clinical evaluation process must include assessment of all factors. External impingement in overhead athletes is often secondary to other underlying problems, some of which may be distant from the site of symptoms and may act in combination to create the impingement symptoms. Internal impingement is also a syndrome and appears to be associated with glenohumeral internal rotation deficit, biceps peel-back, excessive scapular protraction, and rotator cuff injury, all of which must be treated and rehabilitated. The clinical examination for chronic shoulder injuries must include a battery of tests because no single test has been shown to be sufficiently specific, sensitive, and accurate to be used independently. Nonsurgical treatment should address all of the physiologic and biomechanical alterations that may be found in the clinical examination. Surgical treatment is becoming more well defined, but it is still based on accurate determination of the type and extent of pathology, skillful use of fixation devices and débridement tools, repair of all injured tissues, and activity-specific rehabilitation.

Annotated Bibliography

Rotator Cuff Function Relating to Normal Shoulder Biomechanics

Hirashima M, Kadota H, Sakurai S, et al: Sequential muscle activity and its functional role in the upper extremity and trunk during overarm throwing. *J Sports Sci* 2002;20:301-310.

The authors of this article used sophisticated electromyography and force evaluation to show a sequential pattern of muscle activation in throwing that starts in the lumbar and trunk muscles, proceeds to the parascapular muscles, and then involves the rotator cuff muscles.

Lee SB, Kim KJ, O'Driscoll SW, Morrey BF, An KN: Dynamic glenohumeral stability provided by the rotator cuff muscles in the mid-range and end-range of motion: A study in cadavera. *J Bone Joint Surg Am* 2000;82:849-857.

This biomechanical study demonstrated that the rotator cuff muscles work primarily as joint compressors in midranges of joint motion. Force couple activation also contributed to joint stability in the end ranges.

Etiologic Factors for Rotator Cuff Tendinopathy

Carpenter JE, Flanagan CL, Thomopoulos S, Yian EH, Soslowsky LJ: The effects of overuse combined with intrinsic or extrinsic alterations in an animal model of rotator cuff tendinosis. *Am J Sports Med* 1998;26:801-807.

This study demonstrated that extrinsic factors alone did not cause significant rotator cuff injury in an animal model but required some type of overuse as well.

Mehta S, Gimbel JA, Soslowsky LJ: Etiologic and pathogenetic factors for rotator cuff tendinopathy. *Clin Sports Med* 2003;22:791-812.

This review article evaluates the intrinsic and extrinsic factors in rotator cuff injury causation and reviews basic science knowledge of internal strains developed in the tendons during arm motion.

Yuan J, Wang MX, Murrell GAC: Cell death and tendinopathy. *Clin Sports Med* 2003;22:693-701.

This article presents new information about the process of apoptosis (programmed cell death) and how cyclic strain could be a major causative factor in initiating apoptosis. The authors report that apoptotic cells are twice as common in injured tendons than in normal tendons.

External Impingement in Throwing Athletes

Cools AM, Witvrouw EE, DeClerq GA, et al: Scapular muscle recruitment patterns: Trapezius muscle latency with and without impingement symptoms. *Am J Sports Med* 2003;31:542-549.

This article documents alterations in parascapular muscle activation patterning in patients with external impingement symptoms. The authors report that the lower trapezius exhibits longer latency before activation, creating an imbalanced force couple for scapular and shoulder control.

Internal Impingement in Throwing Athletes

Burkhart SS, Morgan CD, Kibler WB: The disabled throwing shoulder: Spectrum of pathology. Part I: Pathoanatomy and biomechanics. *Arthroscopy* 2003;19:404-420.

The first part of this three-part article reviews the pathoanatomy and biomechanics of shoulder injuries based on a mechanism of altered joint mechanics caused by acquired posterior capsular/muscular contracture. The authors report that capsular tightness creates altered motion and labral and rotator cuff injuries as a result of peel-back and hypertwist.

Savoie FX, Field LD, Atchinson SA: Anterior superior instability with rotator cuff tearing: SLAC lesion. *Orthop Clin North Am* 2001;32:457-462.

This article describes the clinical presentation, examination findings, and treatment of the superior labrum anterior cuff lesion.

Superior Glenoid Labral Tears

Burkhart SS, Morgan CD, Kibler WB: The disabled throwing shoulder: Spectrum of pathology. Part II: Evaluation and treatment of SLAP lesions in throwers. *Arthroscopy* 2003;19:531-539.

The second part of this three-part article reviews the evaluation and treatment of shoulder injuries based on a mechanism of altered joint mechanics caused by acquired posterior capsular/muscular contracture. The authors report that capsular tightness creates altered motion and labral and rotator cuff injuries as a result of peel-back and hypertwist.

Clinical Examination for Patients With Rotator Cuff Tendinopathy, Impingement, and Labral Injury

Tennent TD, Beach WR, Meyers JF: A review of the special tests associated with shoulder examination: Part I. The rotator cuff tests. *Am J Sports Med* 2003;31:154-160.

Tennent TD, Beach WR, Meyers JF: A review of the special tests associated with shoulder examination: Part II. Laxity, instability, and superior labral anterior and posterior (SLAP) lesions. *Am J Sports Med* 2003;31:301-307.

This two-part review article documents and demonstrates all of the published clinical examination tests to help understand shoulder injury and presentation. None of the tests are sensitive enough to be diagnostic on their own; however, taken together they can provide a great deal of information about the pathology.

Nonsurgical Treatment

Burkhart SS, Morgan CD, Kibler WB: The disabled throwing shoulder: Spectrum of pathology. Part III: The

SICK scapula, scapular dyskinesis, the kinetic chain, and rehabilitation. *Arthroscopy* 2003;19:641-661.

The third part of this three-part article reviews the scapular dyskinesis, the kinetic chain, and the rehabilitation of shoulder injuries based on a mechanism of altered joint mechanics caused by acquired posterior capsular/muscular contracture. The authors report that capsular tightness creates altered motion and labral and rotator cuff injuries as a result of peel-back and hypertwist.

Surgical Treatment

Burkhart SS: A stepwise approach to arthroscopic rotator cuff repair based on biomechanical principles. *Arthroscopy* 2000;16:82-90.

This article provides a detailed framework for understanding rotator cuff tear type and treatment based on the biomechanics of the tendon reaction to tearing and the biomechanics of tissue repair and strength.

Fealy S, Kingham P, Altchek DW: Mini-open rotator cuff repair using a 2 row fixation technique: Outcomes analysis in patients with small, moderate, and large rotator cuff tears. *Arthroscopy* 2002;18:665-670.

This article documents good to excellent results using a mini-open repair technique with two rows of anchors, thereby enlarging the footprint contact area.

Ruotolo C, Nottage WM: Surgical and nonsurgical management of rotator cuff tears. *Arthroscopy* 2002;18:527-531.

This article discusses the clinical presentation, symptoms, and surgical indications for patients with rotator cuff injury. The authors found that poor prognostic findings for successful nonsurgical treatment included tears greater than 1 cm, the presence of symptoms for more than 1 year, and "severe" weakness on first presentation.

Severud EL, Ruotolo C, Abbott DD, Nottage WM: All-arthroscopic versus mini-open rotator cuff repair: A long-term retrospective outcome comparison. *Arthroscopy* 2003;19:234-238.

This article reports on a 2- to 5-year evaluation of treatment outcomes for small, medium, and large rotator cuff tears. University of California at Los Angeles and American Shoulder and Elbow Surgeons scores were not statistically different. There were more reports of restricted motion in the mini-open repair group, but final motion difference was not statistically significant.

Classic Bibliography

Ellman H: Arthroscopic subacromial decompression: Analysis of 1- to 3-year results. *Arthroscopy* 1987;3:173-181.

Happee R, van der Helm FC: Control of shoulder muscles during goal directed movements. *J Biomech* 1995;28:1179-1191.

Jobe CM: Posterior superior glenoid impingement: Expanded spectrum. *Arthroscopy* 1995;11:530-537.

Jobe CM, Pink MM, Jobe FW: Anterior shoulder instability, impingement, and rotator cuff tear: Theories and concepts, in Jobe FW (ed): *Operative Techniques in Upper Extremity Sports Injuries*. St. Louis, MO, Mosby, 1996, pp 164-176.

Kibler WB, Chandler TJ, Pace BK: Principles of rehabilitation after chronic tendon injuries. *Clin Sports Med* 1992;11:661-673.

McQuade KJ, Hwa Wei S, Smidt GL: Effects of local muscle fatigue on three-dimensional scapulohumeral rhythm. *Clin Biomech (Bristol, Avon)* 1995;10:144-148.

Neer CS II: Anterior acromioplasty for the chronic impingement syndrome in the shoulder: A preliminary report. *J Bone Joint Surg Am* 1972;54:41-50.

Uthoff HK, Sano H: Pathology of failure of the rotator cuff tendon. *Orthop Clin North Am* 1997;28:31-41.

Chapter 7

Overuse Elbow Injuries

Marc R. Labbé, MD

Felix H. Savoie III, MD

Introduction

Overuse injuries of the elbow commonly occur in both the athletic and lay populations. These injuries involve a wide spectrum of disorders, including tendinopathies, tendon ruptures, nerve entrapments, osteochondral lesions, and stress fractures. The medical history of a patient with an overuse injury will often include the regular performance of an activity that generates stress within the hard and soft tissues about the elbow. A detailed physical examination is necessary to define the area or structure that is injured and should include not just the involved extremity, but also the entire body. In a study of 485 patients with work-related upper extremity complaints, 78% of the patients protracted their shoulders, 71% routinely held their heads forward, and 70% had signs consistent with neurogenic thoracic outlet syndrome. The authors concluded that although most patients reported pain that was distal in the extremity, the position of proximal body segments was the main contributor to the problem.

Poor proximal extremity posture disrupts the kinetic chain of the entire limb and adds stress to the more distal periarticular tissues. As patients perform routine activities, these soft tissues are subjected to multiple episodes of microtrauma. The healing response is often inadequate in these patients, allowing damaged tissue to accumulate. Symptoms develop that then may persist despite conservative therapy. Scapular protraction and a head-forward position can also add stress to the brachial plexus, which may facilitate a double-crush injury to peripheral nerves. Peripheral nerves that overlie fascia or pass through confined spaces are susceptible to repeated compression with repetitive motions. As injury to the nerve accumulates, patients become symptomatic and often report local pain, dysesthesia, and/or motor weakness. Nonsurgical management will result in resolution of symptoms in most patients with tendinopathy of the elbow and peripheral neuropathy. Surgical intervention, however, may be necessary for optimal function in particular situations or patients with tendon ruptures.

Many recent studies have focused on novel nonsurgical and minimally invasive treatments of these disorders.

Epicondylitis

The term "epicondylitis" refers to a degenerative tendinopathy, which can occur on either the medial or lateral side of the distal humerus. Lateral epicondylitis is often referred to as "tennis elbow," and medial epicondylitis is often referred to as "golfer's elbow." Histologic studies have revealed an incomplete and disorganized healing response in patients with these injuries. In surgically treated patients, the resected tissue displays a mixture of hyalin degeneration and angiofibroblastic hyperplasia, with little evidence of active inflammation. Classically, nonsurgical management has centered on the reduction of inflammation; current nonsurgical management, however, focuses on reducing local tissue stress and encouraging a more vigorous healing response.

Lateral Epicondylitis

Lateral epicondylitis affects between 1% and 3% of the general population. The peak occurrence is during the fourth and fifth decades of life. The dominant arm is involved twice as often as the nondominant arm. The differential diagnosis includes posterolateral rotary instability and radial tunnel syndrome. The key to diagnosis is a careful medical history that includes documentation of the regular performance of any activity that generates stress within the hard and soft tissues about the elbow, and physical examination. Examination typically reveals point tenderness 2 mm anterior to the tip of the lateral epicondyle and pain with resisted wrist and finger extension. Classically, the area of tendinopathy is located at the insertion of the extensor carpi radialis brevis at the lateral epicondyle, but other extensor muscles may be involved. Although termed a tendinitis, the histologic picture is more consistent with a tendinosis.

Nonsurgical Management

The nonsurgical management of lateral epicondylitis typically includes rest, nonsteroidal anti-inflammatory

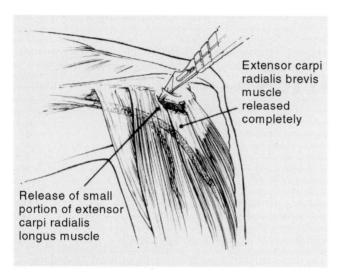

Extensor carpi radialis brevis muscle released completely

Release of small portion of extensor carpi radialis longus muscle

Figure 1 The origin of the extensor carpi radialis brevis muscle is released percutaneously from the anterior aspect of the lateral epicondyle.

medications (NSAIDs), an extension wrist brace and/or counterforce brace, physical therapy, and corticosteroid injections. Several methods of corticosteroid injection have been described, including multiple perforations and scraping of the epicondyle. These techniques attempt to stimulate the healing response by causing local tissue damage. In addition, the scraping method attempts to perform release of the common extensor origin by using the sharp edge of a large bore needle as a knife.

Extracorporeal shock wave therapy (ESWT) has been used to treat a variety of disorders, including gallstones and tendinopathies throughout the body. ESWT involves the application of a large number of focused pressure pulses to the area of maximal tenderness. The proposed mechanisms of action include the stimulation of a local healing response, denervation, and inhibition of pain receptors. Two double-blind randomized controlled studies evaluated the use of ESWT to treat lateral epicondylitis. One used several different machines while patients were under local anesthesia. Three treatments were given within a 6- to 8-day interval between sessions. In another study, patients in the treatment group received 1,500 pulses at monthly intervals for a total of three treatments. No local anesthesia was used. Both studies concluded that ESWT was of no benefit.

Low-level laser therapy (LLT) is another nonsurgical modality that is used to treat epicondylitis. Several proposed mechanisms of action for LLT are improvements in local microcirculation, improved lymphatic flow, and several changes in the local tissue metabolism affecting neural tissues. A multicenter, double-blind, placebo-controlled study tested LLT using three different techniques to treat both acute and chronic cases of medial and lateral epicondylitis. One technique applied

the laser directly to trigger points with the device in contact with the skin. The second technique scanned the area of injury without contacting the skin. The third technique used both methods. No other treatments were given. The treatments were given daily for 5 days and were then tapered, depending on the response. The treatment groups did not show significant improvement over the placebo group.

Using iontophoresis to treat lateral epicondylitis involves the application of a topical steroid cream followed by a low-level electrical current that drives the steroid more deeply into tissues. In a double-blind randomized study, patients received a total of four iontophoresis treatments every other day. Several functional tests were used to measure outcomes. The authors noted no significant differences between the iontophoresis treatment and placebo groups. Another double-blind randomized placebo-controlled study found a significant difference between the two groups on short-term follow up. Patients who underwent iontophoresis treatment improved on visual analog scores and examiner-rated tenderness scores. Patients who completed six treatments within 10 days had greater improvement than those who underwent longer treatment courses. The patients were contacted by telephone 1 month after treatment. There were no additional contacts for longer-term follow-up.

The mainstays of nonsurgical treatment still seem to be the most effective treatments for lateral epicondylitis. ESWT has not been proven effective, but optimal treatment techniques have not been used for evaluation. LLT has shown some positive results, but a standard treatment protocol has not been identified. Evidence is also mounting to document the positive effects of iontophoresis on lateral epicondylitis. Corticosteroid injections have been shown to be of the most benefit in the short-term, whereas physical therapy (for global upper extremity strengthening) has shown better long-term results. These and other therapeutic modalities are often used in concert; when combined with the tendency of lateral epicondylitis to resolve spontaneously, it generally leads to a high rate of symptom resolution.

Surgical Management
Although most patients with lateral epicondylitis do well with nonsurgical management, a significant number do not. Patients with persistent symptoms after several months of appropriate nonsurgical treatment can benefit from surgical intervention. Several surgical techniques have been described to treat lateral epicondylitis. Excision of the degenerated tendon followed by repair, classically described by Nirschl and Pettrone, has been described using both open and arthroscopic techniques. Other methods include percutaneous and open release of the common extensor origin (Figure 1). In one study, percutaneous release yielded excellent results in 26 of 32 elbows (30 patients), with 90% of grip strength

achieved compared with the contralateral side. Three patients had good results and noted elbow pain only with heavy use. Three patients were dissatisfied with the results and classified their outcomes as poor. The percutaneous releases were performed in the operating room with the patient under axillary block or general anesthesia and a tourniquet applied. A transverse incision was made just distal to the epicondyle, and the common extensor origin was released. A similar in-office technique has been described using local anesthesia and a sterile preparation.

Arthroscopic release has shown good early results. In one study, 40 patients (42 elbows) underwent arthroscopic release. Thirty-nine elbows in 37 patients were available for evaluation at an average follow-up of 2.8 years. Thirty-seven of 39 elbows were rated as better or much better, with grip strength averaging 96% of the opposite side. Functional scores averaged 11.1 of 12 possible points. Associated problems were found in 69% of patients. Patients were able to return to work at an average of 2 weeks. No complications were noted.

Medial Epicondylitis

Although not as common as lateral epicondylitis, medial epicondylitis is a common problem among athletes and manual laborers. The pathoanatomy of medial epicondylitis is similar to that of lateral epicondylitis. Repetitive wrist flexion and pronation stresses the origin of the flexor-pronator muscle group. Typical patients include golfers and tennis players who put a lot of topspin on their forehand strokes. Physical examination typically demonstrates pain with resisted pronation and wrist extension and tenderness at the anterior aspect of the medial epicondyle. The differential diagnosis includes medial collateral ligament instability and ulnar neuritis.

Nonsurgical treatments for medial epicondylitis are similar to those for lateral epicondylitis. Corticosteroid injections have been shown to improve symptoms in the short term; however, care must be taken to avoid intraneural injection. Outcomes with conservative therapy are similar to those for lateral epicondylitis, but a small percentage will require surgical treatment. Surgical débridement and repair of the tendon is routinely performed open because percutaneous and arthroscopic techniques would place the ulnar nerve at significant risk.

As with lateral epicondylitis, the majority of patients with medial epicondylitis will respond well to nonsurgical treatment, and the current treatment modalities still seem to be the most effective. Further study is necessary to evaluate the efficacy of ESWT and LLT to treat medial epicondylitis. In patients who do not respond well to nonsurgical treatment, surgical intervention is often successful. Although a variety of surgical techniques are available to treat patients with lateral epicondylitis, including minimally invasive surgery, the options for the surgical treatment of medial epicondylitis are limited. Medial epicondylitis is not at this time amenable to minimally invasive surgical techniques because of the risk of neural injury.

Distal Biceps Tendon Injury

Injuries to the distal biceps tendon are rare. The pathology can range from local tendinitis to partial or, more commonly, complete rupture that is either acute or chronic. The peak incidence of distal biceps tendon injuries occurs between the fourth and sixth decades of life. Rather than report a history of antecedent pain, patients typically recall a single event during which they were resisting a strong extension moment on a flexed elbow and the biceps was then forced into a powerful eccentric contraction that caused the tendon to rupture. Depending on the length of time from injury, a variable amount of swelling and ecchymosis will be present in patients with a distal biceps injury. A defect may be palpable when the biceps aponeurosis is also ruptured and allowing the muscle to retract. Strength testing typically reveals weakness with elbow flexion and significant weakness with supination.

Nonsurgical Management

Tendinitis of the distal biceps can often be treated with rest, NSAIDs, and bracing. Corticosteroid injections should not be used because of the proximity to neurovascular structures and the potential for tendon rupture. Strengthening exercises emphasizing eccentric loading should be gradually incorporated after symptoms resolve. Partial ruptures should be treated with an initial period of nonsurgical management and then an evaluation to determine if any strength or endurance deficits persist. These injuries often continue to be problematic, progress over time, and eventually require surgical intervention. Chronic ruptures can be treated symptomatically with range-of-motion exercises; however, if they limit function, surgical correction should be considered.

Surgical Management

The surgical repair of a distal biceps tendon rupture has been described using a variety of techniques. A muscle-splitting two-incision or one-incision approach can be used. Although the one-incision approach reduces the risk of proximal radioulnar synostosis, a slightly higher incidence of injury to the posterior interosseous nerve (PIN) has been reported in patients treated with this technique. The tendon can then be fixed to the surface of the prepared radial tuberosity or inserted into a bone tunnel or bony trough. Suture anchors are commonly used when the tendon is repaired to the tuberosity (Fig-

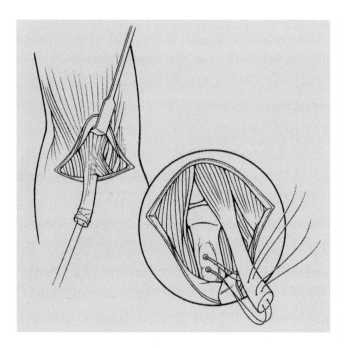

Figure 2 The stump of the distal biceps tendon is identified through a small transverse incision and tagged with a suture. Two suture anchors are placed into the radial tuberosity after it has been prepared for tendon reattachment.

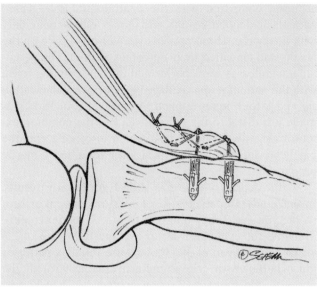

Figure 3 The sutures from the anchors are passed through the biceps tendon, securing it to the tuberosity.

ures 2 and 3), and transosseous sutures are commonly used when the tendon is repaired in a bony trough. Fixation in a bone tunnel can be done using either a tenodesis screw or Endobutton (Acufex Microsurgical, Mansfield, MA).

Multiple reports have shown good short-term return of flexion and supination strength and endurance with all of the various techniques. One long-term study of eight patients who underwent distal biceps tendon repair using the two-incision technique showed less favorable results at an average follow-up of 6 years. One patient developed proximal radioulnar synostosis, and three other patients lost greater than 30° of supination. Six of the eight patients were satisfied with the surgical outcome, even though they had less strength than the other arm and could perform less total work than they could with the other arm. The tendon can also be sutured to the underlying brachialis, which improves flexion strength but still compromises supination strength and endurance.

Recent studies have compared various fixation methods and approaches to determine which may be better. Transosseous suture has been shown to have superior endurance under cyclic loads when compared with two kinds of anchors. Cadaveric specimens were tested at 50 N for 3,600 cycles. Although none of the fixation methods failed, some of the anchors loosened, potentially creating a gap at the tendon-bone interface. The anchors, however, were tested individually and not in pairs. Most authors recommend using two anchors for tendon fixation.

A recent laboratory study compared the classic two-incision technique to a one-incision suture anchor method. Two groups were created based on bone density, which was measured in each specimen. Only one suture anchor was used to fix the tendon to bone. The specimens were then tested for yield and tensile strength to failure. The two-incision technique had higher yield and tensile strength to failure in specimens with higher bone density. No significant differences were detected in samples with lower bone density.

Surgical treatment of a partial distal biceps tendon rupture consists of completing the tear and repairing the tendon. Unfavorable results have been reported with tendon débridement alone. Chronic ruptures represent a distinct surgical challenge. A ruptured tendon that has retracted and is scarred to the surrounding tissues can be difficult to identify and mobilize. In addition, neurovascular structures are at greater risk because they may be captured within the scar tissue. Once isolated, the tendon often will not reach the radial tuberosity. Several successful grafting techniques have been described, including rolled autogenous fascia lata and semitendinosus tendon allografts and allografts using similar tissues.

Controversy still exists regarding the best method of fixation and surgical approach for distal biceps tendon ruptures. Evidence is mounting in favor of a one-incision approach because of the lower incidence of synostosis; however, care must be taken to protect the radial nerve and its branches. When selecting suture anchors to repair the tendon, two should be used. Additional studies are necessary to compare the long-term results of the various techniques.

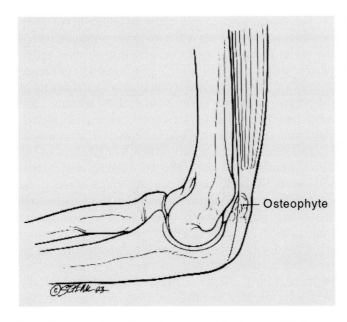

Figure 4 The osteophyte originates from the tip of the olecranon within the substance of the distal triceps tendon.

Triceps Tendon Injury

Overuse injuries of the triceps tendon are common. Most patients with triceps tendinitis present with pain at the tip of the olecranon during resisted elbow extension. Radiographs may reveal calcification within the tendon. The same nonsurgical treatments for distal biceps tendinitis are used to treat triceps tendinitis and will often be curative. Local corticosteroid injection may lead to triceps tendon rupture in patients with triceps tendinitis. Pain that persists despite conservative management can be treated surgically. A posterior approach is used to access the olecranon and triceps tendon, which is reflected to expose the calcified region and excised. Degenerated tendon is excised, and the tip of the olecranon is "freshened" for reinsertion of the tendon (Figures 4 through 6).

Partial or complete rupture of the triceps tendon is a debilitating problem that often requires surgical intervention. Rupture most commonly occurs during eccentric contraction. Patients taking anabolic steroids are at increased risk for triceps tendon rupture because of the relative weakness of the tendon insertion compared with the greatly hypertrophied muscle. Patients with chronic renal failure and renal osteodystrophy can develop calcifications in the periarticular tissues and rupture triceps tendons as well. Primary repair is the procedure of choice and can easily be performed in the acute setting. Chronic triceps tendon ruptures can be difficult to repair when the tendon has retracted and is scarred to the surrounding tissues. Occasionally, a reconstruction must be performed when, after mobilization, it will not reach the olecranon. Allograft Achilles tendon reconstruction has been described with good early success. The anconeus muscle can also be rotated to fill the void

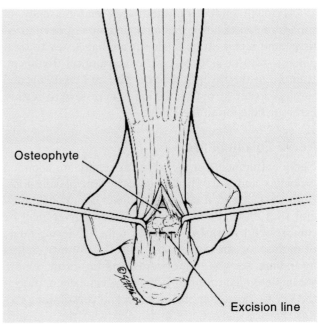

Figure 5 A midline incision exposes the distal triceps tendon, which is reflected away from the osteophyte. The osteophyte is removed with an osteotome, and the bone is prepared for tendon reinsertion.

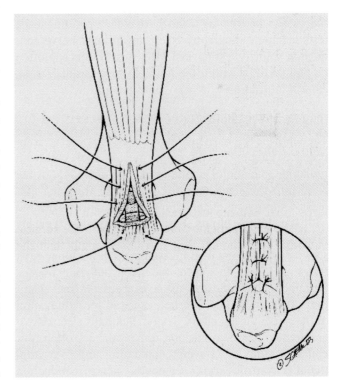

Figure 6 The triceps tendon is repaired to itself and, if necessary, back to the bone with suture anchors or transosseous suture.

if the triceps tendon did not completely detach (allowing the anconeus muscle to remain vascularized). Autologous fascia lata and semitendinosus tendon grafts have also been used to treat triceps tendon ruptures.

Although tendinitis of the triceps tendon usually responds to conservative treatment, excision of devitalized tissue and repair of the tendon is a reliable way to treat patients who do not respond to nonsurgical treatment. Rupture of the triceps tendon is rare and disabling, and surgical repair or reconstruction is necessary to restore extensor function to the elbow.

Nerve Entrapments

Nerve entrapments of the upper extremity are common problems, and a significant source of lost playing time. Both contact and noncontact athletes are at risk. Several sites exist about the elbow where nerves may be compressed by nearby structures, tethered during range of motion, or stretched as a result of deformity caused by trauma. As with other overuse injuries of the elbow, a complete medical history and physical examination is the key to identifying the problem and contributing factors. Several factors are associated with the development of a nerve entrapment syndrome, including health habits (rheumatoid arthritis, diabetes, pregnancy, and hypothyroidism), work habits, female sex, and patient anatomy. A careful assessment of the patient's environment and body posture during play and/or work can further assist in treating contributing factors. Diagnostic tests include radiography, electromyography, nerve conduction velocity testing, and MRI. Test results can often be equivocal or within the normal range despite strong clinical indications of a nerve entrapment.

Ulnar Nerve Compression

The elbow is the most common site of ulnar nerve compression. Patients usually report medial elbow pain with radiating pain and/or numbness on the ulnar side of the hand into the small and ring fingers. In throwing athletes, compression at the elbow is commonly associated with ulnar nerve injury. Physical examination typically reveals a positive percussion test at the cubital tunnel, sensory deficits, and possibly weakness in the ulnar wrist flexor and deep flexors of the small and ring fingers. Sustained elbow flexion often exacerbates the symptoms. Patients should also be evaluated for subluxation of the nerve during elbow flexion. Standard electromyography and nerve conduction test results are often normal. In a study of 21 symptomatic arms and 25 asymptomatic control arms, segmental nerve conduction velocity testing at 2-cm intervals demonstrated improved sensitivity (81%) over standard motor conduction velocity testing using 10- to 14-cm segments across the elbow (24%). The authors concluded that segmental nerve conduction velocity testing significantly improves the detection of ulnar mononeuropathy at the elbow and should be considered when routine test results are negative and clinical suspicion remains high.

The nonsurgical management of ulnar nerve compression consists of cessation of aggravating activities, the use of pads to protect the nerve during other activities, the use of elbow extension splints at night to reduce tension on the nerve, and evaluation and treatment of the valgus overload. Several surgical treatments have been described to treat ulnar nerve compression, including simple decompression and submuscular, intramuscular, and subcutaneous transpositions. Lengthening of the flexor-pronator mass can also be done in conjunction with submuscular transposition. Although there is no clear consensus on which technique is best, better results have generally been achieved with submuscular transposition. A cadaveric study radiographically analyzed the angulation of tungsten-labeled ulnar nerves after subcutaneous and then submuscular transpositions in the area of the flexor carpi ulnaris origin. Statistically significant greater angulations were measured in the subcutaneous group during elbow flexion. The revision of failed transposition remains controversial. Both subcutaneous and submuscular transpositions have been used with good results. In one study, 65% of patients with persistent medial elbow pain after transposition were noted to have abnormalities of the medial cutaneous nerves. Although several surgical techniques for repair of ulnar nerve injury yielded good results, submuscular transposition generally achieved better results.

Median Nerve Compression

Pronator syndrome occurs when the median nerve is compressed at one of several sites around the elbow, including the bicipital aponeurosis, arch of the pronator teres, flexor digitorum superficialis origin, and if present, between a medial supracondylar process and the ligament of Struthers. Tennis players and other athletes who perform repetitive pronation/supination activities are at increased risk. Patients with this condition typically report symptoms similar to carpal tunnel syndrome, including weakness in the thenar muscles and numbness of the radial 3.5 fingers. Patients often have a positive percussion test result in the forearm and a negative Phalen's test result, which helps differentiate the two conditions. A careful physical examination will help determine the site of nerve compression. Nerve conduction velocity studies can be helpful, but they cannot always identify the site of nerve compression above the pronator teres. Decompression of the nerve usually results in a quick recovery.

The anterior interosseous nerve can also be a source of discomfort. Patients with anterior interosseous nerve compression will report vague anterior forearm pain with the loss of thumb to finger end-pinch power. Parsonage-Andrew-Turner syndrome should be considered in patients with bilateral symptoms and those with symptoms that last for at least 3 months. Surgical decompression may facilitate recovery in patients with persistent symptoms.

Radial Nerve Compression

The radial nerve divides proximal to the elbow joint into the PIN and superficial radial nerve. The PIN then passes between the two heads of the supinator where it can be compressed. Symptoms of PIN compression include vague pain, a lack of sensory changes, and weakness in the wrist and finger extensors. As the problem progresses, the wrist will drift radially and drop. Radial nerve compression may be incomplete, involving only a few of the muscles innervated by the PIN. Nerve conduction velocity study results are often diagnostic. Treatment begins with observation and cessation of aggravating activities. Surgical decompression often results in a complete resolution of symptoms.

Radial tunnel syndrome is another neuropathy of the PIN. Patients with radial tunnel syndrome report dorsal lateral forearm pain that often occurs at night. Passive forearm pronation with wrist flexion and resisted forearm supination with wrist extension aggravate symptoms. Pain with resisted middle finger extension during elbow extension (Maudsley's test) has classically been used to aid in the diagnosis of radial tunnel syndrome, which can easily be confused with lateral epicondylitis. One study using cadaveric dissection showed that the origin of the extensor to the middle finger is a separate structure arising from the lateral epicondyle. A concomitant clinical study was performed on patients with recalcitrant tennis elbow necessitating surgical release. Preoperatively, each patient's pain was quantified with a visual analog pain score for wrist extension as well as extension of each of the individual digits. Those patients whose middle finger extension pain scores were at least half of the pain scores generated by wrist extension were noted to have degeneration at the middle finger extensor origin at the time of surgery. The authors concluded that a positive Maudsley's test result might signify tendinopathy at the middle finger extensor origin and not necessarily radial nerve entrapment. Injection of local anesthetic into the radial tunnel should eliminate the pain and produce a temporary wrist drop. For those patients who do not respond to rest and NSAIDs, surgical decompression may be of benefit.

Osteochondral Injuries and Stress Fractures

The hard tissues of the elbow are also at risk for overuse injuries. These injuries are seen more commonly in throwing athletes. The motions involved in throwing create a large valgus moment across the elbow, compressing the radiocapitellar joint. Osteochondral lesions of the capitellum or trochlea may develop, causing lateral elbow pain and mechanical symptoms with activity. The olecranon also impinges against the posterior humerus

and generates significant stress in the bone. Stress fractures of the proximal ulna have been described in professional baseball pitchers.

Patients with osteochondral injuries and stress fractures typically report posterolateral elbow pain during activity. A combination of rest, inflammation reduction, and treatment of the valgus overload followed by gradual return to activity is often the only treatment that is necessary. Surgical intervention may be needed for patients with persistent symptoms.

Summary

Overuse injuries of the elbow can occur at many different sites and in both the hard and soft tissues. The diagnosis of these injuries can be difficult and is based on a good patient history and careful physical examination. As the understanding of the pathology has improved, novel nonsurgical treatments have been proposed. Although some of these treatments appear promising, further testing is indicated to prove their efficacy. Surgical techniques have also improved and trend toward less invasive methods. Care should be taken to avoid iatrogenic neurologic injury when using these techniques.

Annotated Bibliography

General

Pascarelli EF, Hsu Y: Understanding work-related upper extremity disorders: Clinical findings in 485 computer users, musicians, and others. *J Occup Rehabil* 2001;11: 1-21.

The authors report on the physical examination findings of 485 patients with work-related upper extremity problems. Most patients were noted to have significant proximal extremity and body posture problems, which likely contributed to their distal extremity problems.

Epicondylitis

Baker CL Jr, Murphy KP, Gottlob CA, Curd DT: Arthroscopic classification and treatment of lateral epicondylitis: Two-year clinical results. *J Shoulder Elbow Surg* 2000;9:475-482.

This article describes the technique and results for arthroscopic release to treat lateral epicondylitis. The authors report that 95% of elbows were much better or better, and no patients developed neuromas or instability.

Fairbank SM, Corelett RJ: The role of the extensor digitorum communis muscle in lateral epicondylitis. *J Hand Surg [Br]* 2002;27:405-409.

The results of this study suggest that the extensor digitorum communis muscle origin to the long finger is separate from the rest of the fingers and may play an independent role in lateral epicondylitis. This study also shows that Maudsley's test may be an inaccurate method for assessing radial tunnel syndrome.

Gabel GT: Acute and chronic tendinopathies at the elbow. *Curr Opin Rheumatol* 1999;11:138-143.

The author presents an excellent review on tendinopathies of the elbow.

Grundberg AB, Dobson JF: Percutaneous release of the common extensor origin for tennis elbow. *Clin Orthop* 2000;376:137-140.

This article describes the technique and results for percutaneous release of the common extensor origin at the lateral epicondyle. Twenty-six of 32 elbows were rated excellent and 3 elbows were rated as poor. Two patients developed hematomas that resolved.

Haake M, König IR, Decker T, Reidel C, Buch M Müller HH: Extracorporeal shock wave therapy in the treatment of lateral epicondylitis: A randomized multicenter trial. *J Bone Joint Surg Am* 2002;84:1982-1991.

This is a prospective, randomized, blinded, multicenter trail that evaluated ESWT for the treatment of lateral epicondylitis. Because the results were similar for the placebo and treatment groups, the authors concluded that there was no significant benefit to ESWT.

Nirschl RP, Rodin DM, Ochiai DH, Maartmann-Moe C: Iontophoretic administration of sodium dexamethasone phosphate for acute epicondylitis: A randomized, double-blind, placebo-controlled study. *Am J Sports Med* 2003;31:189-195.

The article demonstrates the short-term improvement of patients after receiving iontophoresis to treat acute epicondylitis. The patients who improved most received six treatments within 10 days.

Runeson L, Haker E: Iontophoresis with cortisone in the treatment of lateral epicondylalgia (tennis elbow): A double-blind study. *Scand J Med Sci Sports* 2002;12:136-142.

In this randomized, placebo-controlled, double-blind evaluation of iontophoresis for the treatment of lateral epicondylitis, the authors noted no short- or long-term differences in patients who received the four treatments or placebo.

Simunovic Z, Trobonjaca T, Trobonjaca Z: Treatment of medial and lateral epicondylitis—tennis and golfer's elbow—with low level laser therapy: A multicenter double-blind, placebo-controlled clinical study on 324 patients. *J Clin Laser Med Surg* 1998;16:145-151.

This article compares the treatment of 324 patients who received one of three techniques of LLT for the treatment of medial and lateral epicondylitis or placebo. Because the outcomes of the treatment group did not differ significantly from those of the placebo group, the authors concluded that a combination of scanning and trigger point methods of treatment was the most effective.

Smidt N, van der Windt DAWM, Assendelft WJJ, Deville WLJM, Korthals-de Bos IBC: Corticosteroid injections, physiotherapy, or a wait-and-see policy for lateral epicondylitis: A randomized controlled trial. *Lancet* 2002;359:657-662.

This study compared corticosteroid injection, physiotherapy, and observation in patients with lateral epicondylitis. The corticosteroid injection group improved the most in the short term (3 to 6 weeks), but the physiotherapy group improved more than the other two groups at 12 weeks and 52 weeks.

Speed CA, Nichols D, Richards C, et al: Extracorporeal shock wave therapy for lateral epicondylitis: A double blind randomized controlled trial. *J Orthop Res* 2002;20: 895-898.

This is a prospective, randomized, controlled, double-blind trial of ESWT for the treatment of lateral epicondylitis. The authors report that there was no significant difference in the outcomes of the placebo and treatment groups and that although ESWT has a significant placebo effect, it is of little actual benefit.

Distal Biceps Tendon Injury

Berlet GC, Johnson JA, Milne AD, Patterson SD, King GJW: Distal biceps brachii tendon repair: An in vitro biomechanical study of tendon reattachment. *Am J Sports Med* 1998;26:428-432.

This laboratory study compared one suture anchor to transosseous fixation under cyclic and static loading conditions. The authors report that the transosseous tunnel technique had a higher load to failure compared with a single suture anchor method.

Dürr HR, Stäbler A, Pfahler M, Matzko M, Refior JR: Partial rupture of the distal biceps tendon. *Clin Orthop* 2000;374:195-200.

This is a case review of treatments and outcomes of patients with partial ruptures of the distal biceps.

Pereira DS, Kvitne RS, Liang M, Giacobetti FB, Ebramzadeh E: Surgical repair of distal biceps tendon ruptures: A biomechanical comparison of two techniques. *Am J Sports Med* 2002;30:432-436.

The authors compared transosseous sutures to a single suture anchor in tensile failure to strength. They also controlled for bone mineral density. They report that transosseous repairs were stiffer than single suture repairs and recommend using the traditional Z-incision repair technique.

Ramsey ML: Distal biceps tendon injuries: Diagnosis and management. *J Am Acad Orthop Surg* 1999;7:199-207.

The author presents an excellent review of distal biceps tendon injury diagnosis and management.

Sanchez-Sotelo J, Morrey BF, Adams RA, O'Driscoll SW: Reconstruction of chronic ruptures of the distal biceps tendon with use of an Achilles tendon allograft. *J Bone Joint Surg Am* 2002;84:999-1005.

The authors report on four patients with allograft reconstruction of the distal biceps tendon at an average follow-up of 2.8 years. All four patients had satisfactory results. The authors conclude that Achilles tendon allograft provides an excellent option when performing complex reconstruction of the distal biceps tendon.

Triceps Tendon Injury

Sanchez-Sotelo J, Morrey BF: Surgical techniques for reconstruction of chronic insufficiency of the triceps: Rotation flap using anconeus and tendo achillis allograft. *J Bone Joint Surg Br* 2002;84:1116-1120.

The authors describe the techniques and review the outcomes of reconstructed chronic triceps tendon tears.

Sollender JL, Rayan GM, Barden GA: Triceps tendon rupture in weight lifters. *J Shoulder Elbow Surg* 1998;7:151-153.

The authors of this study report on four weight lifters with triceps tendon raptures, two of whom had received local steroid injections for pain in the triceps. All four patients had taken oral anabolic steroids before injury. Satisfactory results were achieved after surgical reinsertion of the tendon.

Nerve Entrapments

Azrieli Y, Weimer L, Lovelace R, Gooch C: The utility of segmental nerve conduction studies in ulnar mononeuropathy at the elbow. *Muscle Nerve* 2003;27:46-50.

This article describes a nerve conduction velocity study technique that was used to evaluate the ulnar nerve at the elbow. The authors report that segmental nerve conduction studies were much more sensitive than routine ulnar motor and sensory studies.

Berlemann U, al-Momani Z, Hertel R: Exercise-induced compartment syndrome in the flexor-pronator muscle group: A case report and pressure measurements in volunteers. *Am J Sports Med* 1998;26:439-441.

The authors of this article compared the intracompartmental pressure data of a tennis player with much higher flexor-pronator muscle intracompartmental pressures than normal (intracompartmental pressures causing chronic symptoms typically range from 22 mm Hg at rest to 40 mm Hg after 30 minutes of exercise) with intracompartmental pressures measured in six symptom-free volunteers.

Nikitins MD, Ch'ng S, Rice NJ: A dynamic anatomical study of ulnar nerve motion after anterior transposition for cubital tunnel syndrome. *Hand Surg* 2002;7:177-182.

The authors compare the postoperative angulation of the ulnar nerve after subcutaneous and submuscular transpositions in a laboratory postoperative environment. They report that submuscular transposition resulted in less angulation of the ulnar nerve with the elbow in full flexion.

Osteochondral Injuries and Stress Fractures

Koffler KM, Kelly JD IV: Neurovascular trauma in athletes. *Orthop Clin North Am* 2002;33:523-534.

The authors of this article discuss injuries to the neurovascular structures and report that because they are not the most common injuries seen in athletes, they may often be overlooked. Additionally, diagnosis and management may be more difficult because of physician inexperience with these injuries.

Schickendantz MS, Ho CP, Koh J: Stress injury of the proximal ulna in professional baseball players. *Am J Sports Med* 2002;30:737-741.

In this retrospective review, the authors describe a syndrome of osseous stress injury of the proximal ulna in seven professional throwing athletes. They report that plain radiographs of the involved elbows failed to demonstrate any significant findings and that all of the clinically significant lesions were detected using MRI.

Takeda H, Watarai K, Matsushita T, Saito T, Terashima Y: A surgical treatment for unstable osteochondritis dissecans lesions of the humeral capitellum in adolescent baseball players. *Am J Sports Med* 2002;30:713-717.

The authors of this study performed a retrospective review to evaluate the results of surgical treatment with pullout wiring and bone grafting in 11 male baseball players with unstable osteochondritis dissecans lesions of the humeral capitellum. At a mean 57-month follow-up, all patients had obtained pain relief, and all except one had returned to previous throwing levels. Radiographs showed evidence of good healing, and minimal degenerative changes were found in only three joints.

Classic Bibliography

Davison BL, Engberg WD, Tigert LJ: Long-term evaluation of repaired distal biceps brachii tendon ruptures. *Clin Orthop* 1996;333:186-191.

Lorei MP, Hershman EB: Peripheral nerve injuries in athletes: Treatment and prevention. *Sports Med* 1993;16:130-147.

Nirschl RP, Pettrone FA: Tennis elbow. The surgical treatment of lateral epicondylitis. *J Bone Joint Surg Am* 1979;61:832-839.

Chapter 8

Acute Elbow Injuries

Christopher S. Ahmad, MD

Neal S. ElAttrache, MD

Introduction

Injuries related to throwing are common because of the tremendous forces regulated by the elbow that challenge the medial soft tissues, posterior compartment articulation, and lateral compartment articulation. The complex anatomy and biomechanics of the elbow continue to stimulate research to better understand these injuries. Recent advances in the pathomechanics of acute elbow injuries have resulted from basic science anatomy studies and throwing biomechanics studies. The diagnosis of elbow injuries has become more accurate because sports medicine specialists are now more aware of these injuries and more precise physical examination techniques and imaging modalities have been developed. Surgical treatment options for the variety of elbow disorders have also progressed with recent reports documenting improved clinical outcome.

Medial Ulnar Collateral Ligament Injuries

Biomechanical studies of throwing have shown that from late cocking to ball release the elbow rapidly extends from 125° to 25°, with an angular velocity estimated between 2,300° to 5,000° per second^2 and peak accelerations reaching 500,000° per second^2. This tremendous acceleration results in valgus torques that have been estimated between 52 to 120 Nm, which is resisted primarily by the anterior bundle of the medial ulnar collateral ligament (MUCL). The demands on the MUCL have been estimated at 35 Nm in resisting the valgus moments during throwing, and the actual force within the ligament has been estimated at 290 N. Cadaver studies have determined the ultimate failure load of the MUCL under valgus stress to be 22 to 40 Nm and under tensile stress with bone-ligament-bone preparations to be 261 N, which is less than the MUCL forces estimated during throwing. Because these studies demonstrate that the forces generated across the medial elbow with throwing may approach or exceed the tensile strength of the MUCL, it has been proposed that other factors likely contribute to maintaining valgus stability, including direct action of dynamic local muscle forces, con-

straints from the congruous articular geometry, indirect muscle forces acting to compress the congruous articulation, and integrated kinetic chain factors, such as coupled shoulder rotation and forearm pronation just before ball release.

Electromyography analysis has shown that athletes with valgus instability have a decrease in flexor pronator muscle group activity. This finding indicates the presence of either muscular inhibition from painful MUCL instability, primary muscle pathology, or alteration in integrated patterned muscle activation predisposing the MUCL to injury. The flexor-pronator mass anatomy has been described in relation to the MUCL. The humeral head portion of the flexor carpi ulnaris muscle is positioned directly over the anterior aspect of the MUCL during the phase of throwing when valgus loading is the greatest, suggesting a direct muscular contribution to dynamic valgus stability. Similarly, a biomechanical analysis of muscle forces across the elbow found that during cocking and acceleration, the flexor digitorum superficialis and flexor carpi ulnaris muscles are positioned best to provide direct medial elbow support. Local dynamic stability to the elbow is therefore provided by joint compression and also direct pull of the muscles to resist the valgus stress. There are also distant contributors to dynamic stability of the elbow through the production of interactive moments, which are forces at the joints that are produced by the motion and position of adjacent body segments. A biomechanical analysis of throwing skills demonstrated that the largest contribution to the varus acceleration at the elbow (which would be protective against valgus loads) is the interactive moment created by shoulder internal rotation. Based on these findings, flexibility and strengthening of local and distant muscles to enhance valgus stabilization have been recommended.

The overhead throwing athlete with valgus instability usually experiences medial elbow pain during the acceleration phase of throwing. Patients with chronic injuries report a gradual onset of pain that may be present only when throwing greater than 50% to 75% of maximal effort. Patients with acute injuries may report a sud-

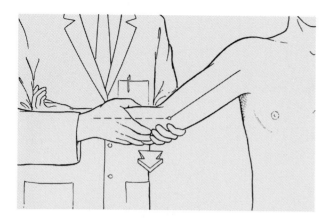

Figure 1 Valgus stress test. Valgus stability is tested with the patient's elbow flexed between 20° and 30° to unlock the olecranon from its fossa and to isolate the anterior bundle as valgus stress (*arrow*) is applied. *(Reproduced with permission from ElAttrache NS, Bast SC, David T: Medial collateral ligament reconstruction. Tech Shoulder Elbow Surg 2001;2:38-49.)*

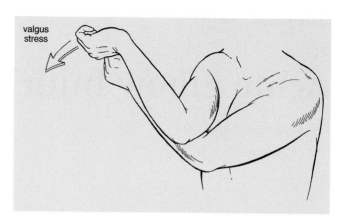

Figure 2 The milking maneuver usually elicits pain localized to the ulnar collateral ligament. *(Reproduced with permission from ElAttrache NS, Bast SC, David T: Medial collateral ligament reconstruction. Tech Shoulder Elbow Surg 2001;2:38-49.)*

den pop, sharp pain, and an inability to continue throwing. Ulnar nerve symptoms are common, especially in the setting of chronic MUCL insufficiency, and include paresthesias radiating to the fourth and fifth digits.

Local physical examination is best performed with the patient seated. Range of motion is assessed and inability to achieve full extension may be secondary to posterior compartment impingement or anterior capsular contracture. Valgus stability is tested using the valgus stress test (Figure 1). Valgus laxity is appreciated by increased medial joint space opening and the absence of a firm end point when compared with the contralateral extremity. Greater appreciation of the instability may be achieved by closing of the medial joint with release of valgus stress rather than opening of the joint with the application of valgus stress.

The milking maneuver is performed by either the patient or the examiner pulling on the patient's thumb to create valgus stress with the patient's forearm supinated and elbow flexed beyond 90° (Figure 2). The subjective feeling of apprehension and instability, in addition to localized pain, is indicative of an MUCL injury. Point tenderness may be elicited directly over the MUCL toward its insertion sites or in the midsubstance. It is important to differentiate an MUCL injury from medial epicondylitis. This is demonstrated by the absence of pain with resisted wrist flexion and pronation. The ulnar nerve should be assessed for subluxation in the cubital tunnel and irritation by attempting to elicit the Tinel sign. In addition, strength of the hand intrinsic muscles and sensation over the fourth and fifth digits should be assessed.

Distant physical examination in patients with elbow injuries should include assessment of the shoulder. Evaluations should include shoulder internal rotation mo-

tion and rotator cuff and shoulder internal rotation strength.

Valgus stress radiographs may be used to document excessive medial joint line opening; openings greater than 3 mm when compared with the radiographs without stress have been considered diagnostic of valgus instability. It has recently been observed, however, that in uninjured baseball pitchers, there is increased medial elbow laxity in the dominant elbow compared with the nondominant elbow. With stress radiography, the opening was small, with increased opening of 0.3 mm compared with the nonthrowing elbow on average.

Conventional MRI delineates the MUCL and is capable of identifying thickening and irregularity within the ligament. Conventional MRI has been 100% sensitive for full-thickness tears but only 14% sensitive for partial tears in one study (Figure 3). Saline-enhanced magnetic resonance arthrography increases the sensitivity in the diagnosis of partial tears. In addition, cadaver studies have determined that magnetic resonance arthrography enhanced with intra-articular gadolinium improves the diagnosis of partial undersurface tears when compared with conventional MRI. Ultrasound imaging has recently been introduced as a diagnostic technique to help demonstrate MUCL pathology, and it has the advantages of being dynamic and noninvasive.

An early MUCL reconstruction technique used a tendinous transection and reflection of the flexor pronator mass with submuscular transposition of the ulnar nerve and creation of humeral tunnels that penetrated the posterior cortex. Since the report describing this technique was published, several authors have described modifications to simplify the technical demands of the reconstruction technique and facilitate reduced handling of the ulnar nerve. Clinical reports on the newer techniques document decreased incidence of ulnar nerve

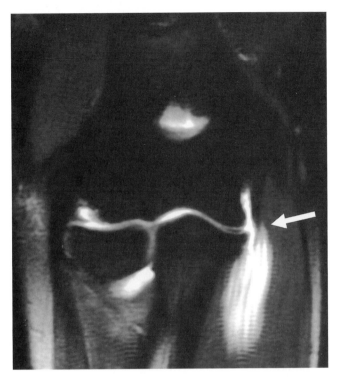

Figure 3 Gadolinium-enhanced MRI scan demonstrating torn ulnar collateral ligament at its ulnar insertion (*arrow*).

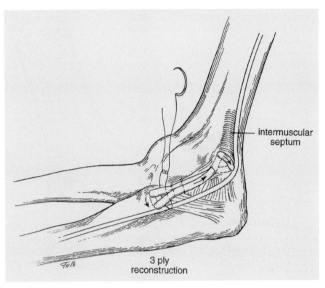

Figure 4 MUCL reconstruction technique with a tendon graft passed through bone tunnels. *(Reproduced with permission from ElAttrache NS, Bast SC, David T: Medial collateral ligament reconstruction. Tech Shoulder Elbow Surg 2001;2:38-49.)*

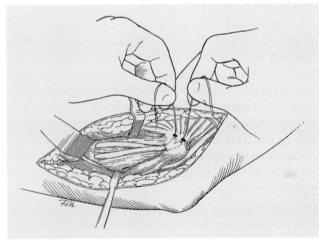

Figure 5 Docking technique for MUCL reconstruction. *(Reproduced with permission from ElAttrache NS, Bast SC, David T: Medial collateral ligament reconstruction. Tech Shoulder Elbow Surg 2001;2:38-49.)*

complications with muscle-splitting approaches to expose the ligament, with or without subcutaneous transposition of the ulnar nerve. Modifications in bone tunnel creation have also been made to redirect the tunnel's more anterior on humeral epicondyle to avoid risk of injury to the ulnar nerve while the graft is passed in a figure-of-8 fashion (Figure 4).

The docking technique modification uses the muscle-splitting approach with drill holes on the sublime tubercle of the ulna, which is similar to the classic technique. Proximally, however, a single unicortical drill hole is created at the humeral origin of the anterior bundle. Small divergent drill holes are then made in the superior cortex for passage of the graft fixation sutures. The graft is passed through the ulnar tunnel, and the free ends are brought into the proximal tunnel, creating a double-stranded graft. The graft is then tensioned, and the sutures are tied over the humeral bony bridge (Figure 5). This technique was developed to facilitate easier graft tensioning and decrease the number of bone tunnels required.

A new technique of MUCL reconstruction has been evaluated in the laboratory that reconstructs the central isometric fibers of the native ligament and achieves fixation in single bone tunnels in the ulna and humeral epicondyle using interference screw fixation. This technique is less technically demanding because the required number of drill holes necessary is reduced from five to two. Less dissection is needed when using a muscle-splitting approach because only a single central tunnel is required rather than two tunnels with an intervening bony bridge on the ulna. With a single tunnel, the posterior ulnar tunnel, which is nearest to the ulnar nerve, is avoided. Finally, graft passage and tensioning is less difficult when using interference screws in a single tunnel (Figure 6). Although the biomechanics of this technique are encouraging, clinical outcome results are not currently available.

MUCL reconstruction is technically demanding with regard to limiting muscular dissection and avoiding ulnar nerve injury. Furthermore, it is challenging to achieve graft isometry, adequate graft tension, and se-

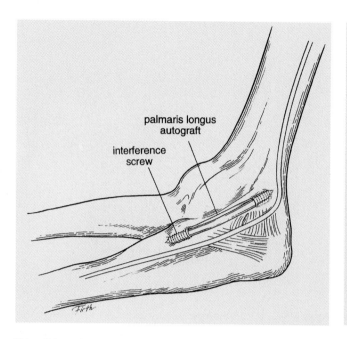

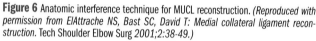

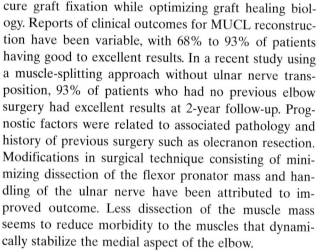

palmaris longus
autograft

interference
screw

Figure 6 Anatomic interference technique for MUCL reconstruction. *(Reproduced with permission from ElAttrache NS, Bast SC, David T: Medial collateral ligament reconstruction. Tech Shoulder Elbow Surg 2001;2:38-49.)*

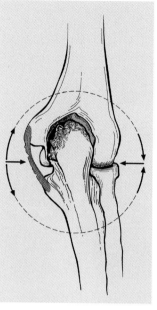

Figure 7 Development of posteromedial olecranon osteophytes from valgus torques. The circle indicates varus/valgus rotation; the curved arrows indicated forces (tension) on the medial side and compression on the lateral side. *(Reproduced with permission from ElAttrache NS, Ahmad CS: Valgus extension overload and olecranon stress fractures. Sports Med Arthrosc Rev 2003;11:25-29.)*

cure graft fixation while optimizing graft healing biology. Reports of clinical outcomes for MUCL reconstruction have been variable, with 68% to 93% of patients having good to excellent results. In a recent study using a muscle-splitting approach without ulnar nerve transposition, 93% of patients who had no previous elbow surgery had excellent results at 2-year follow-up. Prognostic factors were related to associated pathology and history of previous surgery such as olecranon resection. Modifications in surgical technique consisting of minimizing dissection of the flexor pronator mass and handling of the ulnar nerve have been attributed to improved outcome. Less dissection of the muscle mass seems to reduce morbidity to the muscles that dynamically stabilize the medial aspect of the elbow.

Some authors have advocated the use of arthroscopic evaluation of the elbow joint before ligament reconstruction. Arthroscopic assessment of valgus stability may be done by placing valgus stress to the elbow while the arm is positioned at 90° flexion and the forearm is maximally pronated. Normal elbows demonstrate a maximum opening of 1 to 2 mm, whereas elbows with MUCL insufficiency demonstrate an opening greater than 2 to 3 mm. Although an ulnohumeral opening may be appreciated, a cadaveric study demonstrated that the anterior bundle of the MUCL cannot be directly visualized arthroscopically. Arthroscopy does facilitate diagnostic examination of the anterior and posterior compartments, and associated procedures may be performed when necessary, including removal of loose bodies and marginal osteophytes, anterior capsular release, and anterior, posterior, or lateral débridement.

Valgus Extension Overload

During overhead throwing, a combination of valgus and extension forces is generated across the elbow and is resisted by articular, ligamentous, and muscular restraints. Extreme tensile forces generated from valgus torques are resisted primarily by the anterior bundle of the MUCL, whereas the articular constraints of the olecranon in its fossa and the radiocapitellar joint provide secondary stability. Toward full elbow extension, valgus stress is equally resisted by the MUCL, capsule, and articular constraints. Repetitive forceful shearing of the olecranon within its fossa causes posteromedial olecranon osteophytosis, resulting in painful chondromalacia and eventual osteophyte formation (Figure 7). In addition to valgus forces, established arm momentum generated during the acceleration phase of throwing causes elbow extension forces that are resisted by the flexor muscles of the elbow. When deceleration is poorly controlled by the flexor muscle forces, the olecranon traumatically abuts the posterior compartment toward full extension. Thus, the olecranon is subject to injury from both valgus and extension forces, which is described as valgus extension overload.

For isolated valgus extension overload, elbow pain is located on the medial aspect of the olecranon and may be present in both the acceleration and deceleration phases of throwing. Patients may report limited extension from posterior impingement because of osteophytes or locking and catching caused by loose bodies. Physical examination should assess the degree of extension loss. If asymptomatic, motion loss does not affect throwing performance.

Pain may be elicited in the posterior compartment with manual pronation, valgus, and extension forces applied. Crepitus, locking, or catching suggests the presence of a loose body, an osteophyte, or chondromalacia. In addition to assessing the posterior compartment, it is essential to assess the integrity of the MUCL, flexor pronator mass, radiocapitellar articulation, and ulnar nerve for associated injuries. Ulnar nerve subluxation should be noted when symptoms exist or elbow arthroscopy is being planned. Radiographic evaluation should include posterior, lateral, and axial views of the elbow. Posteromedial osteophytes and large loose bodies within the articulation may be identified with axial views. CT and MRI can help further define loose bodies and osteophytes.

Arthroscopy offers the advantages of limited morbidity and complete diagnostic assessment of the elbow. Diagnostic arthroscopy allows evaluation of osteophytes on the posteromedial aspect of the olecranon, loose bodies, and any evidence of chondromalacia. A motorized burr or small osteotome is used to remove osteophytes (Figure 8). It is important to remove only the osteophyte and not normal olecranon. Care should be taken to avoid injury to the ulnar nerve, which lies in close proximity in the cubital tunnel.

In a report on 72 professional baseball players who underwent either open or arthroscopic elbow surgery, posteromedial osteophytes were identified in 65% of patients. Of the patients who underwent olecranon débridement, 25% developed valgus instability and eventually required MUCL reconstruction. This observation suggests that both the olecranon and the MUCL contribute to valgus stability. Therefore, olecranon resection may increase the demand placed on the MUCL in resisting valgus forces during throwing. In a biomechanical study, it was demonstrated that increasing olecranon resection increases elbow valgus angulation. The authors of the study suggested that the kinematic alterations place the MUCL at increased risk for injury.

If MUCL reconstruction is planned in combination with posterior compartment débridement, the posterior compartment may be addressed either arthroscopically before the reconstruction or through an open approach used for the reconstruction. Open capsulotomy is performed just superior to the posterior bundle of the MUCL after mobilizing and protecting the ulnar nerve.

Lateral Ulnar Collateral Ligament Injuries

The lateral ulnar collateral ligament (LUCL) originates on the lateral epicondyle, courses superficially over the annular ligament, and curves posteriorly and ulnarly to insert onto the tubercle of the supinator crest of the ulna. The LUCL lies beneath the fascia covering the supinator and extensor carpi ulnaris muscles. LUCL injury resulting in posterolateral rotatory instability of the elbow can be caused by traumatic elbow subluxation, dis-

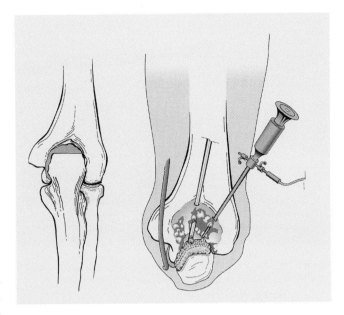

Figure 8 Arthroscopic removal of olecranon osteophytes and posterior compartment débridement. *(Reproduced with permission from ElAttrache NS, Ahmad CS: Valgus extension overload and olecranon stress fractures. Sports Med Arthrosc Rev 2003;11: 25-29.)*

location, or iatrogenic injury to the LUCL complex during lateral elbow surgery, which most commonly is related to the treatment of lateral epicondylitis.

In patients with LUCL injuries, a history of trauma to the elbow usually precedes symptoms of painful clicking or locking of the elbow, which occur during full extension with the forearm in supination. A history of previous surgery to the elbow may also have injured the LUCL. Several physical examination tests have been described to identify posterolateral rotatory instability: the posterolateral rotatory apprehension test or lateral pivot-shift test, posterolateral rotatory drawer test, stand-up test, and push-up test.

The posterolateral rotatory apprehension test is done with the patient supine and the affected extremity overhead. The elbow is supinated, and a valgus moment and axial load are applied while the elbow is flexed (Figure 9). This maneuver elicits apprehension and reproduces the patient's symptoms. The actual subluxation and the clunk that accompanies reduction usually require that the patient be placed under general anesthesia; occasionally, the subluxation and clunk that accompany reduction occur after injecting a local anesthetic into the elbow joint. The actual pivot-shift may be observed as a radial head prominence and formation of a dimple between the radial head and the capitellum. As the elbow is flexed greater than 40°, reduction of the ulna and radius typically occurs with a palpable and visual clunk.

The elbow posterolateral rotatory drawer test is done with the patient supine, the arm overhead, and the elbow flexed 40° to 90°. Similar to a Lachman test for

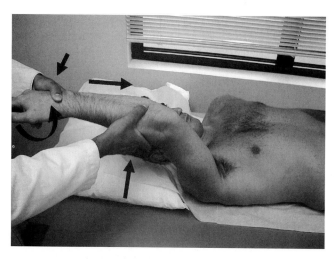

Figure 9 The lateral pivot-shift test of the elbow for posterolateral rotatory instability demonstrating supination, valgus, and axial loads applied at 40° of flexion.

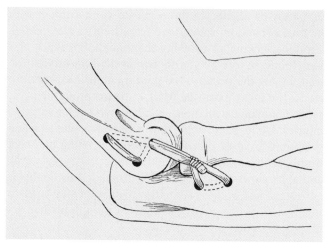

Figure 10 Reconstruction of the LUCL for posterolateral instability. *(Reproduced with permission from O'Driscoll SW, Morrey BF: Surgical reconstruction of the lateral collateral ligament, in Morrey BF (ed): Masters Techniques in Orthopaedic Surgery: The Elbow, ed 2. Philadelphia, PA, Lippincott-Williams & Wilkins, 2002.)*

the knee, the humerus is stabilized and the ulna and radius are translated off the humerus posterolaterally, pivoting around the intact MUCL. The stand-up test is done by having the patient attempt to stand up from a seated position by pushing on the seat with the elbow fully supinated. Reproduction of the patient's symptoms indicates a positive test result. A push-up test is performed by having the patient attempt to do a push-up from the prone position with the forearms maximally supinated and then attempt to do another push-up with the forearms maximally pronated. The test result is positive when symptoms occur with the forearms supinated but not pronated.

A lateral stress radiograph at the point of maximum rotatory subluxation during the pivot-shift test before feeling the clunk can demonstrate the rotatory subluxation required to confirm the diagnosis. Continuous imaging with fluoroscopy during a pivot-shift test may also assist in demonstrating rotatory subluxation. Finally, MRI can be used to help confirm the diagnosis. In one study, MRI demonstrated 100% accuracy in identifying tears of the LUCL that were later confirmed during surgery.

LUCL reconstruction is indicated in patients with persistent symptomatic instability. The reconstruction technique involves isometric placement of a soft-tissue graft at the origin on the lateral epicondyle and supinator crest of the ulna. The supinator crest is identified just distal and posterior to the radial head, and bone tunnels are created using a technique similar to that for MUCL reconstruction (Figure 10). After first creating the ulnar bone tunnels, a suture is then passed and positioned at the most isometric location on the lateral epicondyle for a full arc of motion to indicate the placement of the humeral tunnels. After passing the graft, the graft is tensioned and sutured to itself for fixation.

Osteochondritis Dissecans of the Capitellum

Lateral elbow compartment compressive forces during throwing have been estimated at 500 N. Although the exact etiology is poorly understood, these forces have been theorized to cause alterations in the subchondral blood supply of the capitellum, resulting in osteochondral fragmentation. The condition commonly occurs in gymnasts and adolescent throwing athletes with symptoms of lateral elbow pain during throwing that may be associated with stiffness, catching, or clicking. Imaging with plain radiographs, CT, and MRI assist in classifying the lesions. Nonsurgical treatment consists of a period of cessation from throwing followed by physical therapy as symptoms subside. Nonsurgical treatment is often unsuccessful for patients with large chondral fragments and loose bodies. Surgical treatment options include fragment removal, fragment reattachment, drilling or microfracture, osteochondral grafting, and humeral osteotomy. An arthroscopic classification system has recently been proposed based on the status of the overlying cartilage and stability of subchondral bone (Table 1). An early active range-of-motion and strengthening program should begin as soon as possible postoperatively.

Overall, capitellar osteochondritis dissecans in adolescents appears to be best managed nonsurgically unless there are loose bodies or mechanical symptoms or if extended nonsurgical treatment fails. Arthroscopic débridement, loose body excision, and abrasion chondroplasty appear to offer the best results in terms of reduced surgical morbidity and return of function. The benefit of fixation of loose capitellar osteochondral fragments has not been firmly established. A recent study reported encouraging results with a lateral closing wedge osteotomy of the capitellum for seven baseball players 11 to 18 years of age. The goal of the procedure was to unload the radiocapitellar joint while maintaining the alignment of the ulnohumeral joint. At 7- to 12-year follow-up, six of seven patients had complete relief of pain with return to full activity, all had increased range of motion, all had remodeling of the capitellum, and none had enlargement of the radial head.

Sports-Related Fractures

Olecranon Stress Fractures

Olecranon stress fractures can occur in baseball pitchers, gymnasts, and weight lifters. The pathomechanics of olecranon stress fractures are similar to those of valgus extension overload injuries. Stress injury across the olecranon results from repetitive abutment of the olecranon against the olecranon fossa, traction from triceps activity during the deceleration phase of throwing, and impaction of the medial olecranon onto the medial wall of the olecranon fossa from valgus forces. Based on fracture configuration, olecranon stress fractures are typically classified as either transverse or oblique. Transverse olecranon stress fractures occur when triceps traction and extension forces predominate. Oblique olecranon stress fractures occur when valgus and extension forces predominate, causing olecranon impaction on the medial wall of the olecranon fossa.

Oblique stress fractures may occur in combination with partial MUCL injuries, in which instance physical findings of tenderness are reported over both the olecranon and the MUCL. The pathomechanics of MUCL insufficiency contributing to valgus extension overload syndrome are similar to those of MUCL insufficiency leading to olecranon stress fractures. In the skeletally immature elbow, repeated stresses may result in widening of the olecranon epiphysis. The olecranon epiphysis appears in boys between 9 and 11 years of age and closes between 15 and 17 years of age. Gymnasts and wrestlers are at a unique risk because they perform activities with weight bearing across the elbow and have sudden extension forces associated with triceps demanding maneuvers. Forceful trauma can acutely displace the epiphysis of the proximal olecranon in skeletally immature patients.

Physical examination of patients with olecranon stress fractures typically reveals tenderness over the posterior and posteromedial olecranon. Pain can be elicited with manual forced extension while abuting the olecranon into its fossa or with resistive triceps activity. Limited extension is common in patients with a 10° to 15° flexion contracture. Valgus stress testing and the milking maneuver may elicit pain in both the MUCL and the olecranon.

Standard AP, lateral, and axial radiographs demonstrate a fracture line with sclerosis in patients with olecranon stress fractures (Figure 11). The orientation of either a transverse or oblique fracture should be as-

TABLE 1 | Arthroscopic Classification System for Osteochondritis Dissecans of the Capitellum

Lesion Grade	Lesion Description	Surgical Recommendation
1	Smooth but soft articular artilage	Drilling
2	Cartilage fibrillations or fissuring	Lesions that do not respond to nonsurgical treatment should undergo removal of affected cartilage back to a stable rim and then abrasion chondroplasty
3	Exposed bone with a stable osteochondral fragment	Removal of the osteochondral fragment and abrasion chondroplasty
4	Loose but nondisplaced fragment	Removal of the osteochondral fragment and abrasion chondroplasty
5	Displaced fragment with resultant loose bodies	Abrasion chondroplasty performed with diligence for removal of all associated loose bodies

(Adapted with permission from Baumgarten TE, Andrews JR, Satterwhite YE: The arthroscopic classification and treatment of osteochondritis dissecans of the capitellum. Am J Sports Med 1998;26:520-523.)

sessed. A bone scan can confirm stress fractures in questionable instances of growth plate widening that is not easily identified on plain radiographs. MRI may provide additional detail of the fracture pattern.

Initial treatment requires rest from throwing. Temporary splint immobilization may achieve earlier pain relief. Return to sport is delayed until all symptoms have resolved and radiographic evaluation demonstrates fracture healing. Healing of olecranon stress fractures is slower than regular fracture healing, and restriction from sports for up to 6 months may be required. Electrical bone stimulation may be considered in an attempt to accelerate healing. Athletes who cannot tolerate lengthy healing times or those fractures that fail to heal with nonsurgical treatment may require surgery. Several reports describe success with tension band techniques alone, tension banding with bone grafting, and screw fixation (Figure 12).

Acute Olecranon Fractures

Acute olecranon fractures can occur as the result of direct trauma to the olecranon or extreme triceps forces, such as those that occur during a fall onto the upper extremity with sudden contraction of the triceps. Patients with acute olecranon fractures typically report posterior elbow pain, and physical examination may demonstrate crepitus and a palpable defect in the olecranon. Inability to extend the elbow against gravity indicates discontinu-

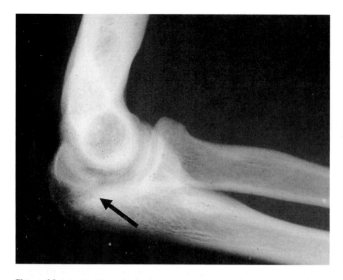

Figure 11 Lateral radiograph showing an olecranon stress fracture (arrow). *(Reproduced with permission from ElAttrache NS, Ahmad CS: Valgus extension overload and olecranon stress fractures. Sports Med Arthrosc Rev 2003;11:25-29.)*

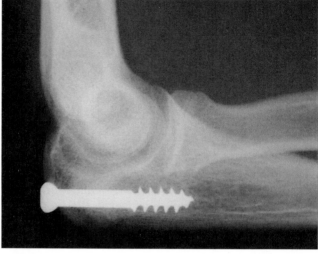

Figure 12 Open fixation with compression screw results in healing of olecranon stress fracture. *(Reproduced with permission from ElAttrache NS, Ahmad CS: Valgus extension overload and olecranon stress fractures. Sports Med Arthrosc Rev 2003;11: 25-29.)*

ity of the triceps mechanism. Radiographs are obtained to identify the fracture pattern, displacement, and presence of comminution. Nonsurgical treatment is indicated for nondisplaced fractures with the arm immobilized in 45° to 90° of flexion. Serial radiographs are obtained to check for fracture displacement that may occur with time. After 3 weeks, stability of the fracture may allow patients to do protected range-of-motion exercises, but excessive flexion must be avoided. Osseous union is usually achieved within 6 to 8 weeks, after which more aggressive range-of-motion exercises are allowed.

Displaced fractures are treated with open reduction and internal fixation, with the goals of restoring elbow extension strength, articular congruity, and elbow range of motion. Tension band wiring with Kirschner wires is commonly performed to repair avulsed olecranon fractures. Plate and screw fixation is indicated for comminuted fractures and fractures that extend beyond the coronoid. Fragment excision with repair of the triceps may be done in elderly patients, but it should be done in athletes to avoid loss of power and stability.

Radial Head Fractures

The radial head is an important valgus stabilizer to the elbow. The mechanism of injury of a radial head fracture is usually a fall onto an outstretched hand that axially loads the radius against the capitellum. Patients with radial head fractures typically report lateral elbow pain. Physical examination usually reveals localized tenderness to the radial head and often a tense effusion from an associated hemarthrosis. Range of motion must be documented. The ipsilateral forearm and wrist should be examined for the presence of associated injuries to the interosseous membrane and distal radioulnar joint.

Valgus stability and tenderness over the MUCL should also be assessed. Aspiration of the hemarthrosis and injection of lidocaine through a direct lateral approach will eliminate pain and allow assessment of a potential mechanical block to motion.

Mason type I radial head fractures have minimal or no displacement and are treated with early mobilization if no mechanical block to motion is identified. Mason type II radial head fractures are marginal fractures with obvious displacement. Aspiration should be performed and range of motion should be assessed for the presence of any mechanical block. When no mechanical block is present, treatment consists of temporary immobilization followed by range-of-motion exercises as symptoms tolerate. When a block to motion is present, treatment consists of open reduction and internal fixation. Small fragments that are not amenable to fixation and cause a block to motion may be excised. Mason type III radial head fractures are severely comminuted and displaced and may be associated with ligamentous injuries. In the absence of ligamentous injury, the radial head may be excised. When an injury to the distal radioulnar joint or interosseous membrane is identified, a radial head replacement should be considered. If the MUCL is injured, it should be primarily repaired or reconstructed.

Capitellum Fractures

Isolated fractures of the capitellum are uncommon. These fractures have been classified into three types: type I fractures are complete and also known as Hahn-Steinthal fractures, type II fractures involve a thin layer of subchondral bone with the articular surface and are also called Kocher-Lorenz fractures, and type III fractures are comminuted. Type I fractures with displacement are treated with open reduction and internal fixation with Herbert screws or standard screws countersunk below the articular surface. For type II and III fractures that are too comminuted or too small to be secured with fixation, excision is performed.

Summary

Recent studies have quantified the complex forces that develop from throwing that place the elbow at risk for injury. More precise physical examination maneuvers and newer imaging techniques have led to greater accuracy in the diagnosis of these elbow injuries. New surgical treatment options for many of these disorders have demonstrated improved outcome, with greater emphasis now placed on reproducing normal anatomy and biomechanics while minimizing muscle dissection and nerve handling.

Annotated Bibliography

General

Ahmad CS, Lee TQ, ElAttrache NS: Biomechanical evaluation of a new ulnar collateral ligament reconstruction technique with interference screw fixation. *Am J Sports Med* 2003;31:332-337.

Cadaveric elbows underwent kinematic testing under conditions of an intact, released, and reconstructed ligament. MUCL reconstruction was performed by creating single bone tunnels at the isometric anatomic insertion sites on the medial epicondyle and sublime tubercles. Palmaris longus graft fixation was achieved with soft-tissue interference screws. The ultimate moment for intact elbows (34.0 Nm) was not significantly different from that of the reconstructed elbows (30.6 Nm). Release of the ulnar collateral ligament caused a significant increase in valgus instability. Reconstruction restored valgus stability to near that of the intact elbow. This technique seems to have adequate fixation strength and returns elbow kinematics to near normal. The technique combines less soft-tissue dissection and less risk of ulnar nerve injury with ease of graft insertion, tensioning, and fixation.

Fleisig GS, Barrentine SW, Escamilla RF, Andrews JR: Biomechanics of overhand throwing with implications for injuries. *Sports Med* 1996;21:421-437.

Elbow kinetics for 26 high-level adult pitchers were calculated using high-speed motion analysis. The requirement of the ulnar collateral ligament to resist valgus torque was estimated to be 34.6 Nm.

Kamineni S, Hirahara H, Pomianowski S, et al: Partial posteromedial olecranon resection: A kinematic study. *J Bone Joint Surg Am* 2003;85:1005-1011.

The kinematic effects of increasing valgus and varus torques and posteromedial olecranon resections were studied in 12 cadaveric elbows. Three sequential resections were performed in 3-mm steps from 0 mm to 9 mm and resulted in stepwise increases in valgus angulation with valgus torque. The authors suggest that excessive removal of normal olecranon in throwing athletes may increase strain on the medial collateral ligament and recommend that bone removal from the olecranon be limited to osteophytes.

Marshall RN, Elliott BC: Long axis rotation: The missing link in proximal to distal sequencing. *J Sports Sci* 2000;18:247-254.

This biomechanical study demonstrates the coupling of internal rotation at the shoulder with pronation of the forearm just before ball impact or ball release. This coupling maximizes centripetal force to the racquet or ball and is the physiologic basis of the varus acceleration to minimize valgus elbow load.

Medial Ulnar Collateral Ligament Injuries

Azar FM, Andrews JR, Wilk KE, Groh D: Operative treatment of ulnar collateral ligament injuries of the elbow in athletes. *Am J Sports Med* 2000;28:16-23.

In this study, 78 throwing athletes underwent MUCL reconstruction with submuscular ulnar nerve transposition. Fifty-nine patients were available for follow-up at 12 to 72 months. Eighty-one percent returned to the same or higher level of competition. One patient had ulnar nerve symptoms that eventually resolved 10 months after surgery.

Ellenbecker TS, Mattalino AJ, Elam EA, Caplinger RA: Medial elbow joint laxity in professional baseball pitchers: A bilateral comparison using stress radiography. *Am J Sports Med* 1998;26:420-424.

This study evaluated differences in medial elbow laxity between the dominant and nondominant extremities in 40 uninjured baseball pitchers with a stress radiography device. With stress, the dominant elbow opened 1.20 mm, whereas the nondominant elbow opened 0.88 mm, which identifies increased medial elbow laxity in the dominant arm in uninjured pitchers.

Eygendaal D, Heijboer MP, Obermann WR, Rozing PM: Medial instability of the elbow: Findings on valgus load radiography and MRI in 16 athletes. *Acta Orthop Scand* 2000;71:480-483.

Sixteen athletes with insufficiency of the MUCL were studied with stress radiographs and MRI. Thirteen elbows showed an increase in the ulnohumeral joint space on dynamic radiography under valgus load. MRI of 10 of these 13 elbows revealed rupture or avulsion of the MUCL. Dynamic radiography under valgus load seems to be of value for the diagnosis of chronic MUCL insufficiency.

Hill NB Jr, Bucchieri JS, Shon F, Miller TT, Rosenwasser MP: Magnetic resonance imaging of injury to the medial collateral ligament of the elbow: A cadaver model. *J Shoulder Elbow Surg* 2000;9:418-422.

MRI was performed on five fresh-frozen cadaveric elbows that had MUCL lesions created. Fat-suppressed T1-weighted sequences enhanced with intra-articular gadolinium were found to provide information regarding inner-surface partial tears and small full-thickness perforations.

Rohrbough JT, Altchek DW, Hyman J: MD, Williams RJ, Botts JD: Medial collateral ligament reconstruction of the elbow using the docking technique. *Am J Sports Med* 2002;30:541-548.

Thirty-six patients with symptomatic MUCL insufficiency underwent the docking technique of MUCL reconstruction that included a muscle-splitting approach without routine transposition of the ulnar nerve and docking the two ends of the tendon graft into a single humeral tunnel. At average follow-up of 3.3 years, 92% of the patients returned to or exceeded their previous level of athletic activity for at least 1 year. The authors recommend the docking technique to allow simplified graft tensioning and improved graft fixation.

Sasaki J, Takahara M, Ogino T, Kashiwa H, Ishigaki D, Kanauchi Y: Ultrasound assessment of the ulnar collateral ligament of the medial elbow laity in college baseball players. *J Bone Joint Surg Am* 2002;84:525-531.

Ultrasonography of the medial aspect of the elbow was performed with gravity stress applied in 30 college baseball players. Medial elbow pain was associated with widening of the medial joint space and the presence of angulation of the MUCL as it bends over the distal-medial edge of the trochlea.

Thompson WH, Jobe FW, Yocum LA, Pink MM: Ulnar collateral ligament reconstruction in athletes: Muscle-splitting approach without transposition of the ulnar nerve. *J Shoulder Elbow Surg* 2001;10:152-157.

Eighty-three athletes with medial elbow instability underwent reconstruction of the MUCL with a muscle-splitting approach without transposition of the ulnar nerve. At 2-year follow-up of 33 athletes, 5% of the patients had transient ulnar nerve symptoms, all of which resolved with nonsurgical management, and 93% of the patients who had not undergone a previous surgical procedure had excellent results.

Lateral Ulnar Collateral Ligament Injuries

O'Driscoll SW: Classification and evaluation of recurrent instability of the elbow. *Clin Orthop* 2000;370:34-43.

This article provides an excellent description of the physical examination for posterolateral rotatory elbow instability.

Osteochondritis Dissecans of the Capitellum

Baumgarten TE, Andrews JR, Satterwhite YE: The arthroscopic classification and treatment of osteochondritis dissecans of the capitellum. *Am J Sports Med* 1998; 26:520-523.

Fourteen excellent results were reported in a group of 17 patients who underwent arthroscopic débridement and abrasion chondroplasty for capitellar osteochondritis dissecans. Fourteen of 17 patients (82%) returned to their preinjury activity levels at an average follow-up of 48 months. No radiographic degenerative changes were noted, but slight residual flattening of the capitellum was seen in eight patients.

Kiyoshige Y, Takagi M, Yuasa K, Hamasaki M: Closed-wedge osteotomy for osteochondritis dissecans of the

capitellum: A 7 to 12 year follow-up. *Am J Sports Med* 2000;28:534-537.

Lateral closing wedge osteotomy of the capitellum was used to treat osteochondritis dissecans of the capitellum in seven baseball players 11 to 18 of age. The goal of the procedure was to unload the radiocapitellar joint while maintaining the alignment of the ulnohumeral joint. At 7- to 12-year follow-up, 6 of 7 patients (86%) had complete relief of pain with return to full activity, all had increased range of motion, all had remodeling of the capitellum, and none had enlargement of the radial head. These results, although promising, remain preliminary because of the small study population.

Takahara M, Ogino T, Sasaki I, Kato H, Minami A, Kaneda K: Long term outcome of osteochondritis dissecans of the humeral capitellum. *Clin Orthop* 1999;363: 108-115.

This study reports the long-term follow-up of 53 patients who underwent either nonsurgical or surgical treatment for osteochondritis dissecans of the humeral capitellum. Poor outcome was observed in 7 of 14 patients treated nonsurgically and 18 of 39 who underwent surgical removal of a loose fragment. Poor outcomes seemed to be related to advanced size and progression of the lesions.

Classic Bibliography

Andrews JR, Timmerman LA: Outcome of elbow surgery in professional baseball players. *Am J Sports Med* 1995;23:407-413.

Baur M, Jonsson K, Josefsson PO, Linden B: Osteochondritis dissecans of the elbow: A long term follow-up study. *Clin Orthop* 1992;284:156-160.

Conway JE, Jobe FW, Glousman RE, Pink M: Medial instability of the elbow in throwing athletes: Treatment by repair or reconstruction of the ulnar collateral ligament. *J Bone Joint Surg Am* 1992;74:67-83.

Davidson PA, Pink M, Perry J, Jobe FW: Functional anatomy of the flexor pronator muscle group in relation to the medial collateral ligament of the elbow. *Am J Sports Med* 1995;23:245-250.

Field LD, Callaway GH, O'Brien SJ, Altchek DW: Arthroscopic assessment of the medial collateral ligament complex of the elbow. *Am J Sports Med* 1995;23:396-400.

Hamilton CD, Glousman RE, Jobe FW, Brault J, Pink M, Perry J: Dynamic stability of the elbow: Electromyographic analysis of the flexor pronator group and the extensor group in pitchers with valgus instability. *J Shoulder Elbow Surg* 1996;5:347-354.

Morrey BF, An KN: Articular and ligamentous contributions to the stability of the elbow joint. *Am J Sports Med* 1983;11:315-319.

Nuber GW, Diment MT: Olecranon stress fractures in throwers: A report of two cases and review of the literature. *Clin Orthop* 1992;278:58-61.

O'Driscoll SW, Bell DF, Morrey BF: Posterolateral rotatory instability of the elbow. *J Bone Joint Surg Am* 1991; 73:440-446.

Potter HG, Weiland AJ, Schatz JE, Paletta GA, Hotchkiss RN: Posterolateral rotatory instability of the elbow: Usefulness of MR imaging in diagnosis. *Radiology* 1997; 204:185-189.

Putnam CA: Sequential motions of body segments in striking and throwing skills. *J Biomech* 1993;26:125-135.

Regan WD, Korinek SL, Morrey BF, An KN: Biomechanical study of ligaments around the elbow joint. *Clin Orthop* 1991;271:170-179.

Schwab GH, Bennett JB, Woods GW, Tullos HS: Biomechanics of elbow instability: The role of the medial collateral ligament. *Clin Orthop* 1980;146:42-52.

Schwartz ML, Al-Zahrani S, Morwessel RM, Andrews JR: Ulnar collateral ligament injury in the throwing athlete: Evaluation with saline-enhanced MR arthrography. *Radiology* 1995;197:297-299.

Suzuki K, Minami A, Suenaga N, Konodoh M: Oblique stress fracture of the olecranon in baseball pitchers. *J Shoulder Elbow Surg* 1997;6:491-494.

Timmerman LA, Schwartz ML, Andrews JR: Preoperative evaluation of the ulnar collateral ligament by magnetic resonance imaging and computed tomography arthrography: Evaluation in 25 baseball players with surgical confirmation. *Am J Sports Med* 1994;22:26-31.

Wilson FD, Andrews JR, Blackburn TA, McCluskey G: Valgus extension overload in the pitching elbow. *Am J Sports Med* 1983;11:83-88.

Chapter 9

Hand and Wrist Injuries

Kevin D. Plancher, MD, MS

Timothy A. Luke, MD

Introduction

The severity of injuries to the hand and wrist is often minimized when they occur in athletes. Whereas athletic participation is often halted when a foot or toe injury occurs, great pressure is frequently imposed on athletes to continue to play after experiencing strains, sprains, ligament or cartilage tears, or fractures of the hand and wrist. This unfortunately compromises the care of many athletes who return to the field of play without an adequate diagnosis or treatment, which can result in long-term complications. As awareness of hand and wrist injuries increases, the magnitude of specific injuries will be treated and the health of the athlete will improve. Therefore, it is important for orthopaedic surgeons to treat these injuries appropriately; to do so, physicians must be aware of the new modalities that are available to treat hand and wrist injuries in athletes and allow for accelerated return to athletic participation.

Epidemiology

Long-term studies have shown that approximately 10% of all athletic injuries involve the hand and wrist. Over a 4-year period, the incidence of hand and wrist injuries as a result of participation in youth and professional football has been reported to be 35% and 15%, respectively. Scaphoid fractures in the general population account for 70% of all wrist fractures (excluding fractures of the distal radius). In gymnastics, the incidence of acute and chronic wrist injuries ranges from 46% to 87%, with injuries occurring more commonly during competition than practice. Rock climbers have a 44.3% incidence of finger, flexor tendon, and pulley injuries. The incidence of upper extremity injuries in adults who participate in athletic activities is reported to be approximately 15%; in the general adolescent population, it is reported to be approximately 39%. The incidence of adult and adolescent athletic injuries of the hand and wrist are reported to be 6% and 9%, respectively, which suggests that athletic participation does not necessarily increase the risk of epiphyseal injuries in adolescents.

Wrist Imaging

Various imaging modalities are available to evaluate sports-related hand and wrist injuries. The medical history, physical examination, and treating physician's experience will help determine whether any additional diagnostic tests are necessary. Diagnostic studies may detect a significant abnormality even though the physical examination may be "normal." Because the presence of an abnormality does not necessarily mean the patient is symptomatic, it is important to treat the patient in accordance with the symptoms and restrict activities accordingly instead of treating the results of imaging studies.

Plain Radiographs

Plain radiographs for injuries of the hand and wrist typically consist of a standard hand series, which includes AP and splay lateral views, and the standard wrist series, which includes zero PA, lateral, and oblique views. If a scaphoid fracture is suspected, an ulnar and radial deviated view and a clenched fist view are added. Special views can help in the detection of unusual injuries of the hand and wrist (Table 1).

Tomography

Tomography provides sectional radiographic images. The main disadvantage of linear tomography is that it can produce artifacts from the edges parallel to the plane of motion. Its advantages over CT, however, are that the equipment is less expensive and images can be obtained in multiple planes. Recent studies have clearly shown that trispiral tomography is more accurate and cost-effective than CT and should be considered the imaging modality of choice for assessing articular step-off in patients with distal radius fractures. Unfortunately, trispiral tomography is not widely available and few technicians know how to operate the equipment for this type of diagnostic imaging.

TABLE 1 | Additional Plain Radiographic Views for Hand and Wrist Injuries

Radiographic View	Rationale
Bora view	Bases of the fourth and fifth metacarpals and carpometacarpal with hamate
Ballcatcher view (Norgaard)	Dorsoradial aspect of the second to fifth phalangeal bases
Brewerton view	Distal articular surface of the second to fifth metacarpals
Eaton stress thumb view	Trapeziometacarpal joint under stress
Hook of hamate view (Papillon)	Hamate hook in its broadest aspect
Carpal tunnel view (Gaynor-Hart)	Carpal tunnel tangential projection
Capitate view	Entire capitate with less foreshortening than a PA view
Pisiform oblique view (Holly)	Pisiform without superimposition of the triquetrum
Modified Roberts hyperpronation thumb view	AP projection of the trapeziometacarpal joint
Carpal boss view	Carpal boss, dorsal bases of the second and third metacarpals

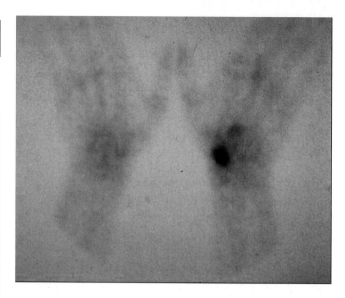

Figure 1 Bone scan of an occult scaphoid fracture.

Bone Scintigraphy

In three-phase bone scintigraphy, the first phase assesses local blood flow, and the second phase (static or blood pool phase) shows the distribution of the tracer within the soft tissue. Delayed-phase images obtained 3 hours after the injection of tracer depicts the local rate of bone turnover (Figure 1). Focal, very intense bone scan abnormalities will provide evidence of fractures; bone scans with subtle findings may not have as predictable results.

Most fractures will show increased activity at 3 days, although many are apparent within the first 24 hours. Delayed-reaction changes are more likely in elderly patients because bone forms more slowly in this population. A diffuse uptake indicates a reactive process or synovitis. A focal uptake indicates a ligament or osteochondral injury. A reduction of uptake or "cold spot" may indicate a cyst or osteonecrosis. Bone scintigraphy may be used 72 hours after an injury to identify or rule out the presence of an occult fracture.

Bone scintigraphy has recently been used to evaluate physiologically active osteochondral problems in patients with unexplained wrist pain. Cyst-like changes seen within the scaphoid are often incorrectly called cysts and may actually be filled with fiber, in which instance they should more appropriately be described as lucent defects. When focal tenderness is associated with these lucent defects, bone scintigraphy may help deter-

mine whether this is a "hot" or active lesion. An active interosseous ganglion cyst may require excision.

Wrist Arthrography

When used for patients with acute trauma in the distal radius, wrist arthrography has been 88% sensitive in correctly diagnosing interosseous carpal ligament and triangular fibrocartilage complex (TFCC) tears. Fibrous or cartilaginous scaphoid unions can also be distinguished with wrist arthrography. A radiocarpal or midcarpal injection can be used. When a pseudarthrosis between the scaphoid fragments is present, arthrography demonstrates opacification of the fracture line and communication between the radiocarpal and midcarpal compartments.

Computed Tomography

It may be difficult to perform direct coronal CT in the acute setting because of pain on movement of the wrist. Most patients with chronic injury can position the arm overhead to allow for adequate data acquisition. Slight extension of the hand removes the distal forearm from most of the coronal images. CT is completed much more rapidly than MRI and therefore is advantageous for patients in discomfort. One of the best ways to examine the scaphoid is to obtain direct CT scans along its long axis using an oblique sagittal view (oblique to the hand but directly sagittal to the long axis of the scaphoid) in a direct coronal plane. Sectioning parallel to the true long axis of the scaphoid has become the gold standard for identifying the humpback deformity of the scaphoid; this view can also identify the shape of the scaphoid after bone grafting to determine whether union has been achieved (Figure 2).

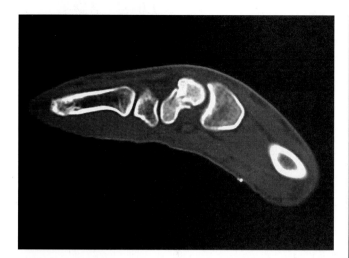

Figure 2 CT scan showing a humpback deformity with sclerotic borders at the non-union site.

Magnetic Resonance Imaging

MRI is more popular with patients than CT because it does not expose patients to ionizing radiation and provides greater soft-tissue detail. Stronger magnets are no longer needed to provide the fine resolution necessary to show small structures such as the scaphoid, and surface coils have improved the overall quality of MRI.

Evaluation of the scaphoid requires sections that are 2 mm thick and taken at 1- to 2-mm intervals. If hardware is present in the wrist, the wrist should be placed parallel to the axis of the hardware as it passes through the scaphoid. A metal screw or wire placed parallel to the gantry can make a metallic streak artifact appear much less obvious. MRI of a healing scaphoid fracture will demonstrate low-signal intensity, which should persist with contrast surrounding a bright signal intensity indicative of marrow edema seen during healing. Sagittal images demonstrate the abnormal morphology of the scaphoid secondary to fracture fragmentation or a humpback deformity.

The articular cartilage of the scaphoid and adjacent surfaces can easily be assessed. Short T1 inversion or fat-suppressed T2-weighted fast spin-echo sequences are more sensitive to hyperemia in the proximal pole of the scaphoid, which may often be misdiagnosed as end stage osteonecrosis (Figure 3) or sclerosis on conventional T1- or T2-weighted images. Tears of the scapholunate ligament can be reliably diagnosed with MRI, whereas tears of the lunotriquetral ligament cannot.

Magnetic Resonance Angiography

MRI provides excellent detail for tumor staging. It also provides extensive information for soft-tissue tumors in the hand and wrist. If ganglion cysts are excluded, the most commonly encountered soft-tissue masses of the

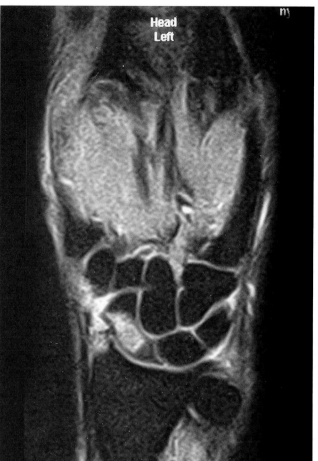

Figure 3 MRI scan showing scaphoid osteonecrosis.

hand and wrist are vascular malformations. Magnetic resonance angiography can demonstrate the vascularity of these lesions and thereby help clinicians formulate treatment options.

Wrist Arthroscopy

Wrist and small joint arthroscopy is ideal for evaluating intra-articular soft-tissue and bony injuries of the hand and wrist. It has been used recently to successfully treat patients with chronic wrist pain, even patients with no evidence of injury during workup. New applications for small joint arthroscopy include arthroscopic wrist capsular release, arthroscopic débridement in wrist arthritis, arthroscopy of the metacarpophalangeal joints, laser-assisted procedures, arthroscopic-assisted scaphoid internal fixation, intra-articular distal radius transcutaneous pin fixation and fracture reduction, repair of radial-sided TFCC tears, stabilization of acute carpal dislocation patterns, and description of anterior portals to allow for a more complete evaluation of the radial carpal joint.

Indications

Arthroscopy may be used for persistent disabling mechanical wrist pain of unknown origin provided the appropriate workup has been completed and no evidence of injury is identified. Judicious use of arthroscopy for this indication is imperative for the integrity of the procedure. Although it has become the gold standard for diagnosing mechanical wrist pain (catching, popping, or clicking in the wrist), arthroscopy is contraindicated for the treatment of dystrophic pain.

Arthritis

Arthroscopic débridement of an arthritic wrist is used frequently as an accepted minimally invasive technique for mature adults with painful wrists who want to prolong participation in sports activities. Patients generally regain motion from the removal of loose bodies as well as a radial styloidectomy. Isolated reports of attempts at arthroscopic proximal row carpectomy demonstrate mixed success. Stiffness after trauma or surgery to the wrist is common, and loss of motion may be reversed with arthroscopic capsular release. Although cadaveric studies of arthroscopic capsular release are limited, success with this technique has been reported, and good improvement in range of motion (17° to 47° of flexion and 10° to 50° in extension) without complications has been noted. A safe zone for neurovascular structures during arthroscopic capsular release has been described, and wrist strength with a capsular release has also been noted.

Laser-assisted arthroscopy with a holmium:yttrium-aluminum-garnet (Ho:YAG) laser is perfectly suited for the wrist because the small probes used during this procedure are efficient in tissue ablation and function in the infrared region of the electromagnetic spectrum at 2.1 nm. Although laser-assisted arthroscopy can be more efficient, the cost is often prohibitive. Volar portals for wrist arthroscopy are now being used more frequently, allowing assessment and treatment of dorsal capsular and articular cartilage defects. Complications noted in the literature have been limited to date.

Radial-Sided TFCC Repairs

The loss of the TFCC may lead to subluxation and dislocation of the distal radial ulnar joint (ie, the ligamentous connections between the distal radius and the ulnar side of the carpus) (Figure 4). Excision of the TFCC in a patient with positive ulnar variance over time leads to an increase in ulnar lunate abutment, erosion of the cartilage, and increasing wrist pain. Excellent results with arthroscopic repair of ulnar-sided TFCC perforations have been reported in at least 84% of patients with Palmer class 1 lesions. The repair of Palmer class 1D or radial-sided lesions are now being reported, and equipment advances have resulted in the development of several new techniques (Figure 5).

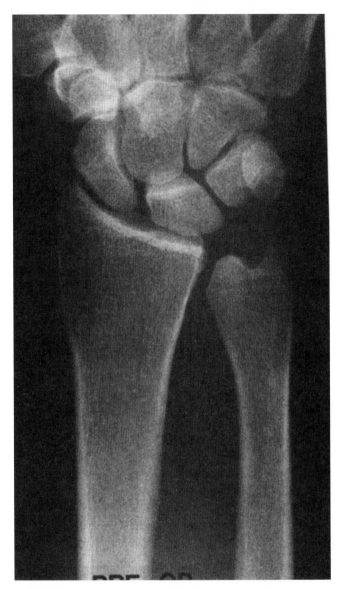

Figure 4 Plain AP radiograph showing a disrupted distal radioulnar joint in a patient who is an avid wind surfer.

Radiocarpal Pathology and Distal Intra-articular Radius Fractures

The identification and treatment of scapholunate and interosseous ligament injuries that occur in association with radial styloid fractures is now routine. This arthroscopic technique minimizes postoperative scarring and returns motion to the wrist faster than an open reduction. In addition, harmful osteochondral flaps and loose bodies not visible on routine radiographs are easily identified. Outcome data from a recent report indicate that limited open reduction may increase the range of motion of the wrist by 20° or more compared with that achieved using a corresponding open reduction. Scapholunate ligament damage occurs when the head of the capitate compresses the scaphoid and lunate space. The scaphoid will inherently flex because of its oblique

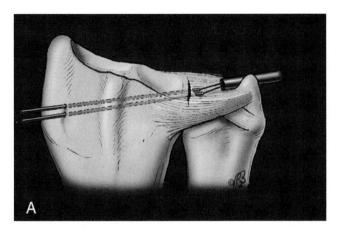

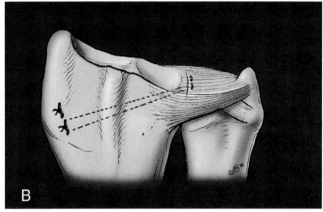

Figure 5 Surgical triangular fibrocartilage complex radial sided repair. **A**, Guides are positioned and verified intraoperatively. **B**, Sutures are passed, and the triangular fibrocartilage complex is secured. *(© 1999 Kevin D. Plancher, MD.)*

position and the loading force applied through the scaphotrapeziotrapezoidal joint. The identification and accurate assessment of associated soft-tissue injuries with early intervention has had a large impact on the final outcome of all patients with intra-articular distal radius fractures.

Arthroscopic-guided reduction and internal fixation of a distal radius fracture should be used not only for young adults, but also for all patients younger than 70 years and those with a distal radius fracture with displacement of greater than 1.0 mm on plain radiographs. Arthroscopic intra-articular distal radius fixation can lead to anatomic restoration of the cartilage and bony surfaces. In one study, mean pain scores were reported as 1.3 (range, 1 to 10), with 88% excellent to good results. Associated injuries included scapholunate ligament tears (85%), TFCC tears (58%), osteochondral lesions (19%), and lunotriquetral ligament tears (6%).

Scaphoid Fractures
Prolonged immobilization can now be avoided when treating patients with nondisplaced scaphoid fractures by using arthroscopically assisted scaphoid reduction; it can also help athletes with nondisplaced scaphoid fractures return to athletic activity more rapidly. Several reports have noted an absence of nonunions with minimal morbidity using this technique. Wrist arthroscopy provides greatly enhanced visualization of the articular surface of the wrist joint and avoids the morbidity associated with wrist arthrotomy.

Ganglia
Several authors have reported on the successful arthroscopic ablation of ganglia. The advantages of arthroscopic ganglionectomy over open excision include increased early range of motion, reduced skin problems, and an apparent decrease in the rate of recurrence.

Carpometacarpal Joints
Arthroscopy of the metacarpophalangeal joint allows direct inspection of the thumb joint for ulnar collateral ligament repairs. Loose bodies can be removed and intra-articular fractures of the metacarpophalangeal joint can be reduced using this technique. Use of a mini-fluoroscopy unit and a 2.3-mm, 30° angled arthroscope permits complete visualization. Arthroscopy of the metacarpophalangeal joint can also help diagnose pathology with minimal soft-tissue disruption.

Complications
Four categories of complications are associated with wrist arthroscopy: (1) complications related to traction and arm position, (2) complications related to the establishment of portals, (3) procedure-specific complications, and (4) miscellaneous complications associated with arthroscopy. Because injury to the metacarpophalangeal or proximal interphalangeal joints can be caused by excessive traction, traction should be limited to 10 lb and four finger traps should be used to distribute the force. Disposable plastic finger traps are gentler on the skin. Exercising extreme care when establishing portal placement and making the incision only through the skin can also help minimize complications, as can spreading of the soft tissue with a hemostat to avoid cutaneous nerve injury. Iatrogenic articular scuffing and chondral lesions can be avoided by using appropriately sized instruments, gentle technique, and proper portal placement.

Complications may be further minimized by using adequate padding and taking care to position the patient to avoid traction injuries to the peripheral nerves of the wrist and forearm. The 6-R portal places the extensor carpi ulnaris and the extensor digiti quinti at risk, whereas the 6-R and 6-U portals both place the transverse branch of the dorsal ulnar sensory nerve at risk. Deep insertion of the scalpel blade should be avoided to protect the cutaneous nerves. Using the safe zone on the

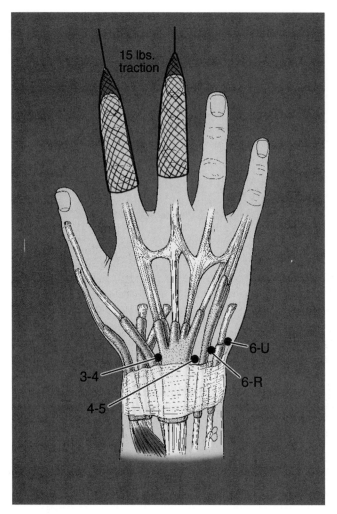

Figure 6 Location of the arthroscopic wrist portals. (© 1999 Kevin D. Plancher, MD.)

radial side of the wrist will help avoid injury to the superficial radial nerve. Although arthroscopic-assisted reduction of internal fixation of the distal radius is increasing in popularity, patients who undergo this procedure must be monitored for compartment syndrome. Distal radius procedures should not be performed within 3 days of the initial injury (Figure 6).

Ulnar-Sided Wrist Pain

Ulna Impaction Syndrome

When the forearm and wrist are in a neutral position, the ulna bears 15% of the load during flexion and extension. This load increases to 24% with ulnar deviation and 37% with pronation. The dorsal triquetrum and hamate are forced toward one another with ulnar deviation. The dorsal articular surfaces are compressed with an extreme range of wrist extension. Movements of pronation and ulnar deviation cause the ulna and triquetrum to impact on each other. These movements lead to an ulna impaction syndrome, which occurs in gymnasts using the pommel horse (males) and the vault

(females). Measured forces were found to be up to two times body weight, with loading rates in excess of five times body weight per second in athletes performing these activities.

Instability

Scapholunate Ligament Instability

Ligament injuries leading to instability of the wrist occur in contact sports such as football, basketball, rugby, and ice hockey or as the result of a high-energy impact or fall from a height. Instability can also be caused by repetitive loading with the wrist in extension, resulting in a pure rotational ligamentous injury called scapholunate ligament instability. Scapholunate ligament instability typically occurs in patients who play tennis or ice hockey. During the fall, the wrist is often injured with extension and loading of the ulna.

Lunotriquetral Ligament Instability

Ulnar-sided wrist pain or dorsal wrist pain over the lunotriquetral ligament with grip weakness, loss of motion, ulnar nerve paresthesias, and a detectable "clunk" on examination are all symptoms of lunotriquetral ligament instability. Tears of the membranous portion of the lunotriquetral ligaments may be a cause of mechanical irritation of the wrist. These membranous tears may cause a lunotriquetral ligament coalition, which is most often asymptomatic. A symptomatic incomplete coalition may be a source of discomfort, in which instance arthrodesis is the treatment of choice.

Lunotriquetral ligament pathology may result from injury to the hypothenar eminence or ulnar variance of ± 2 mm with a distal radius malunion or a resected radial head. Pathoanatomy has shown that complete lunotriquetral ligament tears alone do not cause static volar flexed intercalated segment instability deformities; the dorsal radiotriquetral must be also torn to cause these deformities.

Physical Examination

Physical examination of patients for ulnar-sided wrist pain is easily done, and there are many new tests available to assess patients for this condition. Classic tests include the ballottement test and the Kleinman shear test. In the ballottement test, the lunate is firmly stabilized with the thumb and index finger of one hand while the triquetrum and pisiform are displaced dorsally and palmarly with the other hand; when crepitus, pain, and extreme laxity are present, the test result is positive. The Kleinman shear test is done by stabilizing the dorsal aspect of the lunate just beyond the medial edge of the distal radius with the pisiform loaded in a dorsal direction and creating a shear force at the lunotriquetral joint; when crepitus, pain, and increased motion are present, the test result is positive.

Routine radiographs are often normal in patients with ulnar-sided wrist pain and diagnostic only in patients with advanced volar intercalated segment instability. Plain radiographs will show that Gilula's line is disrupted at the lunotriquetral ligament, and there will be an overlap of the lunate and triquetrum. The carpal height ratio in patients with this injury may be abnormal (normal, 0.54 ± 0.03) with a positive ring sign, but no lunotriquetral or scapholunate ligament gap (pseudogap) may be present.

When arthrography is used, lunotriquetral ligament tears will be confirmed by the leakage of dye from the midcarpal space to the radial carpal joint through the interval, which is normally occluded by the ligament. If this test result is negative, dye should be injected into the radial carpal space to assess leakage to the distal radial ulnar joint, which is diagnostic of a TFCC tear. The sensitivity of MRI for the diagnosis of lunotriquetral ligament tears is 23% to 50%. Nonsurgical treatment consists of a cast or splint.

In acute settings, arthroscopy allows for visualization of partial ligament tears and treatment of symptomatic wrists without gross instability. Débridement with motorized shavers and basket forceps can help restore wrist function. Electrosurgical heat probes, available in small sizes, allow for ablation of tissue rather than excision.

Open surgical treatment is directed at restoring normal carpal kinematics. Ligament repair with suture anchors is a viable treatment with or without capsular augmentation. If a volar intercalated segment instability deformity exists, lunotriquetral ligament repair will not suffice, and a four-quadrant arthrodesis may be considered. Ligament reconstructions have high failure rates. Reconstruction with flexor carpi ulnaris, extensor carpi ulnaris, or other grafts often requires a lunotriquetral ligament arthrodesis with ulnar shortening.

Kienböck Disease

Adults between the ages of 30 and 40 years who participate in repetitive activities in which impact or single traumatic blows to the hand occur (such as the martial arts) are susceptible to microfractures of the lunate. The radius, by extending further than the ulna, subjects the lunate to large compressive and shear forces. Over time, disruption of the blood supply may lead to Kienböck disease, which is defined as osteonecrosis of the lunate.

Physical examination of patients with Kienböck disease typically reveals tenderness to palpation at the radiolunate joint and a decreased range of motion of the wrist in flexion and extension. There is a significant association between the presence of Kienböck disease and negative ulnar variance (Figure 7). Plain radiographs will show radiodensity changes, fracture lines, and can have progressive collapse of the lunate and proximal migration of capitate. MRI is most effective for evaluating medullary circulation and edema. PA and lateral ra-

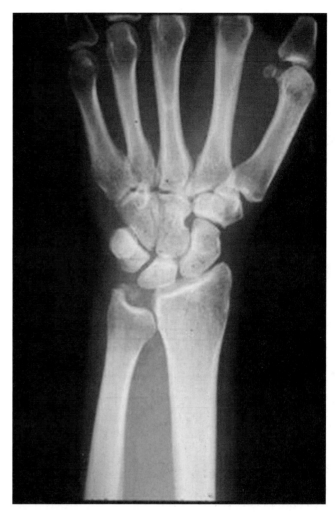

Figure 7 Plain radiograph showing negative ulnar variance.

diographic evidence is used to classify Kienböck disease into the following four stages: in stage I, no radiographic changes in the lunate are visible on plain radiographs; in stage II, sclerosis is visible; in stage III, collapse is visible; and in stage IV, total degeneration is visible.

Treatment includes immobilization for stage I Kienböck disease, and revascularization and ulnar lengthening and/or radial shortening for stage II. Stage IIIA is treated with excision of the lunate and autogenous tendon graft with capitohamate fusion; stage IIIB with a capitohamate fusion, tricaphate fusion, or other limited intercarpal fusions; and stage IV with limited intercarpal fusion, a proximal row carpectomy with or without denervation of the posterior interosseous nerve, or wrist arthrodesis.

Pisotriquetral Osteoarthritis

Osteoarthritis of the pisotriquetral joint, while uncommon, is prevalent in gymnasts. The pisotriquetral view can often detect arthritis between the pisiform and triquetrum joints. This entity can cause local inflammation

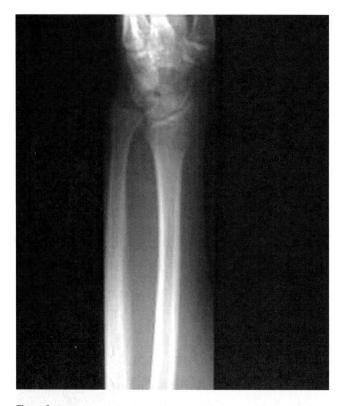

Figure 8 Plain radiograph showing positive ulnar variance.

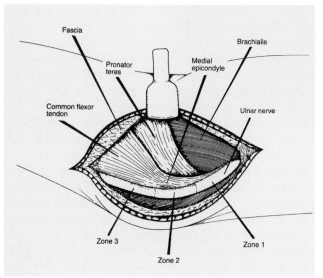

Figure 9 The zones of ulnar nerve distribution of the hand. (© 1996 Kevin D. Plancher, MD.)

of the pisiform in racquet players and may also result in Guyon's canal syndrome. Conservative treatment with steroid injections can alleviate the pain, but care must be taken to avoid injecting the ulnar artery. Excision of the pisiform can lead to resolution of symptoms in patients whose symptoms are refractory to conservative treatment.

TFCC Tears

Symptomatic TFCC tears can significantly improve with débridement. The central portion of the TFCC can be excised or ablated with electrocautery, but the peripheral margins must be preserved to maintain the stability of the distal radioulnar joint. When chondromalacia of the lunate is present on visualization of the ulnar head, it is evidence of ulnocarpal impaction. In such instances, débridement of the TFCC alone will fail if not combined with ulnar shortening (Figure 8). One study reported that patients with TFCC tears who were treated with débridement alone experienced resolution of symptoms after ulnar shortening was done.

Nerve Impingement

Ulnar Nerve Compression at the Wrist

Guyon's canal syndrome (ulnar nerve compression at the wrist) can occur when the ulnar nerve is compressed as it enters the ulnar tunnel or when the superficial or deep branch of the ulnar nerve is compressed in its tun-

nel. The deep branch winds around the hook of the hamate bone and then traverses the palm. Ulnar nerve compression may be caused by ganglia, lipomas, anatomic anomalies, carpal fractures (hook of the hamate bone), local inflammation, or vascular compromise (ie, ulnar artery thrombosis).

Athletic injuries involving Guyon's canal comprise chronic direct compression or acute trauma. Cyclists with "handlebar palsy" or "cyclist palsy" have chronic direct compression or acute trauma to the ulna nerve at the wrist. Repetitive pushing or compression, as occurs in baseball catchers, handball players, and participants in other racquet sports, may also cause Guyon's canal compression. "Push-up" palsy or a missed golf swing or baseball swing that causes a hook of the hamate bone fracture may also result in Guyon's canal compression. Symptoms in patients may vary, depending on whether the injury is the result of a motor, sensory, or mixed lesion. The level of the lesion is located by identifying the exact pattern of motor, sensory, or combined ulnar nerve neuropathy.

Pressure at or proximal to the bifurcation of the ulnar nerve will result in both sensory and motor deficits. Sensory loss in the ulnar nerve distribution and intrinsic muscle weakness or atrophy may also be identified (Figure 9). Testing for a Tinel's sign at the wrist crease may cause paresthesias in the ring and little fingers. Allen's test should be performed to confirm ulnar collateral circulation to the superficial or deep palmar arches (negative results confirm normal circulation). Two-point discrimination should be checked and muscle strength documented. Pressure in Guyon's canal distal to the bifurcation will result in either sensory (superficial branch) or motor (deep branch) deficits.

Plain radiographs can be used to rule out masses, hook of the hamate bone fractures, or other bony abnormalities. CT is the gold standard for identifying hook of the hamate bone fractures. Electromyograms of both the ulnar and median nerves may be helpful. A difference in conduction velocity of only 1 millisecond is considered significant, and changes will assist in identifying the location of a lesion in Guyon's canal (distal or more proximal area of compression).

Surgical treatment is indicated if conservative measures fail. Surgical management requires transection of the volar carpal ligament to decompress the canal, which permits visualization of the superficial branch and main trunk of the ulnar nerve. Dissection is continued to the branch of the adductor digiti quinti minimi, whereupon the pisohamate ligament is released up to the deep branch of the ulnar nerve. Care must be taken during surgery to avoid injury to the palmar cutaneous branch of the ulnar nerve. Neuroma formation must also be avoided, and failure to reach Guyon's canal in its distal third can be associated with continued entrapment neuropathy.

Tendinopathy

Flexor Carpi Ulnaris
Localized swelling over the flexor carpi ulnaris tendon is common in athletes who participate in squash, badminton, and golf. Tenderness over the tendon with pain elicited on passive wrist extension or resisted palmar flexion will confirm the diagnosis. On rare occasions, when a corticosteroid injection and splinting have failed to relieve symptoms, surgery is necessary to excise calcific deposits or lyse adhesions.

Extensor Carpi Ulnaris
Subluxation and tendinitis of the extensor carpi ulnaris tendon can occur as the result of a traumatic event in athletes who participate in rowing, badminton, and squash. Subluxation results from forearm hypersupination while the wrist is in ulnar deviation and palmar flexion. Because forceful wrist flexion motion is necessary for these activities, overuse injuries can result, especially in athletes who participate in racquet sports that require rapid deceleration at ball strike. Athletes with a subluxating tendon typically report painful snapping with forearm supination and ulnar deviation of the hand. Pronation of the forearm often restores the tendon to its correct anatomic position. Acute subluxation should be treated in a long arm cast in pronation with slight dorsiflexion at the wrist for 6 weeks. Persistent or chronic symptoms may require surgical intervention to restore the tendon to its anatomic position.

Fractures

Hook of the hamate bone fractures occur as a result of direct force from a bat, racquet, golf club, or ball. Pa-

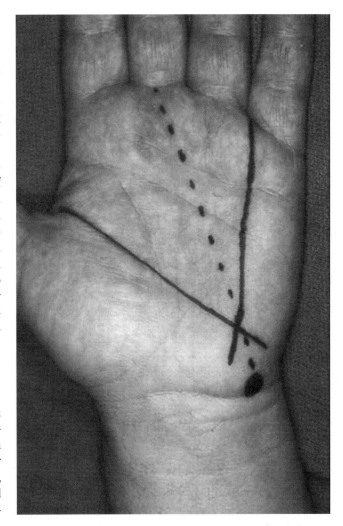

Figure 10 Photograph showing the lines drawn to locate the hook of the hamate bone.

tients with hook of the hamate bone fractures typically report pain localized over the dorsal aspect of the fourth ray (Figure 10). Patients who have been incorrectly diagnosed report chronic symptoms that include numbness and tingling in an ulnar nerve distribution. An athlete with an untreated hook of the hamate bone fracture and chronic symptoms may have a ruptured flexor tendon of the ring or little finger as the only complaint. Plain radiographs, a hamate view, and CT may be necessary to confirm the diagnosis.

Nondisplaced hook of the hamate bone fractures are more common than body fractures. These body fractures are associated with dorsal dislocations of the fourth and fifth metacarpals. Many acute hook of the hamate bone fractures do not heal despite appropriate conservative or surgical treatment. Excision of the hamate bone hook through the fracture site is the most effective method of returning the athlete to competition within 6 to 8 weeks. Displaced fractures of the hamate bone body should be reduced and stabilized with fluoroscopic guidance and a

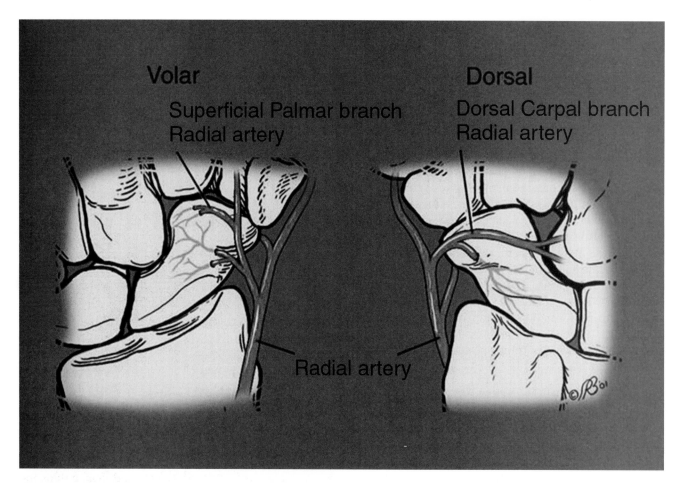

Figure 11 The vascular supply of the scaphoid. (© 2001 Kevin D. Plancher, MD.)

screw. Complications are infrequent unless diagnosis is delayed and the flexor tendon and distal nerve distribution are compromised. An incision that passes directly over the glabrous skin of the hypothenar eminence may result in a tender, painful scar and residual scar tenderness, which can delay the return of full function and the return to athletic activities.

Radial-Sided Wrist Pain

Fractures

Scaphoid
Athletes with proximal pole scaphoid fractures must have these injuries diagnosed early to avoid the complication of a nonunion. Most scaphoid nondisplaced waist fractures heal within 3 months with long arm cast treatment. The amount of displacement of waist fractures is often underestimated by radiographs, and no more than 1 mm of displacement is acceptable. The nonunion rate for proximal pole injuries is unacceptably high with closed treatment. To avoid prolonged immobilization and nonunion, immediate fixation of proximal pole fractures using percutaneous screws is used by most surgeons.

Patients with scaphoid fractures typically report pain and swelling on the radial side of the wrist with tenderness localized to the anatomic snuffbox. Because an injury resulting from minor trauma may be misleading, tenderness in the anatomic snuffbox justifies radiographic imaging to avoid a delay in diagnosis.

The vascular supply of the scaphoid plays a prominent role in the high incidence of scaphoid fracture nonunions (Figure 11). The proximal pole of the scaphoid, which is covered by hyaline cartilage, has a single ligamentous attachment to the deep radial scapholunate ligament providing minimal blood supply. This part of the scaphoid receives its blood supply from interosseous vessels that pass in a retrograde fashion from the waist of the scaphoid. The superficial palmar branch of the radial artery passes volarly along with the dorsal carpal branch of the radial artery and supplies blood to the tubercle and most distal aspects of the scaphoid.

Nonsurgical Treatment
Nonsurgical treatment is indicated for patients with acute and stable fracture patterns. Unless there is considerable deformity and displacement, scaphoid frac-

tures in skeletally immature patients are best treated nonsurgically. Severe osteopenia or stiffness of the wrist is also an indication for nonsurgical treatment. Fractures of the scaphoid tubercle and incomplete fractures of the scaphoid have an excellent prognosis with nonsurgical treatment. Although controversy continues regarding the best position and type of immobilization for this type of fracture, a long arm thumb spica cast for 6 weeks followed by a short arm thumb spica cast for 6 weeks provides optimal immobilization. In athletes with nondisplaced fractures of the wrist, an RTV-11 playing cast (General Electric, Fairfield, CT) may be used effectively to immobilize the patient and allow contact sports participation to continue.

Surgical Treatment

Scaphoid fractures that are displaced more than 1 mm usually require surgical intervention. Failure to reduce these fractures anatomically may result in a high rate of nonunion. Open reduction with a volar approach and fixation with Kirschner wires (K-wires), Herbert screws, or Acutrak screws have all been described. Procedures using the latter two are technically more demanding, but Herbert screws and Acutrak screws have the advantages of providing compression and allowing for early mobilization.

Simple transverse fractures of the waist of the scaphoid are stabilized with a standard palmar approach; if comminution is present, however, bone graft should be used. Newer studies show that synthetic bone substitutes may work better and faster than iliac crest bone grafts, which is the current gold standard of treatment; unfortunately, no long-term prospective studies comparing them have yet been completed. Oblique fractures are extremely unstable, and compression screw fixation should be supplemented with parallel K-wires to achieve a satisfactory reduction. Small proximal pole fractures require internal fixation using a dorsal approach to avoid a high nonunion rate. When fractures of the scaphoid are associated with a dorsal intercalated segmental instability deformity, a dorsal approach may be necessary to reduce and pin the lunate along with the scaphoid fracture. An intercalary graft placed using a palmar approach may be required. Transscaphoid perilunate fracture-dislocations require a classic extended palmar approach to decompress the carpal canal and repair the palmar ligaments. Dorsal approaches may be necessary when any associated ulnar carpal instability is present. Scaphoid fractures treated conservatively that show no evidence of healing after 3 months often require surgical intervention with a bone graft, internal fixation, and accurate reduction.

Arthroscopically Assisted Fixation

Arthroscopically assisted internal fixation is a technically demanding procedure that is used only in select

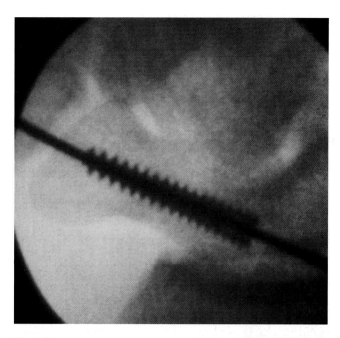

Figure 12 Minifluoroscopy view of the guidewire and cannulated compression screw used in the dorsal percutaneous pinning of a proximal pole fracture.

cases of displaced but reducible fractures. Finger-trap traction applied to the thumb assists in reduction. Diagnostic arthroscopy of the radiocarpal joint is done using standard 3-4 and 4-5 portals. Fracture hematoma should be evacuated and the joint surface and ligamentous injuries assessed. The ulnar midcarpal portal provides the best view of the scaphoid fracture. Fracture reduction, if necessary, is performed via direct manipulation of the distal pole and percutaneous manipulation of the proximal pole through a small volar incision made just radial to the flexor carpi radialis. A cannulated screw is placed over a guidewire for an accurate reduction.

Scaphoid Nonunions

Scaphoid nonunions may be treated with open wedge grafting with iliac crest bone graft, vascularized bone grafting, or dorsal percutaneous approaches when CT shows no evidence of sclerotic edges at the nonunion site. Dorsal percutaneous pinning for proximal pole scaphoid fractures is a safe, reliable, and reproducible procedure (Figure 12). The combination of preserving the ligamentous and tenuous blood supply permits early rehabilitation and results in high union rates and earlier return to athletic activities.

Posttraumatic radiocarpal arthritis may occur despite successful healing of the scaphoid. Salvage procedures such as a proximal row carpectomy have been advocated to treat chronic nonunited fractures, radioscaphoid arthritis, and patients who do not want a long period of immobilization. Partial arthrodesis (scaphocapitate fusion or scaphoid-trapezium-trapezoid fusion) has also been advocated as a salvage procedure for non-unions of the scaphoid.

Infection and disruption of normal cartilaginous surfaces within the wrist joint with the use of intricate jigs are two common complications that can occur during the surgical correction of a scaphoid nonunion. During scaphoid open reduction and internal fixation using a volar approach, care must be taken to avoid damage to the palmar cutaneous branch of the median nerve. Joint stiffness or loss of fixation may result from inappropriate postoperative immobilization. Although range of motion may be limited after extensive surgical exposure, percutaneous fixation techniques show promise for restoration of full wrist motion in most patients.

Distal Radius Fractures

Arthroscopic reduction of displaced intra-articular fractures provides a more precise method of visualizing the fracture reduction than radiographic evaluation. Kirschner wires placed percutaneously are used to elevate depressed articular fragments. Arthroscopic reduction allows anatomic reduction of displaced intra-articular fractures without causing wrist stiffness that often results from open reduction and internal fixation. To allow time for an organized hematoma to form and thereby obtain an unobstructed view, arthroscopic reduction is done 3 to 5 days after a fracture rather than acutely. The forearm must be wrapped with an elastic wrap to prevent extravasation of saline into the forearm and thereby protect the limb from a compartment syndrome.

Tendinopathy

Intersection Syndrome

Intersection syndrome occurs in athletes who participate in repetitive wrist motion activities and experience trauma along with dorsal radial wrist pain. Pain is located 4 to 6 cm proximal to Lister's tubercle. Pathognomonic symptoms consist of swelling, tenderness, and crepitus where the abductor pollicis longus (APL) and the extensor pollicis brevis (EPB) cross over the wrist extensors (the extensor carpi radialis longus and the extensor carpi radialis brevis). Canoeists, rowers, weight lifters, and recreational tennis players are known to have "squeakers" because of the pain and noise present in their forearms.

Nonsurgical treatment consists of rest, splinting, modification of activities, anti-inflammatory medications, and an injection of corticosteroid. A splint, with 10° to 20° of wrist extension, custom-molded to the volar wrist should be worn 24 hours a day for 3 weeks; the patient is then weaned over the subsequent 3 weeks. A 95% success rate has been reported using this method.

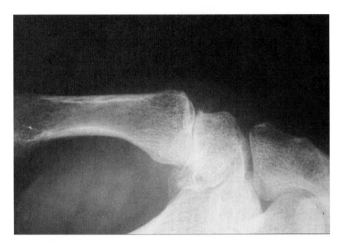

Figure 13 Plain radiograph of a patient with carpometacarpal arthritis.

de Quervain's Disease

de Quervain's disease involves stenosing tenosynovitis of the APL and the EPB tendons. Athletes who participate in racquet sports, golf, fly fishing, and javelin and discus throwing report pain over the radial styloid and tenderness, swelling, and occasionally a triggering or crepitus with a reproducible Finkelstein sign. These sports all require a forceful grip and the repetitive use of the thumb with the wrist in an ulnar-deviated position. Carpometacarpal arthritis or other underlying diseases can result in a false-positive sign. A zero PA, lateral radiograph of the wrist and a hyperpronated view or Roberts' view should be obtained to help identify evidence of carpometacarpal arthritis (Figure 13).

Conservative treatment consists of a custom thumb spica splint, concurrent anti-inflammatory medications, and a corticosteroid injection into the first dorsal compartment. Depending on splint wear, success rates of 62% to 100% have been reported with this type of treatment. Poor results from corticosteroid injection and recurrence of symptoms may occur in up to 30% of patients with longitudinal septums that divide the APL and the EPB into separate subcompartments. Surgical management requires releasing both compartments (multiple slips of the APL, often numbering five and seven) and identifying the EPB within the depths of the wound before closure. Complications from surgery can include damage to the superficial radial nerve, tendinous adhesions, hypertrophic scarring, volar tendon subluxation, and persistence of symptoms.

Flexor Carpi Radialis Tendinitis

Athletes with flexor carpi radialis tendinitis have pain over the volar aspect of the wrist proximal to the wrist crease and overlying the flexor carpi radialis tendon. A provocative test performed by abruptly extending a relaxed wrist to reproduce the pain has been described. Pain also may be elicited on resisted flexion and radial deviation. Chronic synovitis and tendon ruptures may not allow active testing in some patients.

The flexor carpi radialis passes through a synovial tunnel bordered by the scaphoid tuberosity, trapezial ridge, and transverse carpal ligament. Stenosis and synovitis within the fibro-osseous tunnel may occur and occlude the tendon, which occupies 90% of the available space. As the tendon enters this tunnel, it deviates 30° dorsally over the volar pole of the scaphoid to insert at the base of the second and third metacarpals and provides a slip to the trapezial ridge.

Immobilization, anti-inflammatory medication, and a corticosteroid injection may provide pain relief in patients with a primary tendinitis. Chronic processes may be recalcitrant to treatment and often require decompression of the fibro-osseous tunnel. Although complications are rare, rupture of the flexor carpi radialis tendons has been reported. In patients with a flexor carpi radialis rupture, simple débridement of the stump can provide pain relief. A wrist splint placed in neutral rotation postoperatively will often alleviate all the pain.

Hand and Wrist Pain in Athletes
Soft Tissue—Ganglion Cyst
Approximately 85% of patients with ganglion cysts have dorsal ganglion cysts; 15% have volar ganglion cysts. Dorsal ganglion cysts have been treated with needle drainage with varied reports of long-term success. Although the drainage of dorsal ganglion cysts is safe, the same is not true for volar ganglion cysts. Volar ganglion cysts are located at the wrist crease and most commonly originate from the scapholunate and STT joints. Volar aspiration should be avoided because injury of the radial artery may create an iatrogenic false aneurysm with devastating sequelae.

Nerve Impingement—Carpal Tunnel Syndrome
Although carpal tunnel syndrome is infrequently seen in the athletic population, it is the most common type of compressive neuropathy. Carpal tunnel syndrome may be caused by direct trauma, repetitive use, or anatomic anomalies. Athletes who participate in lacrosse, cycling, throwing sports, racquet sports, archery, gymnastics, and wheelchair sports are at increased risk for carpal tunnel syndrome because grip-intensive activities are known to aggravate this condition. Weight lifting can cause hypertrophy of the lumbrical muscle, which can also trigger a compressive neuropathy. Carpal tunnel syndrome can be caused by flexor tenosynovitis and anatomic anomalies, such as the palmaris longus placed within the carpal canal, palmaris profundus, hypertrophic flexor digitorum superficialis, accessory lumbricalis, and a persistent median artery.

Classic symptoms include pain and paresthesias, especially at night, in the radial digits. Athletes will frequently report clumsiness and weakness when performing grip-related activities. In athletes with suspected carpal tunnel syndrome, Phalen's test (sensitive) and Tinel's test (specific) should be done, and grip and pinch strengths should be measured and recorded. It is crucial to exclude the causes of more proximal lesions of nerve compression, such as thoracic outlet syndrome, pronator syndrome, and even cervical radiculopathy. Forty percent of athletes with symptoms of carpal tunnel syndrome have shoulder pain and upper arm pain.

Conservative treatment can include padding over the heel of the hand along with protective gloves to alleviate symptoms. Adjusting the hand and wrist position with rest is important, and the use of forearm guards or lighter bows for an archer can also be helpful. Although corticosteroid injection provides temporary relief in 85% of patients with carpal tunnel syndrome, the lasting effect in all age groups after 1 year is 20% to 24%.

When electrodiagnostic studies show moderate to severe crippling of the median nerve after conservative treatment, surgical intervention is indicated. Limited open, formal open, or endoscopic carpal tunnel release all have limitations. A limited open incision of 1.5 to 2 cm can often provide all the safeguards of an open procedure without the risks of an endoscopic procedure. Postoperatively, patients usually have immediate relief of pain, but not all patients demonstrate immediate improvement in the sensibility of their fingers. The symptoms of severe carpal tunnel syndrome may not resolve for 6 months to 1 year. Swelling at the base of the palm just superficial to the carpal tunnel may take 4 months to completely resolve. Patients may experience aching in the hypothenar eminence (pillar pain) with formal open and endoscopic procedures. Most patients regain 75% to 80% of their grip strength within 3 months.

When the endoscopic technique is used by experienced hand surgeons to treat carpal tunnel syndrome, complications such as mild transient ulnar paresthesias, partial and complete lacerations of the superficial palmar arch and digital nerves, and deep motor branch injuries have been reported. In addition, 19% of patients have been unable to regain full strength after surgical release; the reported rate of recurrence of symptoms is also 19%. Prospective studies have confirmed that the endoscopic procedure is as effective as open release in the relief of paresthesias and nocturnal pain; however, clinical studies have not shown that an endoscopic technique results in earlier return to activities of daily living, quicker recovery of pinch strength, and reduced palmar scar tenderness.

Summary
Sports medicine physicians must appreciate the responsibility to recognize the severity of hand and wrist injuries in athletes. A thorough understanding of the various

types of hand and wrist injuries and their treatment regimes will help physicians provide the most predictable treatment with the fewest complications.

Annotated Bibliography

Wrist Imaging

Desai VV, Davis TR, Barton NJ: The prognostic value and reproducibility of the radiological features of the fractured scaphoid. *J Hand Surg [Br]* 1999;24:586-590.

In this study, the assessment of fracture level comminution and displacement showed moderate inter- and intra-observer reproducibility but not predictability of union of the scaphoid.

Freedman DM, Dowdle J, Glickel SZ, Singson R, Okezie T: Tomography versus computed tomography for assessing step off in intraarticular distal radial fractures. *Clin Orthop* 1999;361:199-204.

The authors report that trispiral tomography is more accurate and cost-effective than CT and should be the diagnostic modality of choice for evaluating patients with intra-articular distal radius fractures.

Grechenig W, Peicha G, Fellinger M, Seibert FJ, Preidler KW: Wrist arthrography after acute trauma of the distal radius: Diagnostic accuracy, technique and sources of diagnostic errors. *Invest Radiol* 1998;33:273-278.

The authors discuss the use of arthrography to diagnose and identify interosseous carpal ligaments and TFCC tears in a posttraumatic wrist.

Kransdorf MJ, Turner-Stephahin S, Merritt WH: Magnetic resonance angiography of the hand and wrist: Evaluation of patients with severe ischemic disease. *J Reconstr Microsurg* 1998;14:77-81.

Magnetic resonance angiography is an exciting new method for evaluating wrist and forearm vasculature. This article reviews magnetic resonance angiography with digital subtraction angiography. It is hoped that management of severe ischemia in the wrist will be aided by this technique once it is developed because magnetic resonance angiography alone is currently unable to provide fine detail.

Linkous MD, Gilula LA: Wrist arthrography today. *Radiol Clin North Am* 1998;36:651-672.

The authors report that wrist arthrography can be a useful device in the hands of a trained radiologist.

Plancher KD: Methods of imaging the scaphoid. *Hand Clin* 2001;17:703-721.

The author discusses the use of special imaging to identify scaphoid fractures and thereby help physicians to treat these fractures in an expeditious and accurate manner.

Scheck RJ, Romagnolo A, Hierner R, Pfluger T, Wilhelm K, Hahn K: The carpal ligaments in MR arthrography of the wrist: Correlation with standard MRI and wrist arthroscopy. *J Magn Reson Imaging* 1999;9:468-474.

The authors compared the use of magnetic resonance arthrography and nonenhanced MRI in 35 patients with refractory wrist pain. Ligament evaluation was possible with high diagnostic confidence in 11% using nonenhanced MRI and in 90% using magnetic resonance arthrography. Wrist arthroscopy was used as a standard of reference. The findings show that magnetic resonance arthrography is more accurate than standard MRI.

Wrist Arthroscopy

Culp R: Wrist and hand arthroscopy. *Hand Clin* 1999;15: 393-535.

In this series of articles covering all aspects of wrist arthroscopy for the novice and advanced surgeon, the latest technique of laser-assisted arthroscopy and metacarpophalangeal arthroscopy are covered. Important complications are discussed in detail by the editor.

Dailey SW, Palmer AK: The role of arthroscopy in the evaluation and treatment of triangular fibrocartilage complex injuries in athletes. *Hand Clin* 2000;16:461-476.

In this up-to-date review of anatomy and function of the TFCC, evaluation and treatment regimes for each type of lesions are discussed. Complications and pearls are also addressed for the novice and advanced arthroscopist.

Doi K, Hattori Y, Otsuka K, Abe Y, Yamamoto H: Intra-articular fractures of the distal aspect of the radius: Arthroscopically assisted reduction compared with open reduction and internal fixation. *J Bone Joint Surg Am* 1999;81:1093-1110.

The authors discuss accurate reduction in intra-articular fractures of the distal radius and report that overall functional results improved as a result of decreased soft-tissue scarring and minimal capsular contracture.

Fontes D: The role of wrist arthroscopy in the management of complex triangular fibrocartilage tears: A report on a series of 124 cases. *La Main* 1998;3:17-22.

In this 6-year retrospective review by a single surgeon, excellent results are reported in 84% of class 1 (Palmer) lesions. The author concludes that ulnar shortening is only indicated in patients with positive ulnar variance who are not responsive to primary arthroscopic treatment.

Grechenig W, Peicha G, Fellinger M, Seibet FJ, Weiglein AH: Anatomical and safety considerations in establishing portals used for wrist arthroscopy. *Clin Anat* 1999;12: 179-185.

The authors safely made eight portals during wrist arthroscopy using external landmarks. This article provides an excellent review of portal placement for a beginning arthroscopist.

Haugstuedt JR, Husby T: Results of repair of peripheral tears in the triangular fibrocartilage complex using an arthroscopic suture technique. *Scand J Plast Reconstr Surg Hand Surg* 1999;33:439-470.

The authors discuss using an arthroscopic suture technique to repair peripheral TFCC lesions and report good objective results in the treatment of patients with class 1 type B (Palmer) lesions.

Mehta JA, Bain GI, Heptinstall RJ: Anatomical reduction of intra-articular fractures of the distal radius: An arthroscopically-assisted approach. *J Bone Joint Surg Br* 2000;82:79-86.

The authors discuss arthroscopic débridement of necrotic scaphoid, lunotriquetral, and scapholunate ligaments and TFCC tears and 31 intra-articular fractures of the distal radius with percutaneous K-wire fixation. Outcomes and recommendations are also discussed.

Plancher KD: Arthroscopic reduction: Internal fixation of the scaphoid. *Atlas Hand Clin* 2001;6:325-339.

The author presents a detailed assessment of using arthroscopic reduction for the internal fixation of the scaphoid.

Ruch DS, Bowling J: Arthroscopic assessment of carpal instability. *Arthroscopy* 1998;14:675-681.

This article reinforces how complex carpal instability and its treatment can be. The need to use arthroscopy to add valuable information that will help treatment regimes for common injuries is discussed. The discussion of specific cases provides good representative examples of the usefulness of wrist arthroscopy.

Taras JS, Sweet S, Shum W, Weiss L, Bartolozzi A: Percutaneous and arthroscopic screw fixation of scaphoid fractures in the athlete. *Hand Clin* 1999;15:467-473.

Using percutaneous or arthroscopically assisted fixation to treat athletes with scaphoid fractures for whom prolonged immobilization is a concern, the authors report rapid return to athletic competition, minimal morbidity, and no nonunions.

Verhellen R, Bain GI: Arthroscopic capsular release for contracture of the wrist: A new technique. *Arthroscopy* 2000;16:106-110.

Arthroscopic capsular release and its technique is described in a cadaver and two patients as a safe and minimally invasive technique that demonstrates good improvement in strength and range of motion at a 6-month follow-up.

Ulnar-Sided Wrist Pain

Tomaino MM, Gainer M, Towers JD: Carpal impaction with the ulnar styloid process: Treatment with partial styloid resection. *J Hand Surg [Br]* 2001;26:252-255.

The authors report that partial resection of the ulnar styloid process is a satisfactory treatment for isolated stylocarpal impaction, but caution that an unstable distal ulna may result if the exposure is inadequate or if the entire styloid process is resected.

Viegas SF, Yamaguchi S, Boyd NL, Patterson RM: The dorsal ligaments of the wrist: Anatomy, mechanical properties, and function. *J Hand Surg [Am]* 1999;24:456-468.

The authors of this article explain in detail the anatomy of the dorsoradial carpal and dorsal intercarpal ligaments. These structures, once thought to not have a large impact in stability of the scaphoid, are discussed as vital structures.

Wolfe SW: Scapholunate instability. *J Am Soc Surg Hand* 2001;1:45-60.

The author discusses the diagnosis and treatment of scapholunate instability.

Radial-Sided Wrist Pain

Hame SL, LaFemina JM, McAllister DR, Schaadt GW, Dorey FJ: Fractures in the collegiate athlete. *Am J Sports Med* 2004;32:446-451.

This study was conducted to determine the demographics and incidence of fractures in collegiate athletes. The authors report that athletes who participated in contact sports experienced the greatest number of fractures. Participation in basketball for men and gymnastics for women posed the greatest fracture risk. Female athletes sustained significantly more stress fractures.

Plancher KD, Faber K: Arthroscopic repair of radial-sided triangular fibrocartilage complex lesions. *Tech Hand Upper Extremity Surg* 1999;3:44-51.

The authors discuss an easy to follow technique to repair radial-sided TFCC perforations. Common complications and a historical perspective are discussed, as well as indications and workup for patients with acute or chronic wrist pain.

Hand and Wrist Pain in Athletes

Werner SL, Plancher KD: Biomechanics of wrist injuries in sports. *Clin Sports Med* 1998;17:407-420.

This article discusses wrist anatomy, biomechanics, and injury mechanisms for the athletic population. Common injuries are discussed in a biomechanical context for impact sports; racquet, stick, and club sports; and apparatus and external contact sports.

Westbrook AP, Stephen AB, Oni J, et al: Ganglia: The patient's perception. *J Hand Surg [Br]* 2000;25:566-567.

The authors of this article argue that it is important to understand the concerns of patients with ganglia and that not every patient who consults with a hand clinic surgeon is seeking or requires surgical excision of the ganglion.

Classic Bibliography

Corso SJ, Savoie FH, Geissler WB, et al: Arthroscopic repair of peripheral avulsions of the triangular fibrocartilage complex of the wrist: A multicenter study. *Arthroscopy* 1997;13:78-84.

Jacobsen MD, Plancher KD: Evaluation of hand and wrist injuries in athletes. *Oper Tech Sports Med* 1996;4: 210-226.

Jones WA, Lovell ME: The role of arthroscopy in the investigation of wrist disorders. *J Hand Surg [Br]* 1996;21: 442-445.

Kukla C, Gabler C, Breitenseher MJ, Trattni GS, Vecsei V: Occult fractures of the scaphoid: The diagnostic usefulness of the indirect economic repercussions of radiography versus magnetic resonance imaging. *J Hand Surg [Br]* 1997;22:810-813.

Nakamura R, Imaeda T, Suzuki K, et al: Sports related Keinbock's disease. *Am J Sports Med* 1991;19:88-91.

Rettig AC, Dipak VP: Epidemiology of elbow, forearm, and wrist injuries in the athlete. *Clin Sports Med* 1995; 14:289-298.

Sennwald GR, Zdravkovic V: Wrist arthroscopy: A prospective analysis of 53 post-traumatic carpal injuries. *Scand J Plast Reconstr Surg Hand Surg* 1997;31:261-266.

Steinberg BD, Plancher KD, Idler RS: Percutaneous wire fixation through the snuffbox: An anatomic study. *J Hand Surg [Am]* 1995;20:57-62.

Tiel-van Buul, van Beek EJ, Broekhuizen AH, Bakker AJ, Bos KE, van Royen EA: Radiography and scintigraphy of suspected scaphoid fracture: A long-term study in 160 patients. *J Bone Joint Surg Br* 1993;75:61-65.

Trumble TE, Gilbert M, Vedder N: Ulnar shortening combined with arthroscopic repairs in the delayed management of triangular fibrocartilage complex tears. *J Hand Surg [Am]* 1997;22:807-813.

Weiss AC, Akelman E, Lambiase R: Comparison of the findings of triple-injections cinearthrography of the wrist with those of arthroscopy. *J Bone Joint Surg Am* 1996;78:348-356.

Chapter 10

Rehabilitation Principles: Kinetic Chain Therapeutic Exercise Application and Progression

John McMullen, MS, ATC

Introduction

Complete rehabilitation of upper extremity injuries is vital for the successful return to athletic participation. Biomechanical analyses of throwing and swinging sports activities demonstrate the importance of kinetic chain principles in the performance of these activities and the protection of upper extremity anatomy. The requisite force to generate arm velocity is most efficiently generated by the sequential muscle activation and segmental movement of the legs, trunk, and arm. These segments then contribute to the deceleration of the arm in the follow-through phase of these sports activities.

The therapeutic exercise component of complete upper extremity rehabilitation should include these kinetic chain principles by integrating multiple segments into exercise patterns. This integrated exercise approach helps stimulate appropriate segmental movement, reestablish appropriate motor patterns, and establish the necessary stability in proximal segments to allow full mobility in the upper extremity. Appropriate movement and stability in the lower extremity, hips, trunk, and scapula, as well as the healing of injured or repaired tissue, mark progression through these types of exercises.

The Role of Kinetic Chain Therapeutic Exercise

Kinetic chain considerations are important in all therapeutic exercise, and this is especially true in upper extremity rehabilitation. In the performance of repetitive upper extremity sports activities, strength or motion deficits at particular segments can often be masked in the short term by compensation at other segments. With repetition, however, these compensations will usually be revealed by a decrease in performance or manifestation of an injury at the shoulder or elbow.

Although rehabilitation of the injured tissue is the primary goal of therapeutic exercise, neglecting the contributions of other segments in the movement sequence creates an incomplete rehabilitation program. For exam-

ple, adequate glenohumeral internal rotation protects the throwing shoulder and elbow of a baseball pitcher and decreases with repetitive pitching. Mechanically, the contribution of this internal rotation potential can be further diminished in the presence of weak contralateral hip abductors. The weak hip abductors cause an unstable base against which this internal rotation can occur. If this stride leg hip adducts through the acceleration phase of the pitch, the spine angle can change, forcing the scapula and arm to compensate. The compensation in these distal segments can mechanically reduce the contribution of shoulder internal rotation to the total movement, exposing the glenoid labrum, capsule, or medial elbow to excessive stress. Therefore, upper extremity therapeutic exercises focus on local functional deficits and also must be attentive to the other segments of the kinetic chain and include them in the exercise design as much as possible.

Integrating multiple segments into rehabilitative exercises can proprioceptively facilitate appropriate motion in the involved extremity. This integration requires careful exercise design to apply appropriate loads, avoid unwanted compensations by dominant muscle groups or segments, and avoid unwanted stresses on healing tissue. Exercises introduced early in the rehabilitation program can emphasize proximal kinetic chain segments and sequential movement of these segments while involved tissue heals. These movement patterns can later include the involved tissue in the upper extremity, and range of motion and load can progress as healing and function allows. The "shoulder dump" is an exercise that is introduced early in the rehabilitation program and involves the legs, hips, trunk, and scapula moving reciprocally from a flexed/medially rotated posture to extended/neutral or laterally rotated posture. During the "shoulder dump" exercise, body weight shifts from the forward, flexed contralateral leg to the extended ipsilateral leg; this exercise can be done with the involved arm still in a sling (Figure 1). This movement pattern stimulates sequential segment and joint movement throughout the

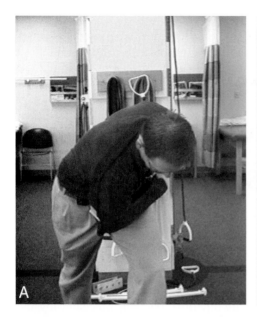
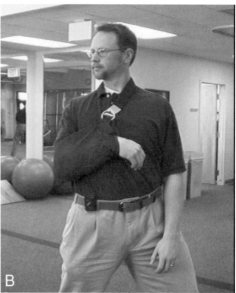

Figure 1 The start (**A**) and end (**B**) position of the "shoulder dump" exercise with the involved arm still in a sling.

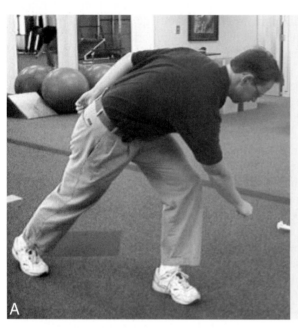
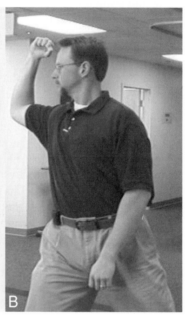

Figure 2 The start (**A**) and end (**B**) position of a "shoulder dump" with arm motion. The end position includes shoulder abduction and external rotation, a progression of the exercise that may be contraindicated early in the rehabilitation program.

kinetic chain and enhances scapular motion, particularly scapular retraction with thoracic spine extension, without active motion of the healing upper extremity.

Potential Obstacles to Kinetic Chain Movement Patterns

Anatomy

Anatomic considerations in using integrated movements therapeutically include the status of the healing tissue, soft-tissue restrictions, and joint restrictions. Early in the rehabilitation program, exercises should not overstress healing tissue or suture lines. Although this is an elementary precaution, particularly for patients who have recently undergone surgery, the facilitating nature of in-

tegrated movements can produce motion that exceeds isolated, active limits and, potentially, safe boundaries. A progression for the extended posture of "shoulder dump" described previously includes 90° of shoulder abduction and 90° of external rotation (Figure 2). This degree of shoulder abduction and external rotation is unsafe for several weeks immediately after a surgical procedure such as an anterior shoulder repair, in which instance arm motion must be limited to safe ranges while repaired tissue heals.

The shoulder girdle is particularly vulnerable to soft-tissue restrictions such as myofascial restrictions, muscular tightness, muscular trigger/tender points, and ligamentous tightness. These movement restrictions often require a combination of manual therapy and stretching techniques to allow normal motion. Common areas of contractile tightness and tenderness are along the medial border of the scapula (rhomboids), at the superior medial angle of the scapula (levator scapulae), in the teres minor/infraspinatus, and in the muscular attachments at the coracoid process (pectoralis minor, short head of the biceps). If not addressed in the course of therapy, these restrictions can limit scapular and glenohumeral motion, enable compensatory muscle activity, and inhibit normal muscle activation patterns. After adequate healing of injured or repaired tissue, appropriate joint mobilizations and passive stretching of the glenohumeral joint can effectively reduce this common ligamentous restriction. Stretching and mobilization of restricted contractile tissue should begin as early as possible and continue throughout the therapeutic treatment.

Mobility and posture of the spine are important factors in upper extremity biomechanics. To achieve full scapular retraction, as in the cocking phase of baseball pitching, thoracic spine extension is necessary. A kyphotic posture and facet restrictions or poor dissociation of the pelvis and lumbar and thoracic spine can ultimately inhibit scapular motion. Specifically, posterior tilt and external rotation of the scapula are limited, creating an environment for internal impingement or subacromial impingement at the shoulder and excessive medial stress on the throwing elbow. Again, manual therapy techniques and aggressive stretching may be necessary to provide the spine mobility that is required for full scapular motion. These techniques will not disturb the healing shoulder or elbow and should begin early in the rehabilitation process.

Muscle Interaction

Another potential problem in developing kinetic chain exercises involves the relationship between the muscles of the shoulder girdle. Scapular stabilizing muscles tend to work in force couples to actively stabilize the scapula, coordinate scapulohumeral motion, and establish optimum length-tension relationships. Postural or tonic muscles, such as the levator scapulae and upper trapezius, tend to dominate phasic muscles, such as the lower trapezius and serratus anterior. This imbalance, along with the low irritability threshold of the tonic muscles, contributes to scapular dyskinesia and periscapular pain. Muscle reeducation using closed kinetic chain exercises to stimulate co-contractions around the shoulder and integrated movement patterns without extrinsic loads are necessary early in the rehabilitation process. In the presence of these active muscle imbalances, it is very difficult to strengthen weak muscles because of the proprioceptive difficulties, poor muscle activation patterns, pain, and muscle spasm they cause.

Compensatory Movements

In upper extremity activities, there are several potential causes of compensatory segmental movement. Range of motion, muscle strength, or muscle endurance may be deficient at the shoulder or at a more proximal kinetic chain segment. Pain may cause an athlete to avoid a particular position, and the revised movement pattern creates the need to compensate by adding or removing a particular component of the original movement pattern. Occasionally, athletes will experience short-term success with a high-risk technique but a mechanically sound technique should enhance performance while maximizing anatomic protections. Effective and complete upper extremity rehabilitation will establish functional motion and strength throughout the kinetic chain and eliminate muscle imbalances that inhibit normal upper extremity function and protect the involved tissue.

Types of Exercises

Four basic types of integrated kinetic chain exercises should be built into all upper extremity rehabilitation protocols: closed kinetic chain, facilitated active motion, resistive active motion, and plyometric/sport-specific exercises. Gradual progressive sport-specific exercises are introduced during the final stage of rehabilitation; therapeutic exercise progression can be initiated immediately when a functional rehabilitation approach is used.

Closed Kinetic Chain Exercises

Closed kinetic chain exercises are a versatile type of exercise used throughout the rehabilitation program. They range from low to high load and zero to full motion. Closed kinetic chain exercises stimulate co-contractions in the scapular and rotator cuff muscles, load scapular stabilizers, and facilitate active motion. In all closed kinetic chain exercises, there is an axial load through the long axis of the upper extremity. Increasing the axial load can progressively challenge contractile tissue, but the closed kinetic chain environment strictly controls for degree and plane of elevation. For most upper extremity athletic activities, the ultimate goal is open kinetic chain function; the primary role of closed kinetic chain exercises in upper extremity rehabilitation is as a means to achieve full, normal active motion.

In the early phase of rehabilitation or any time stabilizing co-contractions are desirable, the distal segment is relatively fixed as in weight shifting, rhythmic stabilization, or weight bearing with gentle perturbation. These are extremely safe exercises because posture, elevation, load, and joint alignment are all controlled.

One type of closed kinetic chain exercise allows proximal segment motion while the distal segment remains fixed. Quadriped rocking (Figure 3) or moving the torso away from the weight bearing hand on a table or countertop creates glenohumeral motion without the

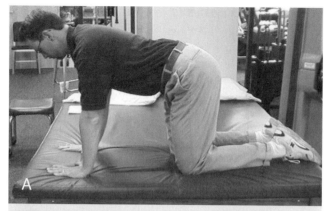

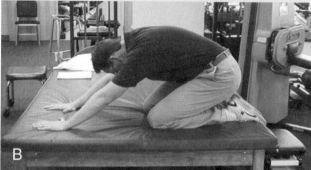

Figure 3 The start (**A**) and end (**B**) position of quadriped rocking to facilitate scapulohumeral coordination in the flexion plane above 90°.

upward shear from deltoid activation. Although this type of closed kinetic chain exercise works well when glenohumeral motion is permitted, rotator cuff demand should be minimized. The axial load provides the glenohumeral compression, reducing the demand on the rotator cuff to maintain glenohumeral congruency. The athlete safely controls the joint motion through body movement rather than arm movement.

In another type of closed kinetic chain exercise, the distal segment moves. Wall or table slides (Figure 4) maintain an axial load, but the sliding hand creates active arm motion relative to the torso. Done while standing, the axial load still protects against humeral head translation; posture, proximal segment movement, degree of elevation, and plane of elevation are easily controlled. This is an excellent type of closed kinetic chain exercise to transition into open chain active arm motion at greater degrees of elevation.

Facilitated Active Motion Exercises
Facilitated active motion exercises use proximal segment motion to stimulate and facilitate motion in the target tissue. Often performed in diagonal movement patterns, this type of exercise can facilitate any plane of movement for the target tissue. The "shoulder dump" is a good example of this type of exercise and, as described previously, targets the scapula when the arm is in a sling. When arm motion is added, it becomes a familiar diagonal pattern of proprioceptive neuromuscular facilitation. Exaggeration of the complementary motion in proximal kinetic chain segments better facilitates the desired arm motion. The hips and trunk provide most of the proprioceptive input in these movements, and the movements should be reciprocal. Coordinating the arm motion with the lower extremities, trunk, and scapula enhances active arm motion. Normalizing the facilitating movements increases the intrinsic demand on upper extremity musculature but keeps the kinetic chain muscle activation pattern in place.

Resistive Active Motion Exercises
As segmental control and motion increases, facilitated active motion exercises are progressed by adding resistance.

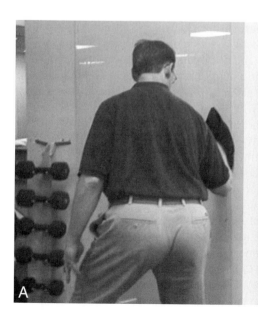

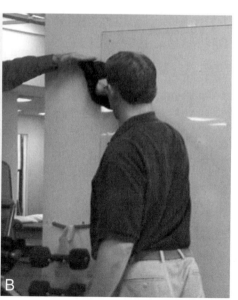

Figure 4 The start (**A**) and end (**B**) position of a diagonal wall slide. The hand slides on a wall to a designated target in coordination with body movement.

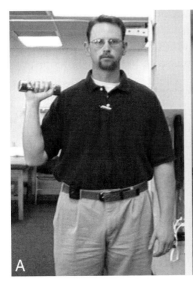
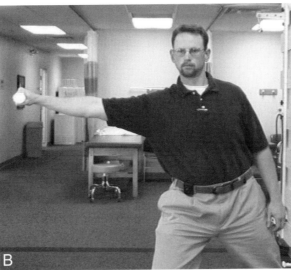

Figure 5 The start (**A**) and end (**B**) position of a lateral dumbbell punch. Complementary weight shifting and body movement is permitted.

These exercises are typically open kinetic chain exercises and involve some degree of active glenohumeral motion. The quality of scapular motion during these exercises is a good indicator of glenohumeral elevation limits. The elevated upper extremity represents an intrinsic load to the scapular muscles, and if this load becomes excessive, scapular motion compensation and dyskinesis may develop to achieve the desired elevation. Even in integrated movement patterns, active glenohumeral elevation is limited to ranges of good scapular control. The introduction of extrinsic loads via dumbbells, medicine balls, or exercise tubing is appropriate when the addition of arm elevation to a movement pattern does not negatively affect the quality of movement. The reduction of the facilitating proximal segment motion, addition of extrinsic resistance, and widening of the range of glenohumeral motion are all methods of progressing resistive active motion exercises for the upper extremity.

Sport-specific movements and movement planes of emphasis influence the invention of exercise movement patterns. Because most sports activities involve some component of rotation, diagonal movement patterns are frequently used. If secondary subacromial impingement is a problem because of anterior tilting of the scapula or poor thoracic spine extension, movement patterns emphasize the sagittal plane. Poor control of the medial scapular border or a lateral scapular slide that contributes to internal or subacromial impingement indicates the need to emphasize frontal plane movement patterns in the exercise program.

Because many athletic shoulder injuries result from repetition of motion, muscular endurance throughout the coordinated movement of the shoulder girdle is important. Isolated rotator cuff strengthening exercises,

performed with good postural control, can develop this locally but do little for coordinated functional thoracoscapulohumeral motion. Dumbbell punches (Figure 5), performed reciprocally at various degrees of elevation and in various planes, place functional demands on the rotator cuff and scapular muscles. The rotator cuff must control glenohumeral translation as the humerus and scapula move through a range of motion. Punches can begin downward, keeping the lever arm short and concentrically working the shoulder girdle muscles in the retraction phase of the movement. The greatest rotator cuff demand occurs when punching at 90°, where the lever arm is the longest. Overhead punches, or presses, require good glenohumeral range of motion and significantly load the scapular muscles.

Plyometric/Sport-Specific Exercises

Plyometric exercise prepares the athlete for a progressive return to play. The movement patterns become increasingly consistent with those of the ultimate sport activity. Performed at slower speeds, these exercises emphasize stabilization and control while promoting proper body mechanics, especially in the more proximal segments of the kinetic chain. As the speed of exercise becomes more functional or comparable to the speed of the actual sport activity, muscles work in the stretch-shortening sequence of most sports activities. The ballistic nature of plyometric exercises usually delegates them to the later stages of upper extremity rehabilitation, after full range of motion and good strength and control have been established. Appropriate stabilization and motion in proximal segments are important because these exercises lead the athlete to a progressive return to sport activity.

TABLE 1 | Return to Throwing Progression*

Distance (feet)	Repetitions (Throws)	Sets
60	25	2
60	25	3
90	25	2
90	25	3
120	25	2
120	25	3
150	25	2
150	25	3

*Each set should begin with a period of warm-up throwing.

(Adapted with permission from Wilk KE, Arrigo CA, Courson R, et al: Preventive and Rehabilitative Exercises for the Shoulder and Elbow. Birmingham, AL, American Sports Medicine Institute, 1991, pp 1-37.)

Return to Play Progressions

After appropriate healing time and demonstration of normal range of motion, strength, and functional movement of the kinetic chain, the athlete begins a progressive return to sport activity. This progression is the final component to rehabilitation. To develop the proper biomechanics and endurance for repetitive overhead activities, a gradual, progressive sport-specific rehabilitation program is required. In most cases, this includes input from coaches and medical and rehabilitation professionals.

These programs vary greatly according to sport. Some begin with basic element movements or by breaking the primary activity into component movements to ensure proper mechanics. For example, the baseball pitcher will begin with full body, flat-ground throwing before pitching from a mound because the intensity of this type of throwing is less intense than pitching. The intensity and duration of the exercise throwing will progressively increase before mound pitching begins. Table 1 provides a sample of this type of throwing progression. In this program, because the athlete throws only hard enough to cover the prescribed distance, the distance determines the intensity or velocity of the throws. The repetitions progressively increase before the intensity or distance increases. Like all exercise programs, pain, ability to complete prescribed repetitions and soreness after exercise guide the progression. The athlete moves through the program by completing the prescribed number of throws and remaining pain free and with little or no soreness after exercise. Other sports require similar rehabilitation programs, and all progressive return to sport programs depend on the individual athlete's injury and skill level.

Therapeutic Exercise Progression

With a functional approach, therapeutic exercise can begin immediately in the rehabilitation process. The early emphasis is on thoracic posture and proximal segment motion and strength while protecting healing tissue. This is especially true for the scapula because it is the site of many functional compensations and muscle imbalances. Integrated hip, trunk, and scapular movement patterns are possible during the phase of arm and shoulder protection. Closed kinetic chain stabilization exercises safely stimulate co-contractions of the scapular musculature while limiting rotator cuff activation and glenohumeral translation. When healing permits active glenohumeral motion, closed kinetic chain exercises can progress to proximal then distal segment motion with an axial load, if necessary. The axial load reduces the load on the rotator cuff, allowing active motion that a weakened rotator cuff may otherwise limit. The axial load also reduces the risk of glenohumeral translation and compensatory dyskinetic scapular motion by providing a centralizing force through the glenohumeral joint.

The establishment of complete scapular motion should precede concentrated scapular strengthening. This begins with facilitated kinetic chain movement patterns and possibly manual therapy techniques. As scapular range of motion and control increase, progressive loading of these muscles begins. Appropriate scapular motion must coordinate with any arm elevation in these integrated motion exercises. Active local strengthening at the glenohumeral joint in ranges of poor scapular control leads to increased scapular dyskinesis, compensatory motion, and ineffective strengthening.

The clinical monitoring of spinal posture, resting scapular position, scapular kinematics through several repetitions of single plane elevation, and lateral scapular slide can indicate the status of scapular control. Patients should exhibit neutral cervical and thoracic posture and have equal scapular position and motion when compared bilaterally. They should be able to demonstrate full active scapular retraction, adduction, and posterior tilt without arm elevation and rhythmic upward rotation of the scapula with arm elevation. The inability to achieve full retraction is an indicator for therapeutic exercise emphasizing scapular motion. If there is dyskinesis with arm motion, scapular control exercises are necessary. In either case, loading glenohumeral musculature in ranges of poor scapular motion or control is ineffective, contributes to the dyskinesis, and may contribute to excessive joint translation.

Summary

Progression within a program of integrated, multisegmented, functional exercises accommodates the need for coordinated scapulohumeral motion and strengthening. Early emphasis is on hip, trunk, and scapular motion; stimulating co-contractions around the shoulder girdle through closed kinetic chain exercises; correcting proximal segment deficits; and addressing muscle imbalances and soft-tissue restrictions. Following normal physiologic healing, these early exercises progress to include axially loaded range of motion and open kinetic chain active arm motion. Adding extrinsic loads, reducing the contribution of facilitating proximal segments, and emphasizing proximal stabilization strengthen the entire link system. Exercises can be customized to meet the individual needs of patients and the demands of their sport-specific activities.

Because the exercises focus on proximal motion and control, particularly of the scapula, the clinical evaluation must note progress in these areas. The motion and stability of proximal segments are excellent indicators of preparedness for progression through a therapeutic exercise program. Although rotator cuff weakness may be noted as a clinical manifestation during physical examination, scapular control is necessary before isolated rotator cuff strengthening will be productive.

The actual sport activity becomes a late component of the therapeutic exercise. Reintroduction to repetitive overhead sports activity must be progressive, beginning with basic controlled activities and gradually increasing in complexity, duration, and intensity. This activity usually accompanies the final phases of clinical exercise or a maintenance exercise program. Coaches become part of the rehabilitation team at this point, providing sport-specific biomechanical feedback and regulating the amount of activity. As with all other therapeutic exercise, quality of movement, pain, and soreness after exercise regulate the progressive return to activity.

Annotated Bibliography

The Role of Kinetic Chain Therapeutic Exercise

Marshall RN, Elliott BC: Long-axis rotation: The missing link in proximal-to-distal segmental sequencing. *J Sports Sci* 2000;18:247-254.

The longitudinal-axis rotations of humeral internal rotation and forearm pronation occur late in the tennis serve movement and are major contributors to terminal velocity. This adds detail to the proximal-to-distal segmental sequence model.

McMullen J, Uhl TL: A kinetic chain approach for shoulder rehabilitation. *J Athl Train* 2000;35:329-337.

The authors describe an approach to shoulder rehabilitation that includes kinetic chain principles, full body movement patterns, and closed kinetic chain exercises. The article provides evidence that basic principles of proprioceptive neuromuscular facilitation and kinetic chain biomechanics form the foundation of this type of rehabilitation.

Potential Obstacles to Kinetic Chain Movement Patterns

Burkhart SS, Morgan CD, Kibler WB: The disabled throwing shoulder: Spectrum of pathology. Part I: Pathoanatomy and biomechanics. *Arthroscopy* 2003;19:404-420.

The first part of a three-part series in which the authors present a concept of the "dead arm syndrome" in throwing athletes, including biomechanics, pathoanatomy, kinetic chain considerations, surgery and rehabilitation. The series draws the microinstability model into question based on arthroscopic evidence, clinical observation, and biomechanical data. This installment focuses on glenohumeral joint mechanics through the throwing motion and the shoulder at risk.

Burkhart SS, Morgan CD, Kibler WB: The disabled throwing shoulder: Spectrum of pathology. Part III: The SICK scapula, scapular dyskinesis, the kinetic chain, and rehabilitation. *Arthroscopy* 2003;19:641-661.

The final part of a three-part series in which the authors present a concept of the "dead arm syndrome" in throwing athletes, including biomechanics, pathoanatomy, kinetic chain considerations, surgery and rehabilitation. The series draws the microinstability model into question based on arthroscopic evidence, clinical observation, and biomechanical data. This part of the series focuses on physical and biomechanical adaptations and deficits and kinetic chain rehabilitation considerations.

Kibler WB: The role of the scapula in athletic shoulder function. *Am J Sports Med* 1998;26:325-337.

This is an excellent review of scapular function and dysfunction in athletic activities. Methods of shoulder and scapula examination are described.

Lukasiewicz AC, McClure P, Michener L, Pratt M, Sennett B: Comparison of 3-dimensional scapular position and orientation between subjects with and without shoulder impingement. *J Orthop Sports Phys Ther* 1999;29:574-586.

This study illustrates the relative importance of scapular position and motion in shoulder function.

Types of Exercises

Hinterwimmer S, Von Eisenhart-Rothe R, Siebert M, et al: Influence of adducting and abducting muscle forces on the subacromial space width. *Med Sci Sports Exerc* 2003;35:2055-2059.

This study demonstrates that isometric adducting muscle forces lead to increased subacromial space when compared with isometric abducting muscle force. Closed kinetic chain exercise progressions use this humeral head depressor effect of the adducting muscle activity demonstrated in this study.

Kibler WB: Management of the scapula in gleno-humeral instability. *Tech Shoulder Elbow Surg* 2003;4: 89-90.

This is a discussion of the role of the scapula in shoulder dysfunction and glenohumeral instability. The author assesses methods to evaluate scapular position and motion and provides examples of rehabilitative exercises and progressions.

Kibler WB: Shoulder rehabilitation: Principles and practice. *Med Sci Sports Exerc* 1998;30:S40-S50.

This article presents a well-organized description of shoulder rehabilitation principles and the specific application of those principles.

Uhl TL, Carver TJ, Mattacola CG, Mair SD, Nitz AJ: Shoulder musculature activation during upper extremity weight-bearing exercise. *J Orthop Sports Phys Ther* 2003;33:109-117.

This is an electromyographic study examining shoulder muscle activation in various weight-bearing, or closed kinetic chain, postures. The study demonstrates a direct linear relationship between the amount of axial load through upper extremity and shoulder muscle activity.

Classic Bibliography

Fleisig GS, Barrentine SW, Escamilla RF, Andrews JR: Biomechanics of overhand throwing with implications for injuries. *Sports Med* 1996;21:421-437.

Putnam CA: Sequential motions of body segments in striking and throwing skills: Description and explanations. *J Biomech* 1993;26:125-135.

Voss DE: Proprioceptive neuromuscular facilitation. *Am J Phys Med* 1967;46:838-898.

Young JL, Herring SA, Press JM, Casazza BA: The influence of the spine on the shoulder in the throwing athlete. *J Back Musculoskeletal Rehabil* 1996;7:5-17.

Zattara M, Bouisset S: Posturo-kinetic organisation during the early phase of voluntary upper limb movement: 1. Normal subjects. *J Neurol Neurosurg Psychiatry* 1988;51:956-965.

Section 3

Injuries of the Lower Extremity

Section Editor:
Ben K. Graf, MD

Chapter 11

Hip and Groin Injuries

Steve A. Mora, MD

Bert R. Mandelbaum, MD

J.W. Thomas Byrd, MD

Introduction

Hip and groin pain in the athlete can result in significant loss of playing time, extensive rehabilitation time, and early retirement from competition. The task of diagnosing and managing hip and groin pain represents one of the greatest challenges in sports medicine. This is especially true in patients with chronic symptoms that are generalized and ambiguous. Therefore, to avoid misguided treatment strategies and to ultimately ensure treatment success, knowledge of a broad differential diagnosis is needed and a methodic diagnostic approach must be followed.

Muscle and Tendon Injuries

Apophyseal Avulsion Injuries

An avulsion fracture is a fracture through an apophyseal cartilage plate caused by a large distraction force. This type of fracture is essentially a Salter-Harris I fracture through the anterior-superior iliac spine, anterior-inferior iliac spine, and ischial tuberosity apophysis. An apophysis is a secondary center of ossification that contributes to peripheral growth but not longitudinal growth. Avulsion fractures occur almost exclusively in athletic adolescent patients within the age range of 11 to 17 years and in such sports as soccer, track, football, and baseball. These fractures most often occur during running or sprinting. Of all pediatric pelvic fractures, avulsion fractures are the most common.

An avulsion fracture typically occurs when a large distraction force is generated from a sudden forceful concentric or eccentric contraction of the muscle group that attaches onto the apophysis. Rarely, these fractures may also be caused by a forceful direct blow. In young patients, there is failure at the apophyseal cartilage interface rather than at the tendon or muscle as in adults. Fractures of the anterior-superior iliac spine are caused by contractions of the sartorius and tensor fascia lata muscles, whereas fractures of the anterior-inferior iliac spine are caused by contractions of the straight head of the rectus femoris muscle (Figure 1). Sprinting and swinging a baseball bat will usually avulse the sartorius

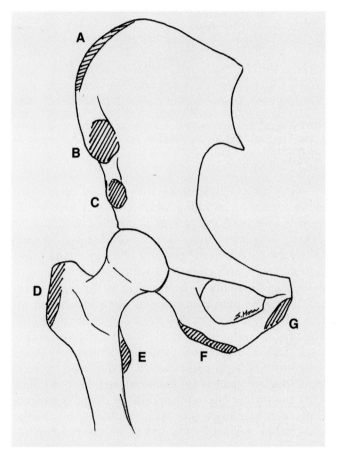

Figure 1 Potential sites for apophyseal fractures and muscle attachments of the pelvis. A = iliac crest (internal and external obliques), B = anterior-superior iliac spine (sartorius and tensor fascia lata), C = anterior-inferior iliac spine (rectus femoris), D = greater trochanter (gluteus medius), E = lesser trochanter (iliopsoas), F = (most common) ischial tuberosity (semimembranous, semitendinosus, and biceps femoris), G = adductors and gracilis.

and tensor fascia lata muscle insertions on the anterior-superior iliac spine. This mechanism occurs when the hip is extended and the knee is flexed. Fractures of the ischial tuberosity are the most common overall and are a result of semitendinosus, semimembranosus, and adductor muscle contractions. Hurdlers are at increased risk of these fractures.

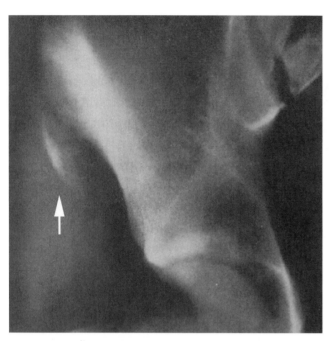

Figure 2 An oblique view of the pelvis showing an acute fracture of the anterior-superior iliac spine (*arrow*). Fractures with subtle displacement are best seen on oblique radiographs.

As a consequence, these fractures are most commonly observed in young athletes after a sudden extreme physical effort, such as a sprinting, hurdling, or kicking. Frequently, there is an associated pop or snap felt by the patient at the moment of injury. Acute lower extremity, hip, and groin pain with restricted range of motion and inability to bear weight is the typical presentation. The pain is aggravated when making an attempt to contract or stretch the avulsed muscle group. The area over the avulsion site may be swollen, ecchymotic, and tender. Rarely, avulsion fractures may cause temporary meralgia paraesthetica. A displaced apophysis is usually apparent on plain radiographs, but CT or MRI can further characterize difficult cases. In patients with anterior-inferior iliac spine avulsions, an oblique plain radiograph projection may be necessary to appreciate subtle displacement (Figure 2). If the apophysis is not yet calcified, then the clinical diagnosis of apophyseal fracture can be presumptively made. Frequently, apophyseal fractures are misdiagnosed as groin strains, hamstring strains, or contusions. A robust formation of callus is usually seen with normal healing. For patients in whom the athletic history is ambiguous or the acute event is forgotten, the formation of abundant callus and periosteal new bone may lead to the misdiagnosis of Ewing's tumor or osteomyelitis and result in unnecessary biopsies.

Treatment is usually conservative and consists of rest and protected weight bearing with crutches followed by a supervised rehabilitation program. Most authors have reported excellent results following nonsurgical treatment despite the fact that the radiographic findings at the end of healing are abnormal because of the large bridging callus formation. Conservative treatment begins with rest and protected weight bearing. Without adequate protection, a symptomatic nonunion may result; therefore, no weight bearing or protected weight bearing for up to 3 weeks or until early callus forms is recommended. A gradual increase in muscle and joint mobilization should be followed by a progressive resistance program. To prevent reinjury, it is important that complete fracture union and complete muscular rehabilitation be achieved before allowing the patient to return to sports. It may be desirable to have a physical therapist perform isokinetic muscle testing to evaluate a patient's progress and make further treatment decisions. In one study, 24 of 27 patients returned to their preinjury status within 4 months after following a closely supervised progressive rehabilitation program. Two patients had a delayed return to preinjury status by 8 months, and one patient had local aching but continued to function competitively. Similarly, asymptomatic nonunions or asymptomatic partial unions may also lead to good clinical results and not require surgery.

The most common complication of nonsurgical treatment is exostosis-like formation at the fracture site, which may lead to mechanical symptoms. If a loss of function is anticipated from a displaced fracture in a high-level athlete, then surgery may be contemplated. Following a displaced nonunion or malunion, impairment may be brought about as a consequence to a shortened musculotendinous contractile unit. The contractile properties of the muscle are altered in such a way that a maximum force cannot be achieved because of the shortened muscle length. There are reports of using open reduction and internal fixation to treat these injuries, but these are few and no improvement in outcome has been shown. In most patients, surgery should not be considered as the primary treatment option. Indications for open treatment and internal fixation include fractures with greater than 3 cm of displacement, painful nonunions, and patients who demand shorter convalescence and/or the highest level of function. Surgery may shorten the convalescent period, reduce the period of immobilization, and allow a competitive athlete to resume athletic activity more promptly. Surgical treatment consists of open treatment and internal fixation with cerclage wiring and/or screw fixation. Potential complications, which are the same as those associated with adult pelvis fractures, can be potentially serious and include cutaneous nerve injury, misguided hardware, hemorrhage, infection, and hip joint damage. Complete recovery, return to sports, and no long-term sequelae can be anticipated following most apophyseal fractures regardless of the nonsurgical or surgical treatment chosen.

Hip Pointers

In athletic competition, muscle contusion injury is a frequent and potentially debilitating condition. A hip pointer is a type of contusion and specifically refers to an injury to the subcutaneous iliac wing and surrounding structures. The injury is caused by a direct blow and often occurs in contact sports such as hockey, rugby, and football. Other adjacent structures may be injured, including the tensor fascia lata, external oblique muscle, and femoral trochanter. Hematomas are common and can dissect between the gluteus muscle and the iliac crest, causing excruciating pain.

Typically, the athlete presents with pain, ecchymosis, muscle spasms, and exquisite tenderness at the impact site. A hematoma may present as a fluctuant mass and may not be initially visible. Although the diagnosis of a hip pointer has traditionally been made clinically, imaging studies such as ultrasonography and MRI are becoming increasingly important in both identifying and delineating the extent of injury. In patients with significant trauma, AP and oblique pelvis radiographs are important to rule out an iliac wing fracture or, in the adolescent patient, an apophyseal avulsion fracture.

The initial treatment for hip pointers consists of rest from activities that aggravate the injury, a short course of nonsteroidal anti-inflammatory drugs (NSAIDs), and ice. Animal studies have shown that NSAIDs do not compromise the basic process of myofiber regeneration after an injury, but supportive controlled clinical studies are not yet available. Injection of corticosteroids (such as methylprednisolone) into the injured muscle may be beneficial in limiting inflammation over the short term but may cause irreversible damage to healing muscle over the long term, including disordered fiber structure and a marked diminution in force-generating capacity; therefore, corticosteroid injections are not routinely recommended. Aspiration of a large painful hematoma will improve symptoms and possibly improve recovery time, and a progressive physical therapy program aimed at regaining hip motion, stretching, and strengthening will typically lead to complete recovery within 2 to 4 weeks. Complications of hip pointers include myositis ossificans traumatica, muscle fibrosis, and delayed muscle soreness.

Snapping Hip Syndrome

Coxa saltans is a term used to describe the snapping hip syndrome. Snapping hip syndrome is usually classified as internal or external. In both types, the symptoms are characterized as an audible soft-tissue snapping, popping, or clicking that occurs while taking the hip through a range of motion. Although the snapping is not always associated with pain, it may become a nuisance. The more common external type is caused by snapping of either the posterior border of the iliotibial band or the an-

terior border of the gluteus maximus over the greater trochanter of the femur. The snapping symptoms typically occur when the hip is brought into adduction with knee extension, causing the iliotibial band to tighten. Pain is caused by mechanical irritation and/or greater trochanteric bursitis. The differential diagnosis for pain over the greater trochanter should also include degenerative joint disease of the hip (including the sacroiliac joint) and radiating pain from spinal pathology.

The internal type of snapping hip syndrome is presumed to be caused by the iliopsoas tendon tightly gliding over the iliopectineal line of the pelvis or the femoral head of the hip joint. The internal type is most commonly seen in ballet dancers. The snapping is over the hip joint and therefore should be differentiated from intra-articular pathology, such as loose bodies or labral tears of the hip joint. The symptoms are usually worse when the hip is fully loaded, such as during running or weight training.

The history and physical examination usually will consistently point toward the diagnosis in most patients. The patient may be able to voluntarily reproduce the snapping with hip flexion and extension or flexion with external rotation and abduction while allowing the examiner to palpate the snap over the anterior hip joint. Plain radiographs will rarely show abnormal calcification near the lesser trochanter. Conventional and dynamic sonography will consistently and economically confirm the pathologic snapping structure in both types of snapping hip syndrome. MRI is useful for ruling out other pathologic conditions that can mimic snapping hip, such as tumors or intra-articular hip lesions.

Both internal and external types of snapping hip syndrome respond to initial treatment consisting of rest, activity modification, avoidance of intentional snapping, stretching and strengthening of the iliopsoas and iliotibial band, NSAIDs, and occasionally to steroid injections. For refractory cases of external snapping hip, a variety of surgical procedures have been used, including Z-plasty, excision, longitudinal incision, ellipsoid excision, and fixation of the iliotibial band. In patients in whom the pain is caused exclusively by trochanteric bursitis, a bursectomy (either open or endoscopic) has been described. The surgical treatment of internal snapping hip syndrome is aimed at either relieving the tension across the iliopsoas tendon or completely releasing it from its insertion onto the lesser trochanter. Complete tenotomy of the tendon using a cosmetic medial approach may lead to postoperative hip flexion weakness. Although fractional lengthening of the iliopsoas tendon at its musculotendinous junction using a modified iliofemoral approach may negate the prevalence of hip flexion weakness, it can also introduce less desirable effects, such as a noncosmetic scar and increased risk to the femoral nerve. The results following surgical release are reported to be excellent and have allowed most patients to return to competitive athletics. Complications of surgical release include cutaneous nerve damage, femoral nerve damage, infections, and hemorrhage.

Iliopsoas Tendinitis

Painful areas of tendon are commonly ascribed the term tendinitis. When the iliopsoas tendon becomes painful, it is frequently referred to as iliopsoas tendinitis. Although tendinitis implies the presence of inflammation, histologic studies of suspected inflamed tissues do not show the characteristic signs of an inflammatory response (few inflammatory cells and little formation of granulation tissue). The histologic appearance is more consistent with a degenerative condition (increased fibroblasts, increased vascularity, disorganized matrix, fatty mucoid features). Therefore, a more accurate term for this condition may be iliopsoas tendinosis.

Although patients with iliopsoas tendinosis are frequently diagnosed as having groin strain or hip flexor strain, iliopsoas tendinosis is actually difficult to distinguish from other local groin injuries, such as pectineus muscle strains, adductor muscle strains, and anterior abdominal wall strains. When iliopsoas tendinosis is associated with the sensation of anterior hip snapping, the condition is referred to as the snapping hip syndrome or coxa saltans.

Patients usually present with unilateral pain and/or snapping over the anterior hip that is accentuated when the hip joint is put through a range of motion. Tenderness and a palpable snap may be present over the iliopsoas tendon, and the pain is accentuated with resistive hip flexion. The diagnosis is readily made and usually based solely on the history and physical examination. However, subtle clinical presentations may prove to be perplexing; therefore, the clinician should be aware of the broad differential diagnosis for groin pain and pubalgia. Imaging studies other than plain radiographs are rarely necessary in patients with an obvious snapping hip. Bursography and tenography have largely been supplanted by sonography and MRI. Conventional and dynamic sonography can help identify iliopsoas tendinitis, bursitis, synovitis, and tendon subluxation. Magnetic resonance arthrography may demonstrate intra-articular hip pathology, such as loose bodies or labral tears. The treatment for iliopsoas tendinosis is the same as the treatment for snapping hip syndrome.

Piriformis Muscle Syndrome

The piriformis muscle syndrome is characterized by extrapelvic sciatic nerve compression in the area of the greater sciatic notch of the pelvis. The symptoms of piriformis muscle syndrome are nonspecific, and include pain and dysesthesias in the gluteal region and radiating to the hip or posterior thigh and sometimes in a radicular pain pattern down the leg. The patient may experience cramping, burning, or aching in the buttock or posterior thigh, making the symptoms indistinct from those of a hamstring tear or intra-articular hip problems. The name deep gluteal syndrome has recently been applied in the sports medicine literature to describe the constellation of symptoms. The symptoms are thought to be caused by entrapment of one or more divisions of the sciatic nerve, gluteal nerves, posterior femoral cutaneous nerve, and pudendal nerve by the piriformis muscle or alternatively by the obturator internus/gemelli muscular complex. Uncommon anatomic variants of the sciatic nerve as it courses along the piriformis muscle are believed to be contributory factors; however, this association is not grounded in diagnostic studies or surgical observation. One such variant is the bipartite piriformis muscle with the peroneal division of the sciatic nerve coursing between and through its muscle belly. Pathologic changes of the piriformis muscle such as inflammation, edema, tight fibrous bands, and hypertrophic changes can affect the sciatic nerve as it courses nearby. Lesions around the greater sciatic notch, such as tumors, infections, inferior gluteal artery aneurysms/pseudoaneurysms, a persistent sciatic artery, and inflammation of the sacroiliac joint, can lead to sciatic nerve dysfunction (Figure 3).

Piriformis muscle syndrome should be suspected in patients with sciatica and/or posterior gluteal/thigh pain and nondiagnostic MRI scans of the spine. The radicular pain may also be reproduced by passively raising the straightened leg and dorsiflexing the ankle (Lasègue's sign). Flexion, adduction, and internal rotation of the hip will frequently exacerbate the symptoms. Although the neurologic examination can reveal abnormalities such as abnormal reflexes and motor weakness, deficits are rare.

Because athletes frequently expose themselves to trauma, microtrauma, and overuse, muscular injuries and stress fractures should be an important part of the differential diagnosis. The differential diagnosis also includes hamstring injuries, labral tears, chondral lesions, intra-articular loose bodies, degenerative arthritis of the hip or sacroiliac joint, masses, and trochanteric bursitis. In patients with radiculitis, more common causes such as lumbar stenosis, central spinal stenosis, lateral recess stenosis, herniated nucleus pulposus, and discogenic pain should be investigated with appropriate imaging studies.

Historically, imaging studies have been nondiagnostic. Pelvic CT and MRI are used primarily for ruling out pathologic lesions such as space-occupying lesions, hematomas, muscle-tendon tears, and intra-articular hip problems. Occasionally, MRI or CT will identify an abnormal hypertrophic piriformis muscle. Nuclear medicine scintigraphy has limited diagnostic benefits. Electrodiagnostic studies are the only diagnostic modality that can objectively document functional impingement of the sciatic nerve by the piriformis muscle. Several investigators have found prolongation of the F response and the H reflex in the sciatic nerve distribution. These findings are accentuated when the patient's hip is placed in the flexed, adducted, and internally rotated position. Abnormally prolonged segmental somatosensory potentials have also been demonstrated in patients with piriformis muscle syndrome. Fluoroscopically assisted or electromyographically assisted anesthetic injections may confirm the diagnosis by immediately alleviating the symptoms.

Once the diagnosis of piriformis muscle syndrome is made, several treatment options are available for piriformis muscle syndrome. The treatment algorithm begins with rest, NSAIDs, muscle relaxants, and a physical therapy program aimed at stretching and strengthening the piriformis muscle and short external rotators of the hip. There is no consensus as to which exercise program is most beneficial. In recalcitrant cases, a piriformis muscle anesthetic and corticosteroid injection will not only confirm the diagnosis but serve as treatment. An alternative to the piriformis muscle injection is a caudal epidural injection for anesthetic/steroid introduction around the sciatic nerve roots. Botulinum toxin has also been selectively injected into the piriformis muscle with limited success. The length of time spent on conservative treatment should be individually based. Surgical exploration and release of all impinging structures is recommended in recalcitrant cases of piriformis muscle syndrome. Surgical treatment consists of sectioning the muscle at its tendinous origin, release of fibrous bands or compressing vessels, and external sciatic neurolysis. Because the impinging lesion may not be the piriformis muscle, it is important to do a methodic exploration of the area and release as necessary. Before contemplating surgery, the surgeon should review the diagnostic steps leading to the diagnosis and, if necessary, additional or repeat investigations should be performed before surgical treatment. Surgical exploration and decompression of the piriformis muscle with or without neurolysis carries several potential risks, including significant injury to vascular and neural structures, wound seroma, infected hematoma, hemorrhage, and nerve injury.

Pubalgia

Athletic pubalgia refers to chronic groin and lower abdominal pain caused by an incompetent abdominal wall. Other terms used to describe this condition include sports hernia, sportsman's hernia, Gilmore's groin, and hockey groin syndrome. Pubalgia is common in sporting activities such as hockey, soccer, rugby, sprinting, and hurdles, which demand sudden forceful contracture or rotation of the hip and lower abdomen. The pathomechanics are thought to be caused by eccentric loading of the abdominal muscles, core weakness, overload, and imbalance. The symptoms can become chronic and se-

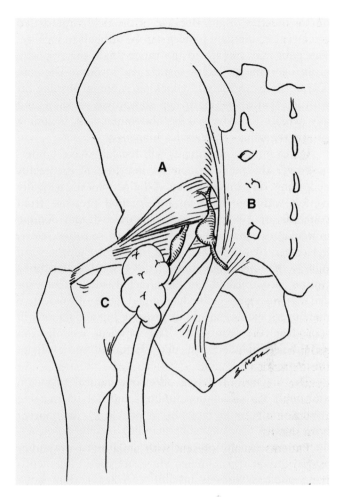

Figure 3 Potential areas for sciatic nerve compression in piriformis muscle syndrome. A = anomalous relationship among a bifid piriformis muscle splitting the sciatic nerve into the peroneal and tibial divisions, hypertrophied and inflamed piriformis muscle, and fibrous bands dividing the muscle; B = inflammation of the sacroiliac joint, pseudoaneurysm/aneurysm of the inferior gluteal artery or persistent sciatic artery; C = mass lesions, such as tumors or infections.

verely debilitating, resulting in significant time away from competitive athletics and potentially ending professional athletic careers.

The main cause of pubalgia is believed to be nonpalpable, small, direct and indirect hernias or microscopic tears or avulsions of the internal oblique muscles. The principal intraoperative pathology is described in the literature as including torn external oblique aponeurosis, torn conjoined tendon, conjoined tendon torn from the pubic tubercle, dehiscence between conjoined tendon and inguinal ligament, and the absence of an inguinal hernia. Other pathologic findings include thinning of the transversalis fascia and entrapment of the ilioinguinal nerve.

Because there are numerous causes for groin pain, a focused history and physical examination are crucial. The athlete characteristically presents with recurrent exertional pain in the pubic symphysis area and adjacent to the insertion of the abdominal musculature and adductor muscles origin. Because of the richly innervated groin region, the pain pattern can be difficult to localize. The pain may radiate to the inner thigh, the opposite groin, or to the ipsilateral testicle and scrotum. The pain is typically exacerbated by kicking, running, pushing off with ice skates, making a slap shot, torso rotation, and any activity that stresses the abdominal wall, including sit-ups, sneezing, or a Valsalva maneuver.

On examination, patients will typically have tenderness over the pubic symphysis, insertion of the rectus abdominis, and inguinal ring. A bulge may occasionally be felt with increased intra-abdominal pressure from coughing, or a palpable gap over the external oblique musculature may be present. The most sensitive test is performed by placing the small finger through the scrotum so that close palpation of the suspected structures can be accomplished. On the affected side, the superficial inguinal ring may be dilated and tender. Provocative maneuvers such as sit-ups or resistive hip adduction will reproduce the symptoms. The physical examination should also include a testicular examination to evaluate for masses.

The diagnosis is based on strong clinical suspicion and physical examination findings and not on imaging studies. Plain radiographs are valuable for diagnosing other causes of groin pain, including osteitis pubis, adductor muscle cortical avulsions, and stress fractures. Single-limb stance flamingo views are useful for identifying pubic symphysis instability. A technetium bone scan may also provide information to help narrow the differential diagnosis. Herniography has been used for identifying nonpalpable hernias in Europe, but it has not been used much in the United States. Ultrasonography has also shown promise for detecting inguinal canal and posterior-wall deficiencies. MRI is best for evaluating soft-tissue injuries such as adductor tears or stress fractures, but it usually produces no evidence of injury in patients with pubalgia. A diagnostic injection of local anesthetic (without steroid) into the point of maximal tenderness along the external oblique is a useful diagnostic option.

Conservative treatment includes relative rest, NSAIDs, physical therapy, and gradual return to athletic activities. A corticosteroid injection into the abdominal musculature is not recommended. The physical therapy program should be based on an active training program, core strengthening, and eliminating muscular imbalances between abdominal and hip musculature. Surgical exploration should take place only if 9 to 12 weeks of physiotherapy fails to relieve symptoms. Surgical treatment is highly successful and includes restoring and reinforcing the normal anatomy with or without a synthetic mesh and ablation of the ilioinguinal nerve, if necessary. Surgically treated patients are allowed to return to athletic activities after 8 weeks, and approximately 90% of athletes will make a successful return to athletic activity following the surgery.

Efforts have been made to identify groin injury risk factors and implementation of prevention strategies, especially in soccer and hockey where groin strains are frequently encountered. Risk factors are thought to include hip adductor weakness, improper warm-up, poor conditioning, and previous groin injury. A prospective controlled intervention study evaluated the effects of a soccer injury prevention program on the total number of injuries sustained in control and intervention groups over a 1-year period. The exercises were specifically designed to improve flexibility of the trunk, hip, and leg muscles; coordination; and endurance. The prevention program also raised coach and player awareness of injuries and promoted the spirit of fair play. Comparison of the intervention and control group revealed a decreased number of total injuries per player, including groin strains. Unfortunately, the sample size in this study was too small to make a comparative analysis of specific injuries.

Adductor muscle weakness was examined in another prospective study that evaluated a therapeutic intervention for the prevention of adductor strains in professional ice hockey players. Players whose adductor-to-abductor muscle strength ratio was less than 80% were considered to be at risk for groin injury. At-risk players participated in a 6-week therapeutic exercise program emphasizing hip adductor muscle strengthening. The program consisted of concentric, eccentric, and functional strengthening of the adductor muscles. The incidence of adductor strains per 1,000 players was 0.71 in the intervention group versus 3.20 in the control group. This study demonstrated that a therapeutic intervention of strengthening the adductor muscles appears to be an effective method for preventing adductor strains.

Hamstring Injuries

Hamstring strains commonly occur in many sports, including soccer, football (American and Australian Rules), sprinting, water skiing, and any other activity requiring rapid acceleration and deceleration. In Australian Rules football, 34% of hamstring strains are recurrent, resulting in significant loss of playing and practice time. Because these injuries are associated with such a high rate of chronicity, recurrence, and sporting disability, identification of athletes at risk and prevention efforts are being emphasized.

The hamstring muscle group consists of the biceps femoris (short and long head), semitendinosus, and semimembranosus. The hamstring muscles are two-joint muscles that extend the hip and flex the knee joint. The long head of the biceps femoris, semitendinosus, and semimembranosus originate from the ischial tuberosity of the pelvis and are innervated by the tibial branch of the sciatic nerve. The short head of the biceps femoris originates along the linea aspera of the distal femur and receives its innervation from the peroneal portion of the sciatic nerve. Distally, the biceps femoris attaches to the fibular head and the lateral condyle to the femur, posterolateral capsule, iliotibial tract, and proximal lateral tibia. The semimembranosus has various attachment sites into the posteromedial corner of the knee joint capsule and proximal tibia. The semimembranosus contributes to the formation of the posterior oblique ligament and enhances valgus stability during knee flexion. The semitendinosus merges with the gracilis tendon and the sartorius to form the pes anserinus complex of the proximal medial tibial metaphysis.

Most patients with hamstring strains report acute posterior thigh pain or tightness, usually at the moment of a strenuous activity such as sprinting. The injury is thought to occur when the hamstring is resisting knee extension or at heel strike. The hamstring strain is a result of eccentric elongation, with failure occurring at the musculotendinous unit of muscle proximal to the insertion into bone. The acute pathophysiologic response is initiated by an inflammatory cascade that concludes with fibrous scar formation and muscle regeneration. The proximal long head of the biceps femoris is most frequently injured, and the majority of hamstring strains are partial-thickness tears.

Studies attempting to identify hamstring strain risk factors are few. Even fewer are the number of studies examining the effects of intervention. The risk factors that have been most closely examined are a history of a previous posterior thigh injury, strength imbalance (weakness), and hamstring muscle tightness (loss of range of motion). Most studies have consistently identified a previous hamstring injury as an important risk factor. Athletes with hamstring injuries often return to athletic competition before reaching maximal recovery and thereby place themselves at risk for reinjury. If hamstring strength parameters are corrected, the risk of reinjury has been shown to be less. Hamstring weakness or strength imbalance has also been shown to be a possible risk factor, although a consensus has not been reached. A recent prospective study revealed a significant association between preseason hamstring muscle weakness and subsequent injury. This cohort study analyzed preseason hamstring/quadriceps concentric peak torques in 37 professional Australian Rules football players and followed these athletes over the course of a football season. The best predictors of injury were found to be the ratios of hamstring-to-quadriceps muscle and limb-to-limb differences in hamstring strength. Players are at risk of hamstring injury if they have hamstring-to-quadriceps muscle ratios (at 60° per second) of less than 0.61 or hamstring-to-opposite hamstring muscle ratios (at 60° per second) of less than 0.92 on either limb. The authors recommend that these athletes complete a ham-

string muscle strengthening program and then repeat concentric isokinetic testing to evaluate their progress. Other authors also recommend correcting hamstring to quadriceps ratios to a desired ratio of 0.60. There are no prospective clinical trials testing the effects of intervention for hamstring strains.

The majority of acute hamstring tears are treated successfully with rest, ice, compression, and elevation (for the first 5 to 7 days), followed by a progressive functional rehabilitation program directed at complete restoration of flexibility and strength before returning the athlete to competition. There is no consensus on the most effective rehabilitation program for patients with hamstring strains. Because injuries usually occur at the point of maximal hamstring muscle stretch (heel strike), some authors advocate the implementation of eccentric exercises (exercises in which the muscle develops force while elongating). In patients with a complete hamstring rupture, nonsurgical treatment has yielded less than satisfying results; therefore, some authors have advocated surgical treatment. A review of 12 patients with severe hamstring injuries revealed persistent and significant functional impairment, especially during vigorous activities, and 5 patients with complete hamstring ruptures were incapable of running or participating in agility sports. The results following surgical repair using suture anchors, a knee flexion harness for 4 weeks, and a supervised rehabilitation program led to satisfactory results. Isokinetic muscle testing revealed an overall average of 91% return of hamstring muscle strength, and patients returned to athletic activity at an average of 6 months after surgery.

Pelvis and Hip Joint Injuries
Stress Fractures of the Pelvis
Stress fractures of the pelvis are most commonly seen in sports involving chronic repetitive motion such as distance running. Stress fractures may occur in the sacrum or the pelvic rami, particularly at the junction of the ischium and inferior pubic ramus. The symptoms are characterized by worsening pain with activity that subsides with cessation. As with most stress fractures, radiographs may show no evidence of an injury until bone remodeling occurs in response to the fracture. Bone scanning is sensitive at detecting these lesions and is relatively inexpensive. Although MRI has comparable sensitivity, it may be more specific for the nature of the lesion. Because these lesions can mimic neoplasms, it is important to consider this in the differential diagnosis; however, it is equally important not to misdiagnose a pelvic stress fracture as a neoplastic process.

Pelvic stress fractures are generally stable and respond effectively to conservative management. The principal treatment involves modifying the athlete's activities below the threshold of symptoms. This may require a pe-

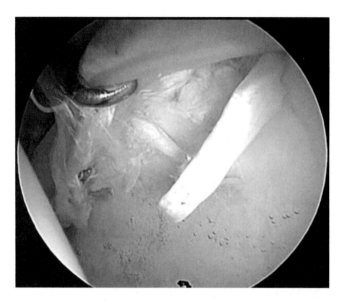

Figure 4 Arthroscopic view from the anterolateral portal demonstrates a comminuted tear of the anterior labrum that is partially retracted by the probe in a 21-year-old collegiate hockey player with mechanical left hip pain. (Copyright © J.W. Thomas Byrd, MD.)

riod of protected weight bearing until patients are pain free. Low-impact exercises should be implemented to maintain conditioning while allowing the fracture to heal. A full recovery is expected, but it may take 3 to 5 months. For multiple or recurrent stress fractures, investigation for an underlying cause of osteopenia is necessary, and physicians should be especially aware of the possible presence of the female athlete triad.

Stress fractures of the femoral neck warrant closer scrutiny. Athletes with stress fractures of the femoral neck can report symptoms of muscle pain that may be migratory and ill-defined. An index of suspicion is paramount because of the potentially disastrous consequences if untreated lesions progress to overt fractures. Medial-sided lesions occur on the compressive surface, which demonstrates more inherent stability and can generally be treated conservatively. Surgical intervention is reserved for patients who remain symptomatic despite conservative measures or when the lesion is large and extends most of the way across the femoral neck. Lateral stress fractures occur on the tensile surface and are considered fractures at risk. These lesions are best managed with early surgical intervention consisting of multiple screw fixation of the femoral neck.

Osteitis Pubis

Osteitis pubis is a painful inflammatory process involving the pubic symphysis. Among athletes, it is most commonly caused by repetitive microtrauma of the joint and is typically associated with activities requiring repetitive kicking or hip abduction/adduction motion, such as soccer, hockey, and Australian Rules football. Breakdown may occur as the result of subtle pelvic instability, and it

has been postulated that this can be accentuated in the presence of athletic pubalgia when there is loss of the stabilizing effect of the conjoined attachment site of the rectus abdominis, pelvic floor musculature, and hip adductors.

Osteitis pubis can develop as the result of nontraumatic causes as well, and this should be kept in mind when assessing this problem in athletes. Nontraumatic causes include infectious and inflammatory processes, often in association with urologic or gynecologic disorders. Again, it is imperative not to overlook these other potential causes when managing an athlete with osteitis pubis.

Athletes with osteitis pubis often report ill-defined muscular symptoms, especially spasm of the hip adductors, which is secondary to the inflamed pubic symphysis. Careful examination will characteristically reveal tenderness localized directly over the pubic symphysis. In patients with chronic symptoms, radiographs may demonstrate degenerative changes within the joint. Bone scanning will typically show increased activity in this region, and MRI may reveal surrounding edema.

Osteitis pubis usually responds successfully to conservative treatment, but complete recovery may take many months. Management includes oral anti-inflammatory medications and activity modification to minimize the offending activities. Judicious use of a corticosteroid injection within the pubic symphysis may be appropriate for patients who do not respond to conservative treatment, but it should not be used as a substitute for avoidance of offending activities during the acute phase of pain. Surgery is rarely indicated for patients with osteitis pubis, and the results of surgical intervention for this condition are uncertain. Various surgical procedures have been proposed for treating osteitis pubis, ranging from simple débridement or adductor tenotomy to resection or fusion.

Hip Joint Pathology
Labral Tears
Labral tears are the most common hip joint lesions encountered in athletes (Figure 4). Labral tears are often attributed to a twisting injury, although the mechanism described may be as variable as the severity of the causative event. The labrum is often susceptible to tearing because of underlying degeneration or abnormal joint morphology, such as in patients with acetabular dysplasia. Predisposing factors should be suspected when the reported injury seems relatively trivial. Senile changes, including degeneration, are known to occur with age and are almost uniformly present in an elderly population. Labral tears occur at its junction with the acetabular articular cartilage. Although labral tears may be isolated tears of the labrum, in at least 50% of patients, there is also a variable amount of associated articular damage.

Of the various diagnostic modalities available for detecting intra-articular pathology, MRI has shown the greatest promise in detecting lesions of the labrum. The sensitivity of MRI can be enhanced by using gadolinium arthrographic techniques. As these studies become more sensitive, however, the chance of false-positive interpretations also increases. Abnormal MRI appearance of the labrum has been reported in asymptomatic volunteers, and the incidence of abnormal signals increases with age. It is also likely that many asymptomatic athletes may start to show imaging evidence of disease during the course of a long competitive career.

Arthroscopy is the procedure of choice for treating persistently symptomatic lesions. Although results are typically favorable, arthroscopy is not uniformly successful in the treatment of labral tears. The best results have been reported among athletes, but in general populations, the success of labral débridement has ranged from 68% to 80%. The extent of associated articular damage is often the limiting factor in the success of this procedure. Published series describe resecting the damaged portion of the labrum while preserving as much of the healthy portion as possible. This is important to minimize the risk of future degenerative changes or potentially destabilizing the joint. Successful results with reparative techniques have not yet been reported. There are only a few technical challenges to repairing the labrum, but the greater barrier is the limited understanding of the pathomechanics of these lesions, which makes it difficult to determine which tears are potentially repairable and have a reliable chance of healing.

Chondral Damage
Acute articular damage is increasingly recognized as a source of disabling hip pain, especially in athletes. The mechanism of injury is often a direct blow to the greater trochanter, as can occur as the result of a fall or collision (Figure 5). In healthy young athletes with strong bones and little adipose tissue over the trochanter to cushion the effects of a blow, rather than fracturing the femoral neck, the force is delivered unchecked into the articular surfaces. This can result in an area of full-thickness articular loss caused by shear forces on the medial aspect of the femoral head or chondronecrosis in the superomedial weight-bearing portion of the acetabulum. Athletes with chondral damage usually recall the specific injury, but the symptoms are often not disabling, and the nature of the problem only becomes evident when athletes fail to fully recover. The location of articular breakdown caused by generalized wear occurs at the articular labral junction of the acetabulum and is usually associated with tearing of the labrum.

Chondral defects are usually difficult to detect using MRI and magnetic resonance arthrography. However, with acute articular damage from an impact load, there may be an accompanying area of altered signal in the

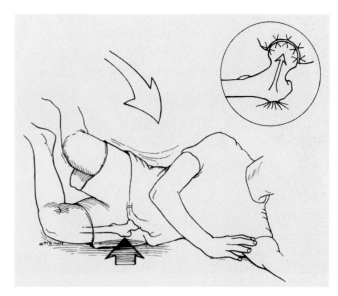

Figure 5 Illustration showing how a direct blow to the greater trochanter is more likely to result in acute articular damage in physically fit young adult athletes. Because this population of athletes has strong bone structure and there is little adipose tissue to cushion the blow, the force is transferred unchecked to the hip joint. Elderly or osteoporotic patients are more likely to simply fracture the proximal femur, and young children are more likely to injure the growth plate. (Copyright © J.W. Thomas Byrd, MD.)

subchondral bone, especially on the femoral side. These findings may mimic the findings of osteonecrosis, but the area and pattern of involvement is distinctly different. The area of involvement is more medial, and the pattern of altered signal emanates more from the subjacent area of impact (Figure 6).

Excision of unstable fragments associated with acute articular damage is often successful in eliminating mechanical symptoms. For the more common lesions that occur at the articular labral junction, chondroplasty to stabilize the articular damage is an important part of the procedure. Microfracture has been reported for some grade IV articular lesions. It is likely that other cartilage restoring techniques will play a role in the repair of chondral defects, but their efficacy has yet to be defined. Chondroplasty of diffuse articular damage associated with degeneration provides unpredictable results; thus, radiographs should be carefully scrutinized for evidence of underlying arthritis.

Disruption of Ligamentum Teres
In one study, lesions of the ligamentum teres were the third most common problem encountered among athletes undergoing hip arthroscopy. Rupture of the ligament is known to occur in association with dislocation of the joint, but it is increasingly recognized to occur as the result of simple twisting injuries as well. This clinical entity has only recently been reported. Investigative studies have demonstrated that lesions of the ligamentum teres are difficult to diagnose, but diagnostic tech-

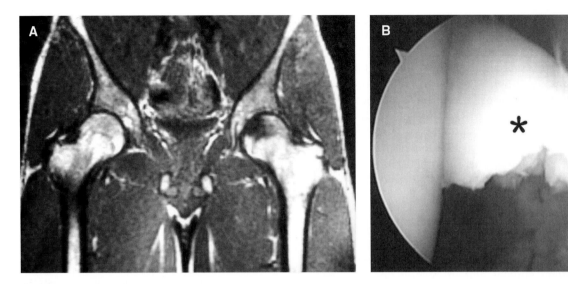

Figure 6 A, Coronal T1-weighted MRI scan demonstrates characteristic signal changes in the medial head subjacent to the area of articular impact in a 20-year-old collegiate basketball player who experienced a direct blow to the trochanter with resultant painful popping of the left hip. **B,** Arthroscopic view from the anterolateral portal demonstrates an unstable grade IV articular flap (*asterisk*). (Copyright © J.W. Thomas Byrd, MD.)

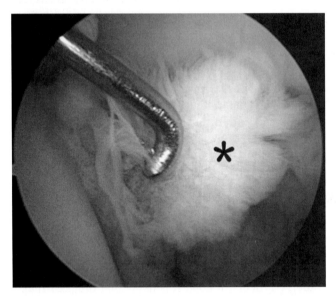

Figure 7 Arthroscopic view from the anterolateral portal demonstrates the ligamentum teres avulsed from its femoral attachment site (*asterisk*) in a 15-year-old high school cheerleader who experienced a twisting injury to her left hip and who has a subsequent 2-year history of painful catching. (Copyright © J.W. Thomas Byrd, MD.)

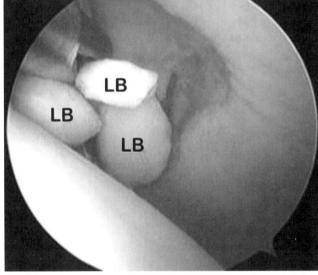

Figure 8 Arthroscopic view demonstrates free-floating loose bodies (LB) in a 19-year-old recreational basketball player with a history of Legg-Calvé-Perthes disease as a child who developed acute catching and locking symptoms in his left hip. (Copyright © J.W. Thomas Byrd, MD.)

niques undoubtedly will improve with the increasing awareness of this type of injury. Athletes with lesions of the ligamentum teres have been found to respond remarkably well to arthroscopic débridement of the disrupted fibers that are entrapped within the joint causing pain (Figure 7).

Loose Bodies
Retrieval of symptomatic loose bodies represents the clearest indication for arthroscopy (Figure 8). The importance of loose body removal has been well documented in the literature, and arthroscopy offers an ex-

cellent alternative to traditional open surgical techniques. Although free fragments caused by trauma are usually readily identified, arthrographic techniques are sometimes required to confirm the diagnosis. Loose bodies caused by disease such as synovial chondromatosis can be more elusive and often require arthroscopy to confirm the diagnosis.

Evaluation and Treatment of Hip Joint Pathology
The evaluation of a patient with hip pain focuses on whether the source of symptoms is intra-articular and thus potentially amenable to treatment with arthroscopy.

TABLE 1 | Characteristic Features of Hip Joint Pathology

Straight plane activity is relatively well tolerated.

Torsional/twisting activities are problematic.

Prolonged hip flexion (sitting) is uncomfortable.

Pain/catching occurs when going from flexion to extension (rising from seated position).

More difficult to walk on inclines than level surfaces.

TABLE 2 | Examination Findings

Groin, anterior, and medial thigh pain

C-sign characteristic of interior hip pain (hand gripped above greater trochanter)

Log-rolling of leg back and forth (most specific indicator of intra-articular pathology)

Forced flexion/internal rotation or abduction/external rotation (more sensitive measure of hip joint pain; reproduces symptoms that patients experience with activities)

Characteristic features of hip joint pathology are summarized in Table 1. In general, a history of a specific traumatic event is a better prognostic indicator than a patient who simply develops the insidious onset of hip pain. Onset of symptoms in the absence of injury implies a degenerative process or predisposition to damage that is less likely to be corrected by arthroscopic intervention. Mechanical symptoms such as sharp, stabbing pain, locking, or catching are also a better prognostic indicator of a potentially correctable problem.

Common examination findings are summarized in Table 2. Although the hip receives innervation from branches of L2 to S1 of the lumbosacral plexus, its principal innervation is the L3 nerve root, which is why irritation of the joint may result in anterior groin and radiating medial thigh pain (it follows the L3 dermatome). Posterior pain is rarely indicative of an intra-articular process, but if clinically suspected, it can be confirmed with a fluoroscopically guided intra-articular injection of anesthetic that should provide temporary alleviation of the pain. The C-sign is characteristic of hip joint pathology. The patient cups the hand above the greater trochanter with the thumb over the posterior aspect and gripping the fingers into the groin. It may appear as if the patient is describing a lateral problem with the iliotibial band or trochanteric bursitis, but this maneuver is actually performed to describe deep interior joint pain.

The log roll test is the most specific test for intra-articular pathology. Gently rolling the thigh internally and externally rotates only the femoral head in relation to the acetabulum and capsule, while not stressing any of the surrounding extra-articular structures. More sensitive maneuvers include forced flexion combined with internal rotation (also referred to as the impingement test) and abduction combined with external rotation. These maneuvers normally cause some discomfort and results must be compared with those of the unaffected hip. More importantly, it should be determined whether the maneuver recreates the type of pain the patient experiences with activities. An accompanying click or pop may be elicited, but this can occur for various reasons; again, more importantly, it should be determined whether this maneuver recreates the patient's symptoms.

Radiographs are an integral part of any assessment of hip joint pathology and should include at least an AP pelvis view of both hips and a lateral view of the affected hip. Radiographs demonstrate poor sensitivity for most intra-articular lesions, but they should be carefully studied for evidence of degenerative disease, preexisting morphologic conditions of the hip (such as dysplasia, impingement, and Perthes' disease), osteonecrosis, lesions in the surrounding pelvis, or asymmetric findings compared with the uninvolved hip. High-resolution MRI has shown promise in detecting intra-articular pathology, but this diagnostic modality requires a 1.5 Tesla magnet and surface coil with a small field of view images of the involved hip. The most reliable indicators are often indirect findings, including effusion, paralabral cysts, and subchondral cysts. Gadolinium arthrography combined with MRI demonstrates superior sensitivity in detecting numerous intra-articular lesions, but its specificity is less certain, with some reports of an increased incidence of false-positive interpretations. In general, these studies are best in showing evidence of labral pathology and poor in showing evidence of lesions of the articular surface. The intra-articular contrast injection should include a long-acting anesthetic (such as bupivacaine) as part of the diluent. Whether patients experience temporary alleviation of their symptoms from the intra-articular anesthetic is the most reliable indicator of the joint being the source of the problem. Following the injection, it is important to have patients perform activities that normally create symptoms to assess the response.

Numerous intra-articular lesions of the hip encountered in athletes can benefit from arthroscopic intervention. In fact, the arthroscope has aided in appreciating the nature and prevalence of many intra-articular disorders that previously went unrecognized and untreated. With this knowledge, clinical assessment skills are starting to improve. Few conditions absolutely obligate arthroscopic intervention. Most clearly, arthroscopy is indicated when hip joint symptoms persist despite a trial of conservative treatment, including activity modification. Among athletes, the most common lesion to be encountered and the lesion most readily diagnosed using

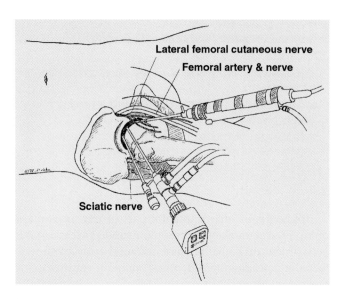

Figure 9 Illustration showing that the relationship of arthroscopy portals to the major neurovascular structures is the same whether the patient is positioned supine or lateral. The three standard portals are shown, including two lateral (anterolateral and posterolateral) and one anterior portal. The femoral artery and nerve lie well medial to the anterior portal. The sciatic nerve lies posterior to the posterolateral portal. Small branches of the lateral femoral cutaneous nerve pass close to the anterior portal. Injury to this structure is avoided by proper technique in portal placement. The anterolateral portal is established first because it lies most centrally in the safe zone for arthroscopy. (Copyright © J.W. Thomas Byrd, MD.)

MRI is damage to the acetabular labrum. Labral pathology, however, has been documented among asymptomatic volunteers, signal changes may begin to occur from the cumulative effect of a prolonged athletic career, and there are numerous examples of athletes who report injuries with MRI evidence of pathology and those injuries then become asymptomatic without surgical intervention. Nonetheless, when managing competitive athletes, time and speed of recovery are often factors that must be considered in the decision-making process.

Hip arthroscopy requires a method for distracting the joint to access the intra-articular structures. The procedure can be performed effectively with the patient in the supine or lateral decubitus position (Figure 9). Some surgeons prefer the familiar orientation of the supine position, which is typically used when managing hip fractures, whereas others prefer the lateral position, which is typically used during total hip arthroplasty. Although the supine approach is advantageous because of the simplicity of patient positioning, the lateral approach may be better for severely obese patients.

A technique of hip arthroscopy without traction is most useful for addressing the extra-articular but intracapsular portion of the joint. Access is facilitated by flexion of the hip, which relaxes the capsule. This is especially advantageous for addressing synovial disease and loose bodies. After completing arthroscopy of the intra-articular region with distraction, traction is released, allowing inspection of the peripheral region.

Challenges to arthroscopy are imposed by the constrained ball and socket architecture of the joint, the deep surrounding soft-tissue envelope, and dense capsule with limited compliance. This increases the risk of iatrogenic intra-articular damage and instrument breakage compared with other joints and thus emphasizes the importance of using a meticulous technique in the procedure and careful patient selection. The reported complication rate ranges from 1% to 6%, with most of these complications being minor or transient. Although direct trauma to the major neurovascular structures should be avoidable, it has been known to occur, especially with inexperienced surgeons. Various neurapraxias have also been described, but most are transient. Neurapraxia of the pudendal nerve resulting from compression is the most common concern, but this is avoided by generous padding and careful positioning of the perineal post as well as minimizing both the traction force and duration of the procedure. Even with these precautions, neurapraxia has occasionally been reported. There are numerous other infrequently encountered but potentially serious complications. Arthroscopy, although properly indicated for a variety of conditions, should not be casually considered to treat patients with ill-defined hip pain.

Summary

Sports-related disorders of the hip and groin are common, with numerous intra-articular and extra-articular sources. With an improved understanding of these disorders, the history and physical examination will usually provide sufficient clues for establishing the differential diagnosis. Investigative studies can be helpful but may not be reliable for some conditions. Thus, the clinician must be careful not to be dissuaded by potentially false-negative findings or lured by false-positive interpretations. Also, several problems may coexist in the hip region, further challenging the clinician's assessment skills.

Annotated Bibliography

Muscle and Tendon Injuries

Anderson K, Strickland SM, Warren R: Hip and groin injuries in athletes. *Am J Sports Med* 2001;29:521-533.

The authors provide a short and concise review on commonly encountered groin conditions affecting athletes.

Beiner JM, Jokl P, Cholewicki J, Panjabi MM: The effect of anabolic steroids and corticosteroids on healing of muscle contusion injury. *Am J Sports Med* 1999;27:2-9.

The authors studied the effects of an anabolic steroid (nandrolone decanoate) and corticosteroid (methylprednisolone) in a rat muscle contusion model. Although corticosteroids demonstrated a possible benefit in the acute setting, this was offset by a detrimental effect on healing muscle over the long term.

Benson ER, Schutzer SF: Posttraumatic piriformis syndrome: Diagnosis and results of operative treatment. *J Bone Joint Surg Am* 1999;81:941-949.

The authors retrospectively reviewed the clinical findings, surgical management, and outcome for 15 instances of piriformis syndrome in 14 patients who underwent sciatic nerve neurolysis. At an average follow-up of 38 months, 11 excellent and 4 good results were obtained. All patients returned to work or usual activity at an average of 2.3 months postoperatively. Complications included a wound seroma and infected hematoma.

Croisier JL, Forthomme B, Namurois MH, Vanderthommen M, Crielaard JM: Hamstring muscle strain recurrence and strength performance disorders. *Am J Sports Med* 2002;30:199-203.

In this prospective study, the authors identified athletes with a previous hamstring muscle injury and a muscle imbalance. The athletes followed a rehabilitation program specific to their predetermined strength profiles. After following the rehabilitation program, the strength parameters of most of the athletes normalized, and none sustained a hamstring reinjury.

Dobbs MB, Gordon JE, Luhmann SJ, Szymanski DA, Schoenecker PL: Surgical correction of the snapping iliopsoas tendon in adolescents. *J Bone Joint Surg Am* 2002;84:420-424.

The authors describe fractional lengthening of the iliopsoas tendon in adolescent patients using a modified iliofemoral approach. At an average follow-up of 4 years, all patients returned to their usual preoperative level of activity, there was no subjective hip flexion weakness, and only one patient had a recurrence of snapping. All patients reported that they would have the operation again. Two patients experienced transient postoperative sensory paresthesias along the lateral femoral cutaneous nerve distribution.

Fishman L, Dombi G, Michaelsen C, et al: Piriformis syndrome: Diagnosis, treatment, and outcome. A 10-year study. *Arch Phys Med Rehabil* 2002;83:295-301.

This study of 918 patients with piriformis syndrome (1,014 legs) was conducted to attempt to validate a definition of piriformis syndrome based on prolongation of the H-reflex with hip flexion, adduction, and internal rotation and to assess the effectiveness of conservative therapy and surgery to relieve symptoms and reduce disability.

Gilmore J: Groin pain in the soccer athlete: Fact, fiction, and treatment. *Clin Sports Med* 1998;17:787-793.

The author describes groin pain in soccer athletes as a complex management problem that can be caused by groin distribution, direct trauma, osteitis pubis, muscle injuries, fractures, bursitis, hip problems, and hernia and referred pain.

Gruen GS, Scioscia TN, Lowenstein JE: The surgical treatment of internal snapping hip. *Am J Sports Med* 2002;30:607-613.

The authors of this article report that although patients with internal snapping hip can usually be successfully treated nonsurgically, surgical tendon lengthening is a viable approach in those who do not respond to nonsurgical therapy.

Irshad K, Feldman LS, Lavoie C, Lacroix VJ, Mulder DS, Brown RA: Operative management of "hockey groin syndrome": 12 years of experience in National Hockey League players. *Surgery* 2001;130:759-766.

The authors of this article describe the clinical presentation of hockey groin syndrome and describe a surgical approach involving ilioinguinal nerve ablation and reinforcement of the external oblique aponeurosis.

Junge A, Dieter R, Peterson L, Graf-Baumann T, Dvorak J: Prevention of soccer injuries: A prospective intervention study in youth amateur players. *Am J Sports Med* 2002;30:652-659.

This prospective controlled intervention study in soccer players investigated the effectiveness of a prevention program on the incidence of all soccer injuries over a 1-year period. The intervention included specific exercises and education of both players and coaches. Twenty-one percent less injuries were seen in the intervention group compared with the control group. The most benefit was seen in low-skilled teams.

Klingele KE, Sallay PI: Surgical repair of complete proximal hamstring tendon rupture. *Am J Sports Med* 2002;30:742-747.

This retrospective cohort study evaluated a surgical protocol for repairing complete ruptures of the proximal hamstring tendon. The series is the largest to date and evaluates both acute and chronic tears. The surgery and postoperative protocol is well described. Postoperative isokinetic testing revealed 91% return of hamstring strength. Ten of 11 patients were satisfied with their results, and 7 of the 9 active athletes returned to sports participation at an average of 6 months. There was no difference between early and late repairs.

Meyers WC, Foley DP, Garrett WE, Lohnes JH, Mandelbaum BR: Management of severe lower abdominal or inguinal pain in high-performance athletes: PAIN (Performing Athletes with Abdominal or Inguinal Neuromuscular Pain Study Group). *Am J Sports Med* 2000;28:2-8.

The authors reviewed a large series of patients treated surgically for athletic pubalgia and report a high rate of success with rectus abdominis muscle reattachment to the pubis and proximal adductor release for selected cases.

Tyler TF, Nicholas SJ, Campbell RJ, Donellan S, McHugh MP: The effectiveness of a preseason exercise program to prevent adductor muscle strains in professional ice hockey players. *Am J Sports Med* 2002;30:680-683.

In this study, 33 National Hockey League players identified as at risk on the basis of preseason hip adductor strength participated in an intervention program consisting of 6 weeks of exercises to functionally strengthen the adductor muscles. There were three adductor strains in the two seasons subsequent to the intervention compared with 11 adductor strains in the previous two seasons (0.71 versus 3.2 per 1,000 player-game exposures). The authors conclude that therapeutic intervention involving strengthening the adductor muscle group appears to be an effective method for preventing adductor strains in professional ice hockey players.

White KK, Williams SK, Mubarack SJ: Definition of two types of anterior superior iliac spine avulsion fractures. *J Pediatr Orthop* 2002;22:578-582.

The authors of this article discuss a type of anterior-superior iliac spine fracture caused by avulsion of the tensor fascia lata origin. Of the eight patients who were identified with this type of fracture, six had type II sartorius avulsion fractures caused by sprinting in various sports.

Pelvis and Hip Joint Injuries

Byrd JW: Hip arthroscopy in athletes. *Instr Course Lect* 2003;52:701-709.

This article reviews the role of hip arthroscopy among athletes including pathology, pathomechanics, and results of the procedure.

Byrd JW: Hip arthroscopy: Patient assessment and indications. *Instr Course Lect* 2003;52:711-719.

This article provides an overview of the assessment of potential candidates for hip arthroscopy and summarizes the current indications with comprehensive references.

Byrd JW: Hip arthroscopy: The supine position. *Instr Course Lect* 2003;52:721-730.

This article details the merits and technique of hip arthroscopy done with the patient in the supine position.

Dienst M, Gödde S, Seil R, Hammer D, Kohn D: Hip arthroscopy without traction: In vivo anatomy of the peripheral hip joint cavity. *Arthroscopy* 2001;17:924-929.

This article details the technique, anatomy, and merits of hip arthroscopy without traction to access the peripheral compartment of the hip.

Erb RE: Current concepts in imaging the adult hip. *Clin Sports Med* 2001;20:661-696.

This article summarizes current imaging technology available for diagnosing hip joint pathology.

Glick JM, Sampson TG: Hip arthroscopy in the lateral position, in McGinty JB (ed): *Operative Arthroscopy*, ed

3. Philadelphia, PA, Lippincott Williams & Wilkins, 2003, pp 859-865.

This chapter details the merits and technique of hip arthroscopy done with the patient in the lateral decubitus position.

McCarthy JC, Noble PC, Schuck MR, Wright J, Lee J: The watershed labral lesion: Its relationship to early arthritis of the hip. *J Arthroplasty* 2001;16(suppl 1):81-87.

This article highlights clinical and cadaveric observations on labral pathology. The authors report that labral and articular lesions often coexist and are part of the continuum of degenerative disease.

O'Leary JA, Berend K, Vail TP: The relationship between diagnosis and outcome in arthroscopy of the hip. *Arthroscopy* 2001;17:181-188.

This article reports on the relationship between diagnosis and outcome in hip arthroscopy and also demonstrates that the presence of mechanical symptoms is a favorable prognostic indicator.

Classic Bibliography

Byrd JWT: Hip arthroscopy utilizing the supine position. *Arthroscopy* 1994;10:275-280.

Byrd JWT: Indications and contraindications, in Byrd JWT (ed): *Operative Hip Arthroscopy*. New York, NY, Thieme Publishing Group, 1997, pp 7-24.

Ekstrand J, Gillquist J, Liljedahl SO: Prevention of soccer injuries: Supervision by doctor and physiotherapist. *Am J Sports Med* 1983;11:116-120.

Eriksson E, Arvidsson I, Arvidsson H: Diagnostic and operative arthroscopy of the hip. *Orthopedics* 1986;9:169-176.

Frieberg A: Sciatic pain and its relief by operations on muscle and fascia. *Arch Surg* 1937;34:337-350.

Fullerton LR Jr, Snowdy HA: Femoral neck stress fractures. *Am J Sports Med* 1988;16:365-377.

Glick JM: Hip arthroscopy using the lateral approach. *Instr Course Lect* 1988;37:223-231.

Heiser TM, Weber J, Sullivan G, Clare P, Jacobs RR: Prophylaxis and management of hamstring muscle injuries in intercollegiate football players. *Am J Sports Med* 1984;12:368-370.

Holt MA, Keene JS, Graf BK, Helwig DC: Treatment of osteitis pubis in athletes: Results of corticosteroid injections. *Am J Sports Med* 1995;23:601-606.

Jackson DW, Feagin JA: Quadriceps contusion in young athletes: Relation of severity of injury to treatment and prognosis. *J Bone Joint Surg Am* 1973;55:95-105.

Lecouvet FE, VandeBerg BC, Melghem J, et al: MR imaging of the acetabular labrum: Variations in 200 asymptomatic hips. *AJR Am J Roentgenol* 1996;167:1025-1028.

Metzmaker JN, Pappas AM: Avulsion fractures of the pelvis. *Am J Sports Med* 1985;13:349-358.

Noakes TD, Smith JA, Lindenberg G, Wills CE: Pelvic stress fractures in long distance runners. *Am J Sports Med* 1985;13:120-123.

Orchard J, Marsden J, Lord S, Garlick D: Preseason hamstring muscle weakness associated with hamstring muscle injury in Australian footballers. *Am J Sports Med* 1997;25:81-85.

Ryan JB, Wheeler JH, Hopkinson WJ, Arciero RA, Kolakowski KR: Quadriceps contusions: West Point update. *Am J Sports Med* 1991;19:299-304.

Taylor DC, Meyers WC, Moylan JA, Lohnes J, Bassett FH, Garrett WE Jr: Abdominal musculature abnormalities as a cause of groin pain in athletes: Inguinal hernias and pubalgia. *Am J Sports Med* 1991;19:239-242.

Teitz CC, Garrett WE Jr, Miniaci A, Lee MH, Mann RA: Tendon problems in athletic individuals. *Instr Course Lect* 1997;46:569-582.

Chapter 12

Posterior Cruciate Ligament Injuries

Timothy S. Johnson, MD

Andrew J. Cosgarea, MD

Introduction

The understanding of posterior cruciate ligament (PCL) injuries is evolving, yet it still lags behind that of anterior cruciate ligament (ACL) injuries. PCL injuries are less common, more variable in their presentation, and more difficult to treat surgically than ACL injuries. Nonetheless, physicians are beginning to understand the natural history of untreated PCL injuries, and reconstructive surgical techniques have recently improved. The treatment of PCL injuries remains controversial, however, and the most contentious issue involves the indications for surgery.

Basic Science: Structure and Function

Anatomy

The PCL is an intra-articular but extrasynovial ligament. It originates from inside the joint off of the lateral border of the medial femoral condyle. The femoral footprint forms an irregular semicircle where the roof of the intercondylar notch joins the wall. The tibial attachment is located on the posterior cortical surface of the tibia approximately 1 to 1.5 cm inferior to the articular margin. The ligament inserts in the sagittal midline in an extra-articular depression between the medial and lateral tibial plateaus called the PCL facet or fovea. The close proximity of this insertion to the adjacent popliteal neurovascular bundle complicates reconstruction of the ligament. The average length of a PCL is 38 mm, and its average width is 13 mm. The PCL originates in an anterior to posterior orientation on the femur and spirals distally where it attaches to the tibia in a lateral to medial direction. Although the PCL is a continuum of fibers, it is commonly described as two major bundles: an anterolateral bundle and a posteromedial bundle. The name of the bundle describes its insertion site on the femur (anterior or posterior) and the tibia (lateral or medial), respectively (Figure 1). The anterolateral bundle is stronger than the posteromedial bundle and has nearly twice the cross-sectional area.

The blood supply to the PCL comes from the middle genicular artery. Compared with the ACL, the PCL

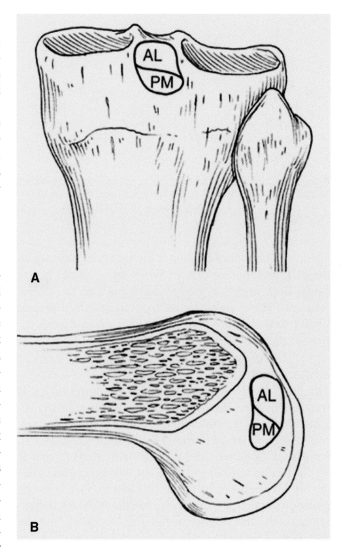

Figure 1 Anatomy of the tibial insertions (**A**) and femoral origins (**B**) of the anterolateral (AL) and posteromedial (PM) bundles. *(Reproduced with permission from Harner CD, Hoher J: Evaluation and treatment of posterior cruciate ligament injuries. Am J Sports Med 1998;26:471-482.)*

blood supply is more generous, which possibly accounts for its improved healing capacity. Along with the two PCL bundles are two meniscofemoral ligaments. The lig-

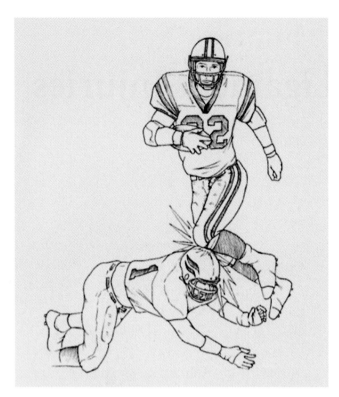

Figure 2 Mechanism of a PCL tear during contact athletics. *(Reproduced with permission from Miller MD, Harner CD, Koshiwaguchi S: Acute posterior cruciate ligament injuries, in Vince KG (ed): Knee Surgery. Baltimore, MD, Williams & Wilkins, 1994, pp 749-767.)*

ament of Humphrey originates on the femur anterior to the PCL and the ligament of Wrisberg originates posteriorly. Both insert on the posterior horn of the lateral meniscus. These act as secondary restraints to posterior tibial translation but may be variably present from patient to patient.

Biomechanics

The PCL is the primary restraint to posterior tibial translation. It resists 85% to 100% of a posteriorly directed force on the tibia when the knee is positioned between 30° and 90° of flexion. Loss of the PCL causes an increase in posterior tibial translation of up to 20 mm at 90° of flexion. The ligament is not isometric during the flexion arc. Because of the differences in anatomic origin and insertion, the anterolateral band tightens in flexion whereas the posteromedial band tightens in knee extension. This reciprocal tensioning in the two bundles during the flexion-extension cycle may explain why surgeons have had difficulty reproducing normal knee kinematics with single-bundle PCL reconstructions.

Diagnosis

Epidemiology

PCL tears have been reported in 1% to 44% of acute knee injuries. Although they may account for an esti-

mated one fifth of all ligament injuries, PCL tears have historically been underdiagnosed because they are frequently asymptomatic. Recent increased interest in PCL injuries has led to an improved understanding of injury mechanisms and clinical evaluation.

PCL injuries occur via several mechanisms. The most common mechanism is a high velocity posteriorly directed force on the proximal tibia when the knee is flexed. This frequently occurs during a motor vehicle accident when a person in the front seat strikes a knee against the dashboard. A similar mechanism can occur at lower velocity during contact sports such as football (Figure 2). The posterior force combined with a varus or rotational force can lead to simultaneous lateral or posterolateral pathology. Another mechanism of isolated PCL tears in sports is a forceful landing onto a flexed knee with the foot plantar flexed. Other indirect mechanisms involving hyperextension and hyperflexion have been described during athletics. Although less common, they are important to recognize because they more frequently lead to combined ligament injuries.

Acutely injured patients most commonly report pain and instability and can often describe the mechanism of injury. Conversely, patients with chronic PCL injuries uncommonly report instability or buckling. They more commonly report discomfort in the knee, particularly when ascending and descending stairs or initiating a run.

Knee Examinations

In addition to observing gait and checking static weight-bearing alignment, a standard assessment for palpable tenderness, range-of-motion alterations, and neurovascular abnormality should be performed. Observation and inspection of the skin after acute PCL injury commonly reveals an abrasion or contusion over the proximal tibia. Patients with isolated PCL tears may present with little pain and only a small effusion. Assessment for concomitant ligamentous insufficiency cannot be overemphasized.

With regard to examining the PCL, the posterior drawer test is the most accurate for assessing PCL injury (Figure 3). This test is performed with the patient supine, the knee flexed at 90° and the foot flat on the examination table. The examiner stabilizes the foot and applies a posteriorly directed load or "drawer" on the proximal tibia. If at the start of the test the examiner cannot palpate the normal 1-cm step-off of the proximal tibia anterior to the femur condyles, then a PCL injury should be suspected. Furthermore, if the posterior drawer yields excessive translation with a soft end point, a PCL injury is almost certain. It is important to avoid internal or external rotation of the tibia during the posterior drawer test because this may yield a false sense of stability.

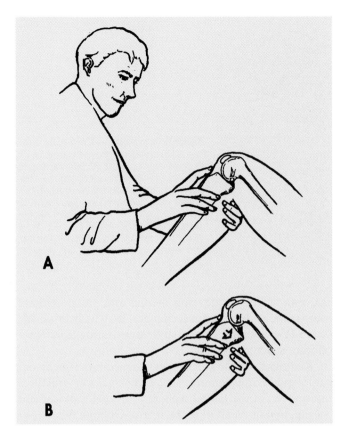

Figure 3 The posterior drawer test. **A,** The examiner stabilizes the foot and assesses the relative position of the tibia to the femoral condyle. **B,** The examiner then applies a posteriorly directed load on the proximal tibia that yields excessive translation consistent with PCL deficiency. *(Reproduced with permission from Miller MD, Harner CD, Koshiwaguchi S: Acute posterior cruciate ligament injuries, in Vince KG (ed): Knee Surgery. Baltimore, MD, Williams & Wilkins, 1994, pp 749-767.)*

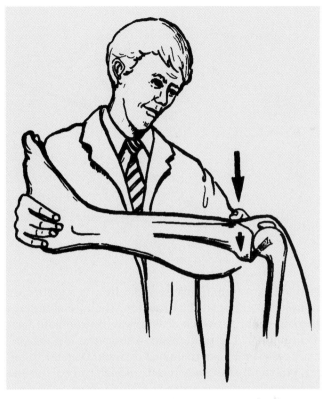

Figure 4 The posterior tibial sag test. Note the abnormal step-off anteriorly of the tibia relative to the femoral condyles with PCL injury. *(Reproduced with permission from Miller MD, Harner CD, Koshiwaguchi S: Acute posterior cruciate ligament injuries, in Vince KG (ed): Knee Surgery. Baltimore, MD, Williams & Wilkins, 1994, pp 749-767.)*

PCL injuries are often incomplete, and palpation of the tibial plateau-medial femoral condyle step-off forms the basis for the most commonly used PCL injury grading system. With a grade 1 posterior drawer, the tibial plateau remains proudly anterior to the medial femoral condyle. With grade 2 tears, the tibial plateau is palpated flush with the condyle; and with grade 3 tears, the plateau is posterior to the condyle. Many authors believe that a grade 3 PCL tear must involve injury to other ligamentous structures, most commonly the posterolateral corner. The KT-1000 arthrometer (Medmetric Corporation, San Diego, CA) objectively quantifies posterior translation and is a useful tool when trying to compare or report surgical results.

The posterior sag test or Godfrey test is also useful in detecting PCL insufficiency. For patients with normal knees, the patient is positioned supine on the examination table, the hip and knee flexed at 90°, and the weight of the leg supported at the heel; the medial tibial plateau rests anterior to the adjacent medial femoral condyle. Loss of this anterior step-off or "sag" of the proximal tibia suggests PCL insufficiency (Figure 4).

The quadriceps active test is another useful test in the assessment of PCL integrity. This test is performed with the patient supine, the knee flexed at 90°, and the foot flat on the examination table. The examiner stabilizes the foot and asks the patient to fire the quadriceps muscle (Figure 5). In PCL-deficient patients, when the quadriceps muscles contract, the examiner will observe reduction of the posteriorly subluxated tibia. Another examination tool is the dynamic posterior shift test, which is performed with the patient's hip and knee flexed at 90°. Starting from a flexed position, the examiner slowly extends the knee until the posteriorly subluxated tibia suddenly reduces with a clunk as the knee reaches full extension. Interpretation of all of these tests is easier in patients with high-grade and chronic PCL tears.

Associated Injuries

The lateral collateral ligament, posterolateral structures, and medial collateral ligament (MCL) are important secondary restraints to posterior tibial translation. They play a minimal role in resisting posterior tibial translation when the PCL is intact but are critical when the PCL is torn. The amount of pathologic posterior displacement increases substantially when these secondary

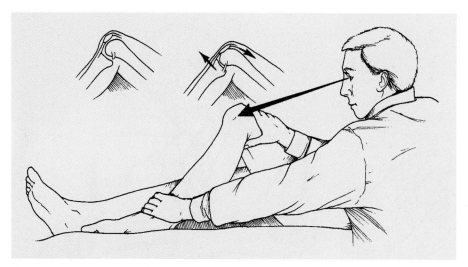

Figure 5 The quadriceps active test. The examiner stabilizes the foot and asks the patient to fire the quadriceps muscle. In PCL-deficient patients, when the quadriceps muscles contract the examiner will observe reduction of the posteriorly subluxated tibia. *(Reproduced with permission from Delee JC, Bergfeld JA, Drez DJ, Parker AW: The posterior cruciate ligament, in Delee JC, Drez D (eds): Orthopaedic Sports Medicine: Principles and Practice. Philadelphia, PA, WB Saunders, 1994, pp 1374-1400.)*

restraints are torn. Conversely, the PCL is a secondary restraint to external tibial rotation. These relationships become important when dealing with concomitant ligament injuries. The posterolateral structures are the primary restraint to external tibial rotation. Damage to the posterolateral structures results in higher forces in the intact native or reconstructed PCL. Similarly, concomitant ACL, lateral collateral ligament, and MCL injuries increase the stress placed on the PCL and must be incorporated into the treatment plan for the PCL injury.

Varus and valgus stress testing at 0° and 30° of flexion are routinely done to detect associated collateral ligament insufficiency. Likewise the Lachman, anterior drawer, and pivot-shift tests are done to rule out an ACL tear. Posterior drawer testing is typically performed in conjunction with anterior drawer testing. Again, it is important to note that the initial step in both anterior and posterior drawer testing is observing the starting position of the proximal tibia relative to the femur. If at the start of the examination, the proximal tibia is subluxated posteriorly, PCL insufficiency may be easily misinterpreted as positive Lachman or anterior drawer test results. Assessment for posterolateral corner insufficiency is crucial if a PCL injury is suspected. Several tests have been described, including the dynamic posterior shift test, the reverse pivot-shift test, and the tibial external rotation test (see chapter 14).

Radiographic Evaluation

A complete radiographic evaluation consisting of AP, lateral, sunrise, and tunnel views is appropriate for any patient after a traumatic knee injury. Avulsion fractures of the PCL tibial insertion are easily identified on the lateral view. Gross posterior subluxation may also be seen on lateral views. Stress lateral radiographs with or without instrumentation demonstrate posterior subluxation (Figure 6, *A*), which may be fixed in the setting of a chronic injury. Patients with chronic PCL tears are

also more likely to develop medial and patellofemoral compartment degenerative changes. Weight-bearing 45° flexed PA views are helpful in demonstrating tibiofemoral joint space narrowing.

Radiographs may also suggest concomitant ligament pathology. Posterolateral structure avulsion fractures can be seen at the lateral collateral ligament attachment on the fibular head (Figure 6, *B*). Oblique views are sometimes helpful to rule out tibial plateau fractures. Calcification next to the medial femoral epicondyle (Pellegrini-Stieda lesion) suggests an old MCL injury (Figure 6, *C*).

MRI is the gold standard for imaging acute PCL injuries because it is highly accurate (Figure 7). MRI can be used to assess the tear location and concomitant ligamentous pathology and to develop a comprehensive treatment plan. Chronic PCL tears may look relatively normal when visualized by MRI. Meniscal tears occur less commonly with PCL tears than ACL tears. This is probably because the pathologic posterior tibial translation decreases the load on the posterior horns of the medial and lateral meniscus. Bone bruises are also seen less commonly with PCL tears than ACL tears.

Bone scanning may be helpful in evaluating patients with chronic PCL injuries who present with pain. Evidence of increased activity in the medial and patellofemoral compartments on a bone scan is consistent with early arthrosis. Symptomatic patients with positive bone scans but without frank arthritis may be appropriate candidates for PCL reconstruction.

Indications for Surgery
Natural History

The natural history of isolated PCL tears is relatively benign. It is not unusual to discover PCL insufficiency as an incidental finding during routine preseason sports examinations. There are few natural history studies in the literature and most involve athletes that suggest that

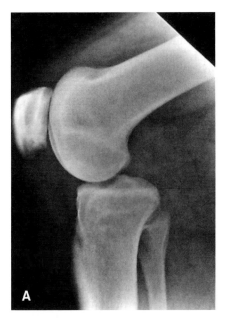
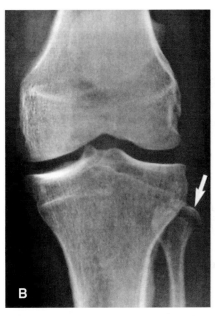
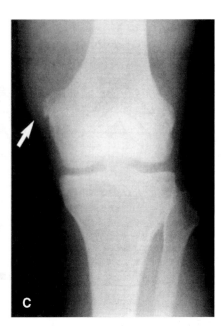

Figure 6 The radiographic appearance of PCL lesions. **A,** Posterior subluxation of the tibia seen on a lateral stress radiograph of a patient with a combined grade 3 PCL and MCL injury. **B,** Avulsion fracture of the fibular head (*arrow*) in a patient with a combined PCL, posterolateral corner, and lateral collateral ligament injury. **C,** Pellegrini-Stieda lesion (*arrow*) indicative of a chronic MCL injury. *(Reproduced from Cosgarea AJ, Jay PR: Posterior cruciate ligament injuries: Evaluation and management. J Am Acad Orthop Surg 2001;9:297-307.)*

the majority of athletes with isolated PCL injury return to sports at the same level of activity without limitation. Although some patients may have residual laxity upon follow-up physical examination and/or KT-1000 testing, this does not appear to correlate with patient satisfaction or the ability to return to sports. Restoring quadriceps strength in the injured limb is a prerequisite to successful return to sports without surgery. The literature regarding the long-term prognosis of isolated PCL injuries is less clear and somewhat variable. However, there have been some reports on the development of early degenerative arthrosis after isolated PCL injury. Grade 3 injuries are of particular concern. Nonsurgical management of multiple ligament injuries with gross laxity has a poorer prognosis than that of isolated injuries and requires surgery more often.

Surgical Intervention

Optimal management of PCL injuries should take into account the patient's age, occupation, overall health, and expectations. The level of energy that caused the injury and the extent of associated injuries are important prognostic factors. A suggested algorithm is shown in Figure 8.

Most authors agree that acute surgical intervention is appropriate when there is a displaced PCL bony avulsion. Likewise, the poor function associated with non-surgically treated combined ligament injuries is significant enough to warrant surgical intervention. The indication for surgery in patients with a chronic isolated PCL tear is evolving and somewhat less clear. Patients with symptomatic isolated PCL injuries who have failed

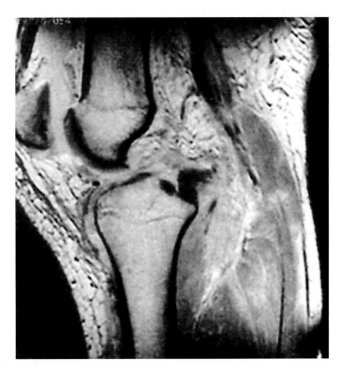

Figure 7 MRI scan of a complete PCL tear. *(Reproduced from Cosgarea AJ, Jay PR: Posterior cruciate ligament injuries: Evaluation and management. J Am Acad Orthop Surg 2001;9:297-307.)*

to respond to nonsurgical management may be good surgical candidates, but this is controversial. Nonetheless, fixed posterior subluxation of the tibia in the setting of a chronic isolated PCL tear should be corrected with a posterior tibial support brace before PCL recon-

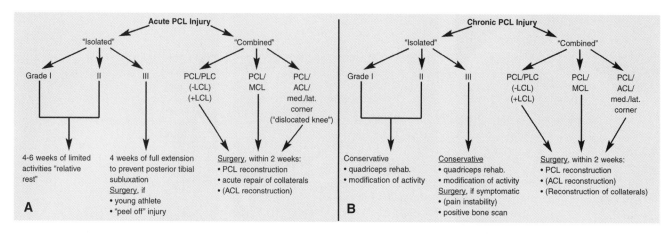

Figure 8 Treatment algorithms for acute PCL injury (**A**) and chronic PCL injury (**B**). *(Reproduced with permission from Harner CD, Hoher J: Evaluation and treatment of posterior cruciate ligament injuries. Am J Sports Med 1998;26:471-482.)*

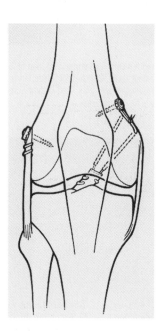

Figure 9 Primary repair of the PCL and lateral collateral ligament. The PCL sutures are passed through drill holes at the avulsion site and tied over a bone bridge. *(Reproduced with permission from Schenck RC: Management of posterior cruciate ligament injuries in knee dislocations. Oper Tech Sports Med 1993;1:143-147.)*

struction to prevent overloading and subsequent failure of the PCL graft.

Surgical Outcomes

Suture repair

Primary repair with sutures is most efficacious when treating ligament insertion site avulsions. Repair is more successful when performed in the acute setting (< 3 weeks). Most avulsions occur from the femoral insertion and are either avulsed or stripped subperiosteally. Repair can be performed using nonabsorbable sutures placed through the avulsed ligament. The sutures are passed through drill holes at the avulsion site and tied over a bone bridge or suture button (Figure 9). The results of suture repair of chronic and midsubstance tears have been generally unsatisfactory, and reconstruction is generally recommended in this setting.

Open Reduction and Internal Fixation Bony Avulsion

Avulsion fractures usually involve the tibial insertion and can be seen on routine lateral radiographs. The avulsion site is exposed through a standard posterior approach with the patient in a prone position. If the bone fragment is large, fixation is accomplished with one or two screws, with or without washers. For smaller comminuted bone fragments, suture fixation through small drill holes may be necessary. The knee is braced in extension, and weight bearing is initially protected for at least 2 weeks. Postsurgical rehabilitation proceeds based on the quality of fixation. Once bony healing occurs at 6 to 8 weeks postoperatively, rehabilitation can proceed more aggressively. As with other knee stabilization procedures performed in the acute setting, postoperative stiffness is more likely. Acute intervention appears to produce better results than later treatment.

Reconstruction

Graft Options

The optimal graft choice for PCL reconstruction is debatable because there are no good studies comparing different graft sources. Commonly used autografts include the patellar tendon, hamstring tendon, and quadriceps tendon. Patellar tendon, Achilles tendon, and tibialis anterior tendon allografts have also been used with success. Allografts are attractive in that they allow surgeons to reduce the duration of an already lengthy procedure. Similarly, allografts spare the patient donor site morbidity, particularly during multiple ligament reconstruction when a large amount of tissue may be required. However, basic science studies do suggest that allograft tissue takes longer to mature.

Transtibial Single-Bundle Reconstruction

Both open and arthroscopic PCL reconstructions have been performed using a single-graft bundle through a single femoral tunnel. Because of the size of the femoral origin, only a portion of the PCL can be reconstructed with a single-bundle technique. Because the anterolateral bundle is larger and stronger than the posteromedial bundle, the femoral tunnel is drilled where the anterolateral fibers of the PCL originate on the femoral condyle.

Surgery is performed with the patient supine. A posteromedial portal is established under direct arthroscopic visualization to gain access to the tibial insertion, which extends well below the posterior joint line. Use of a cannula with a one-way valve can decrease fluid extravasation from the posteromedial portal and facilitate repeated introduction and removal of instruments. A 70° scope can be particularly useful at this point to see over the back of the tibial plateau. The root of the posterior horn of the medial meniscus is an easily identifiable visible landmark that can aid in the positioning of the tibial tunnel. After débriding the tibial stump from the medial portal, a tibial PCL drill guide is inserted through the femoral notch. A guide pin is directed from the anteromedial tibia, just distal and medial to the tibial tubercle, to the posterior tibial cortex in the distal lateral aspect of the PCL footprint (Figure 10). Passage of the Kirschner wire and subsequent drilling should be directly visualized arthroscopically and can also be done under fluoroscopic guidance. A curet or ribbon retractor is used to protect the posterior neurovascular structures during drilling. The rough inner edge of the tibial tunnel is then gently smoothed with a bone rasp.

Biomechanical studies have demonstrated that alteration of the normal PCL femoral attachment sites leads to greater differences in graft tension during knee flexion than alteration of the tibial attachment site. Hence, accurate femoral tunnel placement during PCL reconstruction is critical to restoring normal knee function. When preparing the femoral tunnel, it is helpful to leave the PCL femoral insertion fibers intact so that the outline of the footprint can be readily appreciated. The anterolateral bundle origin is located 8 to 9 mm off the articular margin of the medial femoral condyle in the anterior half of the footprint. This tunnel may be drilled antegrade from the medial side through a small incision midway between the patella and the medial femoral condyle. Alternatively, the femoral tunnel may be drilled retrograde through an accessory inferolateral portal, leaving either a blind tunnel or one that exits through the medial femoral cortex.

The direction in which the graft is passed through the femoral and tibial tunnel is a matter of surgeon preference. Although there are a variety of instruments to assist passing grafts through tunnels, passing the PCL graft around the acute turn or "killer turn" at the back of the tibial plateau remains the most difficult part of the transtibial reconstruction. Femoral and tibial fixation are typically achieved with either metal or bioabsorbable interference screws. Alternatively, a variety of

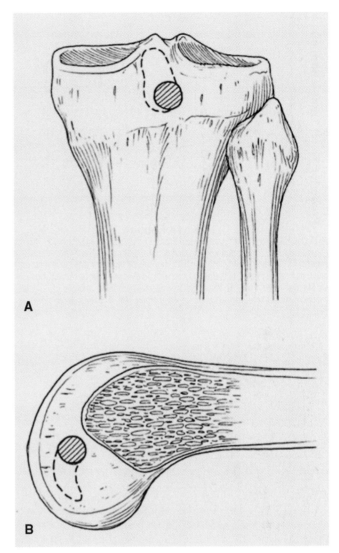

Figure 10 Optimal positions for tibial (**A**) and femoral (**B**) tunnels for single-bundle PCL reconstruction. *(Reproduced with permission from Miller MD, Harner CD, Koshiwaguchi S: Acute posterior cruciate ligament injuries, in Vince KG (ed): Knee Surgery. Baltimore, MD, Williams & Wilkins, 1994, pp 749-767.)*

staples, posts, and spiked washer devices may be used. Restoration of normal PCL biomechanics is most reliably achieved by fixing the graft with the knee at 90° of flexion with an anterior load placed on the tibia. Although it does not restore all the anatomy of the PCL, single-bundle transtibial reconstruction appears to provide satisfactory return of function and strength to the injured limb.

Double Femoral Bundle

The major theoretical advantage of the double-bundle technique is that it replaces both the anterolateral and the posteromedial bundle. Some authors have hypothesized that it is superior to single-bundle techniques, and biomechanical studies have shown that the use of the

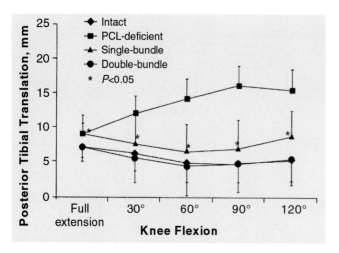

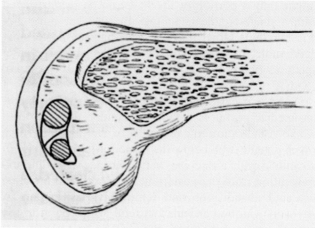

Figure 11 Comparison of posterior tibial translation in knees with an intact, ruptured, and reconstructed PCL. *(Reproduced with permission from Harner CD, Janaushek, MA, Kanamori A, Yagi M, Vogrin TM, Woo SL: Biomechanical analysis of a double-bundle posterior cruciate ligament reconstruction. Am J Sports Med 2000;28: 144-151.)*

Figure 12 Optimal femoral tunnel placement for double-bundle reconstruction. *(Reproduced with permission from Miller MD, Harner CD, Koshiwaguchi S: Acute posterior cruciate ligament injuries, in Vince KG (ed): Knee Surgery. Baltimore, MD, Williams & Wilkins, 1994, pp 749-767.)*

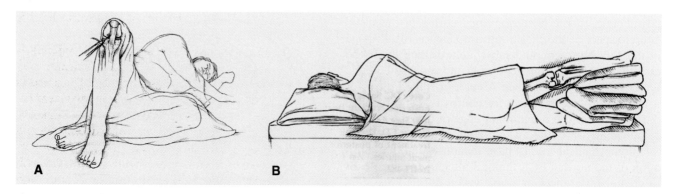

Figure 13 The tibial inlay technique. **A,** Lateral decubitus positioning for initial arthroscopy and femoral tunnel preparation. **B,** The knee is extended and abducted for exposure of the tibial insertion site. *(Reproduced with permission from Berg EE: Posterior cruciate ligament tibial inlay reconstruction. Arthroscopy 1995;11:69-76.)*

additional posteromedial bundle decreased posterior laxity by 3.5 mm (Figure 11). Although the double-bundle technique is conceptually attractive, it is technically more demanding, and clinical results have yet to be published documenting clear superiority.

The double-bundle procedure is identical to the single-bundle procedure through the stage of tibial tunnel preparation. Femoral preparation involves drilling a tunnel into the anterior portion of the femoral footprint for the anterolateral bundle and then drilling a smaller posterior femoral tunnel for the posteromedial bundle (Figure 12). A split Achilles tendon or quadriceps tendon graft can be used to reconstruct the two bundles. Alternatively, a combination of an Achilles tendon or quadriceps tendon graft with a doubled semitendinosus, gracilis, or tibialis anterior graft can be used. Both grafts are routed through a single tibial tunnel. The anterolateral graft is typically fixed at 90° of flexion, and the posteromedial graft is tensioned and separately fixed at 30°.

Tibial Inlay (Onlay)

Several authors have criticized the transtibial approach by theorizing that abrasion of the graft might cause early failure. The site of concern is the "killer turn" where the graft passes acutely around the articular margin of the tibia. The tibial inlay technique was devised to circumvent the technical difficulties caused by using the long tibial tunnel necessary with an anterior approach. Similar to the double-bundle technique, the tibial inlay is conceptually attractive but technically demanding. Clinical results have yet to be published documenting the clear superiority of the inlay technique to other proposed techniques.

Although the procedure may be staged by alternating the patient from the prone to the supine position intraoperatively, the procedure is typically performed with the patient in the lateral decubitus position (Figure 13). Once the initial arthroscopic work is completed, single or double femoral tunnels are drilled. The patient is then repositioned for the posterior approach by extending the knee and placing the leg on bolsters or a Mayo stand. An oblique incision over the medial head of the gastrocnemius muscle allows exposure to develop the interval between the medial head of the gastrocnemius muscle and the semimembranosus muscle. Lateral retraction protects the neurovascular structures and allows access to the posterior capsule. The posterior capsule is incised vertically, and the PCL insertion is visualized. The posterior tibial facet is exposed subperiosteally and prepared for the bone block. A unicortical window can be fashioned to fit the dimensions of the bone block. The popliteus muscle fibers can be undermined if necessary. The graft is inlayed flush and fixed with one or more screws with or without washers. The femoral portion of the graft is then passed through the femoral tunnel for standard fixation. A single- or double-bundle technique may be used.

Tibial Slope

Uncorrected lower extremity malalignment in conjunction with ligamentous reconstruction has been associated with early failure. Abnormal alignment predisposes reconstructed ligaments to abnormal stress and progressive laxity. It is critical to identify and correct asymmetric varus malalignment with a dynamic varus thrust in the setting of combined PCL and posterolateral structure injuries before ligamentous reconstruction. High tibial osteotomy may be the most reliable and reproducible approach to correcting this deformity. Alteration of sagittal tibial slope via osteotomy both with and without ligamentous reconstruction has been proposed as a treatment option for PCL insufficiency. However, there are currently few clinical data to support this treatment approach.

Combined Ligament Surgery

In contrast to isolated PCL tears, patients with multiple ligament injuries who are treated nonsurgically have relatively poor functional outcome. Knee injuries that are severe enough to result in multiple ligament tears are usually the result of a high-energy mechanism. Damage to the secondary restraints leads to a greater degree of laxity and instability in multiple planes. In most patients with this type of injury, surgical treatment of each ligament is necessary to address these combined instabilities (Figure 8).

The combination of PCL and posterolateral structure injury produces much more posterior laxity than either injury alone. Patients are less likely to compensate and more likely to experience functional instability. Failure to address combined ligament injury at the time of surgery leads to a higher failure rate. Persistent posterolateral laxity following PCL reconstruction may increase forces in the graft, predisposing it to ultimate failure. Timing of arthroscopic procedures after high-energy in-

jury is important. Arthroscopic reconstructive procedures are usually safe to perform 2 to 3 weeks after injury at which time the capsule has had time to seal. If substantial fluid extravasation occurs intraoperatively, it may be necessary to abandon arthroscopy and proceed with an open surgical technique. With acute combined ligament injuries an attempt should be made to repair all damaged structures. In the chronic setting or if tissue is inadequate for suture repair, augmentation or reconstruction can be performed (see chapter 14).

Bicruciate ligament injury may represent an unrecognized knee dislocation and has a significantly higher incidence of concomitant neurovascular injuries. After neurovascular injury is ruled out, the knee can be splinted and early rehabilitation initiated. One of the complications of multiple ligament surgery is postoperative arthrofibrosis. Some authors recommend initiating range of motion and delaying surgery for a few weeks or more to decrease this risk. Others advocate doing the reconstruction within 2 weeks, especially if there is any indication of collateral or posterolateral corner pathology. In either case, reconstruction on an elective basis is appropriate to plan the surgical approach.

Treatment of combined PCL and MCL injuries is dictated largely by the extent of medial laxity. A low-grade MCL tear will often heal with brace protection and joint mobilization. When a high-grade MCL tear occurs with a PCL tear the prognosis is worse. Clinically, these patients will have gross valgus instability in full extension. They may be functionally unstable even during simple gait. Acute injuries should be treated with early repair of the parallel and posterior oblique portions of the superficial MCL as well as repair or reconstruction of the PCL. In chronic cases, hamstring autograft or allograft tissue may be needed to reconstruct the MCL, and it is much more difficult for the surgeon to restore normal valgus laxity.

Complications

The most serious intraoperative complication of PCL surgery is iatrogenic neurovascular injury. The popliteal artery is especially at risk for injury during tibial tunnel preparation and graft passage. The most common complication following PCL surgery is residual laxity. Other potential complications include loss of motion, infection, medial femoral condyle osteonecrosis, anterior knee pain, and painful hardware.

Rehabilitation

Nonsurgical

Patients with acute isolated partial (grade 1 or 2) PCL tears can be treated with brief splinting and protective weight bearing to control pain and swelling. Early range-of-motion exercises and quadriceps strengthening are started when pain permits. It is wise to avoid open-chain hamstring exercises because these may exacerbate posterior subluxation. Recovery of strength and motion generally occurs quickly and return to sport is allowed once the knee is pain free with full range of motion and quadriceps strength close to that of the contralateral side. Many patients are able to return to sports in 4 weeks. The use of functional braces may facilitate early return to athletic activities, but it has limited success in patients with persistent symptoms.

Nonsurgical treatment of an acute grade 3 PCL tear is controversial because of the possibility of unrecognized posterolateral corner damage resulting in further subluxation. Nonetheless, when treating grade 3 injuries nonsurgically, it has been recommended that the knee be splinted in full extension for 2 to 4 weeks before initiating a rehabilitation program. In the unusual pediatric case, cast immobilization may be indicated. Immobilization in extension decreases tension on the anterolateral bundle fibers and minimizes the antagonistic effect of the hamstring muscles. Subsequent rehabilitation is similar to that described above.

Postoperative

Postoperatively, patients are placed in a hinged knee brace locked in full extension. Patients are allowed to bear weight as tolerated with crutches. Early rehabilitation focuses on restoration of range of motion and isometric quadriceps strengthening. The brace is typically discontinued 6 weeks after surgery, and closed-chain exercises are emphasized. Patients may return to sports after restoration of full motion and equal quadriceps strength, typically between 9 and 12 months. Postoperative rehabilitation of patients with multiple ligament reconstructions is similar yet includes precautions tailored to protect any other ligaments that were reconstructed.

Knee Dislocation: Evaluation and Management

Knee dislocations can occur as a result of either low-energy or high-energy mechanisms. Purely ligamentous knee dislocations may spontaneously reduce and can be mistakenly overlooked upon initial evaluation. This has led to catastrophic limb loss in some instances as the incidence of popliteal artery disruption is the same regardless of the presentation on initial radiographs. The bicruciate ligament injury is included in this category. The incidence of nerve injury is increased in high-energy injuries compared with that in low-energy injuries. The prognosis of nerve injury is worse if the deficit is present on initial evaluation.

The risk of limb loss associated with knee dislocation is directly related to popliteal artery injury. Early diagnosis and prompt treatment significantly reduce this risk. A high index of suspicion helps to avoid delays in diagnosis and treatment. Initial management involves

expeditious reduction of the knee if it is still dislocated. Vascular examinations before and after reduction are imperative. If pulses are absent after reduction, the patient should be brought to the operating room emergently for vascular repair and placement of a spanning external fixator. Preoperative angiography is not necessary. In high-energy dislocations with associated vascular injury, the surgeon should have a low threshold for performing four-compartment fasciotomy, tendon reattachment, and primary collateral ligament repair.

If perfusion of the limb after closed reduction is borderline or if pulses are asymmetric, urgent angiography should be performed followed by appropriate treatment of the vascular injury. In some medical centers, however, close monitoring of the neurovascular examination is substituted and angiography is not performed routinely. Angiography in the setting of a normal vascular examination after reduction is controversial. Serial monitoring of the pulses with Doppler ultrasonography and ankle-brachial indexes is probably sufficient and more cost-effective, especially because angiography is not always readily available. Most patients will go on to have an MRI evaluation of ligamentous integrity and intra-articular injury. Magnetic resonance angiography is an increasingly popular diagnostic modality for evaluating vascular injury and can conveniently be performed at the same time. In some medical centers, magnetic resonance angiography is comparable to angiography in accuracy, although this is certainly facility-dependent.

Studies of traumatic knee dislocations have failed to provide a consensus regarding the best method of treatment of the ligamentous injuries. In high-energy dislocations with severe soft-tissue injury, a temporary spanning external fixator may be necessary. Upon removal of the external fixator, a repeat examination under anesthesia and manipulation is performed if necessary. An external fixator is not necessary for patients with in low-energy dislocations.

The timing of reconstruction is debatable. Some authors propose early intervention before 2 weeks, whereas some propose delayed intervention after 3 weeks; others recommend staged reconstruction. The decision when to perform surgery should be based on responses to two critical questions: When has the joint capsule disruption healed enough to safely perform an arthroscopic procedure and how long can surgery be postponed before acute repair of the posterolateral structures is no longer feasible? The critical window of opportunity appears to be between 2 and 3 weeks. Regardless of the timing, recent studies suggest that surgical treatment of residual laxity is superior to nonsurgical treatment with immobilization. Restoration of cruciate ligament stability appears to be particularly crucial to tolerating functional rehabilitation. Functional rehabilitation is an important positive prognostic factor.

Summary

PCL injuries commonly occur during sports participation or as a result of a motor vehicle collision. Careful history taking and physical examination will identify most patients with PCL injuries. Most authors recommend nonsurgical treatment for isolated grade 1 or 2 PCL tears. This involves initial splinting in extension followed by range-of-motion and strengthening exercises. Recovery of quadriceps strength is necessary to compensate for posterior tibial translation and return to preinjury activity levels. Grade 3 injuries may not be as benign as originally thought, and surgical intervention is somewhat controversial. Surgical treatment is generally reserved for acute combined ligament injuries, acute bony avulsions, or symptomatic chronic high-grade PCL tears. Single-tunnel reconstruction techniques moderately improve posterior laxity. Newer double tunnel and tibial inlay techniques offer significant theoretical advantages, but studies examining the outcomes of these procedures are limited, and results are only preliminary. When multiple ligaments are damaged, each ligament requires individual surgical treatment.

Annotated Bibliography

Basic Science: Structure and Function

Markolf KL, Zemanovic JR, McAllister DR: Cyclic loading of posterior cruciate ligament replacements fixed with tibial tunnel and tibial inlay methods. *J Bone Joint Surg Am* 2002;84:518-524.

This in vitro study of cyclic loading of PCL reconstructions compared the tibial tunnel technique to the tibial inlay technique. The authors concluded that the inlay technique of PCL replacement was superior to the tunnel technique with respect to graft failure, graft thinning, and permanent increase in graft length.

McAllister DR, Markolf KL, Oakes DA, Young CR: McWilliams: A biomechanical comparison of tibial inlay and tibial tunnel posterior cruciate ligament reconstruction techniques: Graft pretension and knee laxity. *Am J Sports Med* 2002;30:312-317.

This in vitro biomechanical study of PCL reconstructions compared the tibial tunnel technique to the tibial inlay technique. The authors concluded that there was no biomechanical advantage of one technique over the other.

Mejia EA, Noyes FR, Grood ES: Posterior cruciate ligament femoral insertion site characteristics: Importance for reconstructive procedures. *Am J Sports Med* 2002;30: 643-651.

This is a descriptive anatomic study of the PCL femoral origin using cadavers. The authors emphasize that to accurately reproduce the anatomy of the femoral attachment at the time of reconstruction more than one measurement system is required.

Miller MD, Cooper DE, Fanelli GC, Harner CD, LaPrade RF: Posterior cruciate ligament: Current concepts. *Instr Course Lect* 2002;51:347-351.

This is a concise review of PCL anatomy, biomechanics, assessment of injury, and treatment.

Oakes DA, Markolf KL, McWilliams J, Young CR, McAllister DR: Biomechanical comparison of tibial inlay and tibial tunnel techniques for reconstruction of the posterior cruciate ligament: Analysis of graft forces. *J Bone Joint Surg Am* 2002;84:938-944.

This in vitro biomechanical study compared the tibial inlay technique to the transtibial technique of PCL reconstruction. The authors concluded that neither technique for PCL reconstruction had a substantial advantage over the other with respect to generation of graft forces.

Diagnosis

Bergfeld JA, McAllister DR, Parker RD, Valdevit AD, Kambic H: The effects of tibial rotation on posterior translation in knees in which the posterior cruciate ligament has been cut. *J Bone Joint Surg Am* 2001;83:1339-1343.

The authors observed posterior translation of the tibia in PCL-deficient cadaveric knees as a function of tibial internal and external rotation.

Fanelli GC: Treatment of combined anterior cruciate ligament-posterior cruciate ligament-lateral side injuries of the knee. *Clin Sports Med* 2000;19:493-502.

The author of this article discusses the assessment, diagnosis, and treatment of the ACL/PCL-posterolateral corner injured knee.

Miller MD, Bergfeld JA, Fowler PA, Harner CD, Noyes FR: The posterior cruciate ligament injured knee: Principles of evaluation and treatment. *Instr Course Lect* 1999;48:199-207.

This is an excellent review of PCL evaluation and management.

Shelbourne KD, Davis TJ, Patel DV: The natural history of acute, isolated, nonoperatively treated posterior cruciate ligament injuries: A prospective study. *Am J Sports Med* 1999;27:276-283.

This is a prospective study of the natural history of acute, isolated, nonsurgically treated PCL injuries in 133 athletes. The results suggest that athletically active patients with acute isolated PCL tears treated nonsurgically achieved a level of objective and subjective knee function that was independent of the grade of laxity.

Shelbourne KD, Jennings RW, Vahey TN: Magnetic resonance imaging of posterior cruciate ligament injuries: Assessment of healing. *Am J Knee Surg* 1999;12: 209-213.

In this study, MRI was used to evaluate patients with PCL injuries who were treated nonsurgically. The mean follow-up was 3 years. The authors concluded that most PCL injuries healed in continuity without surgical intervention.

Strobel MJ, Weiler A, Schulz MS, Russe K, Eichhorn HJ: Fixed posterior subluxation in posterior cruciate ligament-deficient knees: Diagnosis and treatment of a new clinical sign. *Am J Sports Med* 2002;30:32-38.

The authors of this article describe fixed posterior sublux-ation of the tibia in the setting of PCL injuries. They treated their patients with a posterior tibial support brace to correct the subluxation prior to ligament reconstruction. The authors concluded that fixed posterior subluxation should be detected by stress radiographs and corrected before reconstruction to avoid overloading the PCL graft.

Indications for Surgery

Badhe NP, Forster IW: High tibial osteotomy in knee instability: The rationale of treatment and early results. *Knee Surg Sports Traumatol Arthrosc* 2002;10:38-43.

Fourteen patients with knee instability and varus alignment were treated with tibial osteotomy with or without ligament reconstruction. The authors reported encouraging results and recommended a high tibial osteotomy along with ligament reconstruction in patients with complex ligamentous injuries with varus alignment.

Clancy WG Jr, Bisson LJ: Double tunnel technique for reconstruction of the posterior cruciate ligament. *Oper Tech Sports Med* 1999;7:110-117.

This article is a review of the surgical technique for double tunnel PCL reconstruction.

Klimkiewicz JJ, Petrie RS, Harner CD: Surgical treatment of combined injury to anterior cruciate ligament, posterior cruciate ligament, and medial structures. *Clin Sports Med* 2000;19:479-492.

This article outlines the principles involved in evaluating and managing combined ligament injuries.

Surgical Outcomes

Cooper DE: Treatment of combined posterior cruciate ligament and posterolateral injuries of the knee. *Oper Tech Sports Med* 1999;7:135-142.

This is a review of the surgical technique for combined PCL posterolateral corner reconstruction.

Harner CD, Janaushek MA, Kanamori A, Yagi M, Vo-grin TM, Woo SL: Biomechanical analysis of a double-bundle posterior cruciate ligament reconstruction. *Am J Sports Med* 2000;28:144-151.

The authors experimentally evaluated cadaveric single-bundle versus double-bundle PCL reconstruction and compared the resulting knee biomechanics with those of the intact knee. They concluded that a double-bundle reconstruction can

more closely restore the biomechanics of the intact knee than can the single-bundle reconstruction.

Harner CD, Janaushek MA, Ma CB, Kanamori A, Vo-grin TM, Woo SL: The effect of knee flexion angle and application of an anterior tibial load at the time of graft fixation on the biomechanics of a posterior cruciate ligament-reconstructed knee. *Am J Sports Med* 2000;28:460-465.

In this cadaveric biomechanical study of graft fixation at varying degrees of flexion, the authors concluded that fixation of the graft with the knee in flexion and with an anterior tibial load will best restore intact knee biomechanics.

Kantaras AT, Johnson DL: The medial meniscal root as a landmark for tibial tunnel position in posterior cruciate ligament reconstruction. *Arthroscopy* 2002;18:99-101.

In this article, the authors emphasize using the root of the posterior horn of the medial meniscus as a landmark for tibial tunnel placement during PCL reconstruction.

Kim SJ, Shin SJ, Cho SK, Kim HK: Arthroscopic suture fixation for bony avulsion of the posterior cruciate ligament. *Arthroscopy* 2001;17:776-780.

The authors of this article discuss an original arthroscopic technique using suture fixation for the treatment of tibial PCL avulsion fractures.

Kim SJ, Shin SJ, Kim HK, Jahng JS, Kim HS: Comparison of 1- and 2-incision posterior cruciate ligament reconstructions. *Arthroscopy* 2000;16:268-278.

This clinical study compared the results of the one-incision technique and the conventional two-incision technique for the arthroscopic treatment of PCL injuries.

Margheritini F, Rihn J, Musahl V, Mariani PP, Harner C: Posterior cruciate ligament injuries in the athlete: An anatomical, biomechanical and clinical review. *Sports Med* 2002;32:393-408.

The authors of this article provide a thorough discussion of the basic science and a clinical review of PCL injuries in athletes.

Rehabilitation

Harner CD, Hoher J: Evaluation and treatment of posterior cruciate ligament injuries. *Am J Sports Med* 1998;26:471-482.

This is a review of surgical techniques of PCL reconstruction based on anatomic and biomechanical studies.

Knee Dislocation: Evaluation and Management

Ohkoshi Y, Nagasaki S, Shibata N, Yamamoto K, Hash-imoto T, Yamane S: Two-stage reconstruction with autografts for knee dislocations. *Clin Orthop* 2002;398:169-175.

The authors of this article report short-term clinical outcomes of a two-stage reconstruction of the dislocated knee using autologous tissue in nine knees.

Potter HG, Weinstein M, Allen AA, Wickiewicz TL, Helfet DL: Magnetic resonance imaging of the multiple-ligament injured knee. *J Orthop Trauma* 2002;16:330-339.

The authors of this article provide a retrospective evaluation of the utility of combined MRI and magnetic resonance angiography for assessing multiple ligament knee injuries.

Richter M, Bosch U, Wippermann B, Hofmann A, Krettek C: Comparison of surgical repair or reconstruction of the cruciate ligaments versus nonsurgical treatment in patients with traumatic knee dislocations. *Am J Sports Med* 2002;30:718-727.

The authors compared the results of cruciate ligament repair or reconstruction with those of nonsurgical treatment after knee dislocation in 89 patients. They concluded that surgical repair or reconstruction of the cruciate ligaments was superior to nonsurgical treatment and identified functional rehabilitation as the most important positive prognostic factor.

Classic Bibliography

Berg EE: Posterior cruciate ligament tibial inlay reconstruction. *Arthroscopy* 1995;11:69-76.

Boynton MD, Tietjens BR: Long-term followup of the untreated isolated posterior cruciate ligament-deficient knee. *Am J Sports Med* 1996;24:306-310.

Burks RT, Schaffer JJ: A simplified approach to the tibial attachment of the posterior cruciate ligament. *Clin Orthop* 1990;254:216-219.

Clancy WG Jr, Shelbourne KD, Zoellner GB, Keene JS, Reider B, Rosenberg TD: Treatment of knee joint instability secondary to rupture of the posterior cruciate ligament: Report of a new procedure. *J Bone Joint Surg Am* 1983;65:310-322.

Cooper DE, Warren RF, Warner JJP: The posterior cruciate ligament and posterolateral structures of the knee: Anatomy, function, and patterns of injury. *Instr Course Lect* 1991;40:249-270.

Covey CD, Sapega AA: Injuries of the posterior cruciate ligament. *J Bone Joint Surg Am* 1993;75:1376-1386.

Cross MJ, Powell JF: Long-term followup of posterior cruciate ligament rupture: A study of 116 cases. *Am J Sports Med* 1984;12:292-297.

Dandy DJ, Pusey RJ: The long-term results of unrepaired tears of the posterior cruciate ligament. *J Bone Joint Surg Br* 1982;64:92-94.

Delee JC, Bergfeld JA, Drez DJ, Parker AW: The posterior cruciate ligament, in Delee JC, Drez D (eds): *Orthopaedic Sports Medicine: Principles and Practice*. Philadelphia, PA, WB Saunders, 1994, pp 1374-1400.

Fanelli GC, Giannotti BF, Edson CJ: Arthroscopically assisted combined posterior cruciate ligament/posterior lateral complex reconstruction. *Arthroscopy* 1996;12:521-530.

Fowler PJ, Messieh SS: Isolated posterior cruciate ligament injuries in athletes. *Am J Sports Med* 1987;15:553-557.

Frassica FJ, Sim FH, Staeheli JW, Pairolero PC: Dislocation of the knee. *Clin Orthop* 1991;263:200-205.

Fu FH, Harner CD, Johnson DL, Miller WD, Woo SL: Biomechanics of knee ligaments: Basic concepts and clinical application. *Instr Course Lect* 1994;43:137-148.

Hughston JC, Bowden JA, Andrews JR, Norwood LA: Acute tears of the posterior cruciate ligament: Results of operative treatment. *J Bone Joint Surg Am* 1980;62:438-450.

Jackson DW, Corsetti J, Simon TM: Biologic incorporation of allograft anterior cruciate ligament replacements. *Clin Orthop* 1996;324:126-133.

Keller PM, Shelbourne KD, McCarroll JR, Rettig AC: Nonoperatively treated isolated posterior cruciate ligament injuries. *Am J Sports Med* 1993;21:132-136.

Miller MD, Harner CD, Koshiwaguchi S: Acute posterior cruciate ligament injuries, in Vince KG (ed): *Knee Surgery*. Baltimore, MD, Williams & Wilkins, 1994, pp 749-767.

Nikolaou PK, Seaber AV, Glisson RR, Ribbeck BM, Bassett FH III: Anterior cruciate ligament allograft transplantation: Long-term function, histology, revascularization, and operative technique. *Am J Sports Med* 1986;14:348-360.

Noyes FR, Barber-Westin SD: Surgical restoration to treat chronic deficiency of the posterolateral complex and cruciate ligaments of the knee joint. *Am J Sports Med* 1996;24:415-426.

Parolie JM, Bergfeld JA: Long-term results of nonoperative treatment of isolated posterior cruciate ligament injuries in the athlete. *Am J Sports Med* 1986;14:35-38.

Racanelli JA, Drez D Jr: Posterior cruciate ligament tibial attachment anatomy and radiographic landmarks for tibial tunnel placement in PCL reconstruction. *Arthroscopy* 1994;10:546-549.

Shelbourne KD, Nitz PA: Posterior cruciate ligament injuries, in Reider B (ed): *Sports Medicine: The School Age Athlete*. Philadelphia, PA, WB Saunders, 1991, pp 317-331.

Skyhar MJ, Warren RF, Ortiz GJ, Schwartz E, Otis JC: The effects of sectioning of the posterior cruciate ligament and the posterolateral complex on the articular contact pressures within the knee. *J Bone Joint Surg Am* 1993;75:694-699.

Shino K, Inoue M, Horibe S, Nagano J, Ono K: Maturation of allograft tendons transplanted into the knee: An arthroscopic and histological study. *J Bone Joint Surg Br* 1988;70:556-560.

Torg JS, Barton TM, Pavlov H, Stine R: Natural history of the posterior cruciate ligament-deficient knee. *Clin Orthop* 1989;246:208-216.

Chapter 13

Anterior Cruciate Ligament Injuries

Michael D. Gordon, MD

Mark E. Steiner, MD

Introduction

The anterior cruciate ligament (ACL) continues to be the center of much debate in the orthopaedic community. Treatment of injuries to the ACL has involved a continuous evolution of techniques from extra-articular, nonanatomic procedures to the current arthroscopically assisted techniques. It is estimated that over 100,000 ACL reconstructions are performed in the United States annually.

ACL Structure and Function

The ACL is composed of two bundles (anteromedial and posterolateral) that provide the primary restraint to anterior tibial translation throughout the arc of knee motion. The ACL also provides a secondary restraint to varus and valgus rotations. Recent studies in human cadaveric knees have shown the ultimate tensile load and stiffness of the human femur-ACL-tibia complex to average 2,150 N and 242 N/mm, respectively. The ACL also plays a vital proprioceptive role, with 1% of its volume being occupied by nerve-related structures.

The anterior border of the ACL insertion is just posteromedial to the anterior horn of the lateral meniscus, and its posterior border is approximately 2 mm anterior to the posterior cruciate ligament (PCL). The femoral insertion is an ovoid along the posteromedial aspect of the lateral femoral condyle. The ligament is surrounded by a synovial layer, making it an intra-articular and extrasynovial structure. Histologic studies have demonstrated that at the time of ACL rupture the residual stump develops a "synovial cap" that limits its reparative potential.

Predisposition and Prevention

Multiple studies have evaluated risk factors for ACL injury with the hope of targeting individuals for appropriate preventive treatment. Female athletes clearly have a higher rate of noncontact ACL injuries (Table 1). This was first identified more than 20 years ago, but it has become more apparent with the increased participation of women in organized athletics (see chapter 35). The ACL injury rate for women is approximately twice the men's rate in soccer and approximately four times the men's rate in basketball. Several authors have identified a decreased protective role of dynamic knee stabilizers (quadriceps and hamstring muscles) as contributing to ACL injury in women. Independent of muscle strength, female athletes have a diminished ability to resist anterior shear with muscle cocontraction. Other studies have identified that even with corrections for body weight, the average size of the ACL is smaller in females than in males. There are also data to suggest that the female ACL might be at greater risk during different stages of the menstrual cycle. Multiple studies have measured the intercondylar notch width, and some have demonstrated that a narrow notch contributes to ACL injuries. It has been observed that a narrow notch often coexists with a smaller ACL; however, a recent study again suggests that a smaller notch alone can produce critical stenosis and ligament impingement.

Preseason training focused on proprioceptive conditioning, muscle cocontraction, neuromuscular training, and muscle strengthening has been shown to decrease the rate of ACL injuries in women. Female athletes tend to land on a knee that is in greater extension than that of their male counterparts. Combined with a valgus motion during landing, this position places high tensile forces on the ACL and can result in ACL injury. Training programs have successfully taught female athletes proper landing mechanics, resulting in decreased injury rates. Proprioceptive training alone has been shown to diminish ACL injury rates in male soccer players. Recently, a warm-up program focused on proprioception resulted in decreased ACL injuries in high school and college women's soccer players. Changes in athletic shoes and artificial playing surfaces have also appeared to diminish ACL injuries. The use of braces to prevent ACL injuries continues to be controversial. Functional ACL braces may help prevent medial collateral ligament (MCL) injuries but not ACL injuries. Improvements in ski bindings and teaching injury mechanisms to advanced skiers has been shown to diminish injury rates.

TABLE 1 | Factors Contributing to Increased Noncontact ACL Injury in Women

A decreased protective role of dynamic knee stabilizers (quadriceps and hamstring muscles)

A diminished ability to resist anterior shear with muscle cocontraction

A smaller ACL than in men

Different stages of the menstrual cycle may increase risk to the ACL

A narrower intercondylar notch than in men

Diagnosis and Associated Injuries

The history and physical examination are the primary tools for diagnosing injuries to the ACL. In a relaxed patient with a normal contralateral knee, the accuracy of a Lachman test to diagnose an ACL tear is even higher than that of an MRI. Instrumented testing can supplement a clinical examination and reliably detect a tear if there is greater than a 3-mm difference in side-to-side testing with a maximum manual force. The most important role for instrumented laxity measurement is to provide reproducible data for objective measurements in outcome studies. MRI can also provide useful information, particularly about any concomitant pathology that may be encountered at the time of surgery or that may be factored into a patient's treatment plan. MRI is highly sensitive for diagnosing bone edema (contusions), other ligament injuries, and meniscal injuries. Currently, MRI technology is focused on improving techniques for detecting chondral lesions.

Partial tears of the ACL are more difficult to detect clinically. The Lachman test may demonstrate increased anterior translation with a firm end point, and the pivot shift may be notable for a "pivot glide." MRI may demonstrate an abnormal continuity of ACL fibers, suggesting partial injury. It has been generally observed that injuries with greater than 50% of the ligament in continuity have resulted in stable knees without need for reconstruction.

Meniscal Injuries

The menisci function as secondary stabilizers of the knee by providing a buttress to anterior tibial translation, and they are commonly injured at the time of an ACL tear. At acute ACL reconstruction, nearly 50% of meniscus tears have been found to be repairable, and they have a greater healing rate than in non-ACL injured knees. Isolated stable tears of the lateral meniscus posterior to the popliteus can be left untreated at the time of ACL reconstruction. If a knee is "locked" with a displaced meniscus in the acute setting, repair of the meniscus can be performed followed by a delayed ACL reconstruction when full knee motion has returned. It is also an option to repair both the meniscus and the ACL after a brief rehabilitation period if motion and particu-

larly extension have returned. Further injury to the meniscus and poorer meniscal healing are caveats to the one-stage procedure. The standard postoperative ACL reconstruction rehabilitation protocol does not need to be altered if a meniscus repair is performed.

The ACL and menisci clearly function symbiotically as a recent long-term study demonstrated. The authors found that if both menisci were intact up to 15 years after ACL reconstruction, then the final follow-up knee scores were equivalent to those for the contralateral leg. If either or both menisci were irreparably injured, the scores were significantly worse at final follow-up, and the knees were found to be more lax on instrument testing. A cadaveric study that evaluated the biomechanical interdependence of the ACL and menisci demonstrated that removal of the medial meniscus increased the in situ forces in an ACL graft by 33% to 50%. Conversely, the resultant forces on the medial meniscus with anterior tibial translation doubled after the ACL had been sectioned.

Combined Collateral Ligament Injuries

Combined ACL and MCL injuries are commonly encountered, particularly in contact sports. Patients often have greater loss of motion with combined collateral ligament injuries than with an isolated ACL injury. ACL reconstruction should be delayed until there is a return of full extension and close to full flexion. The decision to repair, reef, or reconstruct the MCL is based on a surgeon's experience and the extent of the injury. A preoperative MRI scan can help define the extent of the injury. Greater valgus motion places greater stress on the ACL and can predispose an ACL reconstruction to failure; however, 2 to 3 mm of increased valgus motion is probably not detrimental to isolated ACL reconstruction. The critical amount of medial joint line opening that necessitates MCL repair or reconstruction has not been determined and may relate to the overall laxity, alignment, and demands on the knee. Excess valgus laxity can contribute to the failure of ACL reconstruction by resulting in excess anterior translation in the acute healing stage or acute graft rupture on return to sports.

The lateral collateral ligament (LCL) or posterolateral corner structures are often injured in conjunction with an ACL rupture. It is critical that these injuries be detected by clinical examination, MRI, or examination under anesthesia as reports have suggested that up to 50% of failed ACL reconstructions are caused by missed posterolateral corner injuries. Techniques to quantify lateral injury include stress radiographs at the time of surgery and arthroscopic visualization of the lateral compartment. The lift-off or separation of the lateral compartment under varus stress indicates that the lateral structures should be repaired or reconstructed. Difficulties with range of motion have been less common with the repair of lateral structures than medial structures. Because acute repair of the lateral side is often more successful than late reconstruction, early diagnosis and treatment of ACL-LCL injuries is generally recommended.

Articular Cartilage Injuries and Bone Contusions

When an ACL is injured, the tibia shifts anteriorly and the femoral condyles compress the posterior tibia plateau, resulting in bone and articular cartilage lesions, most of which occur laterally. The incidence of these injuries has been reported to be between 16% and 23%. At the time of surgery, these injuries can range from simple softening of the articular surface to full-thickness cartilaginous defects with subchondral fractures. A recent MRI follow-up study of patients with ACL tears and MRI-documented bone contusions found that severe osteochondral lesions were still present on MRI scans up to 2 years after a successful reconstruction. Most MRI abnormalities resolve by 3 months and are not clinically significant.

ACL Injuries in Skeletally Immature Patients

The treatment of ACL injuries in children and adolescents with open physes is a controversial topic. The goal is to provide a stable knee and protect the menisci and articular surfaces at least until maturity when a definitive procedure can be performed. In the past, many of these patients were treated with bracing and/or an extra-articular procedure. It has been demonstrated that nonsurgical care for ACL injuries in skeletally immature adolescents results in subsequent meniscal tears and degenerative knee changes in most patients. Whether these changes can be prevented by early reconstruction of the ACL has not yet been determined. In some patients with low-demand activities, however, nonsurgical care has been successful.

There are case reports of ACL reconstructions in the pediatric population leading to partial or complete closure of growth plates and angular deformities or limb-length discrepancies. The placement of hardware laterally into the distal femoral epiphysis has been a particular problem. To avoid epiphyseal injury during ACL reconstruction, recommendations include (1) drilling tunnels as small as possible, (2) placing the tibial hole as central as possible in the tibia to lessen the chance for angular deformity, (3) using soft-tissue grafts preferentially over bone-tendon-bone grafts, and (4) avoiding extra-articular fixation devices that require significant dissection near the physes. It appears that adolescents who are approaching skeletal maturity (age 14 years for females and 16 years for males) may undergo ACL reconstruction with traditional procedures with little chance for significant growth plate injury. In the very young child, success has been reported with hamstring

grafts routed over the anterior tibia and over the top of the lateral femoral condyle. In the older child or younger adolescent, success has been reported with a hamstring reconstruction with the graft placed through a central tibial drill hole and over the top of the femur.

Partial tears of the ACL in children were recently reviewed in 45 patients 17 years of age or younger with an arthroscopically documented partial ACL tear. All patients were treated with a hinged knee brace and placed into a therapy protocol emphasizing hamstring strengthening. Only 31% of the patients required subsequent ACL reconstruction. Factors that were correlated with successful nonsurgical management included skeletal age of 14 years or younger, near-normal Lachman and pivot-shift test results, and at least 50% of the fibers of the ACL being intact.

Rationale for Reconstruction

Although it is accepted that an ACL-deficient knee with a pivot shift is a liability that will limit pivoting motions, the variability of ACL injury examination results is surprising. A recent comparison of knee function in ACL-deficient patients found that there was no correlation between knee laxity as determined by instrumented testing and simple knee functions (ie, walking, jogging, and stair climbing). The long-term concerns with the ACL-deficient knee include secondary injuries to articular cartilage, menisci, and other ligamentous restraints. An intact ACL is meniscal-protective. Conversely, an ACL-deficient knee has an incidence of secondary meniscal tears of 10% to 25% at 5 years. Recent studies from Sweden have evaluated patients with complete and partial ACL tears at 18- to 24-year follow-up. The complete ACL injuries were treated with direct repair that did not eliminate the abnormal laxity, and the partial tears were simply observed. At follow-up, 84% of the knees with complete tears demonstrated slight-to-moderate osteoarthrosis on weight-bearing radiographs. In this group, 45% had at least one reoperation during the follow-up period, primarily to treat meniscal problems. In the group with partial ACL tears (not greater than 50% ligament damage), the authors found that all of the patients maintained excellent knee function and about 50% demonstrated slight-to-moderate radiographic changes.

It has been documented that knees undergoing ACL reconstruction for chronic injuries have more severe meniscal and chondral injuries than acutely reconstructed knees. Some outcome studies in highly selected groups, however, still found minimal differences between ACL-reconstructed and ACL-deficient knees. The weight of the evidence supports successful ACL reconstruction before a return to participation in sports requiring forceful deceleration and cutting movements. Injury to the contralateral ACL after either nonsurgical or reconstructive surgery has been observed in some series to be greater than normal. This may not be the case for skiing athletes, but for athletes who participate in other sports there appears to be increased risk. This has been attributed to an anatomic predisposition to injury and compensatory altered mechanics.

The "rule of thirds" first presented more than 20 years ago described a select group of patients who sought care for symptomatic ACL-deficient knees. After a rehabilitation program, approximately one third of the patients required ACL reconstruction, one third compensated by eliminating activities, and one third pursued recreational activities. Improved surgical outcomes and diminished surgical morbidity have increased the percentage of patients who opt for ACL reconstruction today. It has been demonstrated that age, activity level, and knee laxity correlate with an individual's ability to cope with an ACL injury. Variations in secondary ligaments, alignment, response to physical therapy, proprioceptive sense, and willingness to modify activities are other factors that may have clinical importance. If a patient wishes to return to pivoting sports with a moderate to high level of involvement, then episodes of instability can be anticipated if the patient does not undergo ACL reconstruction. Ultimately, the purpose of ACL reconstruction is to prevent further knee injury and to allow patients to return to their desired levels of activity.

Surgical Timing

Early attempts at ACL reconstruction focused on operating in the acute setting, which resulted in a large number of patients with postoperative arthrofibrosis. This severe complication prolonged the recovery time and often diminished the functional outcome because of chondral injuries, particularly in the patellofemoral joint. A recent emphasis on delaying surgery until the appropriate "environment" has been established in the knee has resulted in a lower incidence of arthrofibrosis. A patient is ready for surgery when full range of motion returns and good quadriceps contraction is present. Although on average this may take 3 weeks to occur, there is considerable variation among patients. Some skiers with proximal ACL tears will have minimal effusions and a full range of motion within days of the injury, whereas some contact-sport athletes will have stiffness lasting from 6 to 8 weeks. A contributing factor to loss of extension is a torn ACL stump that may impinge in the notch. Most of these knees regain normal degrees of extension with physical therapy, but on rare occasion a preliminary arthroscopy may be necessary to resect the scarred stump of ACL and allow full motion.

Nonsurgical Management

The focus of nonsurgical management is on activity modification and appropriate rehabilitation emphasizing proprioceptive training, quadriceps/hamstring strengthening, and cocontraction during deceleration and cutting maneuvers. Patients who successfully complete a rehabilitation program may be able to participate in recreational activities and have minimal morbidity despite abnormal knee motion.

Knee orthoses can help improve the function of some patients with ACL-deficient knees who pursue moderate activities, but some athletes who participate in sports requiring hard cutting and pivoting may derive no benefit from bracing. Bracing may even provide a false sense of security to some athletes. Interestingly, both functional braces and simple knee sleeves improve proprioception through cutaneous and subcutaneous neural pathways. The ability of a functional brace to prevent instability episodes has been demonstrated clinically, but laboratory tests of functional braces have revealed their limits in preventing abnormal anterior tibial translation. At their very best, functional braces may provide a restraint to the anterior shear forces encountered in light recreational activities.

An in-season ACL injury is a special circumstance, particularly in high school and college athletes. One approach is to quickly rehabilitate the athlete and provide a functional orthosis with the goal of returning the patient to athletic activity in the same season. Despite these interventions, a high incidence of meniscal injuries and recurrent episodes of instability result, and the final treatment outcome may be compromised. As a result, many team physicians recommend reconstruction (even in-season), with the goal being to give athletes the best possible knees for the rest of their careers.

Surgical Management

Good to excellent outcomes for ACL reconstruction performed with careful surgical technique range from 92% to 100%. Objective measurements with instrumented devices have found that 74% to 92% of patients will have less than 3 mm of side-to-side difference in laxity. The results of reconstruction of the chronic ACL-deficient knee are diminished because of impaired secondary restraints and concomitant chondral and meniscal injuries. Use of the single- versus double-incision technique does not seem to affect the outcome as long as proper technique and, in particular, appropriate tunnel placement is used. The choice of graft has been heavily scrutinized and does not appear to have any significant effect on functional results. Patellar tendon grafts, hamstring grafts, and allografts have all been reported to result in essentially the same clinical results. A few clinical trials with patients randomized to receive either patellar tendon or hamstring tendon grafts have suggested that greater long-term stability results in those with patellar grafts; this long-term stability is achieved, however, at the expense of morbidity to the extensor mechanism. In most patients, this morbidity resolves within 6 to 12 months after surgery, but pain with kneeling after a patellar tendon harvest may persist. The patellar tendon is still the most widely used ACL graft in the United States, but there may be a trend toward using hamstring grafts, which is fostered by the development of new fixation techniques. Some studies have reported diminished results in female athletes with hamstring tendon graft ACL reconstructions.

Well documented in the literature are reports of anterior knee pain in ACL-deficient knees and after ACL reconstruction. Dynamic anterior translation of the ACL-deficient knee tends to produce evidence of lateral patellar tilt on MRI scans and lateral patellar tracking in laboratory studies. A return to normal patellar tracking after ACL reconstruction would be expected were it not for the morbidity of the procedure itself. Parapatellar fibrosis, loss of motion, and hemarthrosis may all predispose patients to patellar chondral injuries after surgery. The patella and extensor mechanism continue to be the most common sources of pain in the ACL-deficient and ACL-reconstructed knee.

Surgical Technique

The technique of ACL reconstruction has undergone a significant evolution to the current arthroscopically assisted procedure that is favored today. The keys to a successful outcome are listed in Table 2. The pace of rehabilitation depends on biologic healing of the bone-graft interface and the mechanical strength of the fixation method.

Graft Selection

A myriad of choices exist for ACL substitution. Prosthetic replacement or augmentation have fallen out of favor because of material failures and secondary synovitis. Biologic grafts can be either native tissue (autografts) or acquired cadaveric tissue (allografts).

Patellar tendon, quadriceps tendon, and semitendinosus/gracilis bundled tendons are the primary autografts used in ACL reconstructions. Patellar tendon grafts are still the gold standard and have the advantages of bone-to-bone fixation at both ends, high ultimate tensile strength (approximately 2,300 N for a 14 mm-wide graft), and high stiffness (approximately 620 N/mm for a 14 mm-wide graft). When this graft heals to the bone, the entire tendinous portion is essentially anchored and therefore functional. Multistranded grafts require healing of all strands to achieve their potential. The primary disadvantages of patellar tendon grafts are anterior knee pain and early perioperative morbidity; however, several studies have documented post-ACL reconstruction pain to be unaffected by patellar tendon harvest. At least two series of patients have been reported in which the patellar tendon graft was

TABLE 2	The Keys to Successful Outcome for ACL Reconstruction
Proper patient selection
Close to full knee motion with a good quadriceps contraction preoperatively
Placement of accurate bone tunnels
Selection of an appropriate graft
Adequate fixation to allow early rehabilitation

harvested from the contralateral knee. The proposed advantage of this approach is that postoperative stiffness and muscle inhibition are minimized. Proponents suggest that this approach may allow a return to sports participation at 4 months rather than the customary 6 months after reconstruction.

Hamstring tendon grafts have increased in popularity and offer the advantages of increased collagen mass over patellar tendon grafts (65% greater) and high ultimate tensile load (reported as up to 4,100 N). Grafts should have uniform tension on all strands to ensure maximum strength and stiffness. This can be accomplished by tying the sutures of each pair of tendons together and then looping an additional suture between these two groups. Holding on to the last suture will tension all strands equally. The primary disadvantages include concerns with slower tendon to bone healing in comparison with more rapid bone-to-bone healing.

Quadriceps tendon grafts offer the advantages of a high ultimate tensile load (approximately 2,300 N), a donor site with minimal morbidity, and the potential to harvest a bone plug on one end. The primary disadvantages are unfamiliarity with its use, a depth of harvest that is variable, and the same concerns with tendon-to-bone healing as with hamstring grafts.

Multiple allograft choices have become popular, particularly in the revision setting. These include bone-patellar tendon-bone, quadriceps tendon, hamstring tendon, Achilles tendon, and both anterior and posterior tibialis tendons. The advantages to allograft use are less surgical time, less surgical morbidity, faster rehabilitation, and flexibility in graft preparation. The disadvantages include the risk of viral and/or bacterial infection, slower incorporation of allograft tissue, immunologic reactions, and a paucity of long-term outcome data.

Recently, the tissue bank industry has undergone increased scrutiny because of reports of infections related to grafts. The transmission of HIV and hepatitis C to several patients has been reported, and the transmission of bacterial infections to more than 20 patients by infected allografts has now been documented to have occurred within the past several years. At least one death has occurred because of a *Clostridium* infection transmitted by an osteochondral allograft. Tissue harvesting

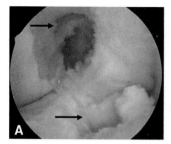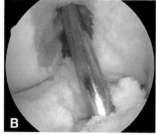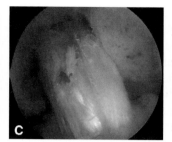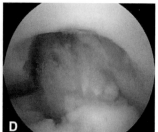

Figure 1 Arthroscopic views of correct tunnel placement and graft position in a right knee. **A,** The arrows identify the tibial and femoral holes before graft passage. The tibial hole is placed just anterior to the PCL and centered between the tibial eminences. The femoral tunnel, drilled endoscopically, lies flush with the posterior cortex at the junction of the roof and lateral wall. **B,** A metal rod traverses the tibial and femoral tunnels with the knee in 90° flexion. The rod demonstrates the obliquity required in the tibial tunnel to correctly place an endoscopic femoral tunnel. **C,** The soft-tissue graft has been passed across the knee. It abuts on the PCL, but it is not distorted by the PCL. Additionally, it does not impinge on the lateral wall of the notch. **D,** When the knee is close to full extension, the graft does not impinge on the roof or lateral wall. A portion anterior and slightly medial to the PCL has been resected to prevent any impingement.

techniques, culture methods before processing, and terminal sterilization methods have been reviewed and cited as areas for improvement. Although tissue bank procedures are proprietary, guidelines have been established by the American Association of Tissue Banks. Many hospitals have elected to obtain grafts only from vendors accredited by the American Association of Tissue Banks.

The role of gamma irradiation continues to be controversial in the preparation of allografts. Common practice in the past was to process tissue with washes and antimicrobial agents and then irradiate grafts to eradicate bacterial and viral contamination, a process called terminal sterilization. More common today is the selective irradiation of donated tissue before processing based on bacterial cultures and the degree of "bacterial burden." Unfortunately, gamma irradiation can weaken grafts and increase deformations of grafts under cyclic loading. Gamma irradiation at levels greater than 4 Mrad can decrease the failure strength of grafts up to 45%, and in a laboratory study the DNA of the HIV virus could still be identified after treatment with 5 Mrad. Nonetheless, irradiation at low doses up to 2.5 Mrad are still used as a compromise. Irradiation at this level may be bacteriocidal and greatly diminish the infectivity of the HIV virus. Gamma irradiation of 2 Mrad had significant biomechanical effects in a recent in vitro study in which a 17% decrease in strength and a 13% decrease in stiffness were documented. Terminal sterilization with ethylene oxide has been discontinued because it can lead to significant synovitis after implantation. Freeze drying is a process that is commonly used with bone allografts because it inactivates viral contamination, but soft tissues are weakened by the process. Cryopreservation is a proprietary process that slowly cools tissues to –135°C; rapid freezing, which cools tissues to –80°C, is used the most by tissue banks. Cryopreservation of ACL allografts may preserve properties that improve incorporation, but mechanical properties are minimally affected compared with traditional freezing.

Multiple studies have documented the slower incorporation of allograft tissue compared with autograft tissue in animal models. Supporting this finding is a recent study in which the retrieval of implanted ACL allografts at autopsy suggested that incorporation may proceed for more than 2 years. Based on these data, surgeons have debated the patient-selection criteria and rehabilitation protocols for allograft implantation. Although several authors have suggested that allograft tissue should not be used in patients with chronically injured knees with more lax secondary restraints, this continues to be a common use of allografts. Outcomes of ACL reconstruction with autografts and allografts have been comparable, perhaps because of a selection bias.

Tunnel Position

One goal of tunnel placement in ACL reconstruction is to approximate the tibial and femoral attachments of the native ACL to minimize changes in graft length and tension throughout range of motion. Functionally, current techniques tend to replace only the posterior portions of the ACL, which is the portion under the greatest tension in extension. Furthermore, it is now well documented that the graft should not impinge in the notch in extension; therefore, the graft should be placed posterior in the tibial footprint. Anatomic measurements indicate that the guide pin for the tunnel should be 6 to 7 mm anterior to the PCL. The shape of the notch also affects the tunnel placement, and the surgeon should evaluate the notch anatomy to determine possibilities for tunnel placements and the need for a notchplasty. In some selected knees, a notchplasty may not be necessary if the tunnel is placed in the posterior footprint of the ACL and the size of the notch is adequate to accommodate the graft (Figure 1). The angle of the tibial tunnel in the coronal plane is also an important variable when the femoral tunnel is drilled through the tibial tunnel. Loss of knee flexion and increased anterior translation have resulted when the tibial tunnel is too vertical. This results in a femoral tunnel that over-tensions the graft in flexion and may impinge the graft in extension. It has been suggested that the tibial tunnel should be at least 15° from the vertical to achieve a correct femoral tunnel. This will produce a starting point that is often in the MCL. In regard to the femoral tunnel, most authors now recommend that it be placed as posterior as possible in the 10:30 to 11:00 o'clock position in a right knee and 1:00 o'clock to 1:30 position in a left knee. A recent cadaveric study suggests that placing the graft more "horizontally" will theoretically provide greater restraint to rotational stress on the knee and ultimately function more like a native ACL. The femoral tunnel can also be drilled from an anteromedial portal with the knee flexed approximately 120°. This avoids the constraint of femoral tunnel placement based on tibial tunnel placement (Figure 2).

There has been a recent resurgence in studies evaluating the role of a double femoral socket reconstruction of the ACL as has been suggested for PCL reconstruction. Theoretically, this would allow for recreation of both bundles of the ACL that could be tensioned individually (anteromedially in flexion and posterolaterally in extension). An in vivo study from Japan found equivalent short-term results between double-socket and single-socket reconstructions. An in vitro study demonstrated clearly better function for anterior tibial translation and transverse rotation with a two-bundle technique.

Initial Graft Tension

Initial graft tension is determined by the following three variables at the time of graft fixation: the manual tension applied to the graft, the angle of knee flexion, and any posterior translation applied to the tibia. Greater tension on the graft will clearly result in greater graft stiffness and less anterior translation. Knee flexion is a variable because most grafts are placed nonisometrically to avoid impingement and therefore grafts tend to tighten in extension. Posterior tibial translation at the time of fixation directly increases graft tension. Concerns with overtensioning the graft and "capturing the knee" dictate that the knee should be in full extension with no applied posterior translation at the time of fixation. Greater tension on the graft and pretensioning the graft are two accepted methods of increasing graft stiffness and tension. It is thought that a graft will not be overtensioned if the knee is in absolute full extension at fixation. There is clear evidence that higher initial graft tensions result in increased stiffness in the graft, which may be present at 2-year follow-up. A cadaveric study found that initial tensions as high as 140 N had no deleterious effects on the biomechanical properties of soft-tissue grafts. If multiple bundle ACL grafts are secured with all limbs of the graft equally tensioned, then the total force applied may not be any greater than is needed for single-bundle bone-tendon-bone grafts.

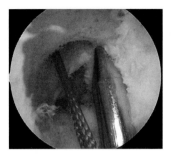

Figure 2 In this arthroscopic view, the metal rod traverses the tibial tunnel and demonstrates the position of an endoscopic femoral tunnel. The femoral tunnel traversed by the suture was drilled from an anteromedial portal. The ability to place a tunnel lower and posterior in the notch is demonstrated by the tunnel drilled from an anteromedial portal.

Graft Fixation

Graft fixation continues to be a rapidly evolving technology that directly changes clinical practice. Initial fixation of ACL grafts is critical to long-term success because a stable construct needs to be maintained until the progression from mechanical to biologic fixation is complete. Ideal fixation has sufficient strength to avoid traumatic failure, sufficient stiffness to restore normal anterior translation, and a location close to the joint line to minimize graft movement within the tunnel and provide resistance to deformation under cyclic loading to prevent instability before graft incorporation.

Multiple techniques have evolved over the past few years on both the tibial and femoral sides. Clearly, interference screw fixation is the gold standard for bone-patellar tendon-bone grafts, and multiple studies have documented that the clinical results are equivalent for bioabsorbable and metal screws. The inside-out placement of an interference screw at the entrance to the femoral tunnel has the benefit of posterior graft displacement, and the method minimizes graft motion within the tunnel. An important technical point in using interference screws is to avoid divergence between the bone plug and the screw. The biomechanical properties of the fixation deteriorate significantly when there is divergence of greater than 15° between the screw and the bone plug.

A criticism of soft-tissue grafts has been the inability to replicate the fixation strength and stiffness of bone plugs and interference screws. However, novel devices and techniques have been developed over the past few years that test well in vitro and appear to function well in vivo. Cross-pin fixation is one such method on the femoral side that provides rigid fixation of soft-tissue grafts; however, cross-pin fixation requires a second incision, and the graft is secured 2 to 4 cm from the femoral tunnel entrance. There is a theoretic potential for a bungee or windshield wiper effect, and clinical follow-up will be necessary to validate this technology. Endobutton (Smith & Nephew, Mansfield, MA) fixation has also demonstrated excellent fixation characteristics, but this method poses an even greater concern with fixation far from the intra-articular region. The addition of a continuous loop to the endobutton may improve its function. Some surgeons have supplemented endobutton fixation with a soft-tissue interference screw to address these concerns.

On the tibial side, soft-tissue fixation is more complex because the bone tends to be less dense and hardware placed on the tibial surface will be more prominent. Forces applied to the graft tend to be more in line with the tibial tunnel and are not mitigated by the bony anatomy. Most fixation techniques do not provide their primary fixation at the joint surface; rather, it is at or near the anterior tibial cortex. Tapered interference screws, nontapered interference screws, screws with washers, and expanding screws (Intrafix, Mitek, Norwood, MA) have all been evaluated. In vitro studies suggest that tapered 35-mm interference screws and expanding screws provide optimal fixation in regards to pullout strength and stiffness. Clinical experience with expanding screws has supported their fixation qualities, but dead space inherent in these devices and the insertion of nonreabsorbable plastic in the tibia may mitigate against their use.

Recent research has also addressed the improvement of graft-to-tunnel healing rate and, in particular, soft-tissue grafts to osseous tunnel incorporation rates. Animal models have been used to evaluate the role of bone morphogenetic proteins (BMPs) in speeding up this process. In both rabbits and dogs, studies have demonstrated that BMP-2 increases the rate and quality of tendon-to-bone healing. The addition of the BMP led to a more normal appearing tendo-osseous junction rather than poorer quality fibrous tissue. In a rabbit study, when loaded to failure, all of the grafts treated with the BMP-2 failed within the intra-articular substance of the tendon, whereas the control grafts failed by pulling out from the tunnel. The two animal studies used different techniques for introducing the BMP: one used a viral vector, and the other wrapped the graft in a collagen sponge. More research is being done on BMP-2 and other growth factors such as fibroblast growth factor, transforming growth factor-β, and platelet-derived growth factor.

Thermal Shrinkage

Thermal shrinkage of soft tissue is a technology that has yet to be clearly validated in clinical orthopaedics. There has been interest in treating partial ACL tears and elongated ACL grafts with thermal energy in lieu of performing a complete reconstruction. Thermal devices have been used to "shrink" capsuloligamentous tissue in the shoulder, and the application of this technology to a lax ACL is a logical extension. The results have been mixed, with several published cases in humans and canines reporting complete disintegration of remaining ACL fibers after thermal treatment. A recent review of 18 partial ACL tears treated with a monopolar device reported that 11 failed at an average of 4 months

follow-up. The seven successful outcomes occurred primarily with acutely injured ACLs. However, another study of 28 patients with partial tears had good results. The rehabilitation required 6 weeks of bracing and no weight bearing including limited motion for 4 weeks. Thermal shrinkage would be contraindicated in the chronically lax ACL and in the previously reconstructed ACL that has become lax. In summary, the usefulness of thermal shrinkage in the treatment of ACL tears is at best controversial.

Rehabilitation

The benefit of closed-kinetic chain exercise programs to the ACL-reconstructed knee has been clearly established as the cocontraction of hamstrings and quadriceps decreases the stress on the ACL graft while allowing for strengthening of the surrounding muscles. As surgical techniques and fixation methods have improved and with greater understanding of knee kinematics, physicians have been able to accelerate the postoperative rehabilitation. It is recognized that ligaments and soft-tissue grafts heal faster when joint motion is allowed and when stress to the healing tissue is applied well below the fixation strength of the construct. It is documented that if rehabilitation in the first 8 weeks after ACL reconstruction is too aggressive, it can result in greater joint inflammation and greater ultimate laxity. Allograft tissues are incorporated at a slower rate than autografts, which has led some surgeons to slightly delay the progression of activity levels when using allografts.

It is generally accepted currently that full range of motion, particularly extension, should be promoted immediately after surgery. Progression to full weight bearing has generally been at 2 weeks or when the patient can comfortably bear weight. Protocols differ significantly between surgeons regarding the use of rehabilitation braces, resistive exercise programs, activity level progression, and functional braces. A return to full activities at 6 months is still common, with the use of a functional brace being optional. The understanding of muscle function after ACL injury and reconstruction continues to evolve. When adequate strength has been restored to the quadriceps and hamstring muscles, a program focused on proprioception training can be initiated. Several studies have evaluated proprioceptive sense about the knee and the response of ACL-deficient knees with and without reconstructions. A recent study found that by 6 months after reconstruction, the threshold to detect motion (a measure of proprioceptive sense) had significantly improved and approached normal. Other studies of ACL-injured knees have found an evolution of quadriceps and hamstring recruitment patterns beyond 6 months from injury. Interestingly, intraosseous metabolic activity measured by bone scanning does not return to normal until almost 18 months after ACL reconstruction. There are data suggesting that knee function may not truly approach normal until approximately 18 months after surgery as well. Return to sport is generally delayed until appropriate knee control is demonstrated and quadriceps strength is equal to or almost equal to that of the uninvolved leg.

Several authors have evaluated the role of physical therapy in decreasing the postoperative morbidity related to graft harvest. Anterior knee pain was for many years thought to be caused by the harvest of the patellar tendon as a graft source; however, more recent reviews suggest that anterior knee pain is multifactorial. These authors demonstrated that by 6 months postoperatively, the return of full extension and normal strength eliminated anterior knee pain that was equal throughout all graft choices.

Revision ACL Surgery

There are estimates that between 3,000 and 10,000 ACL reconstructions fail each year in the United States. Although traumatic rerupture of the ACL graft does occur, errors in diagnosis and surgical technique have been identified as the most common cause of recurrent instability. These include graft impingement, improper tunnel placement, improper graft tensioning, inadequate fixation of the graft, and missed concomitant pathology at the time of surgery (Figure 3). A recent review of a series of 114 consecutive ACL revisions found that 39% were done because of traumatic reinjuries, 30% involved improper graft placement, and 28% involved missed lateral or posterolateral pathology (Figure 4).

The evaluation of a patient with a failed ACL reconstruction must first establish whether the primary problem is pain or instability. Meniscal and chondral injuries may be the primary causes of symptoms. The alignment of the involved leg and the gait pattern should be assessed to ensure that there is no varus malalignment or lateral thrust suggesting that a bony procedure, such as a high tibial osteotomy, may need to be performed separately or in conjunction with an ACL revision. The static stabilizers of the knee also should be evaluated in the same manner as with an acute ACL injury. The failure of an ACL reconstruction should raise the concern for identifying secondary stabilizers of the knee that may be deficient. Although not established, it has been speculated that loss of the medial meniscus can contribute to ACL graft failure by increasing the forces on the graft with anterior tibial translation. An indication for medial meniscal allograft replacement may be revision ACL reconstruction in the absence of the medial meniscus.

The methods of revision surgery can vary considerably among patients, and the ability to use multiple options is necessary (Figure 5). Existing hardware need not be removed unless it interferes with the current surgical plan. The choice of graft for revision surgery is

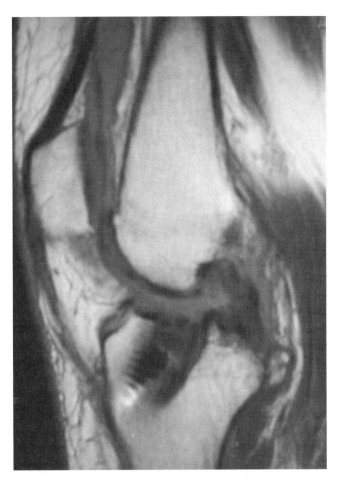

Figure 3 A sagittal MRI scan of a failed ACL allograft demonstrates the lysis often observed with allografts and suggests that graft impingement on the roof of the intercondylar notch contributed to failure.

quite controversial and more limited in many situations because other tissue may have been previously harvested for the primary procedure. The use of grafts including the contralateral bone-patellar tendon-bone, ipsilateral hamstring or patellar tendon, quadriceps tendon, or multiple types of allografts is currently being discussed. Several authors have raised particular concerns over the use of allografts in revision surgery because of the theoretical longer incorporation time. It is suggested that lax secondary stabilizers will lead to greater early stress on a revision graft compared with a primary graft.

The outcomes of ACL revisions do not match those of primary ACL reconstructions. Various authors have reported that 60% to 80% of patients will have improved pain levels and improved overall function, and 50% to 65% will be able to return to active sports participation. The keys to a good outcome are proper recognition of the reason for failure and addressing these issues at the time of surgery and in the rehabilitation period.

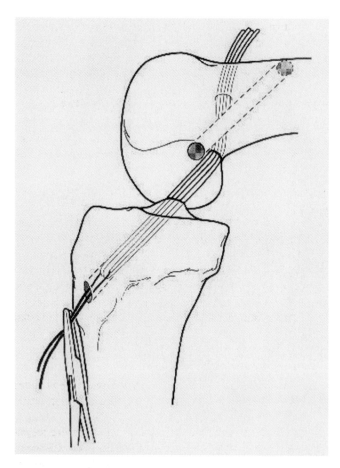

Figure 4 An illustration showing that in a revision ACL the femoral hole can be drilled outside-in from a lateral thigh incision. The tunnel can be placed further posterior and inferior than a standard endoscopic tunnel.

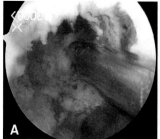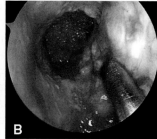

Figure 5 Arthroscopic views of a femoral tunnel in a revision ACL reconstruction. **A,** The femoral tunnel has extensive bone resorption that prevents the placement of a new tunnel in a correct position. **B,** The femoral tunnel has been filled with bone graft, and the reconstruction will be performed in approximately 3 months. *(Reproduced with permission from Kowalk DL, Steiner ME: Anterior cruciate ligament reconstruction using hamstrings for a two-incision technique. Tech Orthop 1998;13:253-261.)*

Annotated Bibliography

ACL Structure and Function

Murray MM, Martin SD, Martin TL, Spector M: Histological changes in the human anterior cruciate ligament after rupture. *J Bone Joint Surg Am* 2000;82:1387-1397.

Ten intact ACLs obtained at the time of total knee arthroplasty and 23 ruptured ACLs were evaluated. The authors found that the human ACL forms a layer of synovial tissue over the ruptured stump that is highly populated with myofibroblasts.

Papageorgiou CD, Gil JE, Kanamori A, Fenwick JA, Woo SL, Fu FH: The biomechanical interdependence between the anterior cruciate ligament replacement graft and the medial meniscus. *Am J Sports Med* 2001; 29:226-231.

This cadaveric sequential sectioning study compared the ability of the ACL, the medial meniscus, and ACL replacement graft to resist anterior tibial translation. The authors report that ACL deficiency doubles the load on the medial meniscus, which returns to normal with an ACL graft in place. A medial meniscectomized knee led to an increase of 33% to 50% of in situ forces on the ACL.

Predisposition and Prevention

Anderson AF, Dome DC, Gautam S, Awh MH, Rennirt GW: Correlation of anthropometric measurements, strength, anterior cruciate ligament size, and intercondylar notch characteristics to sex differences in anterior cruciate ligament tear rates. *Am J Sports Med* 2001;29: 58-66.

This prospective study compares 100 matched high-school basketball players (50 male and 50 female). The authors found that male basketball players had greater quadriceps and hamstring strength and larger ACLs than female basketball players, whereas the notch width index of both groups was equal.

Patel RR, Hurwitz DE, Bush-Joseph CA, Bach BR Jr, Andriacci TP: Comparison of clinical and dynamic knee

Summary

The most recent significant improvement in understanding and treating ACL injuries has been in injury prevention. The mechanisms of ACL rupture have been elucidated, and the biomechanical variants that predispose athletes to injury have been identified. The application of this information will likely reduce ACL injuries in the future. The choice of graft for ACL reconstruction continues to be a dilemma; however, comparable results for ACL reconstruction have been documented with all types of grafts. Each type has unique attributes; consequently, most surgeons use multiple grafts. Correct placement of a graft is still a surgical challenge, particularly when using the endoscopic technique. Unfortunately, ACL reconstruction procedures still result in significant perioperative morbidity and extended rehabilitation. The goal of treatment continues to be to provide a painless knee with stability and normal muscle strength and coordination. The challenge is to perform the reconstructive procedure with high success and minimal morbidity.

function in patients with anterior cruciate ligament deficiency. *Am J Sports Med* 2003;31:68-74.

Forty-four patients with an ACL-insufficient knee were compared with 44 control subjects by gait analysis during walking, jogging, and stair climbing. The authors found that passive measures of knee laxity were not indicative of dynamic knee function and that patients with more normal quadriceps strength were able to perform the activities in a more normal fashion.

Reider B, Arcand MA, Diehl LH, et al: Proprioception of the knee before and after anterior cruciate ligament reconstruction. *Arthroscopy* 2003;19:2-12.

The proprioception of the knees of 26 patients undergoing ACL reconstruction was compared to that of the contralateral knee as an internal control as well as to that of 26 control subjects. Joint position sense and threshold to detection of passive motion were evaluated preoperatively and postoperatively. The authors found that the threshold to detection of passive motion was a more reliable method of testing proprioception and that it improves in the first 6 months postoperatively.

Wojtys EM, Ashton-Miller JA, Huston LJ: A gender-related difference in the contribution of the knee musculature to sagittal-plane shear stiffness in subjects with similar knee laxity. *J Bone Joint Surg Am* 2002;84:10-16.

Male and female volunteers were evaluated for knee stiffness with maximum cocontraction of their hamstrings and quadriceps. The authors found that the male subjects were able to produce a significantly greater increase in shear stiffness of the knee than the female subjects (379% versus 212%).

Diagnosis and Associated Injuries

Costa-Paz M, Muscolo DL, Ayerza M, Mankino A, Aponte-Tinao L: Magnetic resonance imaging follow-up study of bone bruises associated with anterior cruciate ligament ruptures. *Arthroscopy* 2001;17:445-449.

Twenty-one patients with ACL tears and with MRI-identified bone bruises were followed for a minimum of 2 years after ACL reconstruction with repeat MRI. Seventy-one percent had complete resolution of their bone edema, and 29% had persistent evidence of the osteochondral lesion.

Kocher MS, Micheli LJ, Zurakowski D, Luke A: Partial tears of the anterior cruciate ligament in children and adolescents. *Am J Sports Med* 2002;30:697-703.

Forty-five skeletally immature patients with arthroscopically confirmed partial ACL tears were treated with a structured rehabilitation program and followed for a minimum of 2 years. Fourteen patients underwent subsequent reconstructions, and this was associated with tears that were greater than 50%, predominantly posterolateral tears, a grade B pivot shift, and older chronologic and skeletal age.

Shelbourne KD, Gray T: Results of anterior cruciate ligament reconstruction based on meniscus and articular cartilage status at the time of surgery: Five- to fifteen-year evaluations. *Am J Sports Med* 2000;28:446-452.

Objective data on 482 patients and subjective data on 928 patients were collected at a mean of 8.6 years after ACL reconstruction. The authors concluded that long-term subjective and objective results of a successful ACL reconstruction are affected by the status of the menisci and articular surface.

Steiner ME, Koskinen SK, Winalski CS, Martin SD, Haymen M: Dynamic lateral patellar tilt in the anterior cruciate ligament-deficient knee: A magnetic resonance imaging analysis. *Am J Sports Med* 2001;29:593-599.

MRI was used to evaluate patellar tracking abnormalities in 11 patients with ACL ruptures; their contralateral legs were used as controls. There was no difference in patellar alignment when the quadriceps were at rest; however, when the quadriceps were contracted, a significant increase in lateral patellar tilt in the ACL-insufficient knees was noted.

Rationale for Reconstruction

Maletius W, Messner K: Eighteen- to twenty-four-year follow-up after complete rupture of the anterior cruciate ligament. *Am J Sports Med* 1999;27:711-717.

Fifty-six patients with complete ACL ruptures were reevaluated at 12 and 20 years. Eighty-four percent had evidence of changes on weight-bearing radiographs equivalent to those for osteoarthrosis. Forty-five percent had at least one reoperation, primarily for meniscal problems.

Surgical Management

Hamner DL, Brown CH Jr, Steiner ME, Hecker AT, Hayes WC: Hamstring tendon grafts for reconstruction of the anterior cruciate ligament: Biomechanical evaluation of the use of multiple strands and tensioning techniques. *J Bone Joint Surg Am* 1999;81:549-557.

Fresh-frozen hamstring grafts were evaluated as one-, two-, and four-stranded grafts. The authors found that four combined strands that were equally tensioned were stronger and stiffer than all 10-mm patellar tendon grafts that have been described in previous reports.

Haut-Donahue TL, Howell SM, Hull ML, Gregersen C: A biomechanical evaluation of anterior and posterior tibialis tendons as suitable single-loop anterior cruciate ligament grafts. *Arthroscopy* 2002;18:589-597.

In this study, 10 anterior tibialis and 10 posterior tibialis allografts were biomechanically evaluated and compared with published data on a normal ACL, hamstring graft, and patellar tendon graft. The authors concluded that the biomechanical properties of a single loop of anterior or posterior tibialis tendon are either better than or similar to those of the native ACL, hamstring graft, or patellar tendon graft.

Indelli PF, Dillingham MF, Fanton GS, Schurman DJ: Monopolar thermal treatment of symptomatic anterior cruciate ligament instability. *Clin Orthop* 2003;407:139-147.

The authors treated 28 consecutive symptomatically unstable patients with partial ACL tears with a monopolar thermal probe. At minimum 2-year follow-up, 96% had knees were rated as normal or nearly normal both subjectively and objectively. The authors recommended treatment only when patients had less than 6 months of symptoms of instability and greater than 50% of fibers in continuity and it had been at least 6 months since a prior ACL reconstruction.

Kousa P, Jarvinen TLN, Vihavainen M, Kannus P, Jarvinen M: The fixation strength of six hamstring tendon graft fixation devices in anterior cruciate ligament reconstruction, Part I: Femoral site. *Am J Sports Med* 2003;31:174-181.

Six femoral fixation devices were evaluated in porcine femurs with cyclic loading and a single-cycle load-to-failure test. The authors noted that in all tested implants, the majority of residual displacement developed during the first 250 loading cycles of the cyclic-loading regimen, bringing attention to the importance of graft preconditioning.

Kousa P, Jarvinen TLN, Vihavainen M, Kannus P, Jarvinen M: The fixation strength of six hamstring tendon graft fixation devices in anterior cruciate ligament reconstruction: Part II. Tibial site. *Am J Sports Med* 2003; 31:182-188.

Six tibial fixation devices were evaluated in porcine tibias with cyclic loading and a single-cycle load-to-failure test. The authors demonstrated a clear difference in fixation strength among the devices tested.

Martinek V, Latterman C, Usas A, et al: Enhancement of tendon-bone integration of anterior cruciate ligament grafts with bone morphogenetic protein-2 gene transfer: A histological and biomechanical study. *J Bone Joint Surg Am* 2002;84:1123-1131.

This in vivo study examined the use of a viral vector to transfer the *BMP-2* gene into tendon grafts in rabbits. The infected grafts had a significantly improved rate of integration into bone tunnels compared with controls.

Rodeo SA, Seneviratne A, Suzuki K, Felker K, Wickiewicz TL, Warren RF: Histological analysis of human meniscal allografts: A preliminary report. *J Bone Joint Surg Am* 2000;82:1071-1082.

The authors of this histologic analysis concluded that despite the absence of frank immunologic rejection, a subtle immune reaction may affect the healing, incorporation, and revascularization of human meniscal allografts. They also suggest that it is possible that the structural remodeling associated with cellular repopulation may render the meniscus more susceptible to injury.

Vangsness CT Jr: Overview of allograft soft tissue processing. *AAOS Bulletin* 2004;52:33-38.

The author of this article presents an in-depth look at the current problems with allografts and considerations for keeping them safe in the future.

Woo SL, Kanamori A, Zeminski J, Yagi M, Papageorgiou C, Fu FH: The effectiveness of reconstruction of the anterior cruciate ligament with hamstrings and patellar tendons: A cadaveric study comparing anterior tibial and rotational loads. *J Bone Joint Surg Am* 2002; 84:907-914.

The kinematics of the knee with the ACL intact, with the ACL torn, and with the ACL reconstructed were determined in response to an anterior tibial load with and without a combined rotational load. The authors found that the ACL-reconstructed knees were successful in resisting the anterior tibial load, but were not as effective in resisting the combined rotational and anterior load.

Yagi M, Wong EK, Kanamori A, Debski RE, Fu FH, Woo SL: Biomechanical analysis of an anatomic anterior cruciate ligament reconstruction. *Am J Sports Med* 2002;30:660-666.

Ten cadaveric knees were biomechanically tested and the ACLs were then reconstructed using single- and double-bundle techniques. The authors found that the double-bundle technique produced a better biomechanical outcome.

Rehabilitation

Numazaki H, Tohyama H, Nakano H, Kikuchi S, Yasuda K: The effect of initial graft tension in anterior cruciate ligament reconstruction on the mechanical behaviors of the femur-graft-tibia complex during cyclic loading. *Am J Sports Med* 2002;30:800-805.

This ex vivo study evaluated the initial stiffness and ultimate failure loads of several different reconstruction constructs. Higher initial tension was recommended for quadrupled hamstring grafts than for patellar tendon grafts.

Revision ACL Surgery

Noyes FR, Barber-Westin SD: Revision anterior cruciate surgery with use of bone-patellar tendon-bone autogenous grafts. *J Bone Joint Surg Am* 2001;83:1131-1143.

This prospective study was conducted to determine the functional results, patient satisfaction, and graft failure rate after 57 consecutive revision replacements of the ACL with use of a bone-patellar tendon-bone autogenous graft. The authors report significant improvements in the scores for pain ($P < 0.0001$), activities of daily living ($P < 0.01$), sports participation ($P < 0.001$), patient satisfaction ($P < 0.0001$), and overall rating of the knee ($P < 0.0001$). Thirty-three (60%) of the replaced ligaments were functional, 9 (16%) were partially functional, and 13 (24%) failed.

Classic Bibliography

Cosgarea AJ, Sebastianelli WJ, DeHaven KE: Prevention of arthrofibrosis after anterior cruciate ligament reconstruction using the central third patellar tendon autograft. *Am J Sports Med* 1995;23:87-92.

Daniel DM, Stone ML, Dobson BE, Fithian DC, Rossman DJ, Kaufman KR: Fate of the ACL-injured patient: A prospective outcome study. *Am J Sports Med* 1994;22:632-644.

Dodds JA, Arnoczky SP: Anatomy of the anterior cruciate ligament: A blueprint for repair and reconstruction. *Arthroscopy* 1994;10:132-139.

Harner CD, Marks PH, Fu FH, Irrgang JJ, Silby MG, Mengato R: Anterior cruciate ligament reconstruction: Endoscopic versus two-incision technique. *Arthroscopy* 1994;10:502-512.

Harner CD, Olson E, Irrgang JJ, Silverstein S, Fu FH, Silbey M: Allograft versus autograft anterior cruciate ligament reconstruction: 3- to 5-year outcome. *Clin Orthop* 1996;324:134-144.

Janarv P, Nystrom A, Werner S, et al: Anterior cruciate ligament injuries in skeletally immature patients. *J Pediatr Orthop* 1996;16:673-677.

Kannus P, Jarvinen M: Knee ligament injuries in adolescents. *J Bone Joint Surg Br* 1988;70:772-776.

McCarroll JR, Shelbourne KD, Porter DA, Rettig AC, Murray S: Patellar tendon graft reconstruction for midsubstance anterior cruciate ligament rupture in junior high school athletes: An algorithm for management. *Am J Sports Med* 1994;22:478-484.

Noyes FR, Barber-Westin SD: Reconstruction of the anterior cruciate ligament with human allograft: Comparison of early and later results. *J Bone Joint Surg Am* 1996;78:524-537.

Noyes FR, Barber-Westin SD, Roberts CS: Use of allografts after failed treatment of rupture of the anterior cruciate ligament. *J Bone Joint Surg Am* 1994;76:1019-1031.

Noyes FR, Matthews DS, Mooar PA, Grood ES: The symptomatic anterior cruciate-deficient knee: Part II. The results of rehabilitation, activity modification, and counseling on functional disability. *J Bone Joint Surg Am* 1983;65:163-174.

O'Neill DB: Arthroscopically assisted reconstruction of the anterior cruciate ligament: A prospective randomized analysis of three techniques. *J Bone Joint Surg Am* 1996;78:803-813.

Shelbourne KD, Gray T: Anterior cruciate ligament reconstruction with autogenous patellar tendon graft followed by accelerated rehabilitation: A two- to nine-year follow-up. *Am J Sports Med* 1997;25:786-795.

Chapter 14

Collateral Ligament Injuries

C. Benjamin Ma, MD

Stephen Fealy, MD

Introduction

To effectively treat collateral ligament injuries in athletes, orthopaedic surgeons must have a thorough understanding of the medial collateral ligament (MCL) complex (the anatomy, function, diagnosis, and treatment of isolated, combined, and chronic injuries) as well as the various surgical reconstructions and complications associated with these injuries. They must also have a thorough understanding of the lateral structures, including the posterolateral corner of the knee, and knee alignment and its effect on surgical reconstructions of the ligaments. Additionally, orthopaedic surgeons must know how to diagnose and treat collateral ligament injuries of the knee and be familiar with the latest surgical developments.

MCL Complex

Anatomy and Function

The anatomy of the medial aspect of the knee has been well characterized. The medial structures can be divided into three layers (Figure 1). The most superficial layer (layer I) consists of the deep fascia encompassing the patellar tendon anteriorly and the popliteal fascia posteriorly. The sartorius fascia is part of layer I overlying the MCL. Layer II is composed mainly of the superficial MCL. The gracilis and semitendinosus tendons are found between layers I and II. Layer III consists of the medial capsular ligament or deep MCL and the posteromedial capsule. Although these three layers are fairly distinct at the level of the MCL, layers I and II blend anteriorly, and layers II and III blend posteriorly. Surgically, it is difficult to separate layers II and III posteriorly because the two layers blend together to form the posterior oblique ligament (Figure 2). This technical difficulty is often encountered during inside-out meniscal repairs. The MCL complex consists of the superficial and deep MCL as well as the posterior oblique ligament.

The medial structures of the knee are the primary stabilizers for valgus force and act as a secondary stabilizer to anterior translation. They are also important in resisting external rotation. Combined injuries to the anterior cruciate ligament (ACL) and medial structures often lead to anteromedial rotatory instability, which often goes undiagnosed. The ACL and MCL have a codependent relationship because injuries to the MCL can lead to increased forces in the ACL in resisting valgus load and injuries to the ACL can lead to increased forces in the MCL in resisting anterior translation. Robotic studies have shown that the in situ forces in the MCL increase by two to five times for the ACL-deficient knee, indicating their significant role as the secondary stabilizer for anterior translation. Further studies have shown that ACL reconstruction can normalize the in situ forces in the MCL. Conversely, an ACL graft is subjected to significantly higher in situ forces with MCL deficiency during an applied valgus moment. Therefore, the ACL-reconstructed knee with a combined ACL and MCL injury should be protected from high valgus moments during early healing to avoid excessive loading on the graft. Several studies have noted that an ACL-deficient knee in the setting of a chronically lax MCL would require reconstruction of both the ACL and MCL.

Diagnosis of Injuries

Knowing the mechanism of injury is important in the diagnosis of ligament injuries. An isolated valgus moment to the knee is a classic mechanism for MCL injuries. The MCL complex can be examined with stress in the coronal plane. The ligament should be examined with the knee both in full extension and at 30° of flexion. Examination at full extension tests the integrity of the MCL as well as associated capsular and cruciate ligament injuries. Examination at flexion isolates the MCL itself.

When testing the MCL, the patient is examined in the supine position with the hip abducted and the knee gently hanging off the edge of the examination table and flexed at 30°. A valgus stress is applied at the ankle with support on the lateral side of the knee. The examination should be repeated at full extension. Care should be taken to produce a valgus stress, but not internal or external rotation through the leg. The extent of joint

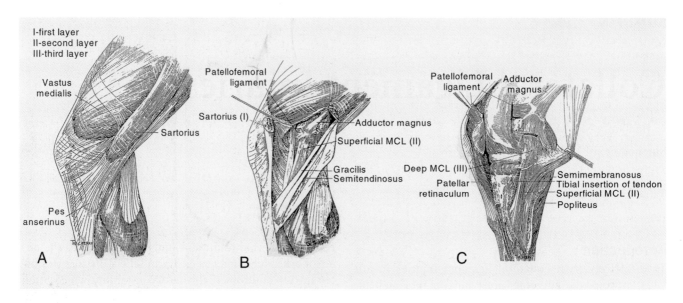

Figure 1 Illustration of the anatomy of the medial side of the knee. **A,** Layer I contains the tensor fascia lata and sartorius tendon. **B,** Layer II contains the superficial MCL; the gracilis and semitendinosus are between layers I and II. **C,** Layer III contains the deep MCL and medial capsule. *(Reproduced with permission from Warren RF, Arnoczky SP, Wickiewicz TL: Anatomy of the knee, in Nicholas JA, Hershman E (eds): The Lower Extremity and Spine in Sports Medicine, ed 2. St. Louis, MO, Mosby-Year Book, 1995, pp 657-693.)*

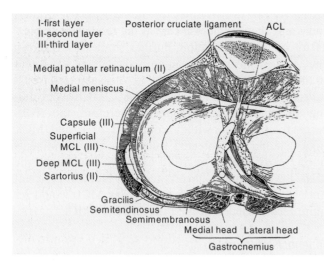

Figure 2 Cross-sectional illustration demonstrating layered approach to the medial side of the knee. *(Reproduced with permission from Warren RF, Arnoczky SP, Wickiewicz TL: Anatomy of the knee, in Nicholas JA, Hershman E (eds): The Lower Extremity and Spine in Sports Medicine, ed 2. St. Louis, MO, Mosby-Year Book, 1995, pp 657-693.)*

space opening during varus and valgus stress should be documented. A primary (grade I) sprain of the collateral ligament signifies stretching of the fibers with localized tenderness but no instability. A second-degree (grade II) sprain has more disruption of fibers and mild to moderate instability. A third-degree (grade III) sprain indicates a complete disruption of the ligament with gross instability. At times, for grade III sprain, because the fibers are completely disrupted, the patient may not experience increased pain with stress even though the knee is unstable.

Palpation along the course of the MCL and joint line can identify the location of injury. MCL tears predominantly occur at the proximal insertion and less commonly at the distal tibial insertion. When a proximal injury of the MCL is present, the examiner should rule out a concomitant injury to the medial patellofemoral ligament. The knee is examined for associated injuries such as cruciate insufficiencies, meniscal pathology, and patellofemoral problems. When examining the medial structures of the knee, it is important to rule out anteromedial instability that can be present with combined injuries of the ACL and MCL. In the skeletally immature patient, stress radiographs should be used to verify that the injury is a true ligament injury and not a Salter-Harris fracture through the distal femoral growth plate.

Plain radiographs can identify avulsion fractures from the femoral insertion of the MCL. Stress radiographs can demonstrate the amount of medial joint space widening. However, diagnosis should be made from physical examination. Coronal MRI scans of the knee are helpful in identifying the location as well as the extent of an MCL injury. Different locations of the MCL injury may change or affect treatment outcome. MRI can help assess knees with multiple knee ligament injuries because the MCL can be displaced intra-articularly and thereby preclude conservative treatment of the MCL while a patient waits for surgical reconstruction of the cruciate ligaments.

Treatment of Isolated MCL Complex Injuries

When injuries to the meniscus, cruciate ligaments, and other structures are excluded, grade I and II injuries of the MCL can usually be treated successfully nonsurgically. Patients are usually treated with crutches until symptoms decrease over the medial aspect of the knee. Patients should bear weight as tolerated, and crutches should be discontinued when symptoms improve. Range-of-motion exercises of the knee should be initiated immediately following injury. Ice, compression, and massage can be used to decrease swelling over the injured site. Anti-inflammatory medicine can be given to decrease pain and swelling. Recent basic science studies have shown that ibuprofen has no adverse effect on MCL healing in an animal model. Good control of swelling can decrease the amount of time for full recovery of motion and strength. Patients' knees are usually protected using hinged braces to dampen the valgus stress on the medial structures to allow healing. They may require a protective brace initially when participating in athletic activities requiring cutting; however, patients can be slowly weaned from brace use as tolerated.

The treatment of grade III MCL injuries can vary. After the diagnosis confirms that a grade III MCL injury is present with no associated ligament or meniscal pathology, a nonsurgical rehabilitation program can be started. The general rule for treatment is to control swelling via a brief period of immobilization. Casting has been used in the past, but it has not shown significant benefit. To protect motion, range-of-motion exercises can be started as the initial swelling subsides.

The location of the MCL injury can affect healing. In general, femoral side injuries tend to heal better than tibial side or midsubstance injuries. Patients with grade III MCL injuries may require a longer period of protected weight bearing because of the severity of their injuries. These patients should be observed closely during the initial 4 to 8 weeks of healing. If valgus instability persists, it may be an indication for early surgical reconstruction.

Treatment of Combined MCL Complex and Other Ligamentous Injuries

Combined ACL and MCL injuries will often not require reconstruction of the MCL. Patients are encouraged to rehabilitate the medial side injury and achieve full range of motion before the ACL reconstruction. Early reconstruction of both the ACL and MCL may lead to motion loss postoperatively. A few studies have demonstrated that if valgus instability is persistent following rehabilitation, reconstruction of both the ACL and MCL is recommended.

Sixty-four patients with combined ACL and MCL injuries with early versus late ACL reconstructions were evaluated in a retrospective study. All MCL injuries were treated nonsurgically with a total of 6 weeks of brace treatment. Twenty-seven patients had ACL reconstruction within 3 weeks of injury, and 37 patients had

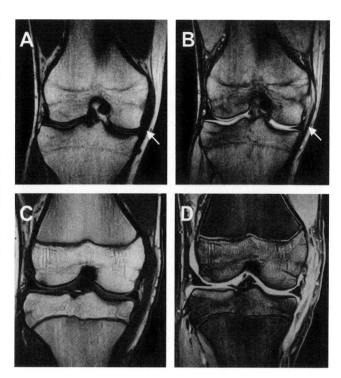

Figure 3 Coronal MRI scans of type I (**A** and **B**) and type III (**C** and **D**) MCL injuries. The superficial MCL, which is depicted as low signal on spin-echo (A, *arrow*) and gradient-echo (B, *arrow*) images, is interrupted by high-signal image at the femoral attachment site in type I MCL injuries. In contrast, interruption of the superficial fiber by high-signal image is visible throughout the length of the fiber in type III MCL injuries. This injury later required surgical stabilization. *(Reproduced with permission from Nakamura N, Horibe S, Toritsuka Y, Mitsuoka T, Yoshikawa H, Shino K: Acute grade III medial collateral ligament injury of the knee associated with anterior cruciate tear: The usefulness of magnetic resonance imaging in determining a treatment regimen. Am J Sports Med 2003:31:261-267.)*

ACL reconstruction at a minimum of 10 weeks following injury. The late ACL reconstruction group had a significantly lower rate of motion loss and repeat arthroscopy for loss of extension than the early ACL reconstruction group. Subjective knee scores were higher for the late ACL reconstruction group. There was no difference in anterior or medial instabilities for both groups.

In a recent study, the significance of the MRI appearance of MCL injuries on the treatment outcomes of combined ACL and MCL injuries was evaluated. Seventeen patients were initially treated nonsurgically with bracing. Eleven patients with restored valgus stability underwent ACL reconstruction only, and six with residual valgus laxity underwent ACL and MCL reconstruction. MRI depicted complete disruption of the superficial layer of the MCL in all 17 patients and disruption of the deep layer in 14. The study demonstrated that restoration of valgus stability significantly correlated with the proximity of the injury to the superficial MCL. Injury was evident over the entire length of the superficial MCL in five patients, and these five patients had residual valgus laxity despite bracing (Figure 3). The location of injury in the superficial layer may be useful in predicting the outcome of nonsurgical treatment of acute grade III MCL lesions combined with ACL injuries.

Combined injuries to the posterior cruciate ligament (PCL) and MCL without injury to the ACL are less common. If significant posterior subluxation is present following injury, both ligaments should be reconstructed acutely. If the joint is well reduced, the MCL can be treated nonsurgically with bracing, and the PCL can be reconstructed when full range of motion is achieved and valgus stability is restored. If valgus instability persists following a trial of nonsurgical treatment, combined PCL and MCL reconstruction is recommended.

Treatment of Chronic Injuries of the MCL Complex

Chronic MCL complex injuries occur when the MCL complex loses its potential for spontaneous healing. This usually occurs 3 to 4 months following the initial injury. For chronic injuries to the MCL complex, the patient can develop associated ligamentous instabilities or secondary limb malalignment. It is important to recognize that this is not true anatomic malalignment, but rather the result of chronic insufficiency of valgus restraints. Long-standing alignment radiographs are needed to rule out malalignment of the limb. If there is valgus deformity of the limb secondary to chronic MCL insufficiency, a concomitant osteotomy may be required at the time of MCL reconstruction.

If the patient has chronic insufficiencies of the MCL and ACL, both ligaments should be reconstructed at the time of surgery. ACL reconstruction alone can reduce the degree of valgus instability. Intraoperative evaluation after ACL reconstruction would most likely demonstrate decreased valgus instability. However, because of the chronic nature of the medial side injury, the MCL complex will not heal, and the ACL graft will experience increased forces and early failure. Deficiencies of the collateral structures can be one of the causes for failure following ACL reconstructions. However, the literature is unclear regarding the recommendation of MCL reconstruction in combined ACL and MCL injuries. In one study, only 8 of 60 patients developed radiographic evidence of instability, which is defined as a medial opening on stress radiographs of more than 2.5 mm. No difference in the amount of instability was reported when the MCL was reconstructed during the index operation.

Surgical Treatment

Bony avulsion injuries of the proximal MCL can be adequately treated with reattachment of the avulsion fracture to the femoral epicondyle. Primary MCL repair can be successful when the midsubstance tissue is not significantly stretched. Preoperative MRI can help determine the extent and location of the injury.

Techniques for surgical reconstructions of the MCL complex have focused on the reconstruction of the superficial MCL. The medial hamstrings can be used for reconstructing the superficial MCL. The semitendinosus can be isolated and brought up to the femoral epicondyle while leaving its distal insertion intact. The semitendinosus can be detached from its musculotendinous junction or left intact. The importance of the MCL reconstruction is to restore valgus stability and to prevent overconstraining the knee. When determining the femoral insertion, the isometric point has to be identified. The isometric point can be identified by placing a guidewire at the medial epicondyle. The semitendinosus is draped over the guidewire, and the excursion of the tendon is noted through a complete range of motion of the knee. The guidewire can then be adjusted anteriorly or posteriorly to achieve isometricity. Once the isometric point is identified, the semitendinosus tendon is fixed to the femoral epicondyle with a soft-tissue washer and a cannulated screw. The MCL can also be reconstructed using an allograft. The Achilles tendon can be used to reconstruct the MCL by fixing the calcaneal bone block at the femoral epicondyle and the tendon at the anteromedial tibia. The tendon should be stapled to the tibia at least 2 to 4 cm below the joint line to avoid overconstraining the knee. The intact superficial MCL inserts distal to the joint line and has a physiologic excursion along the joint line throughout the entire range of motion of the knee. For associated anteromedial rotatory instability, the posterior oblique ligament can be advanced anteriorly when the laxity is more rotatory than valgus. This operation is usually performed in conjunction with a combined ACL and MCL injury in which the ACL is also reconstructed in the same setting.

Complications of MCL Injuries

The biggest complication following MCL injuries is stiffness after injury or reconstruction. This complication is more common with acute reconstruction for combined ACL and MCL injuries. Range-of-motion exercises should be started early during the rehabilitation phase to maintain motion. Incorrect reconstruction can lead to decreased motion of the knee. A common mistake is to fix the reconstructed MCL close to the joint line, which will then capture the knee. It is essential to take the time to achieve isometricity. Calcification or myositis can occur following MCL injuries. Painful Pellegrini-Stieda lesions can develop and lead to pain near the proximal portion of the MCL. Early development of calcification or myositis can be managed with anti-inflammatory medicine or steroid injection. Patients with late sequelae or those who are refractory to treatment may require complete excision and allograft reconstruction of the MCL.

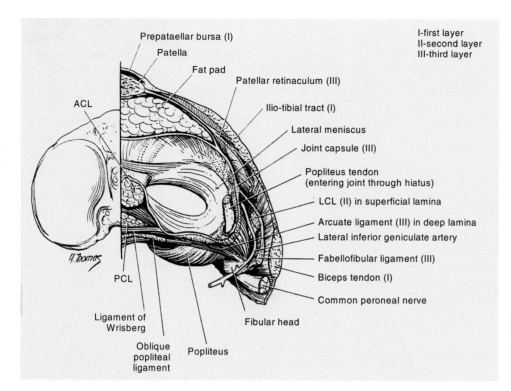

Figure 4 Cross-sectional illustration demonstrating a layered approach to the lateral side of the knee. *(Reproduced with permission from Seebacher JR, Inglis AE, Marshall JL, Warren RF: The structure of the posterolateral aspect of the knee. J Bone Joint Surg Am 1982;64:536-541.)*

Lateral Structures of the Knee

Anatomy and Function

The lateral structures, including the posterolateral corner, comprise a complex anatomic area, consisting of several vital structures that have both static and dynamic capabilities in restraining knee motion. The lateral collateral ligament (LCL), the popliteus muscle and its tendon, the popliteofibular ligament, the popliteomeniscal attachment, the iliotibial tract, and the arcuate ligament all contribute to the complex arrangement of the posterolateral corner of the knee.

The anatomy of the posterolateral corner can also be described using the layer concept. There are three distinct layers of the lateral structures of the knee (Figure 4). The most superficial layer (layer I) consists of the iliotibial tract and the superficial portion of the biceps. Layer II consists of the patellar retinaculum and lateral patellofemoral ligament. Layer III can be divided into the superficial and deep lamina layers. The superficial layer consists of the LCL and fabellofibular ligament. The deep lamina layer consists of the coronary ligament and popliteus hiatus, ending at the arcuate ligament. The popliteofibular ligament is a component of the deep lamina layer of layer III. The posterolateral corner has more variations than the MCL complex. In general, the consistent structures of the posterolateral corner are the LCL, popliteus tendon complex, and popliteofibular ligament. The remaining structures can be variable in existence. The lateral geniculate artery courses between the deep and superficial lamina of layer III and can be injured during sur-

gical approaches to the posterolateral corner. The common peroneal nerve lies beneath layer I posteriorly to the biceps tendon. The common peroneal nerve should be identified and protected during surgical reconstruction of the posterolateral corner.

Although it is known that the LCL is the primary stabilizer for varus load, the importance of the posterolateral structures in controlling external rotation and posterior translation has not been recognized until recently. Several authors have identified the intricate relationship between the posterolateral corner and the PCL. The popliteofibular ligament is an essential element for the stability of the posterolateral corner. The cross-sectional area of the ligament and the maximum strength of the popliteofibular ligament approach that of the LCL. Biomechanical testing demonstrated that the popliteofibular ligament and the popliteus tendon attachment to the tibia are important in resisting posterior translation, primary varus and external rotation, and coupled external rotation. These structures are important in resisting posterior forces at full extension and, when the PCL is sectioned, at all angles.

Besides the popliteofibular ligament, the popliteus tendon is also an important static and dynamic stabilizer of the knee. Cadaveric studies have shown that loading the popliteus muscle can significantly reduce the in situ forces in the PCL by 9% to 36% in the intact knee. In the PCL-deficient knee, posterior tibial translation was shown to be reduced by the popliteus muscle load by up to 36% of the translation caused by PCL deficiency. The results of these studies indicate that the popliteus mus-

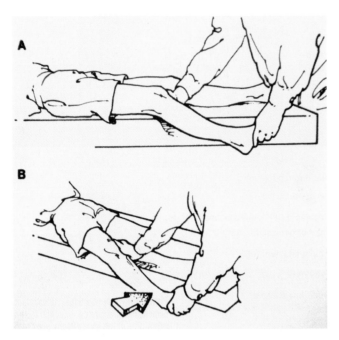

Figure 5 Illustration of a varus stability test with the knee at 30°. With the patient supine and the knee flexed to approximately 30° and the thigh supported by the hand or examination table (**A**), a valgus force is directed to detect opening of the lateral compartment (**B**). *(Reproduced with permission from LaPrade RF, Terry GC: Injuries to the posterolateral aspect of the knee: Association of anatomic injury patterns with clinical instability. Am J Sports Med 1997;25:433-438.)*

cle shares the function of the PCL in resisting posterior tibial loads and can contribute to knee stability when the ligament is absent.

The iliotibial band of tract, which runs between the supracondylar tubercle on the femur and Gerdy's tubercle on the proximal tibia, is also an important stabilizer of the lateral compartment. The most important portion of this structure acts as an accessory anterolateral ligament. During knee flexion, the iliotibial band becomes tight and moves posteriorly, exerting an external rotational and backward force on the lateral tibia. During knee extension, it moves anteriorly and is thus spared in most cases of varus stress and posterolateral injury.

Although injuries to the posterolateral corner can lead to posterior and rotatory instability, studies have shown that combined injuries to the posterolateral corner and PCL resulted in significantly higher patellofemoral joint contact pressure than isolated sectioning of the PCL. These studies illustrate the importance of the complex posterolateral corner on the biomechanics of the knee.

Diagnosis of Injuries

The same principle of examination and grading of the ligaments applies to the diagnosis of posterolateral corner injuries—that is, the determination of the mechanism of injury is essential for diagnosis. The most common mechanisms of injuries to the posterolateral corner

are a blow to the anteromedial aspect of the knee, contact and noncontact hyperextension injuries, and a varus blow to the flexed knee. When diagnosing posterolateral corner injuries, it is important to rule out associated cruciate injuries, especially PCL injuries. Isolated injuries to the posterolateral corner are rare. Combined injuries to the cruciates and the posterolateral corner are usually caused by extreme trauma that may have led to knee dislocation. The examiner should have a high index of suspicion for associated injuries when the posterolateral corner of the knee is injured. The overall incidence of posterolateral corner injuries accounts for 2% of all acute knee ligamentous injuries. One series reported that the LCL was injured in only 23% of all posterolateral corner injuries. The authors recommended that injury to the LCL with increased varus instability should not be the sole criteria for diagnosis and treatment of posterolateral corner injuries. With this type of injury, there is a 15% incidence of common peroneal nerve injuries and up to a 33% incidence of vascular injuries with the dislocated knee. The examiner has to be careful to rule out paresthesia over the dorsum of the foot, weakness with ankle dorsiflexion, and asymmetry in distal pulses in patients with posterolateral corner injuries.

When examining the LCL, an adduction or varus stability test should be done. This test is similar to the valgus stress test, but a varus-directed force and medial placement of the hand counteract the stress (Figure 5). The test is done again with the patient's knee at full extension and at 30° of flexion. Varus instability at 30° of flexion alone indicates injury to the LCL; varus instability at full extension represents associated injuries to the cruciate ligaments and the posterior capsule. Another way of applying varus stress to the knee is by placing the knee in a figure-of-4 position while palpating the LCL directly. Pain along the LCL and lateral joint line opening during this provocative test is a positive finding. These tests should also be done on the contralateral uninjured side for comparison. As with MCL injuries, the amount of lateral side opening is graded as I, II, or III.

The posterolateral corner can be tested with the anterior drawer at 90° with internal tibial rotation. As with the posteromedial capsule, when the posterolateral capsule is torn, the drawer with internal rotation will show an increase in translation when compared with the neutral test. The tibia will also tend to "internally rotate" as the anterior drawer test is being done. The hyperextension recurvatum sign also correlates with injury to the posterolateral corner (Figure 6). With the patient lying supine and relaxed, both legs are held up at extension by the examiner standing at the end of the examination table. In patients with a PCL and posterolateral capsule injury, the knee hyperextends and the tibia rotates externally because of the incompetency of the posterolateral structures. The reverse pivot-shift test should also be done with the tibia rotated externally and the knee

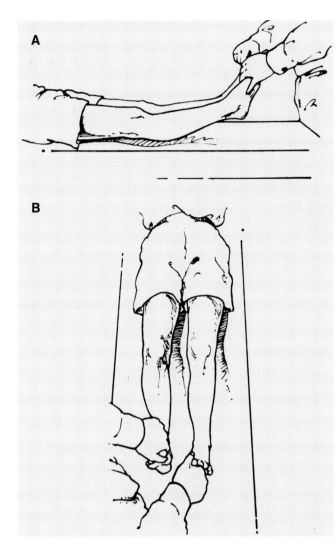

A

B

Figure 6 Illustration of the external rotation-recurvatum test. **A,** The patient is supine with both legs extended. The examiner grasps the great toes of both feet and simultaneously lifts both legs. **B,** A positive test result is indicated by increased recurvatum, varus, and apparent internal rotation of the tibia on the injured leg caused by posterolateral opening of the joint. *(Reproduced with permission from LaPrade RF, Terry GC: Injuries to the posterolateral aspect of the knee: Association of anatomic injury patterns with clinical instability. Am J Sports Med 1997;25:433-438.)*

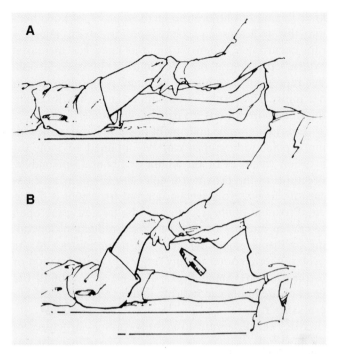

A

B

Figure 7 Illustration of the reverse pivot-shift test. **A,** The examiner lifts the supine patient's leg by grasping the ankle and gently applying abduction and an axial load. **B,** This motion flexes the knee while allowing external rotation of the tibia as a posterior translation force is applied (arrow). As the knee goes into flexion, posterolateral subluxation of the tibia can be palpated. This is in contrast to the pivot-shift maneuver, in which the subluxation is anterior and occurs near extension. *(Reproduced with permission from Laprade RF, Terry GC: Injuries to the posterolateral aspect of the knee: Association of anatomic injury patterns with clinical instability. Am J Sports Med 1997;25:433-438.)*

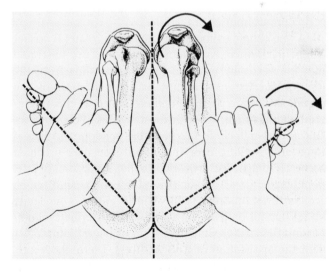

Figure 8 Illustration of the tibial external rotation test or dial test. The test can be performed with the patient supine or prone. The degree of external rotation of the foot relative to the axis of the femur is assessed while palpating the tibial plateau. External rotation is compared with the contralateral side. *(Adapted with permission from Loomer RL: A test for knee posterolateral rotatory instability. Clin Orthop 1991;264:235-238.)*

flexed (Figure 7). As the knee is extended, the tibia reduces with a palpable clunk, indicating that the posterolateral capsule is injured.

To specifically test for combined or isolated injuries to the PCL and posterolateral corner, the rotatory competency of the knee is examined (Figure 8). Both the PCL and posterolateral corner provide restraints to external rotation of the lower leg; however, their importance changes at various knee flexion angles. This test can be done with the patient in the supine or prone position. Both the injured and uninjured knees are examined. The PCL restrains external rotation of the tibia at 90° of knee flexion, whereas the posterolateral corner restrains external rotation at 30° of knee flexion. Therefore, when the injured knee has increased external rota-

tion at 90° of knee flexion but no increase at 30° of knee flexion, this represents an isolated PCL injury. When the injured knee has increased external rotation at 30° of knee flexion but little or no increase at 90° of knee flexion, this indicates an isolated posterolateral injury, a rare occurrence. When the injured knee has increased external rotation at both 30° and 90° of knee flexion, this represents a combined PCL and posterolateral corner injury. The results of this important test will dictate the treatment options for patients with PCL injuries.

For radiographic imaging of posterolateral corner injures, plain radiographs can be obtained to look for avulsion fractures of the fibula or femoral epicondyle. Fractures of the proximal fibula can explain insufficiencies of the posterolateral corner, but treatment is different. Proximal fibula fractures can be treated using open reduction internal fixation or closed reduction depending on displacement, whereas soft-tissue injuries to the posterolateral corner usually require primary fixation or reconstructions. Small flecks of bone seen around the head of the fibula can indicate injuries to the posterolateral corner.

MRI can be useful to identify various structures of the posterolateral corner and act as a road map for surgical reconstruction. A prospective study was performed to determine the accuracy of thin-slice coronal oblique T1-weighted images through the entire fibular head in diagnosing injuries to the posterolateral corner. These images were 90% to 95% accurate in identifying injuries to the LCL and popliteus and biceps tendons. The accuracy of diagnosing of popliteofibular ligament injuries was 68%. MRI can help diagnose injuries to the posterolateral corner as well as associated ligamentous and cartilaginous injuries of the knee.

Arthroscopic evaluation of the posterolateral corner can be performed. An anatomic study has demonstrated that the vertically oriented fibers descending from the inferior surface of the intra-articular portion of the popliteus tendon at the popliteal hiatus is the popliteofibular ligament; however, most injuries of the posterolateral corner include the popliteus tendon, and hematoma and swelling over the lateral side may preclude accurate diagnosis arthroscopically. Avulsion of the popliteus tendon from its femoral insertion can often be seen arthroscopically at the lateral gutter. One study noted that all patients with grade III posterolateral corner injuries had greater than 1 cm of lateral joint laxity with the application of a varus stress. The authors suggested that when an unexpected amount of lateral joint laxity is seen arthroscopically (a "drive-through" sign) in a patient with suspected ligamentous instability, a diagnosis of posterolateral knee complex injury should be considered.

Treatment of Isolated Posterolateral Corner Injuries

The natural history of isolated posterolateral injuries has not yet been characterized. Although some early studies indicated that most professional and recreational athletes with isolated posterolateral corner injuries can have no evidence of impaired function, it has been proposed that recurrent instability with abnormal knee kinematics can lead to early degenerative joint disease. It is also believed that the degeneration can be worse with combined ligamentous injuries. Nonsurgical treatment is usually indicated for partial posterolateral corner injuries. Immobilization of the knee in full extension for 3 to 4 weeks followed by progressive functional rehabilitation similar to that for MCL complex injuries is recommended. In a retrospective study, 7 of 28 patients with acute lateral knee ligament injuries also had isolated injury of the LCL and capsular structures. Five patients with initial varus instability of 1+ who underwent nonsurgical treatment were stable at follow-up. Two patients who underwent nonsurgical treatment (one with a 2+ varus instability and one with a 1+ varus instability) showed no improvement. The authors concluded that conservative treatment is sufficient for patients with mild varus instability (1+) and no additional cruciate ligament injuries.

The role of early surgical intervention to treat isolated posterolateral corner injuries is unclear; however, it is recommended that stability should be restored when patients become symptomatic or before the setting of degenerative changes. For higher-grade posterolateral corner injuries with gross instability, surgical reconstructions can be done. Anatomic repair of the injured structures should be done within 3 weeks of the injury; after that time, these injuries are considered chronic because the ability to perform a primary repair diminishes. Acute repairs with and without augmentation have more favorable results than chronic repairs. The decision to reconstruct or augment with free tissue grafts depends on the quality of the injured ligaments. Avulsion injuries can be repaired directly to bone, whereas repairs of midsubstance ruptures usually do not allow good restoration of functional stability. Acute repair should be performed as soon as possible after injury because individual anatomic structures can be more easily identified before the formation of scar tissue. The common peroneal nerve can also be identified more easily between the injured tissue planes.

Treatment of Posterolateral Corner Injuries and Other Ligamentous Injuries

For the posterolateral corner injury, it is recommended that primary repair should be performed acutely. The reconstruction of the cruciate ligaments should also be performed at the same setting. For patients with multiple knee ligament injuries, early intervention is recommended when there is an injury to the posterolateral corner. Also to be considered are the condition of the patient and overlying skin and other orthopaedic or soft-tissue injuries. A period of immobilization following

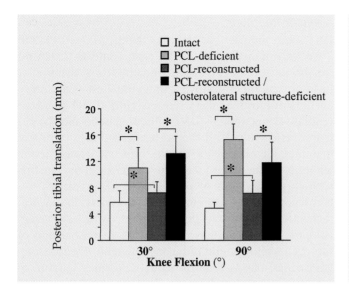

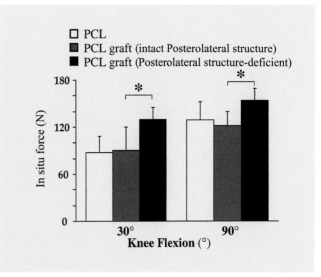

Figure 9 A bar graph illustrating posterior tibial translation (mean ± SD) in response to a 134 N posterior tibial load for intact, PCL-deficient, PCL-reconstructed, and PCL-reconstructed but posterolateral structure-deficient knees. There was significant increase in posterior translation of the PCL-reconstructed but posterolateral structure-deficient knee when compared with the intact knee and PCL-reconstructed knee. * = (P < 0.05). *(Reproduced with permission from Harner CD, Vogrin TM, Hoher J, Ma CB, Woo SL: Biomechanical analysis of a posterior cruciate ligament reconstruction: Deficiency of the posterolateral structures as a cause of graft failure. Am J Sports Med 2000;28:32-39.)*

Figure 10 A bar graph illustrating in situ force in the PCL and PCL graft (mean ± SD) in response to a 134 N posterior tibial load. In situ forces of the PCL graft increase significantly with posterior tibial load if the posterolateral structures are deficient. This may predispose the PCL graft to premature failure. * = (P < 0.05). *(Reproduced with permission from Harner CD, Vogrin TM, Hoher J, Ma CB, Woo SL: Biomechanical analysis of a posterior cruciate ligament reconstruction: Deficiency of the posterolateral structures as a cause of graft failure. Am J Sports Med 2000;28:32-39.)*

surgical reconstruction is necessary, and the patient typically should not bear weight for 4 to 6 weeks. Range-of-motion exercises should begin as soon as possible to avoid arthrofibrosis, which occurs commonly in patients with multiple knee ligament injuries. During the early rehabilitation phase, patients should refrain from any hamstring activity to allow healing of the posterolateral structures. Basic science studies have shown that simulated hamstring activities can lead to increased forces in the posterolateral structures and PCL. Quadriceps activity is protective of the PCL and posterolateral reconstruction.

For patients with multiple knee ligament injuries, it is important to recognize a posterolateral injury in the setting of a PCL injury. Biomechanical studies have shown that in the combined PCL and posterolateral corner injury model, deficiency of the posterolateral structures increased posterior tibial translation of the PCL-reconstructed knee by 4.6 to 6.0 mm (Figure 9). External rotation increased up to 14°, whereas varus rotation increased up to 7°. In situ forces in the PCL graft also increased significantly by 22% to 150% (Figure 10). These results demonstrate that a graft that restores knee kinematics for an isolated PCL deficiency is rendered ineffective and may be overloaded if the posterolateral structures are deficient. A retrospective review of 17 patients with combined PCL and posterolateral corner injuries showed that the group with PCL reconstruction only had significantly lower Tegner and Lysholm scores than the

group that had both PCL and posterolateral corner reconstruction. Patients who did not have posterolateral corner reconstruction reported more residual instability and pain. Therefore, surgical reconstruction of both structures is recommended in the setting of a combined injury.

For patients with combined ACL and posterolateral corner injuries, both ligaments should be reconstructed. Basic science studies have shown that deficiency of the LCL can lead to a significant increase in force on the ACL graft during varus loading. In addition, coupled loading of varus and internal rotation can further increase graft force relative to varus loading alone. Additional sectioning of the popliteofibular ligament and popliteus tendon resulted in similar increases in force on the ACL graft relative to the knee with posterolateral structures intact. The authors concluded that with combined ACL and posterolateral injuries, ACL reconstructions alone will lead to increased graft forces and may lead to premature graft failure.

For patients with multiple knee ligament injuries involving both cruciates and the collateral ligaments, it is generally recommended that all the injured structures should be repaired or reconstructed. The posterolateral injury should be addressed acutely so that primary repair is possible. Both cruciates should be reconstructed at the same setting because the posterolateral reconstruction can fail if the central pivot is not restored with the cruciate reconstructions. Patients with an MCL complex injury can undergo primary repair or reconstruction depending on the tissue quality. Care must be taken not to capture the knee when performing the MCL re-

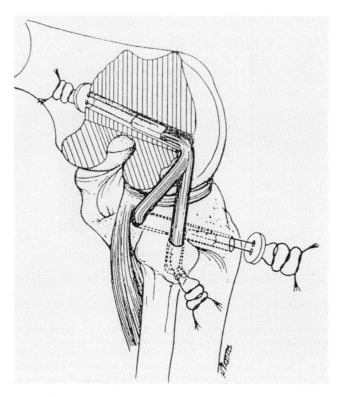

Figure 11 Illustration of double-bundle reconstruction for posterolateral corner injuries. One limb is fixed at the fibular head for reconstruction of the LCL while the other limb is brought to the posterior tibia for reconstruction of the popliteus tendon. *(Reproduced with permission from Bowen MK, Nuber GW: Management of associated posterolateral instability in posterior cruciate ligament surgery, in Drez DD Jr, Delee JC (eds): Operative Techniques in Sports Medicine. Philadelphia, PA, WB Saunders, 1993, pp 148-153.)*

construction in patients with multiple knee ligament injuries. The central pivot should be restored before the MCL reconstruction to allow accurate positioning of the isometric point.

Treatment of Chronic Posterolateral Corner Injuries

For chronic posterolateral corner injuries, patients must be carefully examined and observed for development of other instabilities. The complaints can be variable but may consist of medial knee pain with abnormal stress over the medial compartment. During the physical examination, patients should be evaluated standing and their gait should be observed closely to identify any varus thrust. If genu varus is present, the mechanical malalignment has to be corrected concurrently during ligament reconstruction to avoid premature graft failure. A medial-based opening wedge osteotomy may be preferred over a lateral closing wedge osteotomy to put tension on the lax lateral structures. MRI or flexion weight-bearing radiographs are needed to evaluate the chondral surfaces for chronic injuries. Premature arthrosis, especially in the patellofemoral compartment, may have developed following chronic injuries to the posterolateral corner.

Surgical Treatment

For acute injuries or injuries being treated within 3 weeks, primary repair of the posterolateral structures can be performed. Avulsion fractures from the fibular head or femoral epicondyle can be repaired using suture anchors or intramedullary screws. Injury to the musculotendinous junction of the popliteus tendon can be repaired using sutures. If the posterolateral structures still maintain adequate tissue quality, primary reconstruction without augmentation can be sufficient. For patients with chronic injuries or poor tissue quality, surgical reconstructions are recommended. A variety of surgical reconstructions of the posterolateral corner are available, most of which have focused on reconstruction of the LCL and popliteofibular ligament. Double-loop hamstrings, biceps femoris tendon, Achilles tendon allograft, or bone-patella-bone grafts have all been used for reconstruction.

Careful examination with the patient under anesthesia should be performed to identify the significance of rotatory instability. The LCL and popliteofibular ligament can be reconstructed using a free semitendinosus tendon graft. The fibular head is exposed, and a tunnel is created in an anterior to posterior direction at the area of maximal fibular diameter. A semitendinosus graft is pulled through the fibular tunnel, and both ends of the grafts are pulled into a close-end femoral tunnel. The location of the femoral tunnel should be the isometric point for the lateral structures. A double-bundle reconstruction can be performed using a split Achilles tendon allograft (Figure 11). The allograft is fixed over the femoral epicondyle with screws, and one limb is brought down to the fibula head for reconstruction of the LCL. The second limb is brought posteriorly to the posterior tibia to reconstruct the popliteofibular ligament. This reconstruction allows a more anatomic reconstruction; however, it requires more dissection. Some authors recommend reconstruction of the posterolateral corner using a bone-patella tendon-bone allograft (Figure 12). In one study, the LCL was reconstructed with a 9-mm bone-patellar tendon-bone allograft secured with interference screws in 10 patients with combined PCL and posterolateral corner injuries. Fixation tunnels were placed in the fibular head and at the isometric point on the femur. The cruciate ligaments were reconstructed with autograft or allograft material. Excessive external rotation at 30° of flexion was corrected in all but one knee. The average Tegner score was 4.6, with five patients returning to their preinjury level of activity and four returning to one level of activity lower. The authors suggested that because the 9-mm allograft is significantly bigger than the patient's own LCL, it may serve as a functional substitute for the nearby arcuate and popliteofibular ligament. Further studies are needed to evaluate whether these procedures can provide long-term benefit.

For reconstructions of knees with multiple ligament injuries, a cadaveric study demonstrated that external rotation of the tibia increased significantly when all of the posterolateral structures were cut and when 60, 80, or 100 N of distal traction on the ACL graft was applied. The authors concluded that deficiency of the posterolateral structures of the knee can significantly affect the relative external rotation of the tibia and recommended that for patients with combined ACL and posterolateral corner injuries, the injured posterolateral structures should be repaired first before fixation of ACL grafts. For patients with ACL, PCL, and posterolateral corner injuries, we recommend that the ACL and PCL grafts be passed and fixed on one side of the knee first. The posterolateral corner should then be reconstructed. With the PCL graft tensioned to restore the tibial step-off, the posterolateral corner is tensioned and fixed at 30° of flexion with the knee in neutral rotation. The PCL graft is then tensioned and fixed in flexion while the ACL graft is tensioned and fixed near extension. Restoring the tibial step-off with the PCL graft and controlling rotation with the posterolateral reconstruction allows better tensioning of the ACL graft.

Complications of Posterolateral Corner Injuries

The main complication following posterolateral corner injuries is the failure to recognize the injury. Isolated posterolateral corner injuries are rare. Posterolateral corner injuries are commonly associated with cruciate ligament injuries, especially PCL injuries. Injuries to the posterolateral corner can be difficult to diagnose in the severely traumatized knee. Reconstruction of the cruciate ligaments alone without addressing a grade III injury of the posterolateral corner can lead to high cruciate graft forces and premature failure.

The common peroneal nerve is in close proximity to the posterolateral corner. Injuries to the common peroneal nerve frequently occur after injuries to the posterolateral corner. Careful preoperative evaluation is needed to rule out associated nerve injuries. Paresthesia over the dorsum of the foot and weakness with ankle dorsiflexion and eversion are all signs of common peroneal nerve palsy. The nerve should be identified and protected during reconstructions or repair of the posterolateral corner. For significant trauma, the nerve should be followed distally into the muscle compartments to ensure that it is not tethered following ligament reconstruction.

Posterolateral corner injuries should be recognized and treated early because the results of late reconstruction are less successful. The cruciate ligament reconstructions should be performed simultaneously for combined injuries because the posterolateral corner reconstruction can fail prematurely if the central pivot of the knee is not restored.

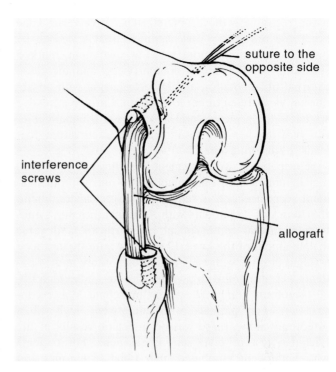

Figure 12 Illustration of reconstruction of the LCL using interference screws. *(Reproduced with permission from Latimer HA, Tibone JE, ElAttrache NS, McMahon PJ: Reconstruction of the lateral collateral ligament of the knee with patella tendon autograft: Report of a new technique in combined ligament injuries. Am J Sports Med 1998;26:656-662.)*

The Effect of Knee Alignment on Ligament Injuries

Knee alignment is important when treating patients with collateral ligament and cruciate ligament injuries. Although knee osteotomies have traditionally been used to treat patients with isolated medial or lateral compartment arthrosis, with further understanding of knee biomechanics, knee osteotomy can now play a role in treating ligament insufficiency and be used in combination with ligament reconstruction.

Chronic cruciate insufficiency can lead to the development of limb malalignment. Chronic ACL injuries have been associated with medial compartment arthrosis as well as varus and hyperextension gait abnormalities. Chronic ACL insufficiency can lead to laxity of the posterolateral structures secondary to chronic stretch. Varus malalignment can be classified as primary-, double-, or triple-varus knee syndrome. Primary-varus knee syndrome refers to tibiofemoral osseous alignment and geometry at the knee, including the added varus alignment that occurs with the loss of medial meniscus and articular cartilage in the medial compartment. Double-varus knee syndrome refers to varus alignment that is caused by two factors: the tibiofemoral osseous alignment and the separation of the lateral tibiofemoral compartment as a result of deficiency of the lateral structures. This is caused by laxity in the lateral soft-tissue restraint with chronic stretch. Triple-varus knee syndrome refers to varus alignment that is caused by three factors: tibiofemoral osseous alignment, marked separation of the lateral compartment, and increased external tibial rotation and hyperextension with an abnormal varus recurvatum lower limb. Chronic excessive stretch to the posterolateral structures or traumatic injuries may further result in the varus recurvatum that leads to this syndrome.

For patients with ligament insufficiency and limb malalignment, limb realignment with and without ligament reconstruction is required for surgical treatment. In a series of 26 patients with ACL insufficiency, symptomatic medial compartment osteoarthritis, and varus malalignment of the knee, 12 patients were treated with a valgus closing wedge high tibial osteotomy, and 14 patients were treated with a valgus closing wedge high tibial osteotomy combined with arthroscopic ACL reconstruction. For patients who underwent high tibial osteotomy alone, there was no effect on results of the Lachman test or pivot-shift phenomena. For patients who underwent combined high tibial osteotomy and ACL reconstruction, the results of the Lachman test were grade I in 11 of 13 patients, and 12 of 13 patients had a negative pivot shift. The results of this study suggest that high tibial osteotomy alone and combined high tibial osteotomy with ACL reconstruction are effective in the surgical treatment of varus, ACL-deficient knees with symptomatic medial compartment arthritis; however, good or excellent results were more often reported with the combined procedure.

In a series of 41 patients with double- or triple-varus knee syndrome, a combination of limb realignment with and without ACL and posterolateral reconstructions was performed. Seventy-three percent of the patients had loss of the medial meniscus, and 63% had marked articular cartilage damage in the medial compartment. All patients were treated with high tibial osteotomy, 83% had ACL reconstructions, and 44% had posterolateral reconstructions. At follow-up, 71% reported reduction in pain and 85% had elimination of giving way episodes; 66% of the patients resumed light recreational activities without symptoms. Correction of varus alignment was maintained in 80% of the limbs. The authors recommended osteotomy in addition to ligament reconstruction procedures in patients with complex knee injury patterns.

The effect of tibial slope has also been studied in the setting of cruciate ligament injuries. Deficiency of the PCL can lead to posterior translation/sag of the tibia, unloading the menisci, and increasing the load to the articular cartilage. A robotic cadaveric study has shown that increasing the tibial slope with an anterior opening wedge osteotomy can reduce the posterior tibial translation by shifting the resting position of the tibia anteriorly. This tibial translation was further reduced when

subjected to axial loads. The results of this study suggest that increasing the slope of the tibia may be beneficial for the patient with the PCL-deficient knee in restoring the resting position and articulation between the femur and tibia.

Summary
Collateral ligaments are commonly injured as isolated or combined injuries. Early recognition and accurate diagnosis is necessary to determine the appropriate treatment. Therefore, it is important that orthopaedic surgeons have an understanding of the treatment of acute and chronic injuries involving the MCL and the lateral structures of the knee. With better understanding of the interdependence of cruciate and collateral ligaments, physicians can be more effective and successful when treating knee ligament injuries.

Annotated Bibliography
MCL Complex
Kanamori A, Sakane M, Zeminski J, Rudy TW, Woo SL: In-situ force in the medial collateral and lateral structures of the intact and ACL-deficient knees. *J Orthop Sci* 2000;5:567-571.

This cadaveric study reports on the changes in in situ forces of the MCL and posterolateral structures of the knee associated with ACL deficiency. The authors report that for the intact knee the in situ forces in the MCL and posterolateral structures were less than 20 N; for the ACL-deficient knee, the in situ forces in the MCL and posterolateral structures were approximately two to five times those in the intact knee. The results of this study demonstrated that, although both the MCL and posterolateral structures play only a minor role in resisting anterior tibial loads in the intact knee, they become significant after ACL injury.

Ma CB, Papageogiou CD, Debski RE, Woo SL: Interaction between the ACL graft and MCL in a combined ACL + MCL knee injury using a goat model. *Acta Orthop Scand* 2000;71:387-393.

The authors of this animal study assessed the effect of ACL and MCL deficiency under various external loading conditions. Their results demonstrated that the ACL graft is subjected to significantly higher in situ forces with MCL deficiency during an applied valgus moment. The authors recommend that the ACL-reconstructed knee with a combined ACL and MCL injury should be protected from high valgus moments during early healing to avoid excessive loading on the graft.

Moorman CT III, Kukreti U, Fenton DC, Belkoff SM: The early effect of ibuprofen on the mechanical properties of healing medial collateral ligaments. *Am J Sports Med* 1999;27:738-741.

This animal study investigated the effect of ibuprofen on the early healing stage after an MCL injury. The rabbits were sacrificed at 14 and 28 days following a 14-day course of either ibuprofen or placebo. There was no statistically significant difference between the values of mechanical properties of the healing MCL in rabbits treated with ibuprofen and those that received placebo.

Nakamura N, Horibe S, Toritsuka Y, Mitsuoka T, Yoshikawa H, Shino K: Acute grade III medial collateral ligament injury of the knee associated with anterior cruciate ligament tear: The usefulness of magnetic resonance imaging in determining a treatment regimen. *Am J Sports Med* 2003;31:261-267.

The authors studied the management of acute grade III MCL injuries with combined ACL injuries. They correlated the ability of the injured MCL to restore valgus stability with the location of the injured fibers. All patients with injuries over the whole length of the superficial MCL experienced residual valgus laxity despite bracing.

Petersen W, Laprell H: Combined injuries of the medial collateral ligament and the anterior cruciate ligament: Early ACL reconstruction versus late ACL reconstruction. *Arch Orthop Trauma Surg* 1999;119:258-262.

In this retrospective study, the effect of acute and late ACL reconstruction in patients with a combined injury of the ACL and MCL was evaluated. All MCL injuries were treated nonsurgically. Patients who underwent late ACL reconstruction (at a minimum of 10 weeks after injury) had a lower rate of loss of motion and repeat arthroscopies for loss of extension.

Lateral Structures of the Knee

Covey DC: Injuries of the posterolateral corner of the knee. *J Bone Joint Surg Am* 2001;83:106-118.

This article provides a detailed review of the anatomy, biomechanics, injury mechanisms, diagnosis, and treatment of injuries to the posterolateral corner of the knee.

Freeman RT, Duzi ZA, Dowd GS: Combined chronic posterior cruciate and posterolateral corner ligamentous injuries: A comparison of posterior cruciate ligament reconstruction with and without reconstruction of the posterolateral corner. *Knee* 2002;9:309-312.

This retrospective study compared the results of reconstructing the PCL in isolation with PCL reconstruction combined with stabilization of the posterolateral corner for patients with combined PCL and posterolateral corner ligament injuries. Both groups significantly improved when compared with preoperative status. The group that underwent PCL reconstruction alone had significantly lower scores compared with those who underwent additional posterolateral corner reconstruction.

Harner CD, Hoher J, Vogrin TM, Carlin GJ, Woo SL: The effects of a popliteus muscle load on in situ forces in the posterior cruciate ligament and on knee kinematics: A human cadaveric study. *Am J Sports Med* 1998;26: 669-673.

This cadaveric study demonstrates the importance of popliteus muscle load on resisting posterior tibial translations. The authors report that loading the popliteus muscle can significantly reduce the in situ forces in the PCL by 9% to 36% in the intact knee; in the PCL-deficient knee, posterior tibial translation was reduced by the popliteus muscle load by up to 36% of the translation caused by PCL deficiency.

Harner CD, Vogrin TM, Hoher J, Ma CB, Woo SL: Biomechanical analysis of a posterior cruciate ligament reconstruction: Deficiency of the posterolateral structures as a cause of graft failure. *Am J Sports Med* 2000;28: 32-39.

This cadaveric study investigated the effects of posterolateral structure deficiency on the kinematics and in situ forces in the PCL-reconstructed knee. PCL reconstruction for isolated PCL deficiency can restore kinematics and in situ forces to levels comparable to those of the intact knee. However, PCL reconstruction with deficiency of the posterolateral structures led to a significant increase in posterior tibial translation when compared with the intact knee. The in situ forces in the PCL graft also increased significantly (22% to 150%) for all loading conditions when the posterolateral structures were cut. The authors recommend that both structures should be reconstructed in the setting of a combined injury.

LaPrade RF, Gilbert TJ, Bollom TS, Wentorf F, Chaljub G: The magnetic resonance imaging appearance of individual structures of the posterolateral knee: A prospective study of normal knees and knees with surgically verified grade III injuries. *Am J Sports Med* 2000;28: 191-199.

This study evaluated the accuracy of MRI in identifying posterolateral knee complex injuries. Thin-slice coronal oblique T1-weighted images through the entire fibular head were used to identify the posterolateral structures. The sensitivity, specificity, and accuracy of imaging approached 90% for injuries to the biceps, LCL, and popliteus origin on femur. The sensitivity, specificity, and accuracy dropped to 68% for identifying injuries to the popliteofibular ligament. The authors conclude that MRI of the knee can be very accurate in identifying injuries to the posterolateral complex.

Latimer HA, Tibone JE, ElAttrache NS, McMahon PJ: Reconstruction of the lateral collateral ligament of the knee with patellar tendon allograft: Report of a new technique in combined ligament injuries. *Am J Sports Med* 1998;26:656-662.

The authors report their experience on reconstructing the LCL using a bone-patellar tendon-bone allograft secured using interference screws for patients with combined cruciate ligament and posterolateral instability. Excessive external rotation at 30° of flexion was corrected in all but one patient's knee. Six patients had no varus laxity, and four patients had 1+

varus laxity. The authors recommend this reconstruction for patients with instability resulting from lateral ligament injuries of the knee.

Li G, Gill TJ, DeFrate LE, Zayontz S, Glatt V, Zarins B: Biomechanical consequences of PCL deficiency in the knee under simulated muscle loads: An in vitro experimental study. *J Orthop Res* 2002;20:887-892.

The authors of this cadaveric study evaluated the significance of simulated quadriceps and hamstring loading on the PCL-deficient knee. They report that combined quadriceps and hamstring loads led to increased posterior tibial translation when compared with isolated quadriceps load. In addition to increase in posterior translation for the PCL-deficient knee, there was an increase in external tibial rotation, which the authors propose can lead to increase patellofemoral joint contact pressure, subsequently leading to long-term degenerative changes of the knee after PCL injury.

Wentorf FA, LaPrade RF, Lewis JL, Resig S: The influence of the integrity of the posterolateral structures on tibiofemoral orientation when an anterior cruciate ligament graft is tensioned. *Am J Sports Med* 2002;30:796-799.

This cadaveric study examined the effect of deficiency of the posterolateral structures on tensioning the ACL graft during ACL reconstruction. The authors report significant external rotation of the tibia when the posterolateral structures were cut and distal traction to the ACL graft was applied. The authors suggest that the injured posterolateral structures should be repaired before fixation of the ACL grafts.

The Effect of Knee Alignment on Ligament Injuries
Giffin JR, Vogrin TM, Zantop T, Woo SL, Harner CD: Effects of increasing tibial slope on the biomechanics of the knee. *Am J Sports Med* 2004;32:376-382.

The authors of this robotic cadaveric study evaluated the significance of increasing the tibial slope on anteroposterior translation and in situ forces in the cruciate ligaments. Their results suggest that increasing tibial slope may be beneficial in reducing tibial sag in a PCL-deficient knee, whereas decreasing slope may be protective in an ACL-deficient knee.

Noyes FR, Barber-Westin SD, Hewett TE: High tibial osteotomy and ligament reconstruction for varus angulated anterior cruciate ligament-deficient knees. *Am J Sports Med* 2000;28:282-296.

In this study, 41 patients with ACL deficiency, lower limb varus angulation, and varying amounts of posterolateral ligament deficiency all underwent high tibial osteotomy; 34 underwent ACL reconstruction, and 18 underwent posterolateral ligament reconstruction. The mean Cincinnati Knee Rating Score significantly improved from 63 preoperatively to 82 postoperatively. Thirty-seven percent of the patients rated their knees to be normal or very good, and 34% rated their knees to be good. The authors recommend osteotomy in addition to ligament reconstructive procedures in knees with complex injury patterns.

Williams RJ, Kelly BT, Wickiewicz TL, Altchek DW, Warren RF: The short-term outcome of surgical treatment for painful varus arthritis in association with chronic ACL deficiency. *J Knee Surg* 2003;16:9-16.

The authors of this retrospective study evaluated the effect of closing wedge high tibial osteotomy on patients with symptomatic medial compartment osteoarthritis. Their results showed that 92% of the patients were able to participate in recreational sports at follow-up after undergoing high tibial osteotomy alone or combined high tibial osteotomy and ACL reconstructions. For those patients who underwent combined high tibial osteotomy and ACL reconstruction, 11 out of 13 had grade I on the Lachman test, and 12 out of 13 had negative results on the pivot shift test. The results of this study suggest that high tibial osteotomy alone and combined high tibial osteotomy and ACL reconstructions are effective in the surgical treatment of varus, ACL-deficient knees with symptomatic medial compartment arthritis; however, good or excellent results were more often reported by patients who underwent the combined procedure.

Classic Bibliography

Anderson DR, Weiss JA, Takai S, Ohland KJ, Woo SL: Healing of the medial collateral ligament following a triad injury: A biomechanical and histological study of the knee in rabbits. *J Orthop Res* 1992;10:485-495.

Gollehon DL, Torzilli PA, Warren RF: The role of the posterolateral and cruciate ligaments in the stability of the human knee: A biomechanical study. *J Bone Joint Surg Am* 1987;69:233-242.

Harner CD, Irrgang JJ, Paul J, Dearwater S, Fu FH: Loss of motion after anterior cruciate ligament reconstruction. *Am J Sports Med* 1992;20:499-506.

Hughston JC, Andrews JR, Cross MJ, Moschi A: Classification of knee ligament instabilities: Part I. The medial compartment and cruciate ligaments. *J Bone Joint Surg Am* 1976;58:159-172.

Indelicato PA: Non-operative treatment of complete tears of the medial collateral ligament of the knee. *J Bone Joint Surg Am* 1983;65:323-329.

Laprade RF, Terry GC: Injuries to the posterolateral aspect of the knee: Association of anatomic injury patterns with clinical instability. *Am J Sports Med* 1997;25:433-438.

Seebacher JR, Inglis AE, Marshall JL, Warren RF: The structure of the posterolateral aspect of the knee. *J Bone Joint Surg Am* 1982;64:536-541.

Skyhar MJ, Warren RF, Ortiz GJ, Schwartz E, Otis JC: The effects of sectioning of the posterior cruciate ligament and the posterolateral complex on the articular contact pressures within the knee. *J Bone Joint Surg Am* 1993;75:694-699.

Veltri DM, Deng XH, Torzilli PA, Warren RF, Maynard MJ: The role of the cruciate and posterolateral ligaments in stability of the knee: A biomechanical study. *Am J Sports Med* 1995;23:436-443.

Veltri DM, Deng XH, Torzilli PA, Maynard MJ, Warren RF: The role of the popliteofibular ligament in stability of the human knee: A biomechanical study. *Am J Sports Med* 1996;24:19-27.

Woo SL, Inoue M, McGurk-Burleson E, Gomez MA: Treatment of the medial collateral ligament injury: Part II. Structure and function of canine knees in response to differing treatment regimens. *Am J Sports Med* 1987;15:22-29.

Chapter 15

Meniscal Injuries

C. Benjamin Ma, MD

Scott A. Rodeo, MD

Introduction

The incidence of acute meniscal tears in the United States has been reported to be up to 61 cases per 100,000 persons per year. Injuries to the meniscus can lead to marked physical impairment. The clinical symptoms of pain, swelling, locking, and loss of motion often require surgical intervention. Arthroscopic treatment of meniscal injuries has become one of the most common orthopaedic surgical procedures in the United States. Although meniscal tears can be symptomatic, the loss of meniscus function can be more detrimental to the long-term function of the knee. Therefore, it is important that physicians treating these injuries understand the basic science of meniscus function and the diagnosis and treatment of meniscal injuries as well as be aware of the historical and recent developments in the treatment of meniscal injuries and current developments regarding meniscus function, meniscal repair, meniscal transplantation, and on going efforts to regenerate meniscus using tissue-engineering strategies.

Basic Science

Anatomy

The menisci are semilunar-shaped, fibrocartilaginous wedges positioned between the round femoral condyle and the relatively flat tibial plateau. The medial meniscus is larger but less mobile than the lateral meniscus. The lateral meniscus has more of a C-shape compared with the kidney-bean shape of the medial meniscus. The medial meniscus translates from 2 to 5 mm in the anteroposterior direction, and the lateral meniscus can translate from 9 to 11 mm during knee flexion and extension. The decreased mobility of the medial meniscus may contribute to the higher incidence of medial meniscus tears. The meniscofemoral ligaments (the ligaments of Humphrey and Wrisberg) arise from the posterior attachment of the lateral meniscus and attach to the medial femoral condyle anterior and posterior to the posterior cruciate ligament. The incidence of the ligaments of Humphrey and Wrisberg are around 50% and 76%, respectively, in cadaveric knees.

The peripheral 20% to 30% of the medial meniscus and the peripheral 10% to 25% of the lateral meniscus contain blood vessels. Radial branches from the medial and lateral geniculate arteries supply the vascular zone of the meniscus (Figure 1). Thus, the majority of the meniscus is avascular and derives its nutrition from synovial fluid diffusion. The vascular anatomy of the meniscus has direct relevance in the treatment of meniscal tears.

Histologic studies have identified the presence of neural elements within the meniscal tissue that are most abundant in the periphery and at the anterior and posterior horn attachments. The number of nerve endings was found to decrease with age. The neural elements are thought to contribute to knee joint proprioception and thus may contribute to the functional stability of the knee. At the extremes of motion, increased tension at the meniscal horns may activate these neural receptors and provide joint position information to the central nervous system. The concentration of the neural elements along the periphery correlates with the findings of a neurosensory mapping study in which probing of the centrally located meniscal tissue in awake patients produced little or no pain awareness, whereas mechanical perturbation of more peripheral tissue and the meniscal capsular tissue resulted in pain.

Biochemistry

The biochemical composition of the meniscus is similar to that of other connective tissues. The meniscus contains scattered cells with abundant extracellular matrix. The meniscus matrix is described as fibrocartilage, although the biochemical composition is more similar to fibrous tissue than cartilage. Water comprises 65% to 70% of the overall weight of the extracellular matrix. The macromolecular framework of the meniscal tissue consists primarily of collagens. Type I collagen accounts for over 90% of the tissue collagen, with a small contribution of types II, III, V, and VI collagen. The meniscus matrix also contains proteoglycans (1% to 2% of dry weight). The glycosaminoglycans that are attached to proteoglycans function to bind water molecules and

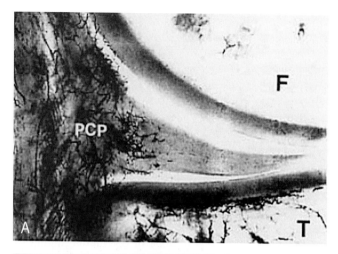

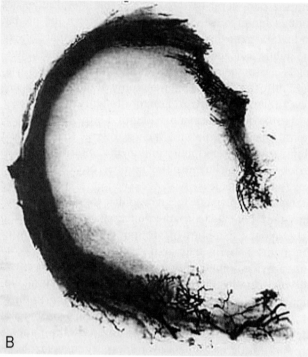

Figure 1 Sagittal (**A**) and axial (**B**) sections of the medial meniscus demonstrating the peripheral vasculature. Branching radial vessels from the perimeniscal capillary plexus (PCP) can be seen penetrating the peripheral border of the medial meniscus. The central portion of the meniscus is avascular. F = femur, T = tibia. (*Reproduced with permission from Arnoczky SP, Warren RF: Microvasculature of the human meniscus. Am J Sports Med 1982;10:90-95.*)

thus provide the compressive properties of the tissue. The meniscal extracellular matrix acts as a porous-permeable solid matrix in which interstitial fluid flow and solid matrix deformation during loading provide the "shock absorber" function of the tissue during weight bearing.

The meniscus has a unique collagen structural orientation that is related to its function. The superficial layer consists of a thin layer of fine fibrils. Below the superficial layer is a layer of randomly aligned collagen bundles. In the deep layer, large circumferentially oriented fibers are anchored by a small number of radially oriented fibers. When an axial load is applied to the knee joint, the meniscus is compressed and displaced away from the joint center, resulting in tensile stress (hoop stress) along the circumferential collagen fibers. The overall biochemical composition and fiber architecture account for the viscoelastic properties of the meniscus.

Biomechanics

The primary function of the meniscus is to distribute loads across the knee joint. Early biomechanical studies have shown that the medial meniscus transmits 50% of the compartment load, whereas the lateral meniscus transmits 70% of the load in the lateral compartment. With the knee in extension, the menisci transmit approximately 50% of joint load, whereas in flexion the menisci are responsible for 85% of load transmission. Partial meniscectomy of the inner one third of the meniscus decreases contact area by 10% and increases peak load by 65%. After total medial meniscectomy, the contact area decreases by 75% and peak load increases by approximately 235%. The results of these biomechanical studies confirm the authors' clinical findings of early degenerative changes in the compartment following meniscectomy.

The meniscus is also important in the stability of the knee. The posterior horn of the medial meniscus acts as a secondary restraint to anterior tibial translation in the anterior cruciate ligament (ACL)-deficient knee. A recent robotic study demonstrated that the resultant force in the medial meniscus of the ACL-deficient knee increased significantly when compared with that in the meniscus of the intact knee. The force experienced by the meniscus increased by a minimum of 52% at full knee extension to a maximum of 197% (50.2 N) in flexion. Medial meniscectomy in the ACL-deficient knee also caused a significant increase in anterior tibial translation in response to the anterior tibial load, ranging from an increase of 2.2 mm at extension to 5.8 mm in flexion. The interdependence of the medial meniscus and the ACL is also supported by the finding that the in situ forces in an ACL replacement graft increased between 33% and 50% after medial meniscectomy in response to a 134 N anterior tibial load. These results indicate that the medial meniscus is at risk of injury in the ACL-deficient knee and support the clinical finding of a high prevalence of medial meniscus tears in knees with chronic ACL insufficiency. Similarly, loss of the posterior horn of the medial meniscus may put the ACL reconstruction graft at risk because of high graft forces.

Epidemiology

According to a European epidemiology study, the incidence of meniscal tears is around 60 to 70 per 100,000 persons. Meniscal tears are more common in males; the male to female ratio ranges from 2.5:1 to 4:1. About one third of all meniscal tears were associated with an ACL injury. The peak incidence was in men age 21 to 30 years and in girls and women age 11 to 20 years. Degenerative types of meniscal tears commonly occur in men in their fourth, fifth, and sixth decades of life. Meniscal pathology in women is relatively constant after the second decade of life. Younger patients are more likely to have an acute traumatic event as the cause of their meniscal pathology.

In patients with acute ACL injuries, lateral meniscus tears occur more frequently than medial meniscus tears (83% versus 17%). In patients with chronic ACL-deficient knees, however, medial meniscus tears are more prevalent. Because of its high rate of tearing in chronic ACL-deficient knees, the role of the medial meniscus as a secondary restraint to anteroposterior translation is thought to be important. Meniscal injury is also frequent in tibial plateau fractures, with 17 of 36 patients (47%) in one study having a meniscal tear associated with the fracture. Additionally, 32% of patients with femoral shaft fractures were shown to have concurrent meniscal injuries. The presence of hemarthrosis should increase the index of suspicion for ligamentous or meniscal injury.

Diagnosis

History and Physical Examination

Accurate diagnosis of meniscal injury begins with a careful history. Traumatic lesions of the menisci are caused most commonly by rotation and axial loading of the flexed knee. An older patient with a degenerative meniscal lesion will usually present with an insidious onset of pain and swelling. There are several typical meniscal tear patterns. Longitudinal or bucket-handle tears are more common in the medial meniscus because it is less mobile and can easily be "crushed" between the condyle and the tibial plateau. One study reported that 78% of medial meniscus tears occur in the posterior horn, possibly because the posterior horn is less mobile and directly loaded in the flexed knee. Radial tears occur more commonly in the lateral meniscus. It has been shown in multiple series that meniscus injuries are commonly associated with ACL injuries. In an acute ACL injury, the lateral meniscus is most commonly torn as the lateral tibial plateau subluxates anteriorly on the lateral femoral condyle. MRI often demonstrates a translational bone contusion ("bone bruise") in the lateral compartment, verifying the transient subluxation of the lateral compartment. In patients with chronic ACL injuries, the incidence of medial meniscus tear increases. As mentioned previously, the posterior horn of the medial meniscus acts as a secondary restraint to anterior tibial translation in the ACL-deficient knee. When the ACL is incompetent, the posterior horn of the medial meniscus is excessively loaded, resulting in injury. These findings

have been confirmed by several clinical studies. Thus, the "unhappy triad" described in the literature (injury to the ACL, medial meniscus and medial collateral ligament as a result of an acute valgus stress injury to the knee) is actually relatively uncommon.

Patients with meniscal tears typically report pain and mild swelling. With a larger tear, patients may report a sensation of locking and/or clicking. These mechanical symptoms may be caused by a posterior longitudinal tear in a meniscus that extends anteriorly. Locking of the knee may or may not cause spontaneous reduction. Small tears of the meniscus will not produce locking, but they may produce a clicking or catching sensation. In contrast to an acute ACL injury, the swelling in the knee following a meniscal injury is usually more gradual in onset. Patients may report recurrent or chronic swelling in the knee following a twisting injury.

The most important physical finding in patients with meniscal tear is localized tenderness along the joint line. The joint line tenderness is likely related to synovitis in the adjacent capsule or synovial tissue. There are several tests that have been described to diagnose meniscal injuries. Most of these tests include provocative maneuvers that trap the meniscus between the femoral and tibial condyles and generate symptoms. The McMurray test is performed with the patient lying supine with the hip and knee flexed to about 90°. With one hand on the knee to apply compression, the other hand holds the foot and maneuvers it from external rotation to internal rotation (Figure 2). If positive, this maneuver can trap the torn meniscus and produce a pop or click that can be felt by the examiner. A variation of this test is the flexion McMurray test. To detect a medial meniscus injury, the patient's knee is held as for the McMurray test. With the foot externally rotated and the knee maximally flexed, the knee is gradually extended and a positive test result occurs when the patient experiences pain and discomfort over the posteromedial joint line. External rotation of the tibia can trap the torn posterior horn of the medial meniscus under the medial femoral condyle. For the lateral meniscus, internal rotation can trap the lateral meniscus under the lateral femoral condyle.

Types of Tears

Meniscal tears can generally be classified as either acute or degenerative. The tear pattern is further characterized by its location, morphology, and stability. The location of the tear is described by dividing the meniscus into posterior, middle, and anterior thirds. The tear should also be described with respect to the vascularity of the meniscus. The common description includes the red-red zone, red-white zone, and white-white zone (Figure 3). A red-red zone tear occurs in the peripheral region of the meniscus close to the meniscal capsular junc-

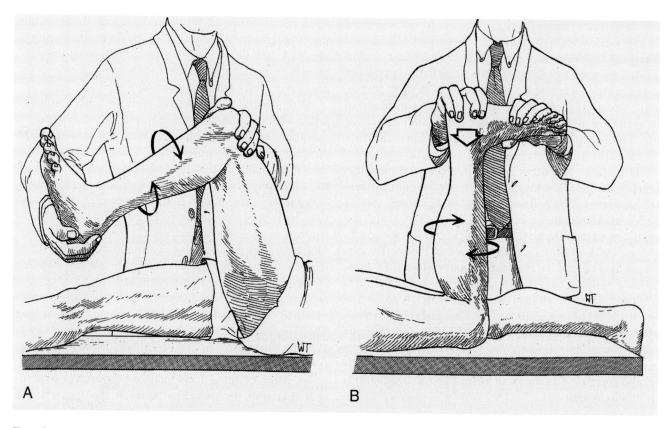

Figure 2 Illustration of the McMurray test (**A**) and the Apley test (**B**). *(Reproduced with permission from Insall JN: Clinical examination of the knee, in Insall JN (ed): Surgery of the Knee. New York, NY, Churchill Livingstone, 1984.)*

tion. A red-white zone tear occurs in the middle part of the meniscus at the junction of the vascular and avascular portion of the tissue. These tears have decreased healing potential. The white-white zone tears occur in the central portion of the meniscus where there is no peripheral blood supply and essentially no healing potential. Accurate identification of the location of a meniscus tear is critical to determine whether repair or meniscectomy is indicated.

Meniscal tears can also be characterized by tear morphology. Common tear patterns include longitudinal, radial, and horizontal tears (Figure 4). Complex tears involve multiple cleavage planes. The tear pattern of the meniscus dictates the treatment options. Vertical longitudinal tears are more amendable to repair, whereas horizontal and complex tears are likely to require meniscectomy.

Magnetic Resonance Imaging

MRI greatly enhances the diagnostic accuracy of meniscus pathology. MRI allows multiplanar imaging of the meniscus, avoidance of ionizing radiation, and the ability to evaluate other surrounding structures. The accuracy of MRI in the detection of meniscal tears is commonly reported at 80% to 90%. The normal meniscus has homogeneous low-signal intensity on all pulse sequences

with MRI. Increased intrameniscal signal intensity may be seen in children because of meniscus vascularity. Increased signal is also produced by age-related meniscus degeneration. Diagnosis of a meniscus tear requires assessment of both intrameniscal signal and morphology. Reliance upon intrameniscal signal alone may lead to a false-positive MRI interpretation. There are four grades of the meniscus appearance on MRI (Figure 5). A meniscus tear can only be diagnosed if high signal extends through either the femoral or tibial surface of the meniscus. Besides signal characteristics, the meniscal appearance is also important in the diagnosis of meniscal tears. The "absent bow tie sign" and "double posterior cruciate ligament sign" indicate a displaced bucket handle tear. For the lateral meniscus, disruption of the popliteomeniscal fasciculi may be accurately diagnosed with MRI (Figure 6). The body of the meniscus itself may be completely normal with injury to the popliteomeniscal fasciculi. This condition can lead to meniscal instability and require surgical stabilization.

Even though MRI is a powerful tool in detecting meniscal pathology, clinicians must rely on the entire clinical picture for treatment. Previous studies have reported a 5.6% rate of false-positive MRI findings in asymptomatic patients between the ages of 18 and 39 years with normal clinical examinations. Other studies

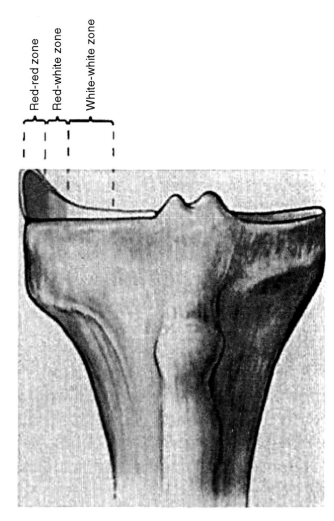

Figure 3 Illustration showing the location of a meniscal tear by its vascular supply. A red-red tear occurs at the peripheral red zone of the meniscus where it is well vascularized. A red-white tear occurs at the transitional red-white zone where the meniscus becomes avascular. The white-white tear occurs at the central avascular white zone of the meniscus. *(Reproduced with permission from Miller MD: Sports medicine, in Miller M (ed): Review of Orthopaedics, ed 3. Philadelphia, PA, WB Saunders, 2000, pp 195-240.)*

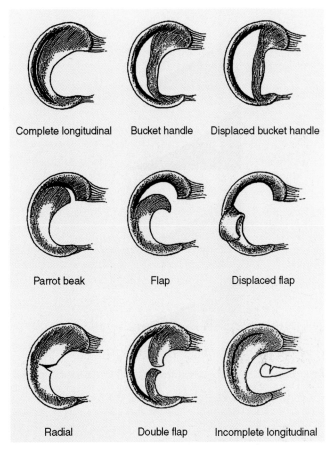

Figure 4 Illustrations of common meniscal tear morphology. *(Reproduced with permission from Tria AJ, Klein KS: An Illustrated Guide to the Knee. New York, NY, Churchill Livingstone, 1992.)*

have shown that in asymptomatic patients, 13% younger than 45 years had positive MRI findings of a meniscus tear and 36% older than 45 years had positive MRI findings.

MRI can be useful to assess meniscal repair. A recent study compared specialized MRI sequences with frequency-selective fat suppression techniques and standard contrast arthrography following meniscal repair. MRI had a high correlation with arthrography in assessing meniscal repair. Second-look arthroscopy also confirmed the ability of MRI to discriminate partial or complete meniscal healing. The study concluded that noncontrast MRI could accurately assess the repaired

meniscus, with accuracy superior to that of contrast arthrography.

Treatment

The treatment of meniscal injuries has been limited to nonsurgical treatment, meniscectomy, or meniscus repair. Recent efforts have included meniscus transplantation or partial meniscus replacement.

Meniscectomy

Historically, complete meniscectomies were performed for the diagnosis of internal derangement of the knee before the recognition of the important function of the meniscus. One study reported long-term (10- to 30-year) follow-up of patients who had undergone complete meniscectomy. Only 45% of male patients and 10% of female patients were symptom free at the time of evaluation. Another study reported a 17-year follow-up of patients who underwent meniscectomy and found degenerative joint disease in 40% of the operated knees versus 6% in the contralateral side. The authors also reported that medial meniscectomies tend to have better results than lateral meniscectomies. Other studies have

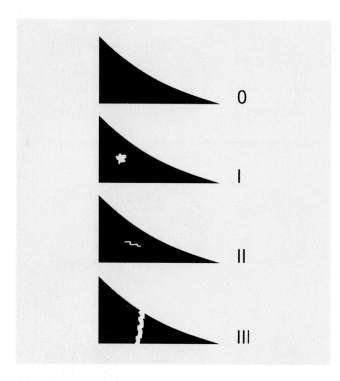

Figure 5 The grading scale for meniscal tears on MRI. Grade 0 is a normal meniscus. Grade I has globular increase signal within the meniscus that does not extend to the surface. Grade II has linear increase signal within the meniscus that does not extend to the surface. Grade III has increase signal that abuts the free edge of the meniscus, indicating a meniscal tear. *(Reproduced with permission from Thaete FL, Britton CA: Magnetic resonance imaging, in Fu FH, Harner CD, Vince KG, Miller MD (eds): Knee Surgery. Philadelphia, PA, Williams & Wilkins, 1998, pp 325-352.)*

verified that degenerative changes proceed more rapidly following lateral meniscectomy than medial meniscectomy. One such study reported that complete lateral meniscectomy resulted in satisfactory results in only 54% of the patients at early follow-up; 16 of 26 patients in this study developed late instability following complete lateral meniscectomy.

Advancements in arthroscopy as well as a better understanding of the importance of meniscal function provided the impetus for the development of partial rather than complete meniscectomy for irreparable meniscal tears. Early reports on arthroscopic partial meniscectomies report 90% good to excellent results in patients with normal stability and no degenerative changes. This decreases to 67% good to excellent results for patients with concomitant ACL injuries or degenerative changes. Recent studies have also demonstrated 95% satisfactory results at 12 years when no degenerative disease is present at the time of surgery; however, in patients with concomitant degenerative disease, only 62% reported satisfactory results at 12 years. Another study with 317 patients and a mean follow-up of 11.5 years reported that 91% of the patients had normal or nearly normal knees (as determined according to the International Knee Document Committee examination) following arthroscopic partial medial meniscectomies. Radiographs

demonstrated a 22.4% increase in joint space narrowing for the operated knee. The risk factors for poor radiographic findings were age older than 35 years, the presence of medial compartment cartilage degeneration before the first arthroscopy, resection of the posterior one third of the meniscus, and meniscal rim resection. Overall, most studies report good long-term clinical and functional results following arthroscopic partial meniscectomy. However, increasing radiographic deterioration is found with long-term follow-up beyond 10 years.

Meniscal Repair

Based on the established important functions of the meniscus and the clinical results of meniscectomy, most clinicians recommend meniscal repair for repairable tears. Although the treatment of meniscal tears should be individualized, the most commonly accepted criteria for meniscal repair include (1) a complete vertical longitudinal tear greater than 10 mm in length; (2) a tear within the peripheral 10% to 30% of the meniscus or within 3 or 4 mm of the meniscocapsular junction; (3) a peripheral tear that can be displaced toward the center of the plateau by probing, thus demonstrating instability; (4) the absence of secondary degeneration or deformity; (5) a tear in an active patient; and (6) a tear associated with concurrent ligament stabilization or a stable knee.

The success of meniscal repair depends on the healing capacity of the meniscal tear, the stability of the repair, and appropriate patient selection. The healing capacity of the meniscal tear depends on the location and chronicity of the tear. A tear in the red-red zone has higher healing potential than a tear in the white-white zone. An acute tear also has higher healing potential than a chronic tear with remodeling. The tear pattern is also important, as a vertical longitudinal tear is more likely to heal than a complex or horizontal tear pattern. A meniscus that has intrasubstance degenerative changes also has inferior healing potential. The stability of the repair depends on the type of repair as well as the stability of the knee. If the knee has a concomitant ligament injury that is not addressed, the meniscal repair is less likely to heal. The type of repair can also influence the healing potential of a meniscal tear. Patient selection is also important as patients younger than 40 years tend to have better healing capacity than older patients, although there are no absolute age limits for meniscal repair.

Studies have reported successful results in more than 90% of patients who had meniscal repairs performed in conjunction with ACL reconstruction, whereas only 50% of patients with stable ACLs who had meniscal repairs performed had successful results when examined using arthroscopy or arthrography. It is postulated that the presence of a hemarthrosis following ACL recon-

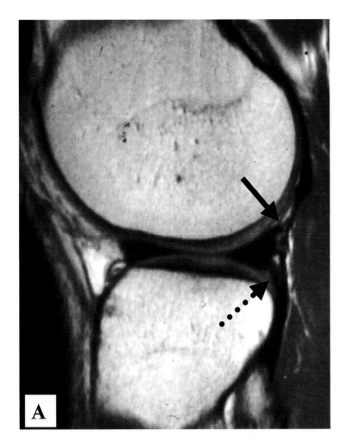
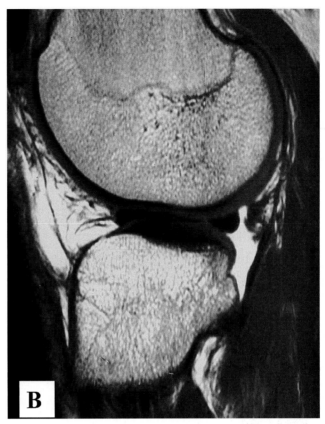

Figure 6 Sagittal MRI scans of the popliteomeniscal fasciculi of the lateral meniscus. **A,** Intact superior (*solid arrow*) and inferior popliteomeniscal (*dotted arrow*) fasciculi. **B,** Ruptured superior and inferior popliteomeniscal fasciculi.

struction improves meniscal healing. A small series reported successful repair of the lateral meniscus in the avascular zone using a fibrin clot. The authors reported that the exogenous fibrin clot may enhance the healing potential of the meniscus even in the avascular portion, likely by providing a scaffold for a reparative response. The fibrin clot also contains serum-derived factors that may improve meniscus healing. One 7-year follow-up study reported that the success rate of arthroscopic meniscal repair was 73%, with 64% of the failures occurring within the first 6 months after repair. The clinical and radiographic evaluation of the patients whose knees were successfully repaired showed that 90% had normal knee function; the remaining 10% had nearly normal function according to International Knee Document Committee grades. A recent study reported the results of arthroscopic repair of meniscal tears extending into the avascular zone in patients age 40 years and older. Seventy-two percent of these patients underwent a concomitant ACL reconstruction. At a mean follow-up of 33 months, 87% of the patients were asymptomatic for tibiofemoral symptoms and had not required additional surgery. In general, most clinicians recommend preservation of meniscal tissue whenever possible.

Meniscal repairs should be performed after adequate preparation of the tear site. The tear edges should be abraded to stimulate bleeding. Anatomic apposition of the tear edges is critical to ensure good healing potential and restoration of biomechanical function. Meniscal repairs can be performed using the open technique, inside-out technique, outside-in technique, and all- inside technique. Long-term survival rate for open meniscal repairs approaches 79%. Only peripheral or meniscocapsular tears are amenable to open meniscal repair. Inside-out meniscal repairs are performed using long needles with attached sutures that are passed across the tear from inside the joint and exit through the joint capsule. A small posteromedial or posterolateral incision is made to retrieve the exiting needles as they pass across the capsule and to protect the posterior neurovascular structures. Outside-in meniscal repair is performed using an 18-gauge spinal needle that is passed across the tear from outside to inside the joint. A No. 0 polydioxanone suture is then passed through the needle and is retrieved inside the joint. A second suture is passed in a similar fashion. A knot may be tied in the end of each suture, after which the knot is pulled back into the joint against the meniscus, thus holding the meniscus in a reduced position (Figure 7). The free ends are tied over the joint capsule. A modification of the technique involves tying the two sutures together and then pulling the knot through the meniscus and capsule,

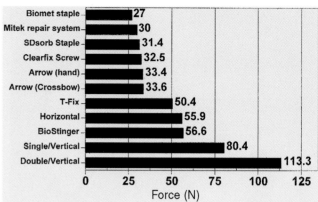

Figure 8 Graph showing the load to failure strength of various meniscal repair devices. *(Reproduced with permission from Barber FA, Herbert MA: Meniscal repair devices. Arthroscopy 2000,16:613-618.)*

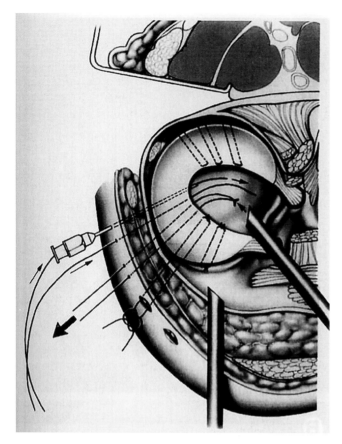

Figure 7 Illustration of outside-in repair of the anterior and middle portion of the meniscus. *(Reproduced with permission from Rodeo SA, Warren RF: Meniscal repair using the outside-to-inside technique. Clin Sports Med 1996,15:469-481.)*

creating a mattress suture across the tear. This suture is then tied outside the capsule to fix the meniscal tear. The outside-in repair technique is especially useful for repairing tears in the middle and anterior horn of the meniscus where access is difficult using the inside-out technique. The outside-in technique is usually not used for far posterior tears (adjacent to the posterior horn insertion) because it is difficult to pass the needle perpendicular to the tear that far posteriorly. For any suture technique, a vertical mattress suture orientation is preferred. The vertical mattress pattern has higher pull-out strength because the sutures capture the circumferential collagen fibers of the meniscus.

All-inside meniscal repairs have been made possible with the development of various implants, including meniscal arrows, darts, screws, and suture devices. All-inside meniscal repair devices are advantageous because they do not require accessory incisions and can save time. However, their effectiveness may decrease when compared with traditional repairs. Biomechanical tests have shown that vertical repairs using sutures have the highest pull-out strength when compared with the all-inside meniscal repair devices (Figure 8). Most of these all-inside meniscal repair devices are made of bioabsorb-

able materials. There have been reports of damage to the overlying femoral condyle from prominent all-inside repair implants and reports of these implants becoming loose bodies. Several recent case reports have documented iatrogenic cartilage injury caused by prominent implants on the meniscal surface. Despite these concerns, recent reports have shown that 80% of patients who underwent meniscal repair with a bioabsorbable arrow were asymptomatic 2 to 3 years following repair. To avoid complications, care must be used to ensure that these implants are well seated in the meniscus and are not left prominent on the meniscus surface.

Meniscal tears often occur in conjunction with ligament injury. Locked meniscal tears are relative surgical emergencies that require reduction and either repair or resection. One study investigated the results of staged repair of a displaced bucket-handle meniscal tear followed by delayed ligament reconstruction once full range of motion was obtained. Fifty-two patients with 55 meniscal repairs were available for follow-up. At reconstruction, 55% appeared healed, 34% were partially healed, and 11% showed no healing. Of 43 tears in the white-white zone, 21 appeared healed, 17 were partially healed, and 5 showed no healing. Of 11 in the red-white zone, 8 appeared healed, 2 were partially healed, and 1 showed no healing. One meniscal tear in the red-red zone appeared healed. At an average follow-up of 4.3 years, 84% of white-white meniscal repairs remained asymptomatic; all repairs in the other zones were asymptomatic. The authors concluded that locked bucket-handle meniscal tears heal at a high rate when repaired as an isolated procedure, even when full weight bearing and activity before ACL reconstruction is allowed and when the tear is in the white-white zone.

Deep knee flexion should be avoided during early rehabilitation after meniscal repair. Biomechanical studies have shown that there is increased stress on the posterior horn of the meniscus with knee flexion. However, no

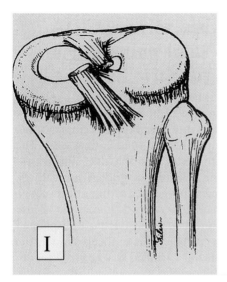
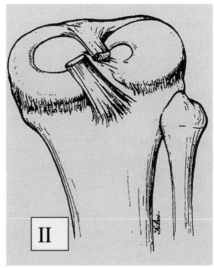
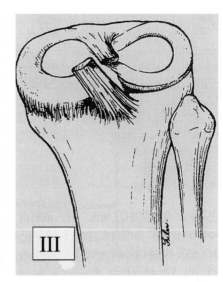

Figure 9 Illustration of the classification system for lateral discoid menisci: type I (complete), type II (incomplete), and type III (Wrisberg ligament). Type III discoid menisci have no posterior attachment to the tibia. The only posterior attachment is through the ligament of Wrisberg toward the medial femoral condyle. *(Reproduced with permission from Neuschwander DC: Discoid lateral meniscus, in Fu FH, Harner CD, Vince KG (eds): Knee Surgery. Baltimore, MD, Williams & Wilkins, 1994, p 394.)*

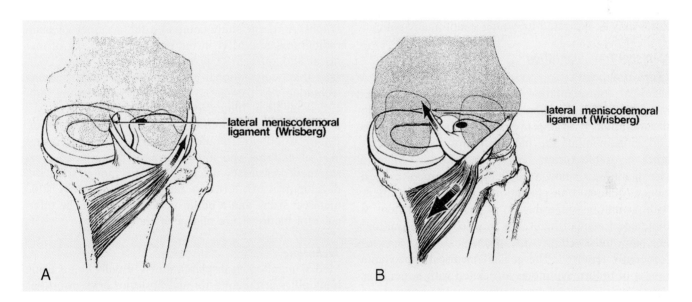

Figure 10 Illustration of type III (Wrisberg ligament) discoid lateral meniscus. **A,** With the knee in flexion, there is no subluxation of the meniscus. **B,** With the knee in extension, the meniscus is displaced into the intercondylar notch by its attachment to the Wrisberg ligament. *(Reproduced with permission from Dickhaut SC, Delee JC: The discoid lateral-meniscus syndrome. J Bone Joint Surg Am 1982;64:1068-1073.)*

studies have measured the stress on a repaired meniscus with various activities (knee motion, weight bearing, etc) or the effect of mechanical stress on meniscal healing.

Discoid Lateral Meniscus

Meniscal injuries in children are rare. Snapping of the knee in a child younger than 10 years often represents an unstable discoid meniscus. Discoid menisci are classified as type I (complete), type II (incomplete), or type III (Wrisberg ligament) (Figure 9). The type III discoid meniscus has no attachment posteriorly to the tibia, being attached only to the medial femoral condyle via the me-

niscofemoral (Wrisberg) ligament. This type of discoid meniscus is unstable and is often symptomatic. With its attachment through the Wrisberg ligament to the medial femoral condyle, the unstable meniscus can be displaced into the intercondylar notch when the knee is in extension (Figure 10). Plain radiographic changes in knees with congenital lateral discoid menisci include subtle widening of the lateral joint space, squaring of the lateral femoral condyle, and cupping of the lateral tibial spine. MRI clearly shows the abnormal meniscus morphology.

No surgical intervention is required for the asymptomatic discoid meniscus that is found incidentally. For symptomatic types I and II discoid menisci, arthroscopic saucerization to a stable peripheral rim is recommended. For type III discoid menisci, efforts should be made to stabilize the posterior rim and recreate the posterior attachments. However, many type III discoid menisci require complete meniscectomy and subsequently lead to early lateral compartment degeneration. Recent studies have reported 83% satisfactory results for patients who underwent partial meniscectomy of a discoid lateral meniscus at a mean follow-up of 58 months. Another study reported that 16 out of 17 patients had a satisfactory outcome following partial or total meniscectomy for a discoid lateral meniscus. However, small osteophytes were present in 8 knees, and early narrowing of the lateral joint space was present in 11 knees. Because most symptomatic discoid lateral menisci occur in young patients, the goal of treatment should be the preservation of functional meniscal tissue. These young patients require long-term monitoring to detect the onset of degenerative changes. Early intervention such as meniscal transplantation or limb realignment procedures may be indicated for young symptomatic patients.

Meniscal Transplantation
Clinical Aspects
Meniscal transplantation has been used for selected meniscus-deficient patients to prevent premature joint degeneration. With improvements in surgical technique and refinement of the indications for this procedure, early favorable results have been reported. Meniscal transplantation is now a viable option for meniscal deficiency. Meniscal transplantation is indicated for patients with symptoms referable to a meniscus-deficient tibiofemoral compartment. The most common symptoms are pain and swelling, with mechanical symptoms less frequently reported. The goal of meniscal transplantation is to reduce symptoms associated with a meniscus-deficient tibiofemoral compartment and to prevent premature compartment degeneration. It is generally not recommended that patients return to high-level competitive athletic activities after transplantation, although this is possible in patients with an otherwise healthy joint. Contraindications for meniscal transplantation include advanced articular cartilage degeneration, instability, axial malalignment, and flattening of the femoral condyle. Transplantation in this group of patients can lead to premature wear of the allograft and graft extrusion. Fresh-frozen and cryopreserved allografts are the most commonly used meniscal transplants. Irradiated meniscal allografts have been shown to decrease failure strength and potentially delayed graft incorporation. Graft sizing is critical for successful meniscal transplantation. Most tissue banks size the meniscus based on radiographic tibial plateau measurements.

Basic Science
Biomechanical studies have been performed to investigate the effect of meniscus transplantation on the contact mechanics of the knee. Contact pressure studies have shown that medial meniscal allograft transplantation in the cadaveric knee reduces maximum and mean contact pressures by 75% compared with a knee after meniscectomy but does not completely restore normal contact mechanics compared with the normal knee. The difference between the intact knee and allograft knee may be related to the difficulty in graft sizing and the difference in mechanical properties of the intact meniscus and allograft meniscus. Animal studies have also demonstrated the protective effect of the transplanted meniscus on hyaline cartilage. In a sheep model, the area of damaged articular cartilage was reduced by approximately 50% in the group treated with transplantation when compared with a meniscectomy group. The authors concluded that the meniscal allograft provides significant although not complete protection against damage to the articular cartilage after meniscectomy.

Meniscal grafts are usually sized using plain radiographs. A recent study compared the accuracy of plain radiographs and MRI in the preoperative sizing of meniscal allografts. MRI proved only slightly more accurate than conventional radiography. Neither imaging technique was completely accurate for measuring individual meniscal dimensions, with only 35% of images measuring within 2 mm of actual meniscal dimensions. Failure to obtain true anteroposterior or lateral images (15° of external and internal rotation) increased measurement inaccuracy when using plain radiographs. The development of alternative techniques for more reliable meniscal sizing and a better understanding of the tolerance for meniscal size mismatch are necessary.

Technique
Medial meniscal transplantation is usually done using bone plugs at the anterior and posterior horn insertions (Figure 11), whereas lateral meniscal transplantation is done using a common bone bridge that connects the anterior and posterior horn insertions (as with the "keyhole" technique) (Figure 12). The allograft is then sutured to the capsule using standard arthroscopic meniscal suturing techniques. A bone bridge is used for the lateral meniscus because of the close proximity of the anterior and posterior horns of the lateral meniscus and the associated difficulty in placing separate bone tunnels for individual bone plugs within such close proximity. Biomechanical studies have shown that the implantation of meniscal grafts with bone plugs resulted in contact mechanics that were significantly closer to normal when compared with fixation with sutures alone without bone plugs. One such study also demonstrated that the contact mechanics of the medial tibial articular surface were not improved by suturing the periphery of

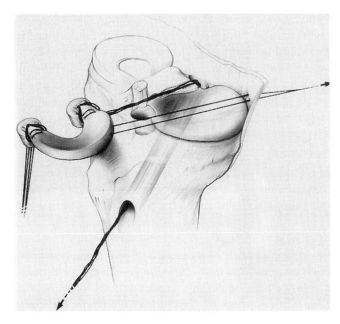

Figure 11 Illustration of medial meniscal transplantation with anterior and posterior bone plugs. *(Reproduced with permission from Fox JA, Lee SJ, Cole BJ: Bone plug technique for meniscal transplantation, in Drez D Jr, Delee JC (eds): Surgical Technique in Sports Medicine. Philadelphia, PA, WB Saunders, 2003, pp 161-169.)*

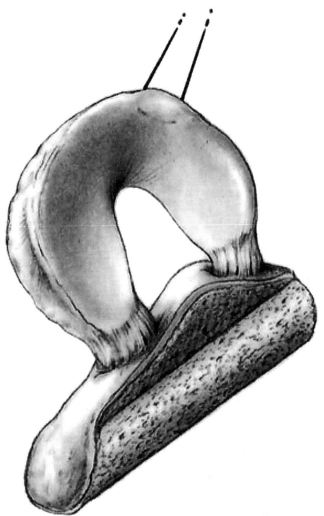

Figure 12 Illustration of lateral meniscal transplantation using the keyhole technique; the graft contains a common bone bridge attached to both anterior and posterior horns. *(Reproduced with permission from Rodeo SA: Meniscal allografts: Where do we stand? Am J Sports Med 2001;29:246-261.)*

the meniscal graft, indicating that accurate placement of the anterior and posterior horn attachment sites is the most important factor in normalizing load distribution and contact mechanics of the meniscal transplant.

Results

There are few published reports on the long-term success of meniscal transplantation. A recent study reported 14-year follow-up on patients who had undergone medial meniscal transplantation and ACL reconstruction for combined anterior knee instability and prior medial meniscectomy. Of the 23 patients, 17 had lyophilized irradiated meniscal allografts and 6 had deep-frozen allografts. The Lysholm score was 84 at 3 years postoperatively and 75 at 14 years postoperatively. Patients with deep-frozen meniscal transplants had better results than patients with lyophilized meniscal transplants. MRI evaluation showed good preservation of the deep-frozen meniscal transplants, even after 14 years. The lyophilized meniscal transplants were noted to be reduced in size during second-look arthroscopy and on MRI scans. When the control groups were compared with the study group, the deep-frozen meniscal allografts were found to be comparable with an intact meniscus, but the lyophilized meniscal allografts were comparable with the control group knees that had undergone meniscectomy.

Another study reported the outcome of meniscal transplantation with and without combined ACL reconstruction in a select group of 31 patients with reports of pain and/or instability at a mean follow-up of 2.9 years.

Eleven patients underwent isolated meniscal transplantation, and 20 patients underwent meniscal transplantation combined with ACL reconstruction. The Activities of Daily Living and Sports Activities Scale scores were 86 and 78, respectively, and the average Lysholm score was 84. There were no significant differences in these scores for the medial and lateral meniscal transplants, those performed with concurrent ACL reconstruction, or the degree of arthrosis at arthroscopy. Twenty-two patients stated they were greatly improved, eight were somewhat improved, and one was without change. All but one patient reported that knee function and level of activity were normal or nearly normal. All but one patient had a negative or 1+ result on the Lachman test. No statistically significant joint space narrowing was observed with plain radiographs over time. The authors concluded that meniscal allograft transplantation with or without combined ACL reconstruction in carefully selected patients with reports of compartmental joint line pain and/or instability appears to provide relief of symptoms and restore relatively high levels of function, particularly during activities of daily living.

A recent study reported on the biopsies of human meniscal allografts. Biopsy specimens were obtained from the human meniscal allografts and adjacent synovial membranes at an average of 16 months following transplantation. Human meniscal allograft transplants were repopulated with cells that appear to be derived from the synovial membrane. The majority of the specimens contained occasional immunoreactive cells (B-lymphocytes or cytotoxic T cells) in the meniscus or synovial tissue. Although there was histologic evidence of an immune response directed against the transplant, this response did not appear to affect the clinical outcome. The presence of histocompatibility antigens on the meniscal surface at the time of transplantation (even after freezing) indicated the potential for an immune response against the transplant. The authors concluded that despite the absence of frank immunologic rejection, a subtle immune reaction may affect the healing, incorporation, and revascularization of the graft.

Tissue Engineering

Besides meniscal transplantation, efforts in tissue engineering have been made to develop an artificial meniscus or scaffolds that will allow tissue regrowth to substitute the function of the normal meniscus. An artificial meniscus using polyvinyl alcohol-hydrogel (PVA-H) has been developed. Biomechanical analysis showed that a PVA-H artificial meniscus with high water content has viscoelastic properties that are similar to the human meniscus. Preliminary rabbit studies using a PVA-H artificial meniscus transplantation reported a decrease in articular cartilage degeneration when compared with meniscectomy. The PVA-H implant did not exhibit any visible wear or breakage at 1 year. The success of this material in a larger animal or in humans is yet to be determined.

Collagen scaffolds have been designed for use as a template for the regeneration of meniscal cartilage. These collagen scaffolds are derived from type I collagen fibers purified from bovine Achilles tendons with chemical treatment. In vitro and in vivo investigations in dogs have demonstrated cellular ingrowth and tissue regeneration throughout the scaffold. A pilot study was performed to determine the safety of the scaffold and its ability to support tissue ingrowth in patients. Patients with an irreparable tear of the meniscal cartilage underwent partial meniscectomy and replacement of the resected area using the collagen scaffold. Preliminary results demonstrated that the scaffold was implantable and safe over the course of a 3-year period. No adverse immunologic reactions were noted using serologic testing. At 3-year follow-up, patients reported a decrease in preoperative symptoms. This preliminary report demonstrated the safety and inert characteristics of the collagen scaffold. Additional studies are needed to evaluate its efficacy in tissue regeneration and replacement of larger meniscal lesions.

Summary

The menisci are important structures with a role in load transmission and stability in the knee, which provides the rationale for current efforts to preserve functional meniscal tissue. Because meniscal repair techniques have improved, they now have lower morbidity and allow repair of a wider range of meniscal tears. Much has been learned from early experience with meniscal transplantation, including the importance of defining the ideal patient candidate and ideal timing for meniscal transplantation. The development of artificial menisci and scaffolds holds great promise and may play a significant role in the management of meniscal injuries in the future. With the improvement in the treatment of meniscal injuries, the early cartilage degeneration and morbidity associated with meniscal tears may be prevented.

Annotated Bibliography

Basic Science

Alhaki MM, Hull ML, Howell SM: Contact mechanics of the medial tibial plateau after implantation of a medial meniscal allograft: A human cadaveric study. *Am J Sports Med* 2000;28:370-376.

This biomechanical study evaluated the change in contact mechanics of the medial compartment of the knee following meniscectomy, autograft transplantation, and allograft transplantation. The results showed that a medial meniscal allograft did not consistently restore normal contact mechanics but did significantly reduce the contact pressure when compared with the knee after meniscectomy.

Allen CR, Wong EK, Livesay GA, Sakane M, Fu FH, Woo SL: Importance of the medial meniscus in the anterior cruciate ligament-deficient knee. *J Orthop Res* 2000; 18:109-115.

The authors evaluated the role of the medial meniscus in stabilizing the ACL-deficient knee and their findings confirm the hypothesis that the resultant force in the medial meniscus is significantly greater in the ACL-deficient knee than in the intact knee when the knee is subjected to anterior tibial loads.

Greis PE, Bardana DD, Holmstrom MC, Burks RT: Meniscal injury: I. Basic science and evaluation. *J Am Acad Orthop Surg* 2002;10:168-176.

This review article provides a comprehensive review on the basic science and diagnosis of meniscal injuries.

Diagnosis

van Trommel MF, Potter HG, Ernberg LA, Simonian PT, Wickiewicz T: The use of noncontrast magnetic resonance imaging in evaluation of meniscal repair: Comparison with conventional arthrography. *Arthroscopy* 1998; 14:2-8.

This was a blinded study to correlate specialized MRI sequences with standard contrast arthrography in the evaluation of meniscal repair. MRI has a high correlation with arthrography in assessing meniscal repair. The authors concluded that noncontrast MRI can obviate the need for arthrography in the assessment of meniscal repair.

van Trommel MF, Simonian PT, Potter HG, Wickiewicz TL: Arthroscopic meniscal repair with fibrin clot of complete radial tears of lateral meniscus in the avascular zone. *Arthroscopy* 1998;14:360-365.

This study presented a small series of repairs on radial tears at the posterolateral aspect of the lateral meniscus using fibrin clot. All 5 menisci healed and showed no further signs of degeneration with second-look arthroscopy. The authors recommended the use of an exogenous clot to stimulate and support a reparative response in the avascular portion of the meniscus when repair is indicated.

Treatment

Aglietti P, Bertini FA, Buzzi R, Beraldi R: Arthroscopic meniscectomy for discoid lateral meniscus in children and adolescents: 10-year follow-up. *Am J Knee Surg* 1999;12:83-87.

This study included 17 patients who underwent arthroscopic lateral meniscectomy for discoid lateral meniscus. With an average follow-up of 10 years, the outcomes of 12 knees were reported as excellent, 4 were reported as good, and only 1 was reported as fair. Radiographic evaluation showed development of minor osteophytes in the lateral compartment of 8 knees and less than 50% narrowing of the lateral joint space in 11 knees.

Barber FA, Herbert MA: Meniscal repair devices. *Arthroscopy* 2000;16:613-618.

This study compared the biomechanical properties of meniscal repairs using traditional horizontal and vertical sutures and various inside-out meniscal devices. The results demonstrated that the double/vertical stitch provided the strongest repair.

Chatain F, Robinson AH, Adeleine P, Chambat P, Neyret P: The natural history of the knee following arthroscopic medial meniscectomy. *Knee Surg Sports Traumatol Arthrosc* 2001;9:15-18.

This study reviewed 317 patients who underwent arthroscopic medial meniscectomy. Ninety-one percent of the patients rated their knees as normal or near normal. Radiographs showed a 22.4% greater excess prevalence of joint space narrowing in operated knees when compared with control knees.

Ellermann A, Siebold R, Buelow JU, Sobau C: Clinical evaluation of meniscal repair with a bioabsorbable arrow: A 2- to 3- year follow-up study. *Knee Surg Sports Traumatol Arthrosc* 2002;10:289-293.

This study presented the results of meniscal repair using bioabsorbable meniscal arrows. At a mean follow-up of 33 months, 20 patients showed signs and symptoms consistent with meniscal tear and underwent partial meniscectomy. The remaining 80% of the patients had average Lysholm score of 92.5 and Cincinnati score of 90.4.

Kobayashi M, Toguchida J, Oka M: Preliminary study of polyvinyl alcohol-hydrogel (PVA-H) artificial meniscus. *Biomaterials* 2003;24:639-647.

This study presents the results of artificial meniscal replacement using PVA-H in the rabbit knee. Articular cartilage had initial regressive changes but did not progress after a certain period. The articular cartilage appears to be preserved even at 1 year after transplantation. No obvious wear or breakage of the PVA-H artifical meniscus was observed. The results suggest that the PVA-H artificial meniscus can compensate for meniscal function in the rabbit meniscectomy model.

Noyes FR, Barber-Westin SD: Arthroscopic repair of meniscus tears extending into the avascular zone with or without anterior cruciate ligament reconstruction in patients 40 years of age and older. *Arthroscopy* 2000;16: 822-829.

This study prospectively evaluated the outcome of the arthroscopic repair of meniscal tears extending into the avascular zone for patients age 40 years and older. At a mean follow-up of 33 months, 87% of the repairs were asymptomatic for tibiofemoral joint pain and had not required additional surgery; 72% had concomitant ACL reconstruction. The authors suggested that for athletically active patients, meniscal tissue should be preserved regardless of age; they based these indications for the procedure on current and future activity levels.

O'Shea JJ, Shelbourne KD: Repair of locked bucket-handle meniscal tears in knees with chronic anterior cruciate ligament deficiency. *Am J Sports Med* 2003;31: 216-220.

This study presents the results for staged surgical procedures of meniscal repair followed by late ligament reconstruction for patients with large locked bucket-handle meniscal tears and chronic ACL deficiency. The study showed that at the time of ligament reconstruction, 89% of the meniscal repairs were healed. Of the 43 tears in the white-white zone, 21 appeared healed, 17 were partially healed, and 5 showed no healing. Of 11 in red-white zone, 8 appeared healed, 2 were partially healed, and 1 showed no healing. The authors concluded that locked bucket-handle meniscal tears heal at high rate when repaired as an isolated procedure, even when full weight bearing and activity before reconstruction are allowed and when the tear is in the white-white zone.

Rodeo SA: Meniscal allografts: Where do we stand? *Am J Sports Med* 2001;29:246-261.

This review article presents the basic science, technique, and results of meniscal transplantation. The author also reviews the clinical indications, contraindications, and graft processing and appropriate sizing issues for meniscal transplantation.

Rodeo SA, Seneviratne A, Suzuki K, Felker K, Wickiewicz TL, Warren RF: Histological analysis of human meniscal allografts: A preliminary report. *J Bone Joint Surg Am* 2000;82:1071-1082.

Biopsy specimens were obtained from the meniscal allografts and adjacent synovial membranes of patients who underwent meniscal transplantation at a mean 16 months earlier. Histologic analysis demonstrated that the cells that repopulated the menisci stained positively with phenotype markers for both synovial cells and fibroblasts. Although there was no evidence of frank immunologic reaction, a number of the specimens stained positive for immunoreactive cells (B lymphocytes and cytotoxic T cells). The authors suggested that despite the absence of frank immunologic rejection, a subtle immune reaction may affect the healing, incorporation, and revascularization of the graft.

Schimmer RC, Brulhart KB, Duff C, Glinz W: Arthroscopic partial meniscectomy: A 12-year follow-up and two-step evaluation of the long-term course. *Arthroscopy* 1998;14:136-142.

This long-term study followed 119 patients with a mean follow-up of 12 years after arthroscopic partial meniscectomy. Although 94.8% of patients with isolated meniscal tears had good and excellent results, only 62% of patients with additional cartilage damage had good and excellent results.

Wirth CJ, Peters G, Milachowski KA, Weismeier KG, Kohn D: Long-term results of meniscal allograft transplantation. *Am J Sports Med* 2002;30:174-181.

This study reported the long-term results of combined medial meniscal transplantation and ACL reconstruction. Seventeen of the 23 patients had a lyophilized meniscal allograft, whereas the remaining 6 patients had a deep-frozen meniscal allograft. The authors reported that at 14-year follow-up, the deep-frozen meniscal allografts were comparable with the intact menisci of the control group, whereas the lyophilized meniscal allografts were comparable with the menisci of the control group that had undergone meniscectomy.

Yoldas EA, Sekiya JK, Irrgang JJ, Fu FH, Harner CD: Arthroscopically assisted meniscal allograft transplantation with and without combined anterior cruciate ligament reconstruction. *Knee Surg Sports Traumatol Arthrosc* 2003;11:173-182.

This study examined clinical and patient-reported outcomes following meniscal allograft transplantation with and without combined ACL reconstruction in a select group of 31 patients with pain and/or instability (34 meniscal allografts). All but one patient reported that knee function and level of activity were normal or nearly normal postoperatively. The authors concluded that meniscal allograft transplantation with and without combined ACL reconstruction in carefully selected patients with compartmental joint line pain and/or instability can provide relief of symptoms and restore relatively high levels of function, particularly during activities of daily living.

Classic Bibliography

Arnoczky SP, Warren RF: Microvasculature of the human meniscus. *Am J Sports Med* 1982;10:90-95.

Burks RT, Metcalf MH, Metcalf RW: Fifteen-year follow-up of arthroscopic partial meniscectomy. *Arthroscopy* 1997;13:673-679.

DeHaven KE, Lohrer WA, Lovelock JE: Long-term results of open meniscal repair. *Am J Sports Med* 1995;23:524-530.

Dickhaut SC, Delee JC: The discoid lateral-meniscus syndrome. *J Bone Joint Surg Am* 1982;64:1068-1073 .

Johnson RJ, Kettelkamp DB, Clark W, Leaverton P: Factors effecting late results after meniscectomy. *J Bone Joint Surg Am* 1974;56:719-729.

McBride GG, Constine RM, Hofmann AA, Carson RW: Arthroscopic partial medial meniscectomy in the older patient. *J Bone Joint Surg Am* 1984;66:547-551.

Northmore-Ball MD, Dandy DJ: Long-term results of arthroscopic partial meniscectomy. *Clin Orthop* 1982;167:34-42.

Northmore-Ball MD, Dandy DJ, Jackson RW: Arthroscopic, open partial and total meniscectomy: A comparative study. *J Bone Joint Surg Br* 1983;65:400-404.

Stone KR, Steadman JR, Rodkey WG, Li ST: Regeneration of meniscal cartilage with use of a collagen scaffold. *J Bone Joint Surg Am* 1997;79:1770-1777.

Tapper EM, Hoover NW: Late results after meniscectomy. *J Bone Joint Surg Br* 1969;51:517-526.

Yocum LA, Kerlan RK, Jobe FW, et al: Isolated lateral meniscectomy: A study of twenty-six patients with isolated tears. *J Bone Joint Surg Am* 1979;61:338-342.

Chapter 16

Patellofemoral Disorders

Matthew G. Friederichs, MD

Robert T. Burks, MD

Introduction

Patellofemoral disorders commonly pose diagnostic and treatment challenges in the orthopaedic practice. Although these disorders have been extensively evaluated, it is still difficult to truly master the complexities of the patellofemoral joint. Nonetheless, physicians treating athletes should understand patellofemoral anatomy, imaging techniques, and the diagnosis and treatment of common patellofemoral disorders.

Structure and Function

The patellofemoral joint experiences significant mechanical load with body movement but is developmentally suited to withstand these natural forces. There is increasing surface area contact with increasing knee flexion, which naturally allows a better distribution of the increased forces that occur when the knee is in a flexed position. Measuring up to 5 mm in thickness, the articular cartilage of the patella is the thickest cartilage in the body. A central ridge divides the patella into a medial and lateral facet. Some anatomists describe an "odd" facet, which is medial to the larger medial facet and articulates with the femur in deep flexion. The inferior quarter of the patella is nonarticular and primarily involved with patellar tendon insertion. The blood supply of the patella is derived from the geniculate artery complex.

The patella is stabilized by both static and dynamic restraints. The patellar tendon, medial patellofemoral ligament, medial retinaculum, lateral retinaculum, and the bony architecture of the patella and the trochlear groove make up the static restraints. Several studies have emphasized the importance of the medial patellofemoral ligament and its role in preventing lateral translation of the patella (Figure 1). It has been shown to comprise 53% to 60% of the resistance to lateral translation. The dynamic stabilizers include the quadriceps muscle, adductor magnus, and the iliotibial band. The vastus medialis and the vastus lateralis are the most important dynamic stabilizers for patellar tracking.

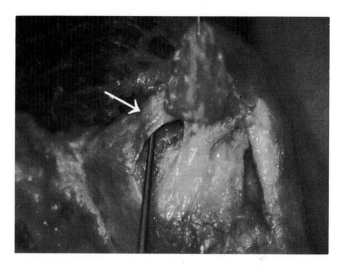

Figure 1 Photograph of a cadaver specimen showing the medial patellofemoral ligament (*arrow*).

Physical Examination

A complete knee examination can only be done when taking into account all of the factors that contribute to alignment, motion, and stability as they relate to the lower extremities. It is important to evaluate the patient while walking as well as standing, sitting, prone, and supine. The standing examination allows for evaluation of varus or valgus alignment of the knee. The ankle joint and subtalar joint should also be evaluated because subtalar pronation, for example, can affect tibial rotation and patellar alignment (Figure 2).

The seated examination is done with the knees flexed at 90°; normal alignment will leave the patella facing directly anterior. Patella alta will result in the patella facing upward because it is sitting more proximally on the trochlea. The 90° tubercle sulcus angle, as defined by a line perpendicular to the transepicondylar axis and a line from the center of the patella to the center of the tubercle, is measured with the patient in the seated position. A normal 90° tubercle sulcus angle is defined as 0°.

Evaluation of the vastus medialis obliquus is also done with the patient's knee in the flexed position; the

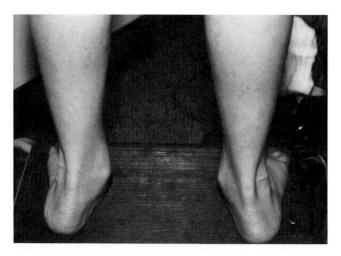

Figure 2 Photograph of a patient with excessive hindfoot pronation on standing examination.

muscle's location and contour can be appreciated as the knee is extended. Extension of the knee from a flexed position also enables the clinician to evaluate for a "J" sign and patella crepitus. The "J" sign is lateral translation in terminal extension and is suggestive of patellar subluxation and malalignment.

The supine position allows for evaluation of patellar mobility in the medial and lateral direction. Grasping both the medial and lateral aspect of the patient's patella and applying a medial or lateral force with the knee in slight flexion assesses patellar mobility. Normal translation should not exceed two quadrants in the medial or lateral direction and should be fairly symmetric in each direction for any given patient.

A quadrant of motion is equal to 25% of the width of that patient's patella. Excessive lateral translation as the result of a hypermobile patella can also be associated with patellar apprehension. The lateral retinaculum is assessed by evaluating patellar tilt. A neutral tilt is defined by the medial and lateral borders of the patella being parallel with the transepicondylar axis when the lateral edge of the patella is lifted or everted as much as possible. A negative angle, which results when the lateral patellar edge remains below the horizontal epicondylar axis during eversion, is indicative of lateral retinacular tightness. This should also be confirmed by having minimal medial translation. It is also essential to palpate both the medial and lateral retinaculum for tenderness. The inferior pole of the patella should be palpated with the patient's knee slightly flexed to evaluate for patellar tendinitis. The classic Q angle is measured in the supine position. The Q angle is measured from the anterior iliac spine to the center of the patella and by comparing this line to a line from the center of the patella to the tibial tubercle. A normal angle is defined as approximately 10° or less in men and 15° or less in women. The classic Q angle is highly variable from ex-

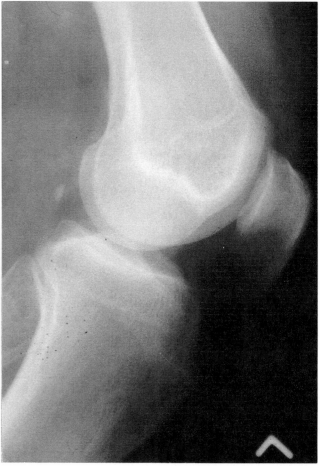

Figure 3 Lateral knee radiograph demonstrating patella baja.

aminer to examiner; although suggestive of maltracking if abnormal, it is not predictive enough to be used as the sole criterion for surgical intervention. The prone position is used to assess hip version and rotation as well.

Radiographic Examination

The radiographic examination starts with a complete series of the knee including AP (or PA), lateral, and axial views. The AP view allows evaluation of the patella for bipartite patella and fractures. The lateral view allows for evaluation of patella alta or patella baja and can also be very sensitive in evaluating malalignment (Figures 3 and 4). Patella height is measured with the Insall-Salvati or the Blackburne-Peel ratio. The Insall-Salvati ratio compares the length of the patellar tendon to the greatest diagonal length of the patella. The Blackburne-Peel ratio compares the perpendicular distance from the lowest articular margin of the patella to the tibial plateau and the length of the articular cartilage of the patella. A normal ratio using both methods is between 0.8 and 1.2. A ratio of less than 0.8 is considered patella baja, and a ratio greater than 1.2 is considered patella alta. The use of a true lateral view also enhances the evaluation of patellar tilt and trochlear morphology (Figure 4). Trochlear dysplasia is suggested when the line representing the depth of the trochlea intersects the anterior cortex on this view. The lateral facet and central ridge can also be evaluated on the lateral radiograph, and patellar tilt can be determined from this view as well. Two different types of axial views have been described in the literature. The Merchant view is obtained with the knee flexed to 45° and the x-ray tube angled at 30° from the horizontal. The Laurin view is obtained with the knees flexed at 30° and the x-ray tube parallel to the tibia with the patient holding the cassette perpendicular to the beam. The congruence angle, a measure of the relationship of the patellar ridge to the trochlear sulcus, is determined from the axial views by measuring the line dividing the sulcus angle and the line from the center of the sulcus angle to the most prominent portion of the patellar ridge. Greater than 16° of lateral subluxation is considered abnormal. It should be noted, however, that this is a static measurement of a dynamic problem.

CT has become more widely used because of its ability to evaluate the patellofemoral joint closer to full extension. Authors have suggested that CT be done because this allows evaluation at multiple angles of flexion. Gun site CT scans, which can help determine important rotational malalignments of the femur and tibia, can play a significant role in diagnosing patellofemoral disorders in certain patients.

MRI has also become a useful tool in the evaluation of the patellofemoral joint and supporting tissues. In patients with acute patellar dislocation, MRI can provide important information about the articular surface and the status of the medial and lateral soft-tissue restraints. In patients with acute dislocation, increased signal is frequently seen in the lateral edge of the trochlea and medial edge of the patella representing bone bruising or perhaps an osteochondral injury.

To complete diagnostic imaging for patients with patellofemoral disorders, bone scanning can be useful to evaluate pain of unknown origin or overuse injuries. Bone scanning can also aid in the diagnosis of reflex sympathetic dystrophy, which is characterized by a significant diffuse uptake in all bony structures around the knee.

Patellofemoral Rehabilitation

Most patellofemoral pain disorders respond to nonsurgical treatment. The goal of therapy is to provide symptomatic relief and allow patients and athletes to return to their desired levels of activity. A good rehabilitation program must take into account not only evaluation of the patellofemoral articulation, but also the entire lower extremity, including the identification of isolated weaknesses around the hip or tightness of the iliotibial band. Patient education, stretching, and strengthening all are

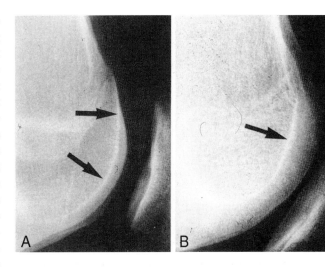

Figure 4 True lateral radiographs demonstrating trochlear morphology. **A**, The double arrows indicate trochlear insufficiency with a very shallow trochlear groove. **B**, The single arrow indicates the depth of a normal trochlear groove. *(Reproduced with permission from Malghem J, Maldague B: Depth insufficiency of the proximal trochlear groove or lateral radiographs of the knee: Relation to patellar dislocation. Radiology 1989;170:507-510.)*

aspects of a successful rehabilitation program. It is important for patients to understand what potentially causes their patellofemoral pain to help them avoid aggravating activities.

Stretching of the quadriceps is best done in the prone position, which keeps the hip in an extended position while flexing the knee. This allows stretching of the rectus, which crosses the hip joint and is in a more relaxed position if stretching of the quadriceps is done with the hip flexed. Quadriceps strengthening is obviously a very important part of trying to obtain a pain-free patellofemoral joint. It is important to identify strengthening exercises that a patient can do painlessly and emphasize those exercises early; other exercises can be added as the patient's symptoms subside. It has recently been shown that hip flexibility and external rotator strength help improve lower extremity alignment and alleviate some of the abnormal stresses across the patellofemoral joint as well.

Management of Specific Patellofemoral Disorders

Patellofemoral Pain With Normal Alignment

Patients often present with debilitating patellofemoral pain without an obvious anatomic abnormality. A recent study identified four risk factors for patellofemoral pain: shortened quadriceps muscle, abnormal vastus medialis obliquus muscle reflex response time, decreased explosive strength, and a hypermobile patella. Although the patellofemoral examination itself may be unremarkable, attention to the entire lower extremity is important in patients with debilitating patellofemoral pain. Some-

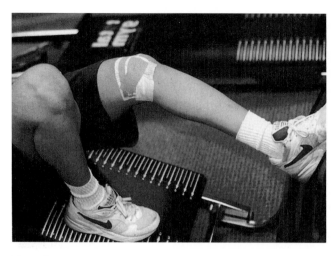

Figure 5 Photograph of a patient who underwent McConnell taping during patellofemoral rehabilitation.

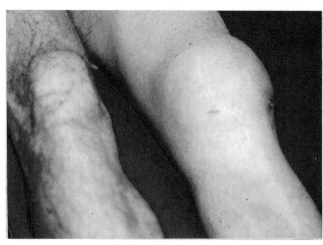

Figure 6 Photograph of a patient with hemarthrosis (left knee) after lateral release.

thing as simple as foot orthotics for some patients with ankle and subtalar abnormalities can make a difference in their perception of patellofemoral pain. Again, most of these patients can be managed with activity modification and a rehabilitation program.

Patellofemoral Pain With Malalignment

Patellar tilt or lateral facet syndrome is common, and it is characterized by a tight lateral retinaculum. This leads to increased joint forces on the lateral facet. In addition to strengthening, the rehabilitation program needs to emphasize stretching of the lateral structures, including retinaculum, vastus lateralis, and iliotibial band. Many patients can obtain relief with the use of McConnell taping (Figure 5) or a patella cut-out brace. McConnell taping has been shown to increase vastus medialis obliquus function and may be beneficial for a strengthening program. However, several studies have shown no added benefit with this technique. It is unclear whether closed- or open-chain exercises are more beneficial, but a recent study suggests closed-chain rehabilitation may have slight advantages in functional results. Terminal extension (open-chain) exercises performed from 20° of flexion to full extension can usually be well tolerated and do not result in excessive patellofemoral load.

Patients should attempt to exhaust all conservative measures before surgical intervention is considered to treat patellofemoral pain with malalignment. In carefully selected patients, a lateral release can provide symptomatic relief. However, lateral release should only be performed in those patients with a tight lateral retinaculum on physical examination. Lateral release is associated with complications. For example, hemarthrosis is a common occurrence and can lead to significant morbidity and delayed rehabilitation. Meticulous hemostasis can help minimize this risk (Figure 6). Studies of patients with reflex sympathetic dystrophy also show an

increased incidence of patients who have a history of patellofemoral surgery of some type. An aggressive lateral release that involves the vastus lateralis tendons can unnecessarily weaken the quadriceps or lead to iatrogenic medial subluxation of the patella. It is important when performing the lateral release to maintain the main vastus lateralis fibers. Most releases need not extend above the superior pole of the patella, and the surgeon should not be guided by the common belief that the lateral border of the patella should be able to be everted 90° to prove an adequate release. This can frequently lead to releasing the patella in a fashion that is too proximal.

Patients with a lateral quadriceps vector can be difficult to treat. Although many patients will respond to a rehabilitation program, some ultimately do require surgical management. Patients without significant arthrosis can be treated with medialization of the tibial tubercle, such as with the Elmslie-Trillat procedure. Patients with patellofemoral arthrosis primarily localized in the lateral facet and lateral trochlea will often respond to transfer of the tubercle both anterior and medially. The typical Fulkerson type osteotomies help unload the lateral and distal patella. Anteriorization such as with the Maquet procedure is fraught with more frequent complications and has not been shown to have superior results in these patients.

Patellar Subluxation

There are many risk factors associated with patellar subluxation, and no one factor dominates in its importance. Patients may have a laterally positioned tubercle, increased Q angle, patella alta, increased valgus alignment of the knee, trochlear dysplasia, and poor quadriceps function to name a few contributory factors. Some patients with patellar subluxation can respond to rehabilitation and patellar braces. Should rehabilitation fail, many procedures have been described for surgical management, including isolated lateral release, formal proximal realignment, and repair or reconstruction of medial supporting structures with or without distal realignment. If a patient has true patellar malalignment and not simply a tight lateral retinaculum, use of an isolated lateral release has resulted in a high failure rate. Proximal realignment alone also has a high failure rate, with the medial advancements weakening the vastus medialis obliquus, the medial reefs stretching out, and sometimes resulting in poor quality medial tissues. Recently, there has been increased emphasis on the importance of the medial patellofemoral ligament. Reconstruction of this ligament has been described and can be very useful, particularly in patients with a dysplastic trochlea, tissue elasticity, failed prior surgery, or other risk factors. Medialization of the tubercle, which decreases the lateral quadriceps vector, has met with good success. In the past, tubercle surgery has raised concerns, but this was primarily with procedures that distalize the tubercle or placed it medial enough on the tibia that it was relatively posterior to its original position. A Trillat type osteotomy of the tubercle is not as prone to result in the arthrosis that can occur with more aggressive tubercle procedures. As already mentioned, if there is any concern about lateral patellofemoral arthrosis, then a Fulkerson type osteotomy can be considered in this setting. Because it is difficult to treat skeletally immature patients with tubercle surgery or medial patellofemoral ligament reconstruction, in addition to a standard proximal realignment, other soft-tissue augmentation procedures have been described for this patient population.

Acute Patellar Dislocation

Acute patellar dislocation is most often a result of an indirect mechanism. The patient will often describe a twisting force on the weight-bearing extremity. Rehabilitation is considered the treatment of choice for acute patellar dislocation despite recurrence rates approaching 50%. A recent study of the nonsurgical management of acute patellar dislocations demonstrated that 58% of patients still experienced limitation in strenuous activity at 6 months after the injury despite not having a recurrent dislocation. Because younger patients and those with risk factors seem to have higher recurrence rates for dislocation, these factors play a role in determining how aggressively surgical management should be considered. The critical lesion in dislocation is disruption of the medial patellofemoral ligament, medial retinaculum, and perhaps even the vastus medialis oblique attachment. Most of the tears of the medial patellofemoral ligament occur at the femoral attachment site, but tears can occur anywhere along its course. Articular lesions occur primarily on the medial patellar facet and lateral trochlea. Fat in the aspirate of a hemarthrosis in a pa-

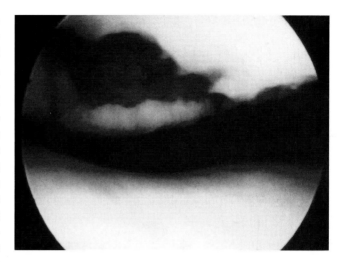

Figure 7 This arthroscopic view of the patellofemoral joint shows an osteochondral defect after acute patellar dislocation.

tient with an acute patellar dislocation is diagnostic of intra-articular fracture. Studies on acute arthroscopic débridement after patellar dislocation have found an approximate 40% rate of osteochondral defects not noted on standard radiographs (Figure 7). MRI can be helpful in this setting to evaluate articular surfaces for loose osteochondral fragments.

Surgical repair of osteochondral injuries in the acute setting is focused on the repair or removal of osteochondral fragments. Repair of the medial retinaculum in the acute setting has been described in the literature, but different authors have found the predominance of injury in completely different locations on the medial aspect of the knee. The medial patellofemoral ligament can be acutely repaired, with recurrence rates described as less than 10%. However, medial repairs done in the acute setting can result in postoperative stiffness and the risk of arthrofibrosis. In many articles, despite successful treatment of instability, pain has been reported to linger, which can be a result of articular damage, persistent maltracking, or scarring from surgery. One study reported a 30% to 50% incidence of anterior knee pain or instability with or without surgical intervention.

Recurrent Patellar Dislocation

Patients with recurrent patellar dislocation usually have malalignment of the extensor mechanism. Although nonsurgical treatment is still a viable option, some of these patients prefer surgical intervention because of the significant downtime from activities and recovery associated with repeated patellar dislocations.

The distal realignment (Trillat) with or without lateral release is an effective treatment of patellar dislocations in skeletally mature patients. Again, a lateral release is done if there appears to be relative tightness of the lateral retinaculum, but a significantly mobile patella certainly does not require a lateral release to be performed. In patients with associated patella alta, a distalization procedure may be indicated to help engage the patella into the trochlear groove in earlier flexion. The tubercle should probably be distalized only to the limit to bring the patella into the upper limits of normal and not overly distalized. Also, with any distalization, the tubercle should be maintained on the anterior aspect of the tibia and not allowed to be moved over onto the medial aspect because this would take the tubercle in a more posterior direction. Fulkerson type procedures can be performed if there is a good articular surface on the proximal and medial aspect of the patella. The distal bony procedure has the advantage of permitting rigid fixation with compression screws, which allows early immobilization and early weight bearing.

When considering distal realignment procedures, a question remains concerning the medial stabilizing soft-tissue restraints. Although a common approach is to add a medial reefing, these frequently stretch out with time even though a patient may be asymptomatic. Many patients with relatively normal patellofemoral anatomy can be treated with a Trillat osteotomy and have good results without attention to the medial structures. However, patients in whom prior surgery has failed or who have significant risk factors making the patellofemoral joint less of a stabilizing factor (such as those with trochlear dysplasia), medial patellofemoral ligament reconstruction is an excellent choice. The advantage of medial patellofemoral ligament reconstruction over repair and reefing of the medial patellofemoral ligament is that the medial patellofemoral ligament is frequently thin and difficult to identify, making specific repair or advancement tenuous. As with ACL reconstruction, ligament reconstruction has some advantages over repair and can actually be done with a minimally invasive approach.

Plica

Plicas are normal remnants of mesenchymal tissue and commonly occur in the suprapatellar, medial, and infrapatellar areas. The incidence of lateral plicas is quite rare. Approximately 90% of all asymptomatic knees have some form of plica; therefore, most plicas are incidental findings. On occasion, plicas can be symptomatic, such as in patients who have experienced a blunt trauma or those who have increased levels of activity or a prior surgery. Plica pain is typically located on the medial aspect of the knee proximal to the joint line over the medial femoral condyle and is exacerbated with activity and possibly by prolonged sitting. Occasionally, patients can have a sense of popping or snapping with flexion associated with a pathologic plica. MRI has been reported to identify plica lesions with high accuracy; however, this is most likely directly related to the qual-

ity of MRI scan and the experience of the reviewer. Standard nonsurgical management, including nonsteroidal medication, ice, and iontophoresis, has been shown to improve symptoms. Surgical management is reserved only for pathologic plica resistant to conservative management. At the time of arthroscopy, pathologic plicas are noted to be thickened and fibrotic, sometimes even torn, such as in patients with a bucket-handle type meniscal tear. Frequently, there is a cartilage irregularity over the proximal medial femoral condyle that can be observed to articulate with the plica when the knee is placed through a range of motion. Surgical treatment consists of resection of the plica with care taken not to remove the adjoining capsule in an attempt to prevent scarring or increased postoperative bleeding.

Patellar Tendinitis

Patellar tendinitis most commonly occurs at the insertion of the patellar tendon at the inferior pole of the patella. Patients with patellar tendinitis usually present with pain, tenderness, and occasionally swelling at the inferior pole of the patella and proximal patellar tendon. This is very common in patients who participate in jumping-intensive activities, such as basketball and volleyball. In athletic populations, quadriceps and hamstring muscle tightness was found to be a significant factor in the development of patellar tendinitis. Patellar tendinitis is a result of recurrent microtrauma at the patellar insertion of the patellar tendon. A tenuous blood supply is believed to be a factor in the development of this entity as well as its poor healing potential. Pathologic sections reveal mucoid degeneration and fibrinous necrosis consistent with degenerative changes in the tendon. Diagnosis is usually based on clinical history and physical examination findings; however, staging and treatment have been described using ultrasound and MRI as adjuncts. MRI staging of patellar tendinitis as defined by McLoughlin is graded by signal intensity, with grades 1 and 2 having high signal and grade 3 having intermediate intensity. A recent study of MRI found sensitivity and specificity to be only 75% and 29%, respectively, when clinical diagnosis was used as the standard. Care should be taken when interpreting MRI scans in older athletes because this particular group has a high rate of false-positive results.

Nonsurgical management consisting of anti-inflammatory medications, stretching, and strengthening yields good results in patients with moderate tendinopathy. Patellar tendon débridement has demonstrated good to excellent results in 70% to 90% of patients in several studies that evaluated the efficacy of the surgical management of patellar tendinitis. Extracorporeal shock wave therapy has recently been used to treat this patient population and has demonstrated similar efficacy to surgical débridement in patients with recalcitrant patellar tendinitis.

Extensor Mechanism Disruption

The extensor mechanism can be disrupted either at the quadriceps tendon or the patellar tendon. Quadriceps tendon rupture is more common in the older patients with preexisting tendon atrophy or damage. Patellar tendon ruptures are more common in younger, more athletic patients. Surprisingly, quadriceps tendon ruptures can be missed in older patients. It is important, therefore, to palpate both the quadriceps tendon and the patellar tendon for defects. The patient should also be able to perform a straight leg raise without any extensor lag on physical examination, and the patella should be checked on radiographs for evidence of patella baja or patella alta, which could help confirm the diagnosis. Repair of the extensor mechanism is mandatory, and the type of repair and rehabilitation will depend on multiple factors, such as patient age, quality of tissue, and coexistent diseases.

Prepatellar Bursitis

Prepatellar bursitis is manifested by subcutaneous swelling anterior to the patella. Inflammation of the prepatellar bursa can be traumatic or perhaps infectious. Treatment of traumatic bursitis can include ice, antiinflammatory medications, compression, and activity avoidance. Aspiration may be necessary to help eliminate significant fluid collection; this can be augmented with steroid injection in an effort to prevent recurrence. A chronic bursitis that does not respond to conservative measures may require bursectomy. Although traditionally done using an open procedure, case reports of arthroscopic excision have been described in the medical literature. Pyogenic bursitis requires adequate débridement and antibiotic therapy with organism-specific coverage.

Accessory Centers of Ossification

When accessory centers of ossification fail to fuse, a bipartite or even tripartite patella can result, a condition that is present in up to 6% of the population. A superolateral ossification center is the most common location. Bipartite patella is often an incidental finding on knee radiographs, but symptomatic lesions, sometimes the result of direct trauma, can occur. These symptomatic lesions will frequently respond to rest and conservative treatment. Symptomatic fragments may be excised without loss of normal function, but with excision the vastus lateralis insertion site should be preserved.

Osteochondritis Dissecans

Although rare, osteochondritis dissecans can occur in the patellar and trochlear groove. As with other osteo-

chondrotic lesions, the exact cause is unknown, but it may be related to trauma. Lesions in a skeletally immature patient may heal with brief immobilization or decreased activities. Lesions that do not seem to respond to conservative treatment or are unstable typically require surgical treatment similar to that used to treat osteochondrotic lesions elsewhere in the knee. If possible, fragment fixation and retention is advantageous, but occasionally excision may be required.

Articular Cartilage Lesions of the Patellofemoral Joint

Articular cartilage lesions of the patellofemoral joint are difficult to manage, and there is no clear treatment algorithm because of the many variables that can be present. Rehabilitation programs similar to those used for patients with standard patellofemoral pain and instability can be effective. Should this fail, surgical management needs to be individualized, taking into account a patient's age and activity level, the location of the lesion, and the degree of joint involvement. Delamination lesions and early degenerative lesions may respond to simple arthroscopic débridement. Degenerative lesions of the lateral facet related to malalignment or lateral compression may respond favorably to lateral release. A recent study on lateral release for patellofemoral arthritis demonstrated a reduction in symptoms in 80% of patients. Standard management used to treat articular lesions encountered elsewhere in the joint (such as those caused by microfracture, abrasion, and drilling) can also be used to treat lesions of the patellofemoral joint. Osteochondral autograft and autologous chondrocyte transplantation have been used recently, but the efficacy of these procedures in treating lesions in the patellofemoral joint does not have the predictability of results that have been reported treating lesions of the femoral condyle. Fulkerson type osteotomies of the tubercle may provide symptomatic relief in patients with primarily distal articular deficits and those with associated subluxation of the patella. Patellectomy may be considered in patients with severe lesions, but this procedure is most effective when the pathology is confined to the patella and the trochlea is relatively normal.

Summary

Despite advances in diagnostic and treatment options, the treatment of patellofemoral disorders continues to be a challenging management area. A careful history and physical examination are essential to understand the underlying pathology in each patient. Because many patellofemoral disorders respond to appropriate rehabilitation and conservative management, this should be the first line of treatment in most patients. When conservative management fails, care should be taken to specifically address the presumed pathology and make further treatment recommendations on a case-by-case basis.

Annotated Bibliography

Structure and Function

Desio SM, Burks RT, Bachus KN: Soft tissue restraints to lateral patellar translation in the human knee. *Am J Sports Med* 1998;26:59-65.

This cadaveric sectioning study demonstrated that the medial patellofemoral was the primary restraint to lateral translation at 20° of flexion and contributed 60% of the total restraining force.

Radiographic Examination

Shalaby M, Almekinders LC: Patellar tendonitis: The significance of magnetic resonance imaging findings. *Am J Sports Med* 1999;27:345-349.

This study compared MRI scans in patients with and without patellar tendinitis. The results demonstrated 75% sensitivity and 29% specificity for diagnosis if physical examination was used as the standard.

Patellofemoral Rehabilitation

Cowan SM, Bennell KL, Hodges PW: Therapeutic patellar taping changes the timing of the vasti muscle activation in people with patellofemoral pain syndrome. *Clin J Sport Med* 2002;12:339-347.

The results of this study demonstrated that patellar taping affected the activation time of the vastus medialis obliquus in symptomatic patients compared with placebo taping during stair stepping tasks. There were no demonstrable changes in asymptomatic subjects.

Witvrouw E, Bellemans J, Lysens R, Danneels L, Cambier D: Intrinsic risk factors for the development of patellar tendonitis in an athletic population: A two-year prospective study. *Am J Sports Med* 2001;29:190-195.

This study evaluated the risk factors for the development of patellar tendinitis in an athletic population. Students enrolled in physical education classes (n = 138) were evaluated at the start of the study for limb alignment and muscle length, strength, and tightness. Nineteen students developed patellar tendinitis confirmed by ultrasound during the 2-year study period. The only significant variable for the development of patellar tendinitis was decreased quadriceps and hamstring flexibility. The authors recommend routine screening and treatment aimed at improving flexibility in this at-risk population.

Witvrouw E, Lysens R, Bellemans J, Peers K, Vanderstraeten G: Open versus closed kinetic chain exercises for patellofemoral pain: A prospective, randomized study. *Am J Sports Med* 2000;28:687-694.

This prospective study compared the efficacy of an all open-chain exercise program with an all closed-chain exercise program over a period of 5 weeks. Both rehabilitation protocols resulted in a decrease in anterior knee pain in study participants. The closed-chained exercise program appeared to have a slight advantage over the open-chain exercise program.

Witvrouw E, Lysens R, Bellemans J, Cambier D, Vanderstraeten G: Intrinsic risk factors for the development of anterior knee pain in an athletic population: A two-year prospective study. *Am J Sports Med* 2000;28:480-489.

This study evaluated the risk factors for the development of patellofemoral pain. Students enrolled in physical education classes (N = 282) were evaluated at the start of the study for motor performance, joint laxity, limb alignment, muscle length and strength, patellofemoral characteristics, and psychologic parameters. Twenty-four students developed anterior knee pain during the 2-year study period. Statistical analysis demonstrated a significant correlation with shortened quadriceps muscle, altered vastus medialis obliquus reflex response time, decreased explosive strength, and a hypermobile patella in patients who developed anterior knee pain.

Management of Specific Patellofemoral Disorders

Aderinto J, Cobb A: Lateral release for patellofemoral arthritis. *Arthroscopy* 2002;18:339-403.

This retrospective study evaluated patients with patellofemoral arthritis after undergoing lateral release. The results demonstrated that 80% of patients had a reduction in pain regardless of the presence of tibiofemoral arthritis.

Al-Duri ZA, Aichroth PM: Surgical aspects of patella tendonitis: Techniques and results. *Am J Knee Surg* 2001;14:43-50.

This retrospective review evaluates the surgical management of "very abnormal" knees. At an average postoperative follow-up of 12 months, 89% of the knees were rated as normal or near normal and 11% were rated as abnormal.

Atkins DM, Fithian MD, Manangi KS, Stone ML, Dobson BE, Mendelsohn C: Characteristics of patients with primary acute lateral patellar dislocation and their recovery within the first 6 months of injury. *Am J Sports Med* 2000;28:472-479.

This prospective study evaluated the characteristics and early recovery period in first-time lateral patellar dislocation patients. All patients were treated nonsurgically with a standardized rehabilitation program for 6 months. Radiographs demonstrated that all patients had lateral patellar overhang, and 50% had patella alta. Sports participation remained limited in 58% of patients at 6-month follow-up. The greatest limitation in activity involved kneeling or squatting.

Coleman BD, Khan KM, Kiss ZS, Bartlett J, Young DA, Wark JD: Open and arthroscopic patellar tenotomy for chronic patellar tendinopathy: A retrospective outcome study. Victorian Institute of Sport Tendon Study Group. *Am J Sports Med* 2000;28:183-190.

This retrospective outcome study on patellar tenotomy demonstrated improved results in 96% of patients who were treated arthroscopically and 81% of patients who were treated with open tenotomy. Forty-six percent of patients in the arthroscopic group and 54% in the open tenotomy group were able to return to full athletic activity. Return to sport averaged

6 months in the arthroscopic group and 10 months in the open tenotomy group.

Panni AS, Tartarone M, Mafulli N: Patellar tendinopathy in athletes: Outcome of operative and nonoperative management. *Am J Sports Med* 2000;28:392-397.

The authors of this study report the results of nonsurgical and surgical management of patellar tendinopathy in 42 athletes with Blazina stage 2 (26 patients) or stage 3 (16 patients) patellar tendinopathy. After 6 months of initial management with nonsteroidal anti-inflammatory drugs, physical therapy, and a progressive rehabilitation program based on isometric exercises, stretching, and eccentric exercises, 33 patients showed symptomatic improvement and were able to resume athletic activity. In nine patients with Blazina stage 3 tendinopathy, nonsurgical management failed, and surgery was done. After a mean follow-up of 4.8 years, clinical results were excellent or good in all patients. In the group treated nonsurgically, results were better in the patients who had stage 2 tendinopathy than in those with stage 3.

Peers KH, Lysens RJ, Brys P, Bellemans J: Cross-sectional outcome analysis of athletes with chronic patellar tendinopathy treated surgically and by extracorporeal shock wave therapy. *Clin J Sport Med* 2003;13:79-83.

This outcome analysis study compared the results of surgical treatment and extracorporeal shock wave therapy for the treatment of chronic patellar tendinitis. The results demonstrate comparable functional outcomes between the two treatment options in patients who were unresponsive to conservative management.

Peters TA, McLean ID: Osteochondritis dissecans of the patellofemoral joint. *Am J Sports Med* 2000; 28:63- 67.

The authors of this study assessed the clinical features of 37 patients with osteochondritis dissecans lesions of the patellofemoral joint and report that treatment generally improved symptoms, but patients with articular cartilage loss experienced persistent patellofemoral crepitus and discomfort.

Classic Bibliography

Aglietti P, Insall JN, Cerulli G: Patellar pain and incongruence: I. Measurements of incongruence. *Clin Orthop* 1983;176:217-224.

Aglietti P, Pisaneschi A, Buzzi R, Gaudenzi A, Allegra M: Arthroscopic lateral release for patellar pain or instability. *Arthroscopy* 1989;5:176-183.

Conlan T, Garth WP, Lemons JE: Evaluation of the medial soft tissue restraints of the extensor mechanism of the knee. *J Bone Joint Surg Am* 1993;75:682-693.

Dainer R, Barrack R, Buckley S, Alexander H: Arthroscopic treatment of acute patellar dislocations. *Arthroscopy* 1988;4:267-271.

Federico D, Reider B: Results of isolated debridement for patellofemoral pain in patients with normal patellar alignment. *Am J Sports Med* 1997;25:663-669.

Fulkerson JP, Becker GJ, Meaney JA, Miranda M, Folcik MA: Anteromedial tibial tubercle transfer without bone graft. *Am J Sports Med* 1990;18:490-496.

Kolowich PA, Paulos LE, Rosenberg TD, Farnsworth S: Lateral release of the patella: Indications and contraindications. *Am J Sports Med* 1990;18:359-365.

Laurin CA, Dussault R, Levesque HP: The tangential x-ray investigation of the patellofemoral joint: X-ray technique. Diagnostic criteria and their interpretation. *Clin Orthop* 1979;144:16-26.

Merchant AC, Mercer RL, Jacobsen RH, Cool CR: Roentgenographic analysis of patellofemoral congruence. *J Bone Joint Surg Am* 1974;56:1391-1396.

Shelbourne KD, Porter DA, Rozzi W: Use of a modified Elmslie-Trillat procedure to improve abnormal patellar congruence angle. *Am J Sports Med* 1994;22:318-323.

Chapter 17

Management of Articular Cartilage Lesions

Jeff A. Fox, MD

Brian J. Cole, MD, MBA

Introduction

With sports participation more common at all ages, articular cartilage injuries are becoming a more common treatment dilemma for the practicing orthopaedist. A myriad of techniques are available to treat these lesions. Although often associated with specific techniques for their management, the truly challenging aspect of managing articular cartilage lesions rests in deciding which procedure to use to maximize the ultimate outcome.

The natural history of chondral lesions remains obscure. A partial-thickness articular cartilage defect will not heal; however, it is not always associated with significant clinical problems. Chondral lesions that penetrate to or through the subchondral bone may fill with fibrocartilage, but fibrocartilage has biochemical properties that are inferior to those of hyaline cartilage. Size is another important variable. On one end of the spectrum, small full-thickness articular cartilage lesions can fill with fibrocartilage and may render a patient asymptomatic. On the other end of the spectrum, large osteochondral lesions are less likely to develop a clinically significant fibrocartilaginous healing response and more frequently result in pain and disability. It is critical to remember that not all chondral lesions cause symptoms and not all symptoms are the result of chondral lesions.

Basic Science: Structure and Function

Articular cartilage is an elaborate mixture of water (65% to 80% of wet weight), collagen (10% to 20% of wet weight), proteoglycans (10% to 15% of wet weight), and chondrocytes (5% of wet weight). The collagen is composed primarily of type II collagen fibers. There are also smaller quantities of collagen types V, VI, IX, X, and XI. Chondrocytes produce the extracellular matrix and are of mesenchymal stem cell origin. The chondrocytes themselves are few in number within the extracellular matrix and have a low rate of cell turnover. The chondrocytes receive nutrients and oxygen from the surrounding synovial fluid by means of diffusion. The function of articular cartilage is to provide a smooth gliding surface that minimizes friction and stress on subchondral bone.

Evaluation of Articular Cartilage Damage

The patient evaluation, one of the most important factors in clinical decision making, consists of history, physical examination, radiographs, and review of previous surgical notes and arthroscopic images.

The patient history will help determine the mechanism of injury. Damage to articular cartilage can be caused by an acute injury and result in a focal, chondral, or osteochondral lesion; osteochondritis dissecans (most common in younger patients); or a degenerative lesion. Patients typically report persistent pain with weight-bearing activities. A thorough physical examination should always be completed to assess knee range of motion, limb alignment, intra-articular effusion, and ligamentous stability.

Radiographs should include standing AP, lateral, Merchant, and 45° flexion PA weight-bearing views. Limb alignment is assessed with full-leg length radiographs. This series of radiographs will show joint space narrowing, osteophytes, cyst formation, and subchondral sclerosis, which are all consistent with osteoarthritis; when present, these are considered relative contraindications for the treatment of articular cartilage lesions. Long-leg alignment radiographs are used to determine where the mechanical axis (ie, a plumb line drawn from the center of the femoral head to the center of the talus) lies. If the mechanical axis bisects the affected compartment, realignment may be necessary. MRI is valuable to assess the status of the knee ligaments and menisci, if unknown. The presence of subchondral edema in the area of a chondral defect may signify overload in that region, but it is not always associated with symptoms. MRI generally tends to underestimate the degree of cartilage abnormalities observed arthroscopically, and there is no uniform consensus regarding the optimal pulse sequence for cartilage imaging. Studies have shown that fat-suppressed imaging is more sensitive than standard MRI for the detection of abnormalities of the hyaline cartilage in the knee. More recently, specialized fast spin-echo MRI sequences with a high-resolution matrix allowed for an accurate assessment of articular cartilage in the knee with little interobserver variability. Although bone bruises that are detected using MRI may be a precursor to an articular cartilage lesion, it is not known how to predict which bone bruises may progress to an articular cartilage lesion or how often.

The role of bone scanning in the assessment of articular cartilage lesions is still being defined. Joint overload that initiates the increased osseous metabolic activity of bone is detectable using scintigraphy. Scintigraphy may be useful in difficult cases in which the source and clinical importance of periarticular symptoms remain in doubt based on the results of the patient's history, physical examination, and radiographic studies. When pain is out of proportion to the clinical presentation, bone scanning can help confirm the existence of increased osseous metabolic activity that is not detectable using other imaging modalities. This increased metabolic activity can be consistent with subchondral activity in the region of a chondral or osteochondral defect.

Nonsurgical Treatment

The first step in the management of articular cartilage lesions is always conservative treatment, which typically begins with the use of various medications or nutritional supplements including acetaminophen, nonsteroidal anti-inflammatory drugs, and glucosamine and chondroitin sulfate. Steroid and hyaluronic acid injections can be helpful in decreasing the symptoms of an articular cartilage lesion, but they are generally of limited benefit to relatively young and active patients. Although physical therapy helps optimize extremity strength and flexibility, it is not highly effective in reducing the symptoms associated with an articular cartilage lesion. When there is an associated malalignment and symptoms are present in the loaded compartment, an unloader brace can help improve symptoms by decreasing the load in the affected compartment. In young and active patients, however, an unloader brace is often not well tolerated.

Surgical Treatment

Débridement and Lavage

Arthroscopic débridement and lavage can temporarily relieve the symptoms of articular cartilage lesions, but the beneficial effects deteriorate over time after the procedure. Most of the literature discusses the results for the treatment of degenerative lesions and rarely includes a population with relatively isolated chondral defects. In older, low-demand patients or those considered less likely to remain compliant with the rehabilitation required of other techniques, however, this may be a first-line option. This technique may be particularly helpful in patients with mechanical symptoms or concomitant meniscal pathology. Typically, only loose cartilage and debris are removed without excessive shaving,

and great care is taken to avoid damaging normal articular surfaces.

Alignment

Any malalignment must be corrected through the judicious use of osteotomies. If malalignment is not corrected, cartilage restoration procedures may fail because the affected compartment will continue to experience increased loads. For patients with varus knee alignment and a lesion in the medial compartment, a medial opening wedge or lateral closing wedge osteotomy should be performed. For patients with valgus knee alignment and a chondral lesion in the lateral compartment, a lateral opening wedge femoral osteotomy or medial closing wedge femoral osteotomy should be performed. For some patients, proximal medial closing wedge osteotomies of the tibia can be used to correct minor degrees of valgus alignment.

Marrow Stimulation Techniques

Marrow stimulation techniques (drilling, abrasion arthroplasty, and microfracture) are effective in treating articular cartilage defects because of the potential for primitive mesenchymal cells to differentiate and produce fibrocartilage repair tissue. Marrow stimulation involves creating a defect in the subchondral bone to allow blood into the cartilage defect to deliver mesenchymal cells and the resultant fibrocartilage formation. Because fibrocartilage primarily consists of type I collagen, it has different biomechanical and structural properties than hyaline cartilage, which primarily consists of type II collagen. The extent and quality of fill is rarely more than 75% of the total volume of the chondral defect. The best results are generally achieved when this technique is used as a first-line treatment for patients with relatively small cartilage defects and for those who are not exceptionally physically demanding on their knees. Drilling of the bone involves using small drills to penetrate through the subchondral bone. Abrasion arthroplasty is performed arthroscopically with a shaver or burr and removes 1 to 2 mm of exposed sclerotic bone down to the vasculature of the subchondral plate. This results in a fibrin clot that later develops into fibrocartilage.

Microfracture was developed in an effort to avoid the heat produced by drilling. Microfracture involves using a small pick to penetrate the subchondral bone, which leaves the majority of the subchondral architecture intact. The first step in this procedure involves creating a well-shouldered lesion that will allow the formation of fibrocartilage. All unstable cartilage should be removed. Animal studies suggest that removing the calcified cartilage with a curet greatly enhances the percentage of defect fill. A surgical awl is then used to create holes placed 2 to 3 mm apart, beginning first at the

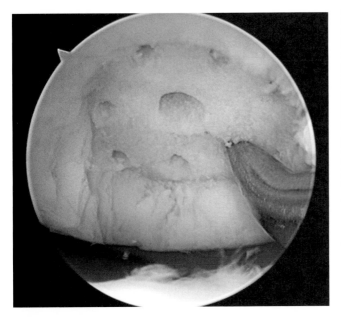

Figure 1 Arthroscopic view of a microfracture of the femoral condyle after the tourniquet has been released, with blood flowing from the penetration of the subchondral bone.

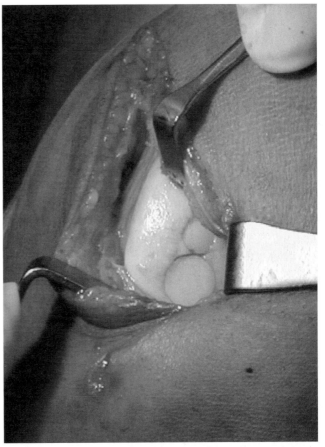

Figure 2 Photograph of an osteochondral autograft with two plugs in place flush with the femoral condyle.

periphery of the lesion (Figure 1). The holes should not be confluent. When fat droplets can be seen coming from the marrow space, the appropriate depth (2 to 4 mm) has been reached. Once the procedure is completed, the tourniquet (if inflated) should be released and the pump pressure turned down to visualize blood and marrow elements coming from each hole. The postoperative rehabilitation program is paramount to the success of this procedure. Patients with femoral condyle and tibial lesions are typically not allowed to bear weight for 6 weeks, whereas patients with patellofemoral lesions are allowed to bear weight initially in extension. Optimally, a continuous passive motion machine is used for 6 hours per day for the first 6 weeks after surgery.

Osteochondral Autograft

Osteochondral autografts survive with intact hyaline cartilage and heal to the surrounding recipient tissue. The key to this procedure is the maintenance of chondrocyte viability. Only living chondrocytes can produce and maintain the extracellular matrix of proper load-bearing capacity. This technique involves transplantation of an osteochondral graft from one region of a joint to another in an effort to restore the damaged articular surface. It is limited by the amount of donor tissue available in the knee. This procedure can be done through a small arthrotomy or arthroscopically. Several commercial systems are available to perform this procedure. When using this technique, it is generally recommended that the lesions are less than 2 cm in diameter (Figure 2). The risk of donor site morbidity increases as more

tissue is harvested. The typical site of harvest is the intercondylar notch and the periphery of the lateral trochlea just proximal to the sulcus terminalis. Although patellofemoral contact does occur in those locations, the clinical significance of this remains unknown.

Fresh Osteochondral Allograft

Fresh osteochondral allografts were first used to restore the articular surface in the early 1900s. As a result of increased graft availability, fresh osteochondral allografts are now used more frequently to treat isolated articular cartilage and osteoarticular defects. Fresh grafts are favored over frozen grafts because chondrocyte survival is diminished after freezing. This is one of the few techniques of cartilage restoration for which long-term (> 15 years) follow-up data are available. Fresh osteochondral allografts are indicated for the treatment of mid- to large-sized lesions with or without subchondral bone involvement in relatively physically demanding patients. Because a subchondral defect is created, the implementation of fresh osteochondral allografts in young patients with superficial and smaller lesions is less commonly indicated.

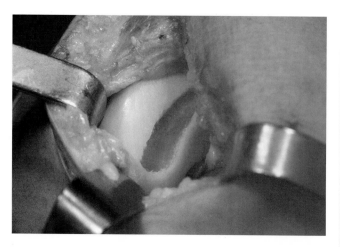

Figure 3 Photograph of a prepared medial femoral condyle lesion (patient is concurrently receiving a medial meniscus transplant).

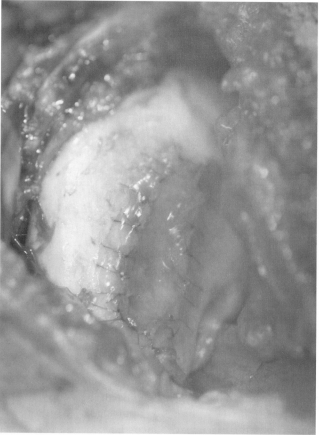

Figure 4 Photograph of a periosteal patch sewn in place, with fibrin glue around the periphery.

In many patients, a medial or lateral peripatellar mini-arthrotomy can be used to expose the lesion. The lesion is assessed to determine the graft shape that would best fit the defect. When possible, an instrumentation system is used to create and harvest a circular graft. Because of the close tolerance between the donor plug and recipient socket that results from this technique, the graft can be press-fit, eliminating the need for supplemental internal fixation. If the lesion is not amenable to a circular graft, a shell graft can be fashioned freehand, typically in a trapezoidal configuration that matches a hand-prepared defect bed using a motorized burr and oscillating saw with cold irrigation. Freehand sizing of a graft is more time-consuming and often requires fixation because the fit is less precise. Recently, there has been concern over the use of allograft tissue. To decrease the risk of disease transmission, it is important to know the source of the graft and the processing technique used. Additionally, grafts that are refrigerated for prolonged periods (> 28 days) have more questionable chondrocyte viability and metabolic activity.

Autogenous Chondrocyte Implantation

Autogenous chondrocyte implantation (ACI) involves culturing chondrocytes and transplanting them into the cartilage defect beneath a periosteal patch. ACI can be used for lesions measuring roughly 2 to 10 cm^2 that are associated with minimal bone loss (6 to 8 mm). This is a two-stage procedure. A biopsy sample must be taken first from either the superomedial edge of the trochlea or the lateral side of the intercondylar notch (the same location where an anterior cruciate ligament notchplasty is performed). The biopsy sample is sent for processing. The biopsy sample can be maintained for 18 months until it is processed and undergoes cellular expansion; after 3 to 5 weeks, it is ready for implantation. The exposure depends on defect location. Patellofemoral lesions are approached through a midline incision, which allows concomitant distal realignment procedures to be routinely performed. Femoral condyle lesions are approached through limited ipsilateral parapatellar arthrotomies (Figures 3 and 4).

Results

To date, it is difficult to derive an evidence-based approach to decision making regarding articular cartilage restoration. The initial studies evaluating abrasion arthroplasty and Pridie drilling included patients with an average age of 50 years and arthritic knees. This population is not comparable to younger patients with symptomatic focal chondral defects treated with osteochondral allografts or ACI, for example. In addition, concomitantly performed procedures often generate nonhomogeneous patient populations. The results of abrasion arthroplasty are unpredictable and generally deteriorate with time. Good results can be expected in 39% to 60% of patients at initial short-term follow-up. One study reported on 73 patients who were treated with abrasion arthroplasty and found that 83% of patients still had "pain present" at 6- to 18-month follow-up.

There have been few published clinical studies on microfracture. One such study recently reported on 71 patients who underwent microfracture and were assessed at 7- to 17-year follow-up; 80% of the patients rated themselves as improved, and patients younger than 35 years had the best outcomes. In an earlier study, some of the same principal authors reported 3- to 5-year results showing that 75% of patients were improved and 20% were unchanged with regard to pain. Regarding activities of daily living and labor, 65% of patients improved, 20% were unchanged, and 13% were worse.

The results of osteochondral autograft transplantation are summarized in Table 1. One study recently reported the 10-year results of 831 patients who underwent osteochondral autograft transplantation; 92% of patients with femoral condyle lesions and 79% of patients with patellar lesions had good to excellent outcomes. Another study reported on a subset of 52 osteochondral autografts in competitive athletes with follow-up greater than 1 year. All patients had Hospital for Special Surgery scores of good to excellent; however, only 63% returned to full athletic participation. Thirty-one percent returned to athletic participation at a lower level. Ninety percent of patients younger than 30 years returned to full athletic participation, whereas only 23% of patients older than 30 years returned to full athletic participation. A multicenter prospective study that compared marrow stimulation techniques to osteochondral allografts in 413 patients reported that osteochondral autografts resulted in significantly better outcomes at 3, 4, and 5 years.

More long-term outcome data are available for osteochondral allografts than any other cartilage defect repair procedure (Table 2). One study reported an initial success rate of 91%; at 10-year follow-up, the success rate was 75%. The treatment of unipolar cartilage defects with osteochondral allografts is considerably more successful than that for bipolar cartilage defects. Treatment of osteochondritis dissecans lesions in adults

using osteochondral allografts is also associated with excellent results.

Published outcome data for ACI now extend to a 9-year follow-up (Table 3). One study reported on 50 patients who were prospectively observed for a minimum of 36 months. Seventy-eight percent of the patients had a previous cartilage repair procedure. Eighty-four percent of the patients had an improvement in their condition, 2% were unchanged, and the condition of 13% declined. One third of these patients had undergone previous marrow stimulation procedures. Another study that included 94 patients with a 2- to 9-year follow-up reported that results varied considerably based on location. When ACI was used to treat articular cartilage lesions of the patella, good to excellent results were reported in 62% of the patients. Later in the series, the authors began performing a distal realignment on these patients, and good to excellent results were then reported in 85% of the patients. Most biopsy specimens revealed the presence of hyaline-like tissue, and immunohistochemical staining for type II cartilage was positive in all biopsy specimens for hyaline-like cartilage. A hypertrophic periosteal healing response with pain and catching occurred in 10% to 15% of the patients be-

TABLE 1 | Osteochondral Autograft Transplantation Results

Author	Type/Location	No. of Patients	Mean Follow-up (months)	Good to Excellent Results (%)
Hangody and Fules (2003)	Femur	461	> 12	92
	Patella/trochlea	93		79
	Tibia	24		87
Kish et al (1999)	Femur	52	> 12	100
Hangody et al (1998)	Femur/patella	57	48	91

TABLE 2 | Osteochondral Allograft Transplantation Results

Author(s)	No. of Patients	Location	Diagnosis	Mean Follow-up (years)	Mean Age (years)	Results (%)		
						Success Rate	Good to Excellent	Failures
Aubin et al (2001)	60	Femur	Multiple	10.0	27		66	20
Bugbee et al (1999)	122	Femur	Multiple	5.0	34	91		5
Chu et al (1999)	55	Femur, tibia, patella	Multiple	6.3	35		76	16
Gross (1997)	123	Femur, tibia, patella	Trauma/osteochondritis dissecans	7.5	35	85		
Garrett (1994)	17	Femur	Osteochondritis dissecans	3.5	20	94		

TABLE 3 | Autologous Chondrocyte Implantation Results

Author(s)	Location	No. of Patients	Mean Follow-up (years)	Results (%)			
				Significant Improvement	Good to Excellent	Fair	Poor
Peterson et al (2002)	Femur	18	> 5		89		
	Osteochondritis dissecans	14	> 5		86		
	Patella	17	> 5		65		
	Femur/anterior cruciate ligament	11	> 5		91		
Minas (2001)	Femur, trochlea, patella, tibia	169	> 1	85			
Micheli et al (2001)	Femur, trochlea, patella	50	> 3	84			
Peterson et al (2000)	Femur	25	> 2		92		
	Patella	19	> 2		65		
	Femur/anterior cruciate ligament	16	> 2		75		
	Multiple	16	> 2		67		
Gillogly et al (1998)	Femur/patella/tibia	25	> 1	88	88		
	Femur/patella	16	3.25		88	–	13
	Patella	7	3		29	43	29

tween 3 and 9 months, and arthroscopic evaluation was required. Graft failure was reported in up to 7% of the patients.

Postoperative Management

Postoperative management is crucial to the success of these procedures. Noncompliance may lead to procedure failure.

Microfracture

The microfracture technique requires a modification of weight bearing and use of continuous passive motion after the surgery. One group of authors recommends 6 hours of continuous passive motion each day for 8 weeks and found better gross healing during second-look arthroscopy in patients who used continuous passive motion when compared with those who did not. If patients are unable to use a continuous passive motion machine, they should do 500 repetitions of knee flexion and extension three times every day. Patients with weight-bearing lesions must not bear weight for 6 to 8 weeks. Patients who have been treated for a trochlear/patellar lesion may bear weight in extension, but they should have their flexion initially limited to about 45° to 60° depending on the flexion angle of defect contact.

Osteochondral Autograft Transplantation

Similarly, the rehabilitation program for patients after osteochondral autograft transplantation relies on early motion and gradual load bearing to ensure chondrocyte survival and continued production of extracellular matrix components. Patients should not bear weight for the

first 2 weeks and should progress to full weight bearing over the ensuing 6 weeks depending on the stability of the implanted grafts. Ergometer exercises typically may begin at 6 to 8 weeks; at 3 months, normal daily activities are typically possible. Some running can begin at 6 months. Athletic activities that involve shear forces can begin at 9 months. Some authors have advocated immediate weight bearing after osteochondral autograft transplantation.

For patients who have undergone osteochondral allograft transplantation, restricted weight bearing is recommended for at least 8 weeks to protect the cartilage surface and to minimize the chance for subchondral collapse during the creeping substitution phase of graft healing. Continuous passive motion is used for 6 to 8 hours per day at 1 cycle per minute as tolerated for the first 4 to 6 weeks. Return to normal activities of daily living and light athletic activity is considered at 4 to 6 months. In general, participation in high-impact sports is not recommended after osteochondral allografting for large articular cartilage lesions because of the risk of graft collapse and potential deterioration in the long-term survival of the graft.

Autogenous Chondrocyte Implantation

For patients who have undergone ACI, the rehabilitation program for the first 6 weeks postoperatively also consists of continuous passive motion for 6 to 8 hours per day. Continuous passive motion has a beneficial effect on the quality of the repair tissue and on the degree of defect fill. Initially, weight bearing should be restricted; however, patients who have undergone ACI to treat

TABLE 4 | Surgical Treatment Options for Chondral Defects

Procedure	Indications	Outcome
Arthroscopic débridement and lavage	Minimal symptoms	Palliative
Marrow stimulation	Smaller lesions, low-demand patients	Reparative
Osteochondral autograft	Smaller lesions, low- or high-demand patients	Restorative
Osteochondral allograft	Larger lesions with bone loss, low- or high-demand patients	Restorative
Autologous chondrocyte implantation	Small and large lesions with and without bone loss, high-demand patients	Restorative
Genetic engineering	Investigational	Restorative

are initiated at 6 weeks. For 3 to 5 months, strengthening exercises continue with wider arcs of motion and increased resistance. Patients who have undergone ACI for trochlear repairs should be restricted from performing deep flexion exercises. The final phase of recovery lasts until there is a full return to activities. This may be as soon as 12 months for patients with small and moderate lesions and as late as 18 months for those with larger lesions or patellofemoral repairs.

Clinical Decision Making

Beyond primary repair, nonprosthetic treatment options for focal chondral defects can be described as palliative, reparative, or restorative (Table 4) (Figure 5). Arthroscopic débridement and lavage is palliative because it provides only temporary relief. Reparative treatment includes marrow stimulation techniques that result in fibrocartilage formation within the defect. Restorative techniques are those that result in cartilage formation that is articular in nature. This includes osteochondral autograft/allograft transplantation, periosteal/perichondrial transplantation, and ACI.

Several factors must be considered before selecting a patient for a particular procedure. Defect size, depth, location, chronicity, response to previous treatments, concomitant pathology, patient age, physical demand level,

trochlear/patellar lesions may bear weight in extension if a distal realignment was not performed. In most patients, an anteromedialization procedure is recommended as concomitant treatment of patellofemoral lesions, and weight bearing is restricted early to minimize the chance for postoperative tibial fracture. Strengthening exercises should focus on quadriceps and hamstring exercises. Short arc closed-chain strengthening exercises

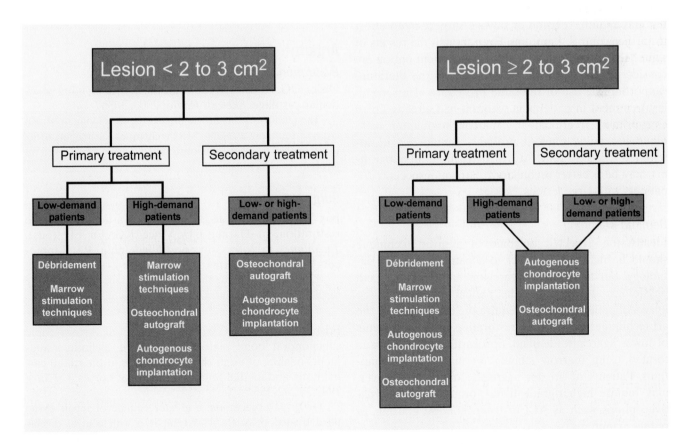

Figure 5 Treatment algorithm for articular cartilage procedures based on size, primary or secondary treatment, and patient demand.

and expectations should all be considered when attempting to match the most appropriate treatment option to the existing pathology. At this particular time, given the complexity of this problem, evidence-based decision making remains an ideal that is yet to be realized.

Chondral Lesion Size

Some generalizations can be made with regard to chondral lesion size, but there are no absolutes. Each technique is surgeon- and situation-specific and varies accordingly. Smaller lesions (< 2 to 3 cm^2) may be amenable to arthroscopic débridement and lavage, marrow stimulation, osteochondral autograft transplantation, and ACI. As the size of the lesion increases (≥ 2 to 3 cm^2), the limits of osteochondral autograft transplantation are approached. Osteochondral allograft transplantation may become a more viable option when the defect is associated with subchondral bone loss. Marrow stimulation techniques have poorer outcomes when used to treat lesions larger than 3 cm^2. ACI is also a viable treatment option for larger lesions.

Primary Versus Secondary Treatment

Some treatment methods, although notably effective, may offer only short- or medium-term symptomatic relief. Thus, patients with symptomatic chondral lesions often may require revision or salvage surgery in an effort to further control symptoms. Even though the results of some techniques used as a primary treatment option are considered limited, there are few data in the literature supporting the use of the same procedure as a secondary treatment in patients in whom it had already failed as a primary treatment. If a marrow stimulation technique has failed once, it probably should not be attempted a second time. ACI or osteochondral allografting may be a better secondary treatment, especially for patients with large lesions.

Demand Matching

Ideally, the expected outcome of a given technique should be matched not only to a patient's specific pathology, but also to the aggregate biomechanical and physiologic demand that the patient imposes on the knee. All patients may not require the use of state of the art techniques for cartilage restoration. In some patients of lower aggregate demand, fibrocartilage repair tissue formed using marrow stimulation may reduce symptoms. Patients of greater aggregate demand, however, may require higher-grade tissue formed using alternative options, such as ACI or osteochondral grafting, to reduce symptoms.

Future Considerations

Genetic engineering is a new strategy for treating chondral injuries. This involves a combination of gene transfer techniques and tissue engineering. In gene therapy, specific genes for growth factors are transferred into the chondrocyte or progenitor cells. Once treated, these cells have the potential to produce the growth factors that are conducive to chondrocyte proliferation. Tissue engineering is based on the creation of biologic substitutes for the repair or regeneration of damaged tissue. The application of this process to treat chondral defects involves the transplantation of viable cells into an appropriate supportive vehicle. ACI is an example of this technique, but the ideal scaffold for cartilage engineering has not yet been identified. It is likely that future considerations will focus on the identification of these scaffolds, reductions in the expenses associated with the production of these technologies, and development of less invasive means to implement cartilage restoration procedures.

Summary

The management of articular cartilage lesions is an evolving treatment continuum. Each patient must be carefully evaluated to determine the most appropriate treatment plan. Clinical and basic science research continues to improve the treatment of articular cartilage lesions in this dynamic area of orthopaedic surgery.

Annotated Bibliography

Evaluation of Articular Cartilage Damage

Disler DG, Recht MP, McCauley TR: MR imaging of articular cartilage. *Skeletal Radiol* 2000;29:367-377.

The authors of this article discuss the development of two types of routinely available MRI techniques for imaging articular cartilage that have demonstrated clinical accuracy and interobserver reliability.

Surgical Treatment

Fox JA, Kalsi RS, Cole BJ: Update on articular cartilage restoration, in Harner CD, Vince KG, Fu FH (eds): *Techniques in Knee Surgery*. Philadelphia, PA, Lippincott Williams & Wilkins, 2003, vol 2, pp 2-17.

The authors describe the current technique for each of the cartilage repair procedures discussed in this chapter.

Frisbie DD, Trotter GW, Powers BE, et al: Arthroscopic subchondral bone plate microfracture technique augments healing of large chondral defects in the radial carpal bone and medial femoral condyle of horses. *Vet Surg* 1999;28:242-255.

On gross observation, a greater volume of repair tissue filled treated defects (74%) compared with control defects (45%). Histomorphometry confirmed that more repair tissue filled treated defects, but no difference in the relative amounts of different tissue types was observed. An increased percentage of type II collagen and evidence of earlier bone remodeling as documented by changes in porosity were found in treated defects compared with control defects. In full-thickness chondral defects in exercised horses, treatment with subchondral bone microfracture increased the tissue volume in the defects and the percentage of type II collagen in the tissue filling the defects when compared with untreated defects. No negative effects of the microfracture technique were observed, and some of the beneficial effects are the basis for the authors' recommendation of its use in patients with exposed subchondral bone.

Results

Aubin PP, Cheah HK, Davis AM, Gross AE: Long-term followup of fresh femoral osteochondral allografts for posttraumatic knee defects. *Clin Orthop* 2001; 391(suppl):S318-S327.

The authors of this study observed 60 patients and report 85% survivorship at 10 years and 74% survivorship at 15 years.

Bugbee WD: Fresh osteochondral allografts. *J Knee Surg* 2002;15:191-195.

The author of this article reports that allografts demonstrated > 75% clinical success in the treatment of focal femoral condyle lesions caused by trauma, chondral injury, osteochondral trauma, osteochondritis dissecans, avascular necrosis, and posttraumatic reconstruction.

Bugbee WD, Convery FR: Osteochondral allograft transplantation. *Clin Sports Med* 1999;18:67-75.

The authors found that the success rate of fresh osteochondral allografting, particularly in isolated femoral condylar defects, compared favorably with other currently available cartilage repair and resurfacing techniques. In their second 100 patients, they found the failure of monopolar allografts to be exceedingly rare in short-term follow-up. Fresh osteochondral allografting also appears to be effective in treating larger osteochondral lesions, for which there are few other attractive alternatives.

Chu CR, Convery FR, Akeson WH, Meyers M, Amiel D: Articular cartilage transplantation: Clinical results in the knee. *Clin Orthop* 1999;360:159-168.

In this study, 55 patients underwent osteochondral allograft transplantation. At 10-year follow-up, 73% of patients reported good to excellent results, and 84% of patients with unipolar disease regained normal use of their knees.

Gillogly SD, Voight M, Blackburn T: Treatment of articular cartilage defects of the knee with autologous chondrocyte implantation. *J Orthop Sports Phys Ther* 1998; 28:241-251.

The authors of this article review the efficacy of available treatment options and the basic science rationale, indications, technique, postoperative rehabilitation, and clinical results of

using cultured autologous chondrocytes to treat focal full-thickness chondral defects of the knee.

Hangody L, Fules P: Autologous osteochondral mosaicplasty for the treatment of full-thickness defects of weight-bearing joints: Ten years of experimental and clinical experience. *J Bone Joint Surg Am* 2003;85(suppl 2):25-32.

The authors of this study report that good to excellent results were achieved in 92% of patients treated with femoral condylar implantations, 87% of those treated with tibial resurfacing, 79% of those treated with patellar and/or trochlear mosaicplasties, and 94% of those treated with talar procedures. Long-term donor-site disturbances, assessed with use of the Bandi score, showed that patients had 3% morbidity after mosaicplasty. Sixty-nine of 83 patients who were followed arthroscopically showed congruent gliding surfaces, histologic evidence of the survival of the transplanted hyaline cartilage, and fibrocartilage filling of the donor sites. Surgical complications included 4 deep infections and 36 painful postoperative hemarthroses. On the basis of these promising results and those of other similar studies, the authors conclude that autologous osteochondral mosaicplasty appears to be a viable alternative for the treatment of small- and medium-sized focal chondral and osteochondral defects of the weight-bearing surfaces of the knee and other weight-bearing synovial joints.

Hangody L, Kish G, Karpati Z, Udvarhelyi I, Szigeti I, Bely M: Mosaicplasty for the treatment of articular cartilage defects: Application in clinical practice. *Orthopedics* 1998;21:751-756.

Since 1992, 227 patients underwent mosaicplasty to treat full-thickness lesions resulting from chondropathy, traumatic chondral defects, and osteochondritis dissecans; the procedure was evaluated in 57 patients at greater than 3 years of follow-up. MRI, CT arthrography, ultrasound, and arthroscopy were used to evaluate the technique. Using the modified Hospital for Special Surgery knee scoring system, 91% of the patients achieved a good or excellent result. The surgical technique, clinical results, and complications are detailed.

Kish G, Modis L, Hangody L: Osteochondral mosaicplasty for the treatment of focal chondral and osteochondral lesions of the knee and talus in the athlete: Rationale, indications, techniques, and results. *Clin Sports Med* 1999;18:45-66.

The authors of this study used autogenous osteochondral grafting mosaicplasty to treat injuries in the athlete population for the 6 years. They discuss the rationale, indications, surgical technique, results, and limitations of mosaicplasty.

Micheli LJ, Browne JE, Erggelet C, et al: Autologous chondrocyte implantation of the knee: Multicenter experience and minimum 3-year follow-up. *Clin J Sport Med* 2001;11:223-228.

Clinician and patient evaluation indicated median improvements in four and five criteria, respectively, in 50 patients at 36 months following ACI ($P < 0.001$). Previous treatment with marrow stimulation techniques and the size of defect did not impact the results of ACI. The most common adverse events reported were adhesions, arthrofibrosis, and hypertrophic changes. Three patients had graft failure and required reimplantation or treatment with alternative cartilage repair techniques. Kaplan-Meier analysis estimated freedom from graft failure was 94% at 36 months postoperatively (95% confidence interval, 88% to 100%). The results of this study indicate excellent graft survivorship using ACI as well as substantial improvement in functional outcome.

Minas T: Autologous chondrocyte implantation for focal chondral defects of the knee. *Clin Orthop* 2001; 391(suppl):S349-S361.

The author of this study evaluated 169 patients who underwent ACI to treat focal chondral defects of the knee. Overall, 87% improved and 13% were considered treatment failures.

Peterson L, Brittberg M, Kiviranta I, Akerlund EL, Lindahl A: Autologous chondrocyte transplantation: Biomechanics and long-term durability. *Am J Sports Med* 2002;30:2-12.

The authors of this study observed 61 patients who underwent autologous chondrocyte transplantation. At a minimum follow-up of 5 years, 50 of 61 patients had good to excellent results.

Peterson L, Minas T, Brittberg M, Nilsson A, Sjogren-Jansson E, Lindahl A: Two- to 9-year outcome after autologous chondrocyte transplantation of the knee. *Clin Orthop* 2000;374:212-234.

Ninety-four patients were evaluated at 2- to 9-year follow-up. Good to excellent clinical results were observed in patients who underwent autologous chondrocyte transplantation for isolated femoral condyle repair (92%), repair of multiple lesions (67%), osteochondritis dissecans (89%), patellar repair (65%), and femoral condyle with anterior cruciate ligament repair (75%). Arthroscopic findings in 53 patients showed good repair tissue fill, good adherence to underlying bone, seamless integration with adjacent cartilage, and hardness comparable with that of the adjacent tissue. Hypertrophic response of the periosteum or graft or both was identified in 26 patients during arthroscopy; 7 patients were symptomatic and their symptoms resolved after arthroscopic trimming. Graft failure occurred in 7 patients (4 of the first 23 and 3 of the next 78). Histologic analysis of 37 biopsy specimens showed a correlation between hyaline-like tissue (hyaline matrix staining was positive for type II collagen and lacked a fibrous component) and good to excellent clinical results. The good clinical outcomes of autologous chondrocyte transplantation in this study are encouraging, and clinical trials are being done to compare the outcomes with those of traditional fibrocartilage repair techniques.

Steadman JR, Briggs KK, Rodrigo JJ, Kocher MS, Gill TJ, Rodkey WG: Outcomes of microfracture for traumatic chondral defects of the knee: Average 11-year follow-up. *Arthroscopy* 2003;19:477-484.

At final follow-up, the Medical Outcomes Study 36-Item Short Form and Western Ontario and McMaster Osteoarthritis Index scores showed good to excellent results. At 7 years after surgery, 80% of the patients rated themselves as "improved." Multivariate analysis revealed that age was a predictor of functional improvement. Over the 7- to 17-year follow-up period (average, 11.3 years), patients age 45 years and younger who underwent the microfracture procedure for the treatment of full-thickness chondral defects without associated meniscus or ligament pathology showed statistically significant improvement in function and indicated that they had less pain.

Clinical Decision Making

Martinek GETV, Fu FH, Lee CW, Huard J: Treatment of osteochondral injuries: Genetic engineering. *Clin Sports Med* 2001;20:403-416.

This article discusses the future of cartilage treatment using genetic engineering.

Classic Bibliography

Curl WW, Krome J, Gordon ES, Rushing J, Smith BP, Poehling GG: Cartilage injuries: A review of 31,516 knee arthroscopies. *Arthroscopy* 1997;13:456-460.

Friedman MJ, Berasi CC, Fox JM, Del Pizzo W, Snyder SJ, Ferkel RD: Preliminary results with abrasion arthroplasty in the osteoarthritic knee. *Clin Orthop* 1984;182: 200-205.

Garrett JC: Fresh osteochondral allografts for treatment of articular defects in osteochondritis dissecans of the lateral femoral condyle in adults. *Clin Orthop* 1994;303: 33-37.

Ghazavi MT, Pritzker KP, Davis AM, Gross AE: Fresh osteochondral allografts for post-traumatic osteochondral defects of the knee. *J Bone Joint Surg Br* 1997;79: 1008-1013.

Gross AE: Fresh osteochondral allografts for posttraumatic knee defects: Surgical techniques. *Oper Tech Orthop* 1997;7:334.

Outerbridge RE: The etiology of chondromalacia patellae. *J Bone Joint Surg Br* 1961;43:742-757.

Rodrigo JJ, Steadman JR, Silliman JF, Fulstone HA: Improvement of full-thickness chondral defect healing in the human knee after debridement and microfracture using continuous passive motion. *Am J Knee Surg* 1994;7:109-116.

Chapter 18

Athletic Ankle Injuries

Annunziato Amendola, MD, FRCSC

Soheil Najibi, MD, PhD

Lisa Wasserman, MD, FRCSC

Introduction

Ankle injuries continue to be one of the most common causes of missed time from participation in athletic activities. Most ankle injuries can be successfully treated by conservative means; however, an understanding of the indications for surgical intervention can facilitate recovery and hasten return to play.

Lateral Ankle Sprains

Anatomy

The lateral ligamentous complex of the ankle joint consists of the anterior talofibular ligament (ATFL), the calcaneofibular ligament (CFL), and the posterior talofibular ligament (PTFL) (Figure 1). A fourth structure, the lateral talocalcaneal ligament (LTCL), is variable and may be found coalescing with the ATFL and/or the CFL. The ATFL is the primary restraint to inversion in plantar flexion. It also resists anterolateral translation of the talus in the mortise. It originates 10 mm proximal to the tip of the fibula, just lateral to the margin of the articular cartilage. It is directed 45° medially toward the talus in the coronal plane and inserts directly distal to the articular cartilage of the talar body, averaging 18 mm dorsal to the subtalar joint. It is the weakest of the lateral ligaments.

The CFL is the primary restraint to inversion when the ankle is in the neutral or dorsiflexed position. The CFL restrains subtalar inversion, thereby limiting talar tilt within the ankle mortise. The CFL originates on the anterior edge of the fibula, 9 mm proximal to the distal tip. It subtends an angle of 133° from the posterior border of the fibula, inserting on the calcaneus 13 mm distal to the subtalar joint and deep to the peroneal tendon sheaths. The PTFL is the strongest of the collateral ligaments and bridges the posterolateral tubercle of the talus to the posterior aspect of the lateral malleolus.

Mechanism and Grading of Injury

The ankle is in a position of instability in plantar flexion and inversion as a consequence of the narrow diameter of the talus posteriorly. The anterolateral joint capsule

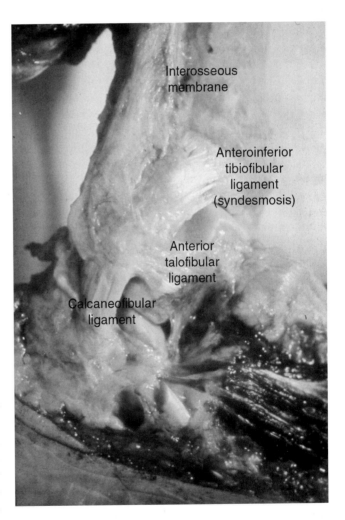

Figure 1 Ligaments of the ankle.

fails first, followed by rupture of the ATFL, and finally the CFL as the arc of injury progresses laterally. The ATFL is involved in 85% of lateral sprains. The CFL is injured concomitantly in 20% to 40% of patients. The PTFL usually is not disrupted.

Grade 1 injuries involve stretching of the ATFL, accompanied by mild tenderness, no evidence of mechanical instability, and ability to bear weight with minimal discomfort. Grade 2 injuries represent a complete tear of the ATFL, usually associated with a partial injury of the CFL. There is moderate tenderness present. Although stability testing may be difficult because of pain, moderate laxity is noted with the anterior drawer test, whereas the results of the talar tilt test remain negative. Grade 3 injuries involve complete rupture of both the ATFL and CFL. Although there is severe tenderness, patients are usually able to bear some weight, albeit with pain and difficulty. The results of the anterior drawer test and talar tilt test are both grossly positive in these patients.

Nonsurgical Treatment

Functional, nonsurgical management remains the treatment of choice for all grades of lateral ankle ligamentous injury. Grades 1 and 2 sprains may be treated with an elastic wrap over a felt horseshoe to minimize swelling and promote rapid return of full range of motion. A short period of weight-bearing immobilization in a removable boot may be necessary. Frequent applications of ice and range-of-motion exercises should be instituted. Once swelling has receded and a good range of motion has been achieved, neuromuscular retraining exercises should begin. These should concentrate on peroneal muscle strengthening and proprioceptive training. A functional brace that controls inversion and eversion is typically used during the strengthening period and prophylactically for high-risk activities thereafter. The treatment of grade 3 injuries is similar, although an extended initial immobilization period in a weight-bearing cast or removable boot for up to 3 weeks may be warranted. In a 1991 literature review of 12 prospective randomized studies comparing surgical and nonsurgical treatment as well as immobilization and functional treatment of grade 3 sprains, the authors concluded that functional, nonsurgical treatment was the method of choice and provided the earliest recovery of range of motion and return to work or physical activity. The incidence of late mechanical instability did not differ among the various treatment protocols.

The use of tape, a brace, or high-top sneakers has been shown to reduce the incidence and possibly the severity of ankle sprains. Although tape is effective when initially applied, it may lose up to 50% of its original support after 10 to 20 minutes of exercise.

Surgical Treatment

There are few indications for acute surgical repair of lateral ligament rupture in the ankle. One recent review, however, found a decreased incidence of late recurrent instability after acute surgical intervention. Some reports advocating acute repairs in ballet dancers may also be found in the literature. Bony avulsion injuries may be treated with surgical repair.

Sequelae of Acute Ankle Sprains and Chronic Lateral Ligamentous Insufficiency

Up to 50% of patients will continue to experience symptoms following an acute ankle sprain. Three common presentations are pain, pain and instability, or instability alone. The most common cause of chronic pain following an ankle sprain is a missed associated injury. Important structures to consider include the anterior process of the calcaneus, the lateral or posterior process of the talus, the base of the fifth metatarsal, the syndesmosis ligaments, the peroneal tendons, and the possibility of an osteochondral lesion of the talar dome. A complex regional pain syndrome may be present. Reports of instability must be probed to determine whether true mechanical instability caused by ligamentous laxity exists. This is differentiated from functional instability related to muscular weakness or pain inhibition reflexes from associated injury. If pain is not present between sprains, true mechanical instability may be the primary problem.

Stress radiographs are not recommended because of the large variability in physiologic values and the lack of correlation with clinical symptoms. Initial treatment of all patients, regardless of the duration of the instability, involves a therapy program of peroneal muscle strengthening and proprioceptive training, combined with the use of a lace-up brace for high-risk activities. This regimen is effective in 90% of patients. The remaining patients are candidates for surgical stabilization. If pain is present between instability episodes and an associated lesion has been identified, it is wise to treat this cause before considering surgical stabilization of the ankle. If no associated lesion is identified, arthroscopy should be performed immediately preceding the lateral repair. The preferred procedure is the Gould modification of the Broström procedure: an anatomic shortening and reinsertion of the ATFL and CFL, reinforced with the inferior extensor retinaculum and distal fibular periosteum. Good or excellent results have been reported in 90% of patients with this procedure.

Nonanatomic reconstructions sacrifice all or part of the peroneus brevis tendon to provide a tenodesis effect across the ankle and subtalar joints. Concerns regarding the loss of the dynamic stabilizing effect of the peroneus brevis and overtightening of the subtalar joint have contributed to their decrease in popularity. Some authors recommend using tendons other than the peroneus brevis or allograft tendon. Tenodesis procedures that attempt to anatomically replace the ATFL and CFL (the Colville procedure) appear to have better functional and radiologic success compared with those that do not replicate the course of the native ligaments (the Watson-Jones procedure and the Evans procedure). Recalcitrant inversion injury in the presence of a varus

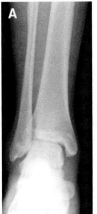
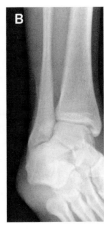
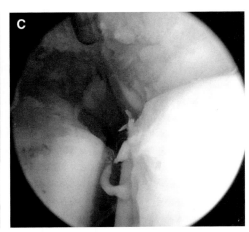
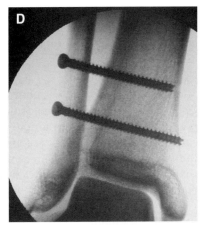

Figure 2 AP (**A**) and mortise (**B**) radiographs showing slight widening of medial and tibiofibular clear spaces. **C,** Arthroscopic view of anteroinferior tibiofibular ligament disruption. **D,** Radiograph showing fixation of the syndesmosis. *(Reproduced with permission from Wasserman L, Amendola A, Saltzman C: Ankle arthroscopy in sports traumatology. Perspectives en Arthroscopie 2004;3:55-60.)*

hindfoot may warrant consideration of supramalleolar or calcaneal osteotomy.

Chronic subtalar instability is believed to be associated with lateral mechanical instability 10% to 25% of patients. The structures considered to be most important in stabilizing the subtalar joint are the CFL, LTCL, interosseous talocalcaneal ligament, and cervical ligament. The mechanism of injury typically involves supination with the ankle in dorsiflexion, or alternatively, the continuation of the arc of injury in a standard inversion ankle sprain. Chronic repetitive stress on the ligaments from athletic activities involving jumping has also been proposed as a mechanism of injury. Controversy continues to surround the diagnosis because positive stress radiographs do not correlate with symptoms. MRI has recently been shown to be accurate in identifying ligamentous injury of the subtalar joint. Initial treatment involves the same rehabilitation protocol as for lateral instability. Surgical treatment involves reconstructing the relevant anatomy.

Syndesmosis Injuries and Medial Ankle Sprains

Anatomy

The distal tibiofibular articulation is secured by the anteroinferior tibiofibular ligament (AITFL), posteroinferior tibiofibular ligament, transverse tibiofibular ligament, and interosseous membrane (Figure 1). The deltoid ligament is composed of a superficial and a deep layer. The superficial layer takes origin from the anterior colliculus and fans out to insert into the navicular, neck of the talus, sustentaculum tali, and posteromedial talar tubercle. The tibiocalcaneal portion is its strongest component and resists eversion of the calcaneus. The deep deltoid is the primary medial stabilizer of the ankle joint. It originates from the anterior and posterior

colliculi of the medial malleolus and inserts into the medial body of the talus.

Mechanism of Injury

Syndesmotic ankle sprain, also referred to as a "high ankle sprain," results from an external rotation or abduction force at the ankle. Less commonly, a severe inversion force may be the cause. Syndesmotic injuries are estimated to be involved in 1% to 10% of all ankle sprains.

Diagnosis

Patients with syndesmotic injuries typically exhibit point tenderness over the AITFL. Estimation of the extent of interosseous ligament injury is made clinically by the proximal extent of tenderness to palpation. Dorsiflexion and external rotation of the ankle usually causes pain. Squeezing the tibia and fibula together at the midcalf level will reproduce pain at the syndesmosis in the presence of an injury.

Standard radiographs of the ankle should be obtained. If these are normal, a mortise view taken with the ankle held in dorsiflexion and external rotation may demonstrate widening of the syndesmosis (Figure 2). This is represented by widening of the medial clear space of greater than 4 mm or widening of the tibiofibular clear space of greater than 6 mm. Syndesmotic sprain may occur without a frank diastasis, even on stress radiographs. Its presence may be confirmed clinically and radiographically by the late appearance of calcification in the interosseous membrane. Chronic syndesmotic injury may be diagnosed clinically by taping the ankle with cloth or silk 2-inch tape. The tape is applied tightly just above the malleoli. The patient is then asked to walk, jump, and run to reproduce the symptoms. If pain is resolved with the tape on, a syndesmotic injury is confirmed. Injury of the deltoid ligament may occur with syndesmotic sprains. Isolated medial ankle sprains are uncommon and usually occur with eversion combined with external rotation of the ankle.

Nonsurgical Treatment

Ankle sprains with syndesmotic involvement typically display a prolonged and notoriously variable recovery period. Immobilization in a non–weight-bearing cast or splint for 2 to 3 weeks is recommended. A functional therapy program using a brace that prevents external rotation stress should then be instituted. These injuries typically resolve within 8 to 12 weeks of injury.

Surgical Treatment

Patients who are refractory to conservative treatment, those displaying diastasis on plain or stress radiographs, and those presenting longer than 3 months since the time of injury should undergo surgical treatment. Two 4.5-mm syndesmosis screws through four cortices are placed. The postoperative plaster splint is removed after 2 weeks; however, non–weight-bearing status is maintained for 6 weeks. The screws are routinely removed after 12 weeks. A recent study challenges the principle of holding the ankle in maximum dorsiflexion while the screws are placed to avoid overtightening. Post-sprain impingement lesions of the syndesmosis may occur. These result from a fascicle of the AITFL that becomes trapped intra-articularly. Treatment involves arthroscopic removal of the fascicle.

Tendinopathies

Achilles Tendon

Anatomy and Physiology

The two heads of the gastrocnemius muscle from the medial and lateral femoral condyles blend with the soleus muscle and form the Achilles tendon, which inserts into the middle third of the posterior tuberosity of the calcaneus. The Achilles tendon, posterior calcaneus, retrocalcaneal bursa (between the calcaneus and Achilles tendon), and adventitial bursa (between the Achilles tendon and skin) are the anatomic structures comprising the posterior heel.

The basic constituent of the tendon is collagen, which accounts for 95% of its dry weight. Approximately 95% is collagen type I, with elastin present only in small amounts. The Achilles tendon lacks a true synovial sheath. Rather, the entire tendon is surrounded by the deep epitenon and superficial paratenon. The paratenon has two layers that are connected by the mesotenon. All of the layers together form the peritendon. The Achilles tendon rotates 30° to 150° before its insertion point. This permits elongation and elastic recoil within the tendon, allowing stored energy to be released during the appropriate phase of gait. Rotation of the Achilles tendon also produces a stress concentration

zone at an area 2 to 6 cm proximal to its insertion as a result of the sawing action of fibers twisting across each other.

The blood supply of the Achilles tendon is from three sources: vessels in the musculotendinous junction, the surrounding mesotenal connective tissue, and the calcaneal osseous insertion. Several authors have documented a decrease in the number of blood vessels in the midportion of the tendon. This corresponds to the most common site of rupture.

Muscle activation results in force transmission to bone via tendons to produce joint movement. The human Achilles tendon can be subjected to considerable loads during locomotion, which can cause the tendon to deform. The load may reach tensile forces of 1,400 to 2,600 N during walking and 3,100 to 5,330 N during running, corresponding to 6 to 8 times body weight. As a result, the tendon is frequently associated with acute and chronic overuse injuries, particularly in runners. Runners with Achilles tendon problems have a significantly lower range of motion of the ankle joint compared with runners without Achilles tendon injuries.

Biomechanical factors and abnormal anatomy may be amplified further to cause pathology if combined with other microtrauma secondary to excessive activity or training errors. This is commonly seen in athletes who participate in sports in which a sudden alteration in activity is undertaken, such as increased uphill training, changing shoes or training surfaces, or switching sports.

History and Physical Examination

In the early phases of injury, patients will report pain following strenuous activities only. This will usually progress to pain with regular activities and sometimes at rest. With respect to sporting activities, information should be obtained regarding warm-up, mileage, intensity, running surface, and shoe wear. Patients with acute ruptures generally present to the hospital emergency department with the classic history of sudden pain with an audible pop and a sensation of being struck by a fellow athlete. Patients with more chronic ruptures tend to give a history that is typically more insidious, with a minor traumatic event followed by decreased functional ability.

The best way to further assess the Achilles tendon is with the patient in the prone position and the feet hanging off the end of the examination table. This allows a systematic assessment of mechanical alignment, palpation of areas of tenderness, nodules, defects in the tendon, and crepitus. Patients with paratenonitis typically display inflammatory signs of swelling, tenderness, and warmth around the tendon. Although patients with tendinosis may have little pain or inflammatory signs, nodular thickening of the tendon is usually present.

Imaging Studies

Plain radiographs should be obtained to confirm the presence of a bony prominence, which is visualized best on the lateral and axial views of the calcaneus as a posterolateral exostosis. Distal calcification should be identified, if present, because it may alter the approach if surgical intervention is undertaken. Ultrasound is useful for demonstrating soft-tissue inflammation, tendinosis, or rupture. MRI is superior in the detection of incomplete tendon ruptures and chronic degenerative changes (Figure 3).

Nonsurgical Treatment

Activity modification including a decrease in training or adoption of a cross-training program is the initial step in treating this condition. Training errors such as sudden increases in intensity, training on hard or sloped surfaces, or the use of worn out shoes must be addressed. Stretching of the heel cord should be instituted. Shoe modifications including a deep heel to control excessive flexible varus or valgus, a nonabrasive heel counter, and adequate shock absorption are essential. Heel lifts may be used on a temporary basis to help in rehabilitation.

The use of corticosteroid injections for treatment of Achilles tendinitis is an area of controversy. Corticosteroids interfere with healing, and intratendinous injection results in weakening of the tendon for up to 14 days. A recent meta-analysis concluded that corticosteroid injections do not play a beneficial role in the treatment of Achilles tendinopathy. The overall incidence of adverse effects with locally injected corticosteroids is about 1%. Most adverse effects are temporary, but skin atrophy and depigmentation can be permanent.

Surgical Treatment

For patients in the earlier stages of paratenonitis alone with no tendinosis, nonsurgical measures are usually successful. Débridement or incision of the paratenon alone has been described. If tendinosis is evident on MRI and conservative treatments have failed, the tendon should be incised longitudinally and areas of degeneration débrided. A longitudinal medial incision avoids the sural nerve. The extent of débridement may leave a localized deficiency in tendon substance, resulting in the need for reconstruction. This may consist of an Achilles tendon turndown flap if a minimal defect is present. A more aggressive reconstruction procedure involving transfer of the flexor hallucis longus (FHL) tendon to the deficiency at the Achilles tendon may be required for patients with acute and chronic ruptures or severe degenerative pathology.

Patients with partial Achilles tendon ruptures will usually respond to a period of protection in a removable walking boot with a heel lift. A primary repair or a reconstructive procedure may be considered if a significant defect exists. The authors of a recent meta-analysis

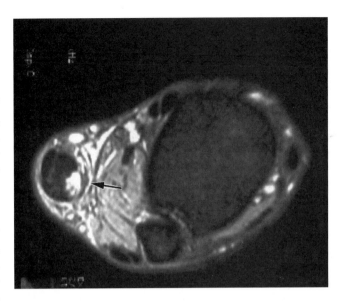

Figure 3 MRI scan showing an area of tendinosis (*arrow*).

concluded that surgical treatment reduces the re-rupture rate at the cost of a 20-fold increase in the complication rate. A tailored approach considering the athletic goals and health of the patient was recommended. Functional bracing has been shown to shorten rehabilitation time postoperatively. Recent evidence indicates that aggressive functional nonsurgical treatment yields good results. A prospective clinical trial comparing functional, nonsurgical rehabilitation and surgical treatment is still lacking. Based on the current literature, it is reasonable to suggest that a surgical treatment plan may be recommended for the experienced surgeon with an active, young, healthy patient who desires a quick return to activity.

Retrocalcaneal Bursitis

The primary function of the retrocalcaneal bursa is to lubricate the tendon during walking and running. Although irritation of the bursa may occur from a bony prominence (Haglund's deformity), isolated bursitis without such a prominence may also occur (Figure 4). Patients with retrocalcaneal bursitis are typically older and have lower activity levels. The presentation is typically acute, with deep pain and visible, tender swelling of the soft tissues medial and lateral to the tendon. Associated warmth and increased pain with dorsiflexion is usually present. Treatment includes rest, ice, a heel lift, and an Achilles tendon stretching program once acute symptoms have receded. If these measures fail, surgery involving resection of the inflamed bursa may be considered.

Haglund's Deformity

In 1928, Haglund first described the enlarged posterosuperolateral calcaneal tuberosity. It has since been associ-

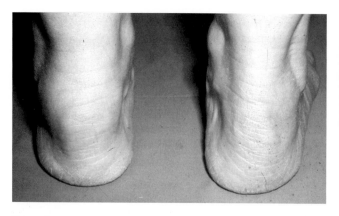

Figure 4 Photograph of a patient with retrocalcaneal bursitis on the left without Haglund's deformity.

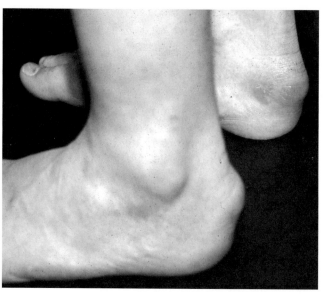

Figure 5 Photograph of a patient with bilateral Haglund's syndrome demonstrating posterior calcaneal prominences.

ated with various shoe types; hence, the names pump bump and winter (skater's) heel. Patients with Haglund's deformity are typically young (between 15 to 30 years of age). A simple pump bump is a chronic irritation of the adventitial bursa causing thickening and pain. The etiology of this condition is usually developmental and aggravated by shoe wear. Patients with pump bump, often younger women, present with localized erythema and focal swelling (Figure 5).

Haglund's syndrome is a triad of retrocalcaneal bursitis, insertional Achilles tendinitis, and adventitial bursitis. An enlarged posterosuperior tuberosity of the calcaneus causes compression of the retrocalcaneal bursa against the Achilles tendon. Swelling is palpable just anterior to the Achilles tendon both medially and laterally. Inflammation, thickening, and degeneration of the tendon occur just proximal to its insertion. There is thickening and swelling subcutaneously as well.

Nonsurgical treatment of Haglund's syndrome is based on relief of friction between the shoe counter, the adventitial bursa, the calcaneus, and particularly the inflamed retrocalcaneal bursa. Activity restriction, including a decrease in hill running, is recommended. Tight posterior heel counters should be modified. Heel lifts decrease pressure on the retrocalcaneal bursa. Stretching and resultant lengthening of the Achilles tendon decreases pressure on the bursa. Ice and anti-inflammatory medication are used as adjunctive treatment.

Surgical treatment includes resection of the bony prominence and all inflamed bursal tissue. For simple posterolateral calcaneal exostosis without extensive retrocalcaneal bursitis and tendon involvement, a small lateral approach for resection of the exostosis alone is used. For severe Haglund's syndrome, the posterosuperior calcaneal prominence must be completely removed. The key to a successful result is resection of an appropriate amount of bone, which should include the entire bony projection plus an additional 0.5 cm. A medial L-shaped incision, lateral incision, medial and lateral in-

cisions, and a central tendon-splitting approach have been described to débride this area. Patients undergoing this surgical procedure must be cautioned that a prolonged recovery period (generally up to 6 to 12 months) is required for resolution of symptoms.

Posterior Tibial Tendon

Anatomy and Physiology

The tibialis posterior muscle originates from the proximal third of the tibia, interosseous membrane, and fibula. Its tendon runs directly behind the medial malleolus, then curves sharply toward its main insertion on the navicular tuberosity. Other tendinous slips insert on the middle three metatarsal bases, cuneiforms, and cuboid. Dye injection studies have demonstrated abundant vascularity of the tendon at the musculotendinous junction and osseous insertion. A zone of relative hypovascularity exists just distal to the medial malleolus.

The primary function of the tibialis posterior muscle is to invert and plantar flex the foot. It is the primary invertor of the hindfoot during the stance phase of gait. It is an important dynamic stabilizer of the arch, and loss of its function has deleterious effects on normal gait.

Posterior tibial tendon injuries are uncommon in young athletes and are usually associated with pes planus. The tendon is subject to great mechanical stress just after heel strike because the hindfoot moves from a position of loaded eversion to inversion. Sports that require rapid changes in direction, including basketball, tennis, soccer, and ice hockey, place increased stress on this structure. The spectrum of disorders in younger athletes includes tenosynovitis, longitudinal tears, or the accessory navicular syndrome, and complete rupture or avulsion is rare. Rupture with collapse of the arch and resultant valgus deformity of the heel is more commonly a disease of attrition, usually occurring in the fourth or fifth decade of life.

Tenosynovitis

The posterior tibial tendon is enclosed in a true synovial-lined tendon sheath. This sheath may become inflamed and hypertrophied, a condition termed "tenosynovitis." Surrounding the tendon is a thin paratenon that has a rich vascular supply. Inflammation of the paratenon is termed "peritendinitis." In cases of chronic peritendinitis, the paratenon may become thickened and constricting. The degeneration of the collagen bundles themselves is termed "tendinosis."

Overuse syndromes, training errors, and direct trauma to the medial aspect of the ankle can result in inflammation and edema within the tendon sheath. On physical examination, tenderness is typically found over the course of the posterior tibial tendon from the medial malleolus to the navicular tuberosity. Often, swelling and fullness are visible in this region. Pain can be elicited along the medial aspect of the ankle by active inversion of the foot against resistance. Single heel rise testing may reproduce the patient's symptoms as well. True inversion weakness is tested manually by applying resistance with the foot in a plantar flexed and everted position. Resisting inversion with the foot in a maximally inverted position recruits accessory invertors such as the tibialis anterior muscle and is less specific for tibialis posterior function.

Treatment of tenosynovitis is aimed at resting the tendon through a combination of decreased training activity, orthotics, and immobilization. Mechanical malalignment of the lower extremity caused by flexible planovalgus feet may benefit from a composite orthotic with a semirigid arch support and slight medial forefoot posting. Gentle stretching to restore or maintain myotendinous unit length should be instituted, followed by strengthening exercises specific to the posterior tibial tendon but inclusive of all muscles crossing the ankle. Strengthening should begin once pain and tenderness have resolved. More severe cases should be treated with a short leg weight-bearing cast for 3 to 4 weeks. This treatment is followed by a period of physical therapy, beginning with range-of-motion exercises and stretching.

Patients who do not respond to this treatment usually have chronic mechanical overload from planovalgus alignment. If malalignment is not present, surgical tenosynovectomy may provide relief. The sheath of the posterior tibial tendon is opened from the medial malleolus to its navicular insertion. A thorough tenosynovectomy is then done. Careful inspection of the tendon often reveals a longitudinal split that is then sutured. Reinforcement with the FHL or flexor digitorum longus (FDL) tendon may be considered. Débridement of thickened paratenon is performed. The spring ligament should be inspected for tears. If the tendon sheath must be opened proximal to the medial malleolus, the overlying flexor retinaculum must be repaired to prevent late tendon dislocation. If planovalgus alignment is present, bony correction may be necessary in association with the soft-tissue surgery.

Posterior Tibial Tendon Rupture

Complete or partial posterior tibial tendon rupture is uncommon in young athletes. The injury occurs to normal tendons that are suddenly overloaded. In athletes with this injury, the disability is marked, unlike in older patients with lower functional demands in whom the tear occurs insidiously. Early diagnosis is imperative if treatment is to be instituted before the onset of flattening of the longitudinal arch.

Physical examination will demonstrate swelling along the course of the posterior tibial tendon with tenderness to palpation. Inversion weakness and inability to rise from one heel are pronounced and cannot be overcome by increased patient effort as in patients with tenosynovitis. When the diagnosis has been delayed, flattening of the longitudinal arch may be noted. Acutely, radiographic evaluation will show no abnormalities except in the unusual case of a tendon avulsion off the navicular tuberosity with a small piece of bone.

Surgical repair and augmentation with a tendon transfer is the treatment of choice for an acute posterior tibial tendon rupture in a young athlete without significant collapse of the arch. If planovalgus alignment is present, bony correction with a medial displacement calcaneal osteotomy, medial column stabilization, or lateral column lengthening may be necessary.

The torn tendon is exposed and a direct repair performed and augmented with a FDL tendon transfer into a drill hole in the navicular. The FDL tendon should be detached just proximal to where it crosses the FHL tendon at the master knot of Henry. Alternatively, the FDL tendon may be used. Pure avulsions of the tendon may be reattached to the navicular tuberosity.

Posterior Tibial Tendon Dislocation

Although acute dislocation of the posterior tibial tendon is a rare occurrence, it is most commonly seen in young adults. On physical examination, patients with this type of injury present with severe pain and swelling in the retromalleolar area, followed by localization of tenderness anterior to the medial malleolus as swelling resolves. Demonstration of tendon dislocation or marked apprehension can be elicited with resisted plantar flexion and inversion of the foot. Strength testing results are typically normal. Plain radiographs will be unremarkable. MRI may reveal the tendon anterior to the medial malleolus. Nonsurgical treatment has been reported to be uniformly unsuccessful.

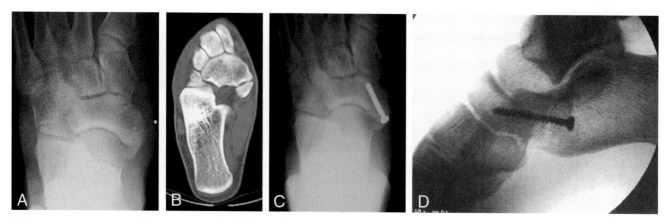

Figure 6 A large accessory navicular on a preoperative radiograph (**A**) and CT scan (**B**) and fixed via open reduction and internal fixation on postoperative AP (**C**) and lateral (**D**) radiographs.

Once the proper diagnosis is established, surgical exploration, relocation of the tendon, and repair or reconstruction of the flexor retinaculum should be done. An assessment of the depth of the retromalleolar groove should be made, and the groove deepened if necessary. An avulsed flexor retinaculum may be directly repaired. Redundant retinaculum is imbricated in a pants-over-vest manner after relocation of the tendon.

The Accessory Navicular

The accessory navicular may be a source of pain for the athlete. It is found in 4% to 14% of the population but becomes symptomatic only in a small portion of this group. The diagnosis of an accessory navicular is based on a careful history and physical examination with radiographic demonstration of the bone. Patients with an accessory navicular often present with erythema overlying the navicular tuberosity with point tenderness in this region. Pain reproduced by resisted inversion is an unreliable indicator. Anteroposterior and lateral radiographs of the foot may not adequately show the accessory navicular; however, the oblique view clearly demonstrates the bone. A technetium bone scan is helpful when the clinical diagnosis is not evident, particularly in cases of bilateral accessory navicular or when pain and tenderness are not specific to a point.

Accessory naviculars are classified as one of three types. Type I is a sesamoid contained within the posterior tibial tendon and comprises 30% of all accessory naviculars. Type II is an ossicle of approximately 8 to 12 mm adjacent to the parent navicular separated by an area of cartilage 1 to 3 mm thick; type II accessory naviculars are most commonly symptomatic. Type III is an ossicle united to the navicular by a bony bridge forming a prominent navicular tuberosity.

Treatment of a symptomatic accessory navicular involves relieving stress on the synchondrosis to allow it to heal. In mild cases in patients with a pronated foot,

an orthotic and arch support with medial heel posting may be used and, once symptoms resolve, continued for a minimum of 6 months. Rigid orthotics should not be used because they increase pressure over the bony prominence of the accessory navicular and worsen the symptoms. Patients with more severe symptoms require cast immobilization. Failure of nonsurgical treatment of type II accessory naviculars is an indication for surgical excision. A 4- to 5-cm longitudinal incision over the distal tendon and bone is made, and the accessory bone is excised. Very large accessory naviculars may benefit from stabilization with fixation rather than excision to maintain mechanical stability and better function of the tendon (Figure 6).

Flexor Hallucis Longus Tendon

The FHL tendon is a bipennate muscle that originates from the lower two thirds of the posterior aspect of the fibula and the interosseous membrane. Proximally, its tendon begins high in the muscle, and distally the muscle extends low on the tendon. The FHL tendon passes posterior to the distal end of the tibia and deep to a retinaculum, a groove created by the medial and lateral tubercles of the posterior talus (Figure 7).

Its course then passes along the medial surface of the calcaneus in a fibro-osseous tunnel under the roof of the sustentaculum tali. As the FHL tendon traverses the sole of the foot on the dorsal and lateral surface of the FDL tendon, both tendons are bound to the vault of the arch by a common tendon sheath, the master knot of Henry. It is at this location, approximately 2 cm lateral to the navicular tuberosity, that the tendons cross, with the FHL tendon progressing medially to the hallux, and the FDL tendon continuing laterally to the lesser toes.

Stenosing tenosynovitis of the FHL tendon is common in ballet dancers. Pain may be localized anywhere along the course of the tendon, including the posteromedial ankle, the master knot of Henry, or between the sesamoids under the base of the first metatarsal. The most common location of pain is behind the sustentaculum tali within its fibro-osseous tunnel. Active plantar flexion of the hallux against resistance typically reproduces the pain. Nodule formation within the tendon may cause triggering of the hallux. Localization of pain to the posterior ankle may be associated with irritation of the tendon from an os trigonum.

Conservative treatment including rest or modified activities (no pointe work for dancers) is usually successful. Patients who do not respond to conservative treatment may undergo surgical release of the tendon's fibro-osseous tunnel.

Peroneal Tendons

Peroneal tendon injuries can occur as a result of direct trauma to the tendons, ankle sprains, and calcaneal fractures. Peroneal tenosynovitis, subluxation, dislocation, and tears have all been reported in athletes and nonathletes. There is often a delay in diagnosis and treatment.

Peroneal Tenosynovitis

Peroneal tenosynovitis has a variety of causes, including inversion injury to the ankle, anomalous extension of the peroneus brevis tendon into the fibular groove, and the presence of a large peroneal tubercle or os peroneum. Stenosing tenosynovitis presents as pain and swelling with tenderness along the path of the peroneal tendons as they course behind the lateral malleolus, around the peroneal tubercle, and under the cuboid. Forced eversion against resistance reproduces the pain. Lateral ankle instability has been shown to be associated with peroneal tenosynovitis. In one case series, 47 of 61 ankles that underwent surgery for chronic lateral ankle instability had coexisting peroneal tenosynovitis.

Treatment of tenosynovitis consists of anti-inflammatory medication, rest, identifying and treating any strength deficits, activity modification, a lateral heel wedge in mild cases, use of an ankle-foot orthosis, and in some instances, immobilization in a short leg cast. An adequate trial of immobilization consists of 6 weeks in a short leg cast or ankle-foot orthosis. Steroid injection around the tendons may be considered. Surgical treatment involving open tenosynovectomy is a consideration for patients with persistent symptoms that are not adequately relieved by conservative modalities. Underlying pathology, such as chronic ankle instability, should also be addressed. A hypertrophied peroneal tubercle that is related to the tenosynovitis can be excised.

Peroneal Tendon Subluxation and Dislocation

Peroneal tendon subluxation or dislocation is an uncommon injury and is frequently misdiagnosed as an ankle sprain. Skiing is the sport most commonly associated with this injury because of a mechanism of acute dorsi-

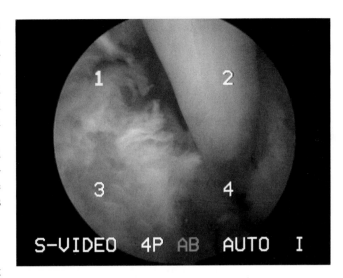

Figure 7 Arthroscopic view of the FHL tendon (quadrant 2) in the fibro-osseous tunnel adjacent to talus (quadrant 1) and calcaneus (quadrant 3). *(Reproduced with permission from Wasserman L, Amendola A, Saltzman C: Ankle arthroscopy in sports traumatology. Perspectives en Arthroscopie 2004;3:55-60.)*

flexion and violent reflex peroneal musculature contraction. Physical examination typically reveals diffuse lateral swelling and ecchymoses in the acute injury setting. Tenderness posteriorly along the course of the peroneal tendons is in contradistinction to an ankle sprain, in which the pain is located anterior and inferior to the lateral malleolus, along the ATFL and CFL. Extreme pain or apprehension with resisted eversion testing of the foot is often a key diagnostic feature.

Treatment of acute injuries is controversial. Nonsurgical management consisting of a short leg, non–weight-bearing cast for 4 to 6 weeks has a 50% success rate. Acute reconstruction involving repair of the retinaculum to bone, with or without deepening of the groove, is the preferred treatment for the young athletic population. Chronic symptomatic injuries respond poorly to conservative measures. Surgical repair options include retinacular repair or reconstruction with local or transferred tissue, groove-deepening or bone-block procedures, or anterior rerouting of the tendons.

Peroneal Tendon Tear

Traumatic rupture of the peroneal tendons may occur in association with ankle fractures and severe sprains. Partial tears and complete ruptures are more commonly associated with established peroneal tenosynovitis. Patients who present with tendon rupture often report preexisting pain and disability. A partial tear should be considered in patients who appear to have tenosynovitis but fail to respond to nonsurgical treatment. Complete tendon rupture can lead to recurrent sprains and ankle instability. Tendon degeneration and complete rupture usually occur in locations where stenosing tenosynovitis is observed, such as the retromalleolar sulcus, peroneal

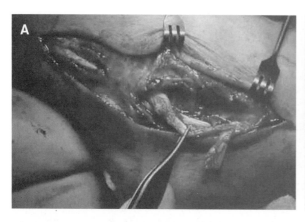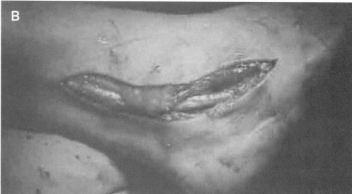

Figure 8 Photographs showing débridement (**A**) and tenodesis (**B**) of a torn peroneus brevis to the peroneus longus proximally and distally.

tubercle, and the cuboid. MRI is helpful in making the diagnosis.

Treatment of longitudinal attritional tears consists of the same nonsurgical management as previously discussed for peroneal tenosynovitis. Failure of conservative treatment is an indication for surgical débridement or repair. Intraoperatively, a partial tear of the peroneus brevis tendon has the gross appearance of a longitudinal attritional tear and typically occurs in the region of the retromalleolar sulcus. The relatively wide peroneus brevis tendon lies deep and anterior to the relatively narrow peroneus longus tendon. Therefore, the peroneus longus tendon may act as a wedge and divide the fibers of the peroneus brevis tendon over the fibrocartilaginous ridge of the posterolateral distal fibula. This mechanism is accentuated by incompetency of the superior peroneal retinaculum. Occasionally, a bucket-handle tear of the peroneus brevis tendon may occur when the tendon is split by the peroneus longus and separated into two parallel portions that converge proximally and distally. If one tendon is unsalvageable, tenodesis of the proximal and distal ends of the ruptured tendon to the intact tendon is recommended (Figure 8). Areas of frank tendinosis should be excised.

Osteochondral Lesions of the Talus

Recognized osteochondral lesions of the talus account for 0.09% of all fractures and 1% of fractures involving the talus. The majority of these injuries, however, are undiagnosed. A recent study showed that at the time of surgery, 71% of patients with ankle fractures and 41% of patients with recurrent lateral ankle instability had talar dome osteochondral lesions.

In the chronic or subacute setting, the presenting symptoms are usually poorly defined and may be coincident with a sprain. Posteromedial lesions are more often atraumatic and deeper, whereas anterolateral lesions are usually traumatic and shallow. CT will delineate the

extent of bony depth of the lesion, and MRI will determine the extent of separation of the overlying cartilage.

Treatment is based on the size, location, and the grade of the lesion as well as the age of the patient. Lesions are classified according to the staging system described by Berndt and Harty as follows: stage I is compression of subchondral bone, stage II is a partially detached lesion, stage III is a completely detached lesion that is nondisplaced, and stage IV is a free osteochondral fragment within the joint. A nonsurgical trial of casting for 6 weeks is indicated for patients with stage I or stage II lesions, as well as those with medial stage III defects. All lesions in skeletally immature patients, other than loose bodies within the joint, should initially be treated with casting. Stage IV and lateral stage III lesions are indications for surgical treatment in adults.

Surgical modalities include excision of the osteochondral fragment, excision and curettage with or without drilling the base of the lesion, cancellous bone grafting, and internal fixation. A recent systematic review of the literature found excision, curettage, and drilling to be most effective, with an 86% success rate.

Newer strategies such as osteochondral transplantation and autologous chondrocyte grafting are showing promise in short- to intermediate-term reports. Osteochondral transplantation, in the form of autograft or allograft plugs, is indicated for patients with osteochondral lesions larger than 1 cm². Autograft is harvested from a non–weight-bearing area of the lateral femoral condyle anterior to the terminal sulcus or intercondylar notch. Donor site morbidity has been minimal based on published reports. For lesions larger than 2 cm², harvest site morbidity becomes prohibitive and the use of allograft tissue is indicated. Allograft tissue should also be used when preexisting knee pain is present. Bulk osteochondral allografting of the talus for involvement of greater than 50% of the joint surface has recently been reported. Autologous chondrocyte transplantation is an option for treating larger lesions. Reports indicate an early success rate of approximately 50%.

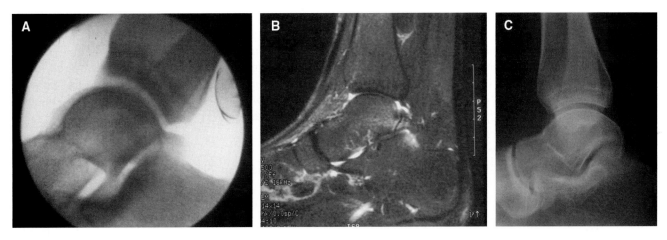

Figure 9 A, Radiograph showing an os trigonum in a left ankle with impingement in plantar flexion posteriorly. **B,** MRI scan demonstrating edema and fluid around the os trigonum. **C,** Radiograph of os trigonum in a right ankle after resection. *(Part C is reproduced with permission from Wasserman L, Amendola A, Saltzman C: Ankle arthroscopy in sports traumatology.* Perspectives en Arthroscopie *2004;3:55-60.)*

Ankle Impingement Syndromes

Anterior Bony Impingement

Anterior ankle impingement syndrome is characterized by anterior ankle pain with limited and painful dorsiflexion. Bony or soft-tissue impingement is a common cause of chronic anterior ankle pain, catching, and subjective feelings of giving way in athletes. The presence of osteophytes has been reported in as many as 45% of football players, and it is common in soccer players, dancers, and other athletes. In general, osteophytes are a manifestation of osteoarthritic changes. In sports ankle trauma, however, bony spur formation may be the result of traction from repetitive microtrauma. The exact cause of the formation of osteophytes is not fully understood. One hypothesis suggests that traction on the joint capsule during maximal plantar flexion movements of the foot, as occurs during kicking a ball in soccer or American football, is the essential cause, resulting in traction spurs. Another hypothesis assumes that the formation of osteophytes is the result of direct damage to the rim of the anterior ankle cartilage in combination with recurrent microtrauma.

Lateral ankle radiographs can reveal evidence of these osteophytes on the anterior tibia and talar neck. These spurs have been described as "kissing osteophytes," implying that the pain associated with the anterior ankle impingement syndrome is caused by impingement of the opposing osteophytes on one another. However, study of the morphology of the tibial and talar osteophytes using radiography and CT has recently shown that tibial and talar osteophytes typically do not overlap. The talar spur peak most often lies medial to the midline, whereas the tibial spur peak lies lateral to the midline. The tibial spur is wider than the talar spur, and the talar spur usually protrudes medially off the edge of the talar neck.

It is possible that both proposed hypotheses are correct. Traction spur formation is a possible mechanism for formation of the anterior lateral tibial spur, and microtrauma of ball impact can be the causative mechanism for the medial talar neck spur. These ankles are not osteoarthritic, and in general, open or arthroscopic débridement is successful.

Posterior Bony Impingement

The os trigonum is the ununited lateral tubercle of the posterior talus. It is present in up to 10% of the population. Impingement of the os trigonum or fracture of a prominent posterior process is rare in athletes, but it may be present in dancers. This has classically been described as posterolateral pain, anterior to the Achilles tendon, occurring in the hyper–plantar flexed position. Radiographs will usually demonstrate evidence of the bony prominence. MRI or bone scanning can demonstrate evidence of edema or increased uptake around the os trigonum (Figure 9).

More commonly, symptoms are the result of irritation of the FHL tendon by the prominent process or os trigonum with repetitive jumping and pivoting maneuvers. Examination typically reveals tenderness posteromedially over the FHL tendon. Pain is reproduced by forced passive plantar flexion of the ankle and by resisted hallux flexion. Pain is not usually severely disabling, and athletes with low-grade symptoms are usually able to participate in athletic activities until the end of the season.

Treatment includes activity modification, local corticosteroid injection of the FHL tendon sheath, bracing, and in recalcitrant cases, débridement and excision of the prominent os trigonum to relieve impingement of the FHL tendon. Results of this procedure are good to excellent in most series with open or arthroscopic methods. An arthroscopic approach in the prone position has recently been described. Prone positioning is believed to decrease the risk to neurovascular structures. In theory, an arthroscopic approach improves visualization and minimizes surgical exposure, leading to earlier recovery and return to play.

Soft-Tissue Impingement of the Ankle

After an ankle sprain, hemorrhage into the joint is followed by traumatic synovitis with thickening and exudation. In most circumstances, the exudate and scar tissue are removed during the repair process. In some ankles, however, there is incomplete resorption of the exudate, and it becomes thickened and hyalinized, resulting in a synovial impingement lesion. Historically, this was referred to in the literature as a "meniscoid" lesion. The hallmark of this condition is anterolateral ankle pain that continues well past the expected healing time of a simple lateral ankle sprain. Weight bearing, forced dorsiflexion, and palpation of the joint line exacerbate the pain, and it is refractory to physical therapy. Other causes of persistent pain must be ruled out.

Radiographs of the ankle will often show normal anatomy of the ankle joint. Magnetic resonance arthrography has been used to assess patients with chronic ankle pain. In one prospective study, 13 patients with anterolateral impingement and 19 control subjects underwent magnetic resonance arthrography of the ankle and subsequent arthroscopic examination. Intraoperative findings were compared with the preoperative magnetic resonance arthrography results. Magnetic resonance arthrographic assessment of the anterolateral soft tissues of the ankle showed an accuracy of 97%, sensitivity of 96%, specificity of 100%, negative predictive value of 89%, and positive predictive value of 100%.

Most patients with soft-tissue impingement do not respond to treatment with intra-articular corticosteroid injection. Arthroscopic débridement of the impingement lesion will resolve the symptoms in most patients. On histologic inspection, the incarcerated tissue will show varying degrees of chronic inflammation, synovial hyperplasia, and fibrosis.

Posteromedial impingement of the ankle, an uncommon lesion, occurs with severe inversion injuries in which the deep posterior fibers of the deltoid ligament are crushed between the medial wall of the talus and the medial malleolus. Initially, the posteromedial symptoms do not predominate, being overshadowed by the lateral ligament disruption, and they usually resolve without specific treatment. Occasionally, however, thick, disorganized, fibrotic scar tissue persists and impinges between the talus and the posterior margin of the medial malleolus. Clinically, patients with posteromedial impingement develop persistent posteromedial activity-related pain. On physical examination, there is deep soft-tissue induration immediately posterior to the medial malleolus, with localized tenderness and reproduction of pain on provocative testing by palpating this site while moving the ankle into plantar flexion and inversion. Open or arthroscopic débridement should be used to treat lesions that fail to respond to an ankle rehabilitation program.

Summary

Ankle injuries can be frustrating for both the athlete wanting to minimize time away from training and the surgeon who is trying to expedite recovery. A rational approach emphasizing a guided rehabilitation program supplemented with surgical intervention when indicated will provide optimal care of patients with these injuries.

Annotated Bibliography

Lateral Ankle Sprains

Frost SC, Amendola A: Is stress radiography necessary in the diagnosis of acute or chronic ankle instability? *Clin J Sport Med* 1999;9:40-45.

This review of eight prospective studies reports that talar tilt and anterior drawer stress radiographs are too variable to determine accepted normal values and therefore not useful in the diagnosis of either acute or chronic lateral instability.

Handoll HH, Rowe BH, Quinn KM, de Bie R: Interventions for preventing ankle ligament injuries. *Cochrane Database Syst Rev* 2001;3:CD000018.

This meta-analysis of 14 randomized trials including 8,279 subjects found a reduction in the incidence of ankle sprains in patients using external ankle support. This was most pronounced in those with a prior history of ankle sprain, although those without a previous history also benefited. No difference in severity of sprains was noted. The protective effect of high-top shoes was not established. There was only limited evidence found in support of disk training exercises.

Kerkhoffs GM, Struijs PA, Marti RK, Blankevoort L, Assendelft WJ, van Dijk CN: Functional treatments for acute ruptures of the lateral ankle ligament: A systematic review. *Acta Orthop Scand* 2003;74:69-77.

This systematic review of nine trials examining nonsurgical treatments found short-term persistent swelling to occur least often with a lace-up brace than a semirigid brace, elastic wrap, or tape. A semirigid brace required a shorter return-to-work period compared with taping.

Messer TM, Cummins CA, Ahn J, Kelikian AS: Outcome of the modified Broström procedure for chronic lateral ankle instability using suture anchors. *Foot Ankle Int* 2000;21:996-1003.

The authors describe a modified Broström technique and report 91% good or excellent results at average 34-month follow-up.

Pijnenburg ACM, Bogaard K, Krips R, Marti RK, Bossuyt PM, Van Dijk CN: Operative and functional treatment of rupture of the lateral ligament of the ankle: A randomized, prospective trial. *J Bone Joint Surg Br* 2003;85:525-530.

At an average 8-year follow-up, patients who underwent surgical treatment for rupture of the lateral ligament of the ankle reported fewer recurrent sprains than those who had functional treatment. The results of anterior drawer testing were less frequently positive and functional scores were higher in the surgical treatment group as well.

Pijnenburg ACM, Van Dijk CN, Bossuyt PMM, Marti RK: Treatment of ruptures of the lateral ankle ligaments: A meta-analysis. *J Bone Joint Surg Am* 2000;82: 761-773.

Twenty-seven trials were included in this meta-analysis. A significant difference with respect to recurrent "giving-way" was found in favor of acute surgical treatment, which was reported to be more effective than functional treatment; functional treatment, in turn, was reported to be more effective than 6 weeks of casting. Residual pain increased in the patients who underwent casting and was equal in the surgical and functional treatment groups.

Verhagen EA, Van Mechelen W, de Vente W: The effect of preventive measures on the incidence of ankle sprains. *Clin J Sport Med* 2000;10:291-296.

This systematic review of eight studies found bracing more effective than taping in reducing the incidence of ankle sprains. Both methods reduced the severity of sprains. The effectiveness of shoes was inconclusive. Proprioceptive training was found to reduce the incidence of ankle sprains in those with recurrent injury to the same incidence as those without a history of injury.

Syndesmosis Injuries and Medial Ankle Sprains

Keefe DT, Haddad SL: Subtalar instability: Etiology, diagnosis, and management. *Foot Ankle Clin* 2002;7: 577-609.

The authors of this study report that diagnosis of subtalar instability is difficult because stress radiographs are technique-dependent and do not reliably correlate with symptoms. For patients who do not respond to initial conditioning exercises, anatomic reconstruction of ligamentous stabilizers is recommended.

Krips R, van Dijk CN, Halasi T, et al: Long-term outcome of anatomical reconstruction versus tenodesis for the treatment of chronic anterolateral instability of the ankle joint: A multicenter study. *Foot Ankle Int* 2001;22: 415-421.

The authors of this study report that the tenodesis group more often had positive talar tilt and anterior drawer stress radiographs, medial joint degenerative changes, and inferior functional results. However, the tenodeses done were the Watson-Jones and Castaing procedures, neither of which re-

creates the anatomic locations of the ATFL and CFL. Of note, more females were in the tenodesis group, and the number of revision cases included in each group was not reported.

Nussbaum ED, Hosea TM, Sieler SD, Inceremona BR, Kessler DE: Prospective evaluation of syndesmotic ankle sprains without diastasis. *Am J Sports Med* 2001;29: 31-35.

For patients with syndesmotic ankle sprains without diastasis, the average time to return to play was 13.4 days. The number of days missed was directly correlated with the interosseous tenderness length and a positive squeeze test.

Tornetta P III, Spoo JE, Reynolds FA, Lee C: Overtightening of the ankle syndesmosis: Is it really possible? *J Bone Joint Surg Am* 2001;83:489-492.

The authors of this study report that reduction of the syndesmosis matters more than the amount of dorsiflexion of the ankle when the syndesmosis screw is placed.

Tendinopathies

Mortensen NHM, Skov O, Jensen PE: Early motion of the ankle after operative treatment of a rupture of the Achilles tendon: A prospective, randomized, clinical and radiographic study. *J Bone Joint Surg Am* 1999;81:983-990.

The authors of this study report that faster return to work and athletic activity was observed in the early motion group; however, there was no difference in calf muscle atrophy between groups.

Myerson MS, McGarvey W: Disorders of the Achilles tendon insertion and Achilles tendinitis. *Instr Course Lect* 1999;48:211-218.

The authors of this article review Achilles tendon disorders and specifically address both acute and chronic injury, various forms of tendinitis, and the pain syndromes of the retrocalcaneal space, including retrocalcaneal bursitis and Haglund's deformity.

Peroneal Tendons

Clarke HD, Kitaoka HB, Ehman RL: Peroneal tendon injuries. *Foot Ankle Int* 1998;19:280-284.

The authors report that the peroneal tendons can be a cause of persistent lateral ankle pain after trauma.

DiGiovanni BF, Fraga CJ, Cohen BE, Shereff MJ: Associated injuries found in chronic lateral ankle instability. *Foot Ankle Int* 2000;21:809-815.

Of 61 patients undergoing lateral ligament reconstruction, peroneal tenosynovitis was found in 77%, anterolateral impingement lesion in 67%, attenuated peroneal retinaculum in 54%, ankle synovitis in 49%, loose body in 26%, peroneus brevis tear in 25%, talar osteochondral lesion in 23%, and medial tenosynovitis in 5%.

Safran MR, O'Malley D, Fu FH: Peroneal tendon subluxation in athletes: New exam technique, case reports and review. *Med Sci Sport Exerc* 1999;31(7 suppl):S487-S492.

The authors of this article report that examination of patients in the prone position facilitates visualization of subluxation. They recommend acute repair of traumatic peroneal tendon subluxation in athletes and report that nonsurgical casting has a 40% to 50% failure rate.

Osteochondral Lesions of the Talus

Giannini S, Buda R, Grigolo B, Vannini F: Autologous chondrocyte transplantation in osteochondral lesions of the ankle. *Foot Ankle Int* 2001;22:513-517.

At 2-year follow-up after using autologous chondrocyte transplantation to treat osteochondral lesions of the ankle, the authors reported that the mean American Orthopaedic Foot and Ankle Society scores of the patients studied improved from 32 preoperatively to 91 postoperatively (range, 0 to 100) with no complications. Chondrocytes and type II collagen were identified in the graft material.

Gross AE, Agnidis Z, Hutchinson CR: Osteochondral defects of the talus treated with fresh osteochondral allograft transplantation. *Foot Ankle Int* 2001;22:385-391.

In this study, six of nine fresh osteochondral allografts were reported to remain in situ at a mean of 11 years (range, 4 to 19 years). The three failures were caused by resorption and fragmentation of the graft.

Hangody L, Kish G, Modis L, et al: Mosaicplasty for the treatment of osteochondritis dissecans of the talus: 2- to 7-year results in 36 patients. *Foot Ankle Int* 2001;22:552-558.

The authors of this study report excellent results in 94% of 34 patients and 2- to 7-year follow-up with no long-term donor site morbidity.

Petersen L, Brittberg M, Lindahl A: Autologous chondrocyte transplantation of the ankle. *Foot Ankle Clin* 2003;8:291-303.

In this study, 14 patients with talar defects and 11 patients with tibial defects were treated with autologous chondrocyte transplantation of the ankle. At a mean follow-up of 45 months, 11 of 25 patients reported good or excellent outcomes and 12 patients considered themselves improved.

Sammarco GJ, Makwana NK: Treatment of talar osteochondral lesions using local osteochondral graft. *Foot Ankle Int* 2002;23:693-698.

Twelve patients were treated with local osteochondral grafts for talar osteochondral lesions. The authors report that the mean American Orthopaedic Foot and Ankle Society scores of these patients improved from 64 preoperatively to 91 postoperatively (range, 0 to 100). The donor site was the ipsilateral medial or lateral talar facet, and the lesions were visualized through an anterior tibial osteotomy. Good graft incor-

poration was noted in two patients who underwent arthroscopy at 6 and 12 months after surgery. No complications occurred at the donor sites or tibial osteotomy sites.

Takao M, Ochi M, Uchio Y, Naito K, Kono T, Oae K: Osteochondral lesions of the talar dome associated with trauma. *Arthroscopy* 2003;19:1061-1067.

In this study, 71% of 92 ankle fractures and 41% of 86 ankles with chronic lateral instability demonstrated evidence of an osteochondral lesion using arthroscopic or MRI assessment.

Verhagen RA, Struijs PA, Bossuyt PM, Van Dijk CN: Systematic review of treatment strategies for osteochondral defects of the talar dome. *Foot Ankle Clin* 2003;8: 233-242.

The authors of this review article assessed 39 studies from 1966 to 2000 that met their inclusion criteria. Fourteen of these studies described the results of nonsurgical treatment; 4 described the results of excision alone; 10 described the results of excision and curettage; and 21 described the results of excision, curettage, and drilling. The success rate was 86% for excision, curettage, and drilling; 78% for excision and curettage; 38% for excision alone; and 45% for nonsurgical treatment.

Ankle Impingement Syndromes

Paterson RS, Brown JN: The posteromedial impingement lesion of the ankle: A series of six cases. *Am J Sports Med* 2001;29:550-557.

One cause of medial pain after an ankle inversion injury may be scar tissue impinging between the posterior margin of the medial malleolus and the medial wall of the talus. The authors postulate that this arises from the deep fibers of the deltoid ligament being crushed at the time of injury. Plantar flexion and inversion of the ankle reproduced the pain in the patients studied, and open débridement successfully resolved symptoms in most patients.

Robinson P, White LM, Salonen DC, Daniels TR, Ogilvie-Harris D: Anterolateral ankle impingement: MR arthrographic assessment of the anterolateral recess. *Radiology* 2001;221:186-190.

The authors of this article report that magnetic resonance arthrography is accurate in assessing the anterolateral recess of the ankle joint; an accuracy of 97%, sensitivity of 96%, specificity of 100%, negative predictive value of 89%, and positive predictive value of 100% were demonstrated.

Sitler DF, Amendola A, Bailey CS, Thain LM, Spouge A: Posterior ankle arthroscopy: An anatomic study. *J Bone Joint Surg Am* 2002;84:763-769.

Posteromedial and posterolateral portals made with the patient in the prone position were shown to be safe by MRI findings correlating with open dissection visualization. The closest anatomic structure to the posteromedial portal was the FHL (average distance, 2.7 mm), whereas the sural nerve was closest to the posterolateral portal, (average distance, 3.2 mm). The tibial nerve was an average of 6.4 mm and the posterior tibial artery an average of 9.6 mm from the posteromedial portal.

Wayne S, Berberian WS, Hecht PJ, Wapner KL, DiVerniero R: Morphology of tibio-talar osteophytes in anterior ankle impingement. *Foot Ankle Int* 2001;22:313-317.

The CT scans of 10 patients undergoing anterior débridement for anterior ankle impingement were retrospectively examined. Tibial osteophytes usually were larger than medial osteophytes and peaked lateral to the midline of the talar dome, whereas talar spurs usually protruded medially off the edge of the talar neck. The osteophytes usually did not overlap each other.

Classic Bibliography

Andrews JR, Drez DJ, McGinty JB: Arthroscopy of joints other than the knee. *Contemp Orthop* 1984;9:71-100.

Bassett FH, Gates HS, Billys JB, Morris HB, Nikolau PK: Talar impingement by the antero-inferior tibiofibular ligament. *J Bone Joint Surg Am* 1990;72:55-59.

Berndt AL, Harty M: Transchondral fractures (osteochondritis dissecans) of the talus. *Am J Orthop* 1959;41:988-1020.

Boruta PM, Beauperthuy GD: Partial tear of the flexor hallucis longus at the knot of Henry: Presentation of three cases. *Foot Ankle Int* 1997;18:243-246.

Boytim MJ, Fischer DA, Neumann L: Syndesmotic ankle sprains. *Am J Sports Med* 1991;19:294-298.

Burks RT, Morgan J: Anatomy of the lateral ankle ligaments. *Am J Sports Med* 1994;22:72-77.

Colville MR, Grondel RJ: Anatomic reconstruction of the lateral ankle ligaments using a split peroneus tendon graft. *Am J Sports Med* 1995;23:210-213.

Conti SF: Posterior tibial tendon problems in athletes. *Orthop Clin North Am* 1994;25:109-121.

Dacruz DJ, Geeson AMJ, Phair I: Achilles paratendonitis: An evaluation of steroid injection. *Br J Sports Med* 1988;22:64-65.

Egol KA, Parisien SJ: Impingement syndrome of the ankle caused by a medial meniscoid lesion. *Arthroscopy* 1997;13:522-525.

Fest T, Dupond JL: Achilles tendon rupture. *Lancet* 1989;2:918.

Frey C, Shereff M, Greenidge N: Vascularity of the posterior tibial tendon. *J Bone Joint Surg Am* 1990;72:884-888.

Haglund-Akerlind Y, Eriksson E: Range of motion, muscle torque and training habits in runners with and without Achilles tendon problems. *Knee Surg Sports Traumatol Arthrosc* 1993;1:195-199.

Kannus P, Renstrom P: Treatment for acute tears of the lateral ligaments of the ankle: Operation, cast, or early controlled mobilization. *J Bone Joint Surg Am* 1991;73:305-312.

Kennedy JC, Willis RB: The effects of local steroid injections on tendons: A biomechanical and microscopic correlative study. *Am J Sports Med* 1976;4:11-21.

Lo IK, Kirkle A, Nonweiler B, Kumbhare DA: Operative versus non-operative treatment of acute Achilles tendon ruptures: A quantitative review. *Clin J Sport Med* 1997;7:207-211.

Mabit C, Boncoeur MP, Chaudruc JM, et al: Anatomic and MRI study of subtalar ligamentous support. *Surg Radiol Anat* 1997;19:111-117.

Marumoto JM, Ferkel RD: Arthroscopic excision of the os trigonum: A new technique with preliminary clinical results. *Foot Ankle* 1997;18:777.

Massada JL: Ankle overuse injuries in soccer players: Morphological adaptation of the talus in the anterior impingement syndrome. *J Sports Med Phys Fitness* 1991;31:447-451.

McComis GP, Mawoczenski DA, Dettaren KE: Functional bracing for rupture of the Achilles tendon: Clinical results and analysis of ground-reaction forces and temporal data. *J Bone Joint Surg Am* 1997;79:1799-1808.

Miller CD, Shelton WR, Barrett GR, et al: Deltoid and syndesmosis ligament injury of the ankle without fracture. *Am J Sports Med* 1995;23:746-750.

Sammarco JG: Peroneal tendon injuries. *Orthop Clin North Am* 1994;25:135-145.

Schonholtz GJ: Arthroscopic surgery of the ankle joint, in Thomas C (ed): *Arthroscopic Surgery of the Shoulder, Elbow and Ankle.* Springfield, IL, Charles C. Thomas Publisher Ltd, 1986, pp 59-72.

Scranton PE, McDermott JE: Anterior tibiotalar spurs: A comparison of open versus arthroscopic débridement. *Foot Ankle* 1992;13:125-129.

Shapiro MS, Kabo JM, Mitchell PW, Loren G, Tsenter M: Ankle sprain prophylaxis: An analysis of the stabilizing effects of braces and tape. *Am J Sports Med* 1994;22:78-82.

Shrier I, Matheson GO, Kohl HW III: Achilles tendonitis: Are corticosteroids injections useful or harmful? *Clin J Sport Med* 1996;6:245-250.

Sitler M, Ryan J, Wheeler B, et al: The efficacy of a semi-rigid ankle stabilizer to reduce acute ankle injuries in basketball: A randomized clinical study at West Point. *Am J Sports Med* 1994;22:454-461.

Van Dijk CN, Tol JL, Verheyen CCPM: A prospective study of prognostic factors concerning the outcome of arthroscopic surgery for anterior ankle impingement. *Am J Sports Med* 1997;25:737-745.

Wapner KL, Pavlock GS, Hecht PJ, Naselli F, Walther R: Repair of chronic Achilles tendon rupture with flexor hallucis longus tendon transfer. *Foot Ankle* 1993;14:443-449.

Wredmark T, Carlstedt C, Bauer H, et al: Os trigonum syndrome: A clinical entity in ballet dancers. *Foot Ankle* 1991;11:404-406.

Chapter 19

Athletic Foot Disorders

Robert B. Anderson, MD

William C. James III, MD

Simon Lee, MD

Introduction

Disorders involving the foot are extremely common among athletes and range from acute, traumatic injuries to chronic, overuse-oriented problems. Overuse injuries in particular occur more commonly as more people participate in strenuous activities into their later years. When evaluating athletes with foot problems, despite the age or level of competition of the athlete, it is important to obtain a detailed history, with careful attention to activity level, training regimen, and shoe wear. With female athletes, it is also important to inquire about diet and menstrual cycles to evaluate for the possible presence of the female athlete triad. A detailed physical examination should follow and include assessment of overall lower extremity alignment, range of motion, neurovascular status, gait, motor strength, and any areas of tenderness or swelling. Shoe-wear patterns can also help assess foot and ankle posture and potential areas of overload.

Hindfoot

Plantar Fasciitis/Heel Pain

Athletes, particularly joggers, routinely experience heel pain. The most common cause is plantar fasciitis, which accounts for about 10% of running injuries; however, there are several other entities with similar presentations that must be differentiated and treated accordingly.

The plantar fascia is a dense band of fibrous tissue originating from the medial calcaneal tuberosity and inserting on the plantar plates of the metatarsophalangeal (MTP) joints and proximal phalanges (Figure 1). Some authors consider it to be contiguous with the Achilles tendon distal to its insertion onto the calcaneus. Repetitive, impact-oriented activity such as jogging can lead to inflammation and microtears of the plantar fascia, most commonly around its origin. Patients will typically report plantar-medial heel pain that is insidious in onset. Classically, pain is most pronounced when first rising from bed in the morning, and when standing after being in a prolonged seated position. Physical examination will demonstrate focal tenderness over the medial calca-

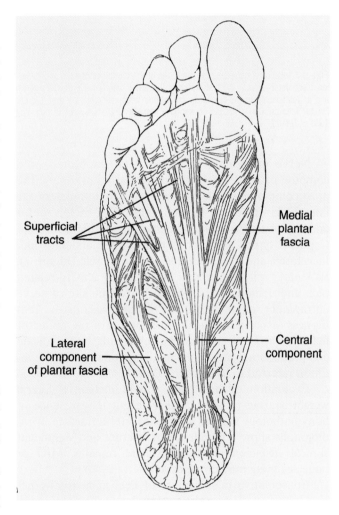

Figure 1 Anatomic components of the plantar fascia.

neal tuberosity. Triceps surae contracture can usually be demonstrated on examination, and it has been implicated as the salient contributing factor in the development of plantar fasciitis. Tenderness over the lateral calcaneal tuberosity with side-to-side compression (squeeze test) should raise suspicion for a calcaneal stress fracture, which can have a clinical presentation very similar to that of plantar fasciitis.

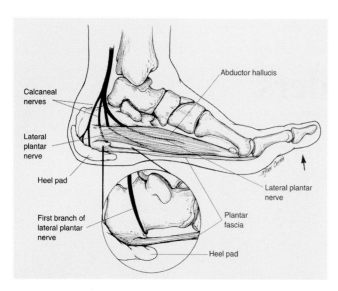

Figure 2 Location of nerves in proximity to the heel. Arrow indicates force of dorsiflexion. Inset, detail showing the first branch of the lateral plantar nerve (Baxter's nerve) and its relationship to the calcaneus and plantar fascia. *(Reproduced from Gill LH: Plantar fasciitis: Diagnosis and conservative management.* J Am Acad Orthop Surg *1997;5:109-117.)*

Nerve entrapment has also been implicated as a common cause of heel pain, particularly in runners. The most common nerve implicated is the first branch of the lateral plantar nerve (Baxter's nerve), a mixed motor and sensory nerve to the abductor digiti quinti, with entrapment typically occurring between the abductor hallucis fascia and the quadratus plantae muscle (Figure 2). Patients typically report lancinating, activity-related pain and demonstrate tenderness over the site of nerve entrapment rather than at the plantar fascia origin. Tenderness associated with the midportion of the abductor hallucis, distal to the sustentaculum tali, may indicate compression neuritis of the medial plantar nerve, a condition referred to as "jogger's foot."

Evaluation of heel pain should include a lateral weight-bearing radiograph to rule out the presence of bony pathology such as a calcaneal stress fracture. If radiographs show no evidence of fracture and significant clinical suspicion of stress fracture remains, MRI or bone scanning may prove useful.

Conservative management of heel pain usually begins with rest, an aggressive Achilles tendon stretching program, accommodative heel cushions/orthoses, and nonsteroidal anti-inflammatory drugs (NSAIDs). Functional biomechanical deficits have been implicated in the development of plantar fasciitis in athletes, and formal physical therapy evaluation and treatment may be useful to address these specifically. If the most pronounced pain occurs in the morning, the patient may also benefit from the addition of a dorsiflexion night splint to stretch the Achilles tendon. Some authors found this to be 80% successful, although others noted a high rate of noncompliance with this modality. Although

steroid injections may be useful in treating plantar fasciitis, they have been associated with an increased risk of plantar fascia rupture. Iontophoresis has also been shown to be of short-term benefit in the treatment of plantar fasciitis, when combined with traditional modalities. One study investigating the effectiveness of iontophoresis involved 40 feet with plantar fasciitis. Twenty feet were treated with traditional modalities, and 20 were treated with a combination of traditional modalities plus iontophoresis with dexamethasone. At 2-week follow-up, the patients treated with iontophoresis had significantly greater improvement than the group treated with traditional modalities alone. One month after treatment, however, both groups demonstrated clinical improvement with no significant difference between them.

In general, conservative modalities are successful in resolving plantar fasciitis in approximately 80% to 90% of patients. Historically, surgical management was the only recourse for those patients who failed to respond to traditional nonsurgical modalities. More recently, however, extracorporeal shock wave treatment (ESWT) has become available as a treatment option. The exact mechanism of ESWT is unknown, but it is thought to increase regional blood flow to the plantar fascia, thus promoting a healing response. Two forms are available: high-energy ESWT and low-energy ESWT. High-energy ESWT involves only a single treatment, but it must be performed with the patient under general or regional anesthesia and typically requires an outpatient surgical suite. Low-energy ESWT is applied in several weekly treatments, but for this procedure patients require no anesthesia and it may be performed in an outpatient office setting. Results of ESWT have been promising. One study investigated 302 patients treated with high-energy ESWT. At 3-month follow-up, the authors noted good to excellent results in 57% of patients, good results in 24%, fair results in 11%, and poor results in 8%. Twenty-two percent of patients required a second treatment. Another study reported on 86 feet in 80 patients who were treated with high-energy ESWT. At 3-month follow-up, 20% of patients reported no pain and 57% reported significant relief. At 6-month follow-up, 59% were pain free and 27% reported significant relief.

Surgical management of recalcitrant plantar fasciitis/heel pain usually involves release of the distal tarsal tunnel with partial plantar fasciotomy. An important component of this surgery is circumferential release of the fascia surrounding the abductor hallucis muscle (Figure 3). Most authors advocate releasing only the medial third of the plantar fascia because complete release has been associated with late collapse of the arch. One study investigated 75 patients (80 heels) treated with distal tarsal tunnel release and partial plantar fasciotomy, and reported good to excellent results in 88%.

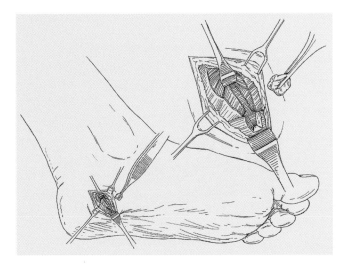

Figure 3 Surgical decompression of Baxter's nerve. The medial approach allows release of the superficial and deep fascia of the abductor hallucis muscle and a partial plantar fasciotomy. Inset, detail showing the medial one third of the plantar fascia segmentally excised. *(Adapted with permission from Pfeffer G: Plantar heel pain, in Myerson (ed): Foot and Ankle Disorders. Philadelphia, PA, WB Saunders, 2000, p 845.)*

Some authors have advocated the use of endoscopic plantar fascia release to treat recalcitrant plantar fasciitis/heel pain. Most use a two-portal technique with cannula insertion across the plantar aspect of the plantar fascia. Common criticism of this technique includes the fact that the deep fascia of the abductor hallucis muscle, which is considered to be one of the primary structures contributing to nerve impingement, is not released. In addition, the exact amount of plantar fascia released is difficult to control. Furthermore, several articles have reported iatrogenic nerve injury associated with endoscopic release. Nonetheless, advocates of the procedure claim that neurovascular structures are at less risk (which has been supported by cadaveric studies) and that patients have shorter recovery times.

Plantar Fascia Rupture

Although uncommon, spontaneous rupture of the plantar fascia has been described in athletes. Patients usually report a tearing sensation or "pop" in the midarch region associated with sudden acceleration. Treatment is supportive and typically involves a period of time in a walking cast or boot, followed by use of an orthotic support. Immediate application of a well-molded short leg walking cast with serial examination at weekly intervals until patients report no tenderness is recommended. Late collapse of the arch has been reported after plantar fascia rupture, but this is a rare occurrence. Also, late sequelae can include lateral column overload and pain, which have been associated with cuboid stress fractures. This overload typically improves over time and may be alleviated with the use of orthotic devices.

Posterior Ankle Impingement/Painful Os Trigonum

The os trigonum represents an ununited lateral tubercle on the posterior aspect of the talus. The trigonal or Stieda process is an abnormally large lateral talar tubercle that often articulates with the calcaneus. The incidence of os trigonum in the general population is approximately 7% to 13%, with 33% to 50% of cases being bilateral. In many patients, os trigona and Stieda processes are asymptomatic and discovered incidentally on radiographs. An os trigonum or Stieda process may become symptomatic, however, following a lateral ankle sprain, as a result of a fracture through the trigonal process (Shepherd's fracture) or soft-tissue impingement (often encountered in dancers). Symptoms include pain in the posterior heel and/or Achilles tendon region or deep posterior ankle pain and may be exacerbated by jumping or dancing en pointe. On examination, tenderness is usually noted along the posterolateral ankle. Pain is usually elicited with full plantar flexion, and pronation and supination in this position may also elicit clicking and reproduce symptoms.

Lateral radiographs will demonstrate the presence of an os trigonum or Stieda process. Plain radiographs may not be helpful, however, in the absence of a fracture or obvious diastasis. Plantar flexion radiographs may demonstrate posterior translation of an unstable os trigonum. If the diagnosis is in question, bone scanning may show increased uptake in the vicinity of the os trigonum. Injection of local anesthetic around the os trigonum may also help confirm the diagnosis.

Initial treatment should consist of relative rest, with avoidance of impact-oriented activity and pointe work. Steroid injection or NSAIDs may also be of benefit. Surgical management for patients who fail to respond to conservative treatment consists of excision of the posterior process or os trigonum through a posterolateral approach.

Flexor Hallucis Longus Tendinitis

When evaluating patients for posterior ankle impingement, it is important to investigate the possibility of flexor hallucis longus (FHL) tendinitis, which can be an associated condition. This entity is especially common among ballet dancers. Distinguishing between FHL tendinitis and posterior impingement may be quite difficult. Pain and tenderness are typically laterally based for patients with posterior impingement, whereas FHL tendinitis usually presents with medial-based pain, tenderness along the course of the FHL tendon, and pain with motion of the hallux. Patients may report a clicking or locking sensation of the hallux, particularly when going from a fully pointed to dorsiflexed position.

Nonsurgical treatment of FHL tendinitis consists of rest, NSAIDs, and physical therapy with phonophoresis and iontophoresis. Surgical management for FHL ten-

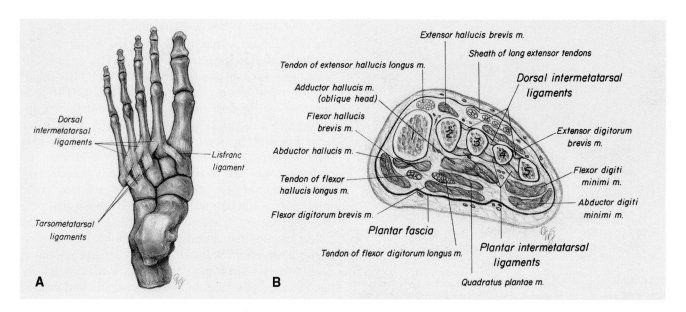

Figure 4 A, Dorsal view of the foot. **B,** Cross-sectional anatomy of the foot at the metatarsal base level. *(Reproduced with permission from Anderson RB: Lisfranc's fracture-dislocation, in Pfeffer GB, Frey CC (eds):* Current Practice in Foot and Ankle Surgery. *New York, NY, McGraw Hill, 1993, pp 129-159.)*

dinitis consists of release of the tendon through a posteromedial approach. If an associated os trigonum or Stieda process is present, it may be removed through the same approach.

Midfoot

Lisfranc Fracture-Dislocation

Background

Jacques Lisfranc, a French surgeon in Napoleon's army, described a technique for amputation through the tarsometatarsal joints, although he never wrote specifically about injuries to these joints. Nevertheless, his name has become synonymous with injuries to these joints. Lisfranc injuries represent fractures or dislocations to any of the tarsometatarsal joints, including the bases of the five metatarsals with their accompanying three cuneiforms and the cuboid. The incidence of Lisfranc injuries is quite rare, averaging about one case in every 5,000 patients injured. Motor vehicle accidents account for the majority of Lisfranc injuries, although athletes, especially football players, have been shown to be at risk from more indirect mechanisms.

The first significant report of Lisfranc injuries was published in 1909. The authors reviewed 30 cases from which they derived a classification system that continues to be the primary method for classifying these injuries today. Over the past 10 years, there has been a renewed interest in Lisfranc injuries. Modifications to the classification system have been made, and advances in CT have helped identify more subtle subtypes of these dislocations, the possibility for proximal extension and variants, as well as to the presence of associated occult injuries.

Anatomy

The tarsometatarsal joints are made up of articulations between the bases of the medial three metatarsals and the three cuneiforms, as well as the lateral two metatarsal bases and the cuboid. The main stabilizer is the second metatarsal base (the "keystone"), which lies nestled between the medial and lateral cuneiforms.

The midfoot is seen as a transverse plantar arch composed of asymmetrically shaped bones on cross section. There are a multitude of stabilizers that provide support to the midfoot and to weight-bearing forces. There are interosseous ligaments that join the bases of the second through fifth metatarsals, and they are larger and more substantial in strength along the plantar aspect of the foot. Although there is no transverse metatarsal ligament between the base of the first and second metatarsals, there is a large, oblique ligament that extends from the base of the second metatarsal to the medial cuneiform (Lisfranc's ligament). The plantar aspect of the tarsometatarsal joints is further reinforced by secondary stabilizers, including the plantar fascia, intrinsic muscles, and extrinsic tendons (Figure 4). The lack of equal supporting fibers to the dorsal aspect of the foot makes this area more susceptible to injuries. The ramus plantares profundus of the dorsalis pedis artery joins the plantar arch between the bases of the first and second metatarsals. This structure, as well as the dorsalis pedis artery itself, is susceptible to injury with a fracture-dislocation at this level.

Mechanism of Injury

The majority of Lisfranc injuries results from trauma and can further be divided into direct and indirect types. The indirect type is more common.

Direct injuries to the tarsometatarsal joint will result in atypical fracture patterns, with a variable degree of bony and soft-tissue injury. Open fractures may occur as well. Often, there is a comminution at the metatarsal base or cuneiform level that occasionally propagates to the tarsal navicular. Compartment syndrome of the foot is one of the complications noted to follow this direct mechanism of injury.

Indirect injuries occur at the anatomically weaker dorsal aspect of this joint. These injuries begin with an axial load applied to the plantar flexed foot. As the forefoot hyperplantar flexes, the weak dorsal tarsometatarsal ligaments rupture. As the injury progresses, the plantar aspect of the metatarsal base may fracture or the plantar capsule may rupture, allowing the metatarsal bases to displace dorsally. If the force of injury is sustained, forces travel proximally through the intercuneiform region, and the dorsal ligaments of Chopart's joints may also rupture.

The direction and degree of metatarsal displacement is determined by the amount of rotation occurring during the injury. Severe abduction and lateral displacement of the metatarsal can lead to a compression fracture of the cuboid ("nutcracker" injury). This fracture, as with a fracture through the base of the second metatarsal, can be considered pathognomonic for Lisfranc injuries.

Classification

Although a classification scheme for Lisfranc injuries was first developed in 1909, the 1982 modification of this system is currently more commonly used. There are three types of Lisfranc injuries as identified with this system: (1) homolateral or total incongruity (all five metatarsals are displaced in the same direction; a fracture through the base of the second metatarsal is common), (2) isolated or partial incongruities (displacement of one or more metatarsals from the others), and (3) divergent (medial displacement of the first metatarsal with lateral displacement of the lateral four metatarsals). In this type of Lisfranc injury, the force of injury can extend to the cuneiforms and the tarsal navicular. Other authors have developed a more recent classification system based on the above scheme that highlights the more proximal variants (Figure 5).

History

It is estimated that approximately 20% of Lisfranc injuries are missed on initial examination. Because many of these midfoot injuries are purely ligamentous, it is mandatory that clinicians have a strong suspicion when evaluating these individuals. Typically, it is the recreational athlete with a twisting injury to the foot for whom radiographs show no evidence of injury who is subsequently diagnosed with a midfoot sprain. There is no age group that is immune to this potential problem.

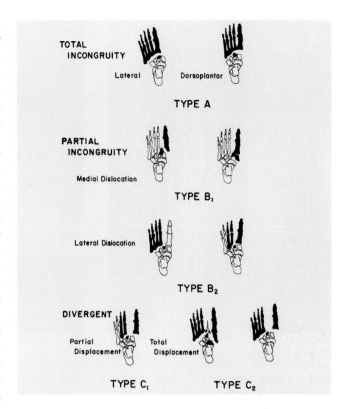

Figure 5 Diagram illustrating the classification of injury types. *(Reproduced with permission from Myerson MS, Fisher RT, Burgess AR, et al: Fracture dislocations of the tarsometatarsal joints: End results correlated with pathology and treatment. Foot Ankle 1986;6:225-242.)*

Therefore, it is mandatory to evaluate patients with chronic midfoot pain for subtle signs and symptoms regardless of the etiology. Patients may have a history of difficulty bearing weight and diffuse pain and swelling.

Physical Examination

A thorough physical examination begins with evaluation of weight bearing, which is typically impossible for patients with even minor Lisfranc injuries. Examination of stance may detect asymmetries, including loss of arch height, an abducted posture to the foot, and a dorsomedial midfoot prominence. Seated examination should elicit any areas of localized tenderness. Frequently, this will be in the region of the Lisfranc ligament. Also, the presence of ecchymosis involving the plantar midfoot, when encountered, is highly suggestive of a Lisfranc injury. Pain may be reproduced with manipulation of the midfoot joints, particularly pronation-abduction and supination-adduction. Because these injuries may not be confined to the tarsometatarsal joint level, joints proximal and distal must also be carefully evaluated. Finally, vascular examination should be done as well as a neurologic examination to assess the function of the deep peroneal nerve to the first web space.

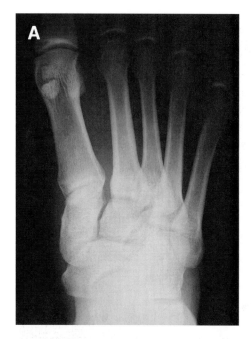
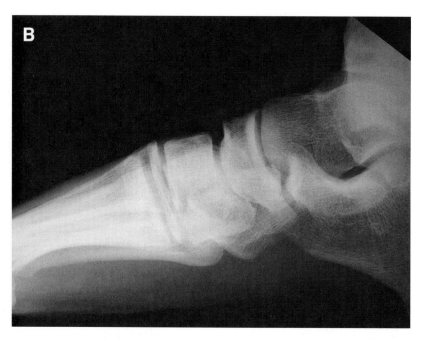

Figure 6 Non–weight-bearing AP (**A**) and lateral (**B**) radiographs of the right foot in a 39-year-old woman who sustained a twisting injury approximately 1 week before presentation. Note the slight diastasis between the first and second metatarsal bases, as well as light dorsal subluxation of the second metatarsal base. No obvious fractures are noted. *(Reproduced from Anderson RB: Missed Lisfranc injury, in Pfeffer GB, Nunley JA, Sanders RW, Trepman E: Advanced Reconstruction: Foot and Ankle. Rosemont, IL, American Academy of Orthopaedic Surgeons, 2004, pp 397-401.)*

Radiographic Examination

AP, lateral, and oblique radiographs of the involved foot are mandatory. These must be weight-bearing films because spontaneous reduction may occur after a ligamentous injury (Figures 6 and 7). In a normal foot, there exists a consistent relationship between the medial margin of the middle cuneiform and the medial aspect of the second metatarsal. On the oblique view, an unbroken line should exist between the medial base of the fourth metatarsal and the medial margin of the cuboid. On the lateral view, an unbroken line should exist between the dorsum of the first and second metatarsals and their corresponding cuneiforms. Also, flattening of the arch is suggestive of midfoot injury. Patients should always be assessed for subtle associated findings, such as compression fractures of the cuboid, second metatarsal base fractures, the presence of a fleck sign (representing a small avulsion fracture of the base of the second metatarsal), lesser MTP joint dislocations, metatarsal head and neck fractures, and intercuneiform diastasis. When in doubt, standing views of the contralateral foot should be obtained for comparison.

Fluoroscopic examination may be useful when weight-bearing radiographs are unobtainable. This technique, however, is dependent on the administration of adequate anesthesia. The maneuver to elicit joint diastasis is pronation-abduction and supination-adduction. A single-limb weight-bearing AP radiograph of the injured foot can be a substitute for a formal stress radiograph.

When evaluating Lisfranc injuries, CT is useful to assess the fracture pattern and plantar comminution. A splay view, which is a coronal view of the midfoot transformed from a mortise configuration to a flattened plane so as to allow detailed examination of each of the tarsometatarsal joints, can be a helpful adjunct.

Bone scanning may be considered in patients with persistent pain and no radiographic evidence of instability. MRI, however, because of its higher specificity, has replaced bone scanning as the diagnostic modality of choice for assessing purely ligamentous injuries, synovitis, and subtle osteochondral injuries.

Treatment

The goal of any treatment is to obtain and maintain anatomic reduction because persistent malalignment greatly increases the risk of late degenerative change and deformity. Therefore, any amount of displacement in a healthy, active patient warrants surgical reduction and fixation. Traditionally, closed reduction and percutaneous pin fixation has been advocated for the treatment of minimally displaced injuries. In recent years, however, there has been a trend to use open reduction to treat all Lisfranc injuries that require surgical stabilization. This allows direct visualization of the fracture fragments as well as removal of interposed soft tissue and debris. Controversy remains regarding the use of screws versus percutaneous pins for fixation. Again, the current trend is to use screws to treat Lisfranc injuries of the first through third tarsometatarsal joints, including a

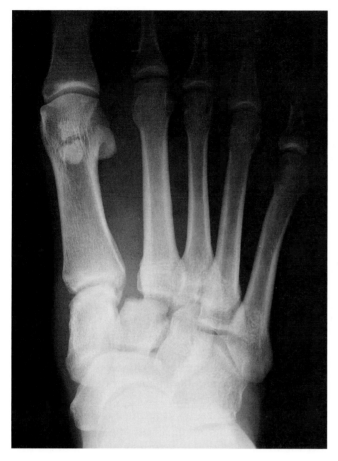

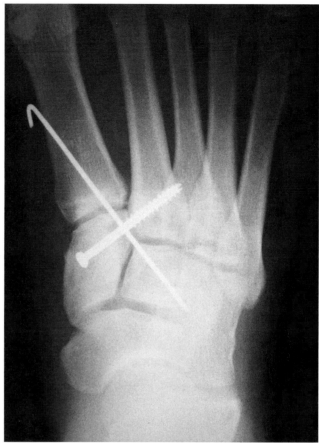

Figure 7 Weight-bearing AP radiograph of the right foot in the same patient demonstrates markedly increased diastasis between the first and second metatarsal bases, along with significant lateral translation of the second metatarsal. Also note the subtle diastasis of the medial and middle cuneiform interspace. Again, no fractures are identified. These findings are consistent with an unstable, ligamentous Lisfranc injury. *(Reproduced from Anderson RB: Missed Lisfranc injury, in Pfeffer GB, Nunley JA, Sanders RW, Trepman E: Advanced Reconstruction: Foot and Ankle. Rosemont, IL, American Academy of Orthopaedic Surgeons, 2004, pp 397-401.)*

Figure 8 The same patient after open reduction and internal fixation. Note the reduction of the second metatarsal base with a home run screw in place, as well as closure of the first and second metatarsals and intercuneiform diastasis. *(Reproduced from Anderson RB: Missed Lisfranc injury, in Pfeffer GB, Nunley JA, Sanders RW, Trepman E: Advanced Reconstruction: Foot and Ankle. Rosemont, IL, American Academy of Orthopaedic Surgeons, 2004, pp 397-401.)*

home run screw from the medial cuneiform through the base of the second metatarsal (Figure 8). The rationale for this is that ligamentous injuries may take 3 to 6 months to heal, which is longer than the life span of a simple pin; 3.5- or 4.5-mm AO cortical screws are most commonly used. To treat Lisfranc injuries of the fourth and fifth tarsometatarsal joints, buttressing with percutaneous 0.062-inch Kirschner wires is typically sufficient.

For competitive athletes, a non–weight-bearing splint is used for 2 weeks postoperatively and then followed by a removable boot (still non–weight-bearing) for another 4 weeks to allow for the initiation of pool therapy with gentle range-of-motion exercises. The patient is then allowed to bear weight in a boot for another 6 weeks, and rehabilitation is continued. At 16 weeks, the patient is allowed to return to competitive play with appropriate protection. A longitudinal arch support with a turf toe plate is used for at least 6 months. For competitive athletes, all screws across the tarsometatarsal

joints are removed at 6 months postoperatively, followed by a 6- to 8-week period of reduced activity (no contact sports). Intercuneiform screws are left in permanently because of the risk of recurrent diastasis.

Forefoot

Turf Toe

Background

Since the term "turf toe" was first used in the literature in 1976, soft-tissue hyperextension injuries to the hallux MTP joint have received increasing attention from physicians, trainers, and athletes. The broad range of injuries that can occur to the hallux MTP joint have historically been lumped under the general category of "turf toe." It is now recognized, however, that in addition to the typical hyperextension-type injury to the hallux MTP joint, there are variations that account for injuries to specific anatomic structures in the capsuloligamentous complex. These injuries can lead to significant functional limita-

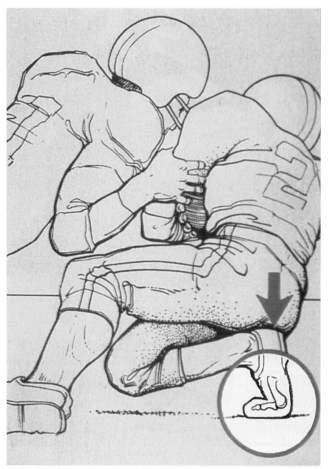

Figure 9 Turf toe is characterized by a dorsiflexion injury of the first MTP joint that damages the plantar structures. *(Reproduced from Sullivan JA, Anderson SJ (eds): Care of the Young Athlete . Rosemont, IL, American Academy of Orthopaedic Surgeons, 2000, p 436.)*

tions, particularly when not recognized early. Loss of push-off strength and late deformities such as clawing or hallux rigidus can follow these ligamentous injuries, often with career-ending consequences. Physicians treating athletes with foot and ankle injuries should be familiar with the spectrum of injuries around the hallux MTP joint, conservative as well as surgical treatment, and late associated sequelae.

Mechanism
Classically, turf toe was thought to be related to shoe-surface interface inequities, and it most commonly occurs in football players participating in athletic activities on artificial turf. The basic mechanism of a turf toe injury is primary hyperextension of the hallux MTP joint with attenuation and disruption of the plantar complex. Typically, an axial load is applied to the heel of a foot in a fixed equinus position, which is quite similar to the mechanism causing Lisfranc injuries of the midfoot (Figure 9). There is a wide spectrum of injury that includes partial tearing of the plantar soft tissues to frank dislocation of the joint. As plantar

rupture occurs, unrestricted dorsiflexion may result in impaction injury of the proximal phalanx on the dorsal articular surface of the metatarsal head.

Numerous variations can occur, depending on the force of the injury and position of the hallux. The most common variation is that created by valgus-directed force, which results in injury to the plantar-medial complex or tibial sesamoid. This type of injury may lead to the development of a traumatic bunion. Hyperflexion injuries to the hallux MTP joint can also occur and have been termed "sand toe." This condition has been reported primarily in beach volleyball players; however, it has also been noted to occur in dancers.

Classification
A classification system for turf toe injuries was described in 1986 (Table 1) and updated in 1999 based on clinical findings and associated treatment (Table 2).

Patient Evaluation
A detailed history and physical examination must be performed. Examination should note hallux alignment as well as any evidence of ecchymosis and swelling. MTP joint range of motion and any evidence of joint instability should also be recorded.

A thorough radiographic evaluation of the hallux MTP joint is mandatory in diagnosing and treating the turf toe injury. Routine radiographs often show no evidence of injury, but they may show small avulsion fractures off of the plantar aspect of the proximal phalanx or at the distal pole of the sesamoids. Capsular avulsions may also be noted. Assessment of sesamoid position using a standing AP radiograph is critical. An AP radiograph of the contralateral foot is recommended for comparison. Any proximal migration of the sesamoid(s) indicates disruption of the plantar complex. Stress dorsiflexion lateral radiographs can assess whether there is normal distal migration of the sesamoids and can also demonstrate diastasis of a bipartite or fractured sesamoid (Figure 10). Formal sesamoid views can help further delineate the presence of a fracture or diastasis.

MRI is recommended for patients with radiographic abnormalities and/or patients with grade II or III injuries. MRI best defines the degree of soft-tissue injury and any associated osseus or articular damage.

Treatment
Little has been written or formalized in the treatment of turf toe injuries. Nonsurgical treatment consists of rest, ice, compression, and elevation as well as analgesics and NSAIDs. A boot or cast can be applied and is typically worn for at least 1 week. A toe spica extension with the hallux in slight plantar flexion may be incorporated. Taping regimens provide compression while limiting motion at the MTP joint. This is most helpful in the treatment of milder injuries in conjunction with shoe-

TABLE 1 | Classification of Turf Toe Injuries

Type of Injury	Classification	Characteristics
Hyperextension (turf toe)	Grade 1—Stretching of the plantar complex	Localized tenderness, minimal swelling, no ecchymosis
	Grade 2—Partial tear	Diffuse tenderness, moderate swelling, ecchymosis, restricted movement with pain
	*Grade 3—Frank tear	Severe tenderness to palpation, marked swelling and ecchymosis; limited movement with pain; positive vertical Lachman's test, if pain allows
	Associated injuries	Medial or lateral injury; sesamoid fracture with bipartite diastasis; articular cartilage and subchondral bone bruise
Hyperflexion (sand toe)	Dislocation—Type I	Dislocation of the hallux with the sesamoids
		No disruption of the intersesamoid ligament; usually irreducible
	Type II	Associated disruption of intersesamoid ligament; usually reducible
	II A	
	II B	Associated transverse fracture of one of the sesamoids; usually reducible
	II C	Complete disruption of intersesamoid ligament fracture of one of the sesamoids; usually reducible

*Grade 3 injuries may represent spontaneously reduced dislocations.

TABLE 2 | Clinical Classification System for Turf Toe Injury

Grade	Objective Findings	Activity Level	Treatment
1	Localized plantar or medial tenderness Minimal swelling No ecchymosis	Continued athletic participation	Symptomatic
2	More diffuse and intense tenderness Mild to moderate swelling Mild to moderate ecchymosis	Loss of playing time for 3 to 14 days	Walking boot and crutches as needed
3	Severe and diffuse tenderness Marked swelling Moderate to severe ecchymosis Range of motion painful and limited	Loss of playing time for at least 4 to 6 weeks	Long-term immobilization in boot or cast versus surgical repair

(Reproduced with permission from Coughlin MJ, Mann RA (eds): Surgery of the Foot and Ankle, ed 7. St. Louis, MO, Mosby, 1999, vol 2, p 1186.)

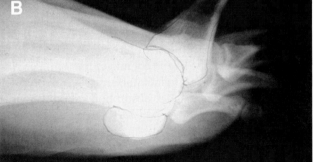

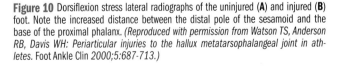

Figure 10 Dorsiflexion stress lateral radiographs of the uninjured (**A**) and injured (**B**) foot. Note the increased distance between the distal pole of the sesamoid and the base of the proximal phalanx. *(Reproduced with permission from Watson TS, Anderson RB, Davis WH: Periarticular injuries to the hallux metatarsophalangeal joint in athletes. Foot Ankle Clin 2000;5:687-713.)*

wear modification and orthoses. Orthoses can either be custom-made or off the shelf; they typically incorporate a rigid forefoot component (turf toe plate).

Steroid injections are not recommended in the treatment of turf toe injuries; however, local anesthetic alone may be useful to address localized pain in a single nerve distribution.

Surgical management is seldom necessary, but it should be considered for a large capsular avulsion with an unstable joint, diastasis of bipartite sesamoid or sesa-moid fracture, retraction of the sesamoids, traumatic or progressive bunion, vertical instability, and the presence of a loose body or chondral injury. The goal of surgery is to restore the anatomy for preservation of function.

Sesamoid Disorders

The sesamoids are particularly vulnerable to overuse disorders in athletes. Pain can be caused by a variety of sources, including arthrosis, chondromalacia, osteochondritis dissecans, stress fractures, and flexor hallucis brevis tendinitis. Neuritic pain has also been reported.

Treatment of most of these conditions is largely supportive (ie, immobilization, activity and shoe-wear modification, NSAIDs, specialized orthotics, and selective injections). Turf toe plates are often helpful. Imaging using bone scanning or MRI is recommended before surgery to confirm the precise location of the pathology. Surgical management typically involves complete or partial resection of the offending sesamoid. A cadaveric study reported a significant loss of effective tendon moment arms with sesamoid excision, which corresponds with the loss of push-off strength usually seen in vivo. Sesamoid excision, therefore, should only be considered when all other treatment options have been exhausted. As an alternative to sesamoid excision, autogenous bone grafting has been advocated for select patients with sesamoid nonunions.

Stress Fractures

Foot and ankle stress fractures are extremely common in athletes. The increased awareness of stress fractures among physicians has also resulted in more stress fractures of the lower extremity being recognized and treated early. Causative factors include poor training techniques, osteoporosis, playing surfaces, shoe wear, and foot and ankle alignment. Bone typically fails when the stress applied exceeds its reparative capacity. The amount of load, the frequency of loading, and the number of repetitions all determine the point of failure. Anatomic variations can help dictate the location of stress fractures. Rigid, cavus feet tend to distribute more force to the tibia and femur and increase the risk of stress fractures in these bones. Patients with varus hindfoot posture are at increased risk for stress fractures involving the lateral column of the foot. Pes planus predisposes athletes to metatarsal stress fractures because of the increased shock absorption within the midfoot and hindfoot.

Patient Evaluation

Evaluation should begin, as always, with a careful history. A high index of suspicion for these injuries will minimize the morbidity of prolonged treatment and recovery. The history should include details of the athlete's training regimen and any recent changes in training regimen and shoe wear. Early in the course of disease, athletes will typically report vague soreness or throbbing pain with specific activity. If athletes fail to seek medical attention or this disease is not recognized, it can result in pain that occurs earlier and more frequently during activity. This may eventually result in

pain outside of athletic activity. Physical examination typically results in a paucity of findings early in the course of the injury. The examination should focus on any focal areas of tenderness and swelling, as well as gait changes, guarding, and/or weakness. Radiographs may show no evidence of injury for the first 3 to 4 weeks after the onset of symptoms. In addition, plain radiographs may be unable to identify some stress fractures in the foot secondary to the complex anatomy and overlapping shadows. In the absence of radiographic evidence of injury, bone scanning has been used to detect stress fractures because it will usually show evidence of a fracture within 48 to 72 hours of symptom onset. MRI is being used more often because it has high sensitivity and specificity and can define both osseous and soft-tissue structures. CT may also be used to evaluate patients with suspected stress fractures of the foot and ankle, but is best used to assess the healing of known stress fractures.

Treatment

Once recognized, most stress fractures of the foot and ankle can be treated with conservative methods. The one exception is a stress fracture of the fifth metatarsal. In high-level athletes, these should almost always be treated with partially threaded cancellous screw fixation with or without bone grafting. When recognized early in the course of the disease, stress fractures involving bones other than the fifth metatarsal should be treated initially with rest. This can simply consist of restriction from the inciting activity or immobilization in a walker boot or cast for a limited period of time. Athletes can be permitted to continue participation in activities that do not elicit symptoms, such as cycling or swimming, to maintain cardiovascular conditioning. Patients with stress fractures that are recognized late and have evidence of fragmentation, displacement, or sclerotic margins should be considered for surgical treatment with open reduction, bone grafting and drilling of the fracture site, and internal fixation.

Distal Fibular Stress Fractures

This fracture is common in long-distance runners and may be mistaken for an ankle sprain, peroneal tenosynovitis, or peroneal tear. Distal fibular stress fractures have been associated with planovalgus feet. In addition, these fractures typically occur in the isthmus of the distal fibula. Treatment usually consists of a walking cast or boot from which the patient is weaned as symptoms allow. Patients with planovalgus feet may also require the use of orthotics when resuming activity.

Stress Fractures of the Medial Malleolus

Fractures of the medial malleolus are rare. Genu varum and tibia vara are associated anatomic variations. Medial malleolus fractures are thought to occur from impingement of the talus on the medial malleolus during dorsiflexion of the tibiotalar joint. If the fracture is non-displaced, a walking cast or boot will usually suffice for treatment. Any displacement, persistent pain, or failure of the fracture to unite after 8 weeks of treatment warrants treatment with open reduction and internal fixation.

Calcaneal Stress Fractures

Calcaneal fractures are typically difficult to differentiate from other posterior heel pathologies. Because radiography cannot effectively identify this entity, bone scanning or MRI is typically required to make a definitive diagnosis. Pain elicited by the squeeze test may be the only specific physical finding. When calcaneal stress fractures are diagnosed early, they may be treated with restriction of the inciting activity and the use of a heel cushion. Later in the disease course, these fractures should be treated with a walking cast or boot and at least 6 weeks of rest. Long-term sequelae are rare.

Navicular Stress Fractures

Navicular stress fractures have recently been receiving increased recognition within the realm of sports medicine. These injuries are typically seen among athletes involved in sports requiring sudden acceleration and deceleration, such as track and field, basketball, and football. Anatomic features predisposing athletes to these injuries (eg, a long second metatarsal or a short first metatarsal) have been reported in the literature. Another feature contributing to these injuries is the unique vascular anatomy of the navicular. It is supplied by peripheral arteries branching from the posterior tibial and dorsalis pedis arteries, which provide an adequate blood supply to the medial and lateral aspects of the navicular. The central portion of the navicular, which is the most common site for stress fractures, is relatively avascular.

Athletes with these injuries will typically have diffuse and poorly defined symptoms. Because pain may be initially referred to the medial arch or the anterior ankle, this entity may be mistaken for anterior tibial tendinitis, midfoot sprain, or a plantar fascial injury. Physical examination may reveal tenderness over the dorsal aspect of the navicular, or symptoms may be elicited by asking the patient to hop on a plantar flexed foot. Patients are often diagnosed late secondary to the paucity of findings as well as no evidence of injury on plain radiographs early in the course of the disease. Although bone scanning is an excellent initial screening tool for this type of injury, MRI or CT may be required to further delineate the injury. Navicular stress fractures typically occur in the central third of the navicular and dorsal to plantar in the sagittal plane. Patients with stress fractures that are partial or complete but nondisplaced and have no evidence of sclerosis should be treated with immobilization and should not bear weight for 6 to 8 weeks. Navicular stress fractures that do not respond to conservative measures and those that are displaced, complete, or have sclerotic margins should be treated with curettage and drilling of the margins and placement of internal fixation across the fracture site, with or without bone graft.

Second, Third, and Fourth Metatarsal Stress Fractures

These fractures rarely displace and are treated supportively. One variant is the so-called "dancer's fracture," involving the base of the second metatarsal, which can occasionally be intra-articular.

Fifth Metatarsal Base Stress Fractures (Jones Fracture)

The Jones fracture is classically described as a fracture within the fifth metatarsal's proximal metaphyseal-diaphyseal junction. This is a watershed area with poor vascularity; fractures in this region have a particularly high rate of nonunion. Although controversy exists as to the appropriate treatment of Jones fractures, most authors agree that noncompetitive athletes with these injuries should be treated with a short leg non–weight-bearing cast for 6 to 8 weeks, followed by protected weight bearing for another 6 weeks.

Surgical treatment is currently recommended for fractures that fail to respond to conservative management or for competitive athletes who require more aggressive rehabilitation and return to play. Fixation usually consists of a partially threaded cancellous screw, either cannulated or solid. Recommended screw sizes range from 4.5 mm to 7.0 mm. If the patient demonstrates lateral column overload with a varus hindfoot, a lateral closing wedge calcaneal (Dwyer) osteotomy should be considered. Postoperatively, the patient should be immobilized for 2 weeks, followed by early range-of-motion exercises and pool therapy. The use of an external bone stimulator may also be considered. Weight bearing should begin at 2 to 4 weeks, and running exercises are permitted at 6 weeks if there is radiographic evidence of healing. Return to play is usually allowed at 8 to 12 weeks, again depending on radiographic and clinical evidence of healing. Nonunions are addressed with repeat fixation with a larger screw (if possible) and autogenous bone grafting.

Summary

Athletic disorders and injuries to the foot are increasing in incidence, which is likely related to training issues, peak performance levels, shoe wear trends, and athletic field composition. Etiologies for these injuries are numerous and can be broadly classified as acute or chronic. Neglected injuries can lead to long-term deformity and dysfunction. Imaging is extremely helpful in diagnosing subtle injuries and should be used early for athletes with chronic discomfort without associated clinical and radiographic findings. Although most of these athletic injuries are overuse related and can be treated with a period of relative rest and activity modification, the physician needs to be mindful of ligamentous injuries with joint diastasis or stress fractures, which require prompt surgical intervention.

Annotated Bibliography

Hindfoot

Berlet GC, Anderson RB, Davis H, Kiebzak GM: A prospective trial of night splinting in the treatment of recalcitrant plantar fasciitis: the ankle dorsiflexion Dynasplint. *Orthopedics* 2002;25:1273-1275.

This prospective study noted that nighttime dorsiflexion splinting of patients with recalcitrant heel pain is successful approximately 80% of the time; compliance, however, is difficult because of patient discomfort.

Chen HS, Chen LM, Huang TW: Treatment of painful heels syndrome with shock waves. *Clin Orthop* 2001;387:41-46.

The authors of this study assessed 80 patients (86 feet) who underwent high-energy shock wave treatment and report that of 54 patients evaluated at 6-month follow-up, 59% had no symptoms and 27% reported substantial improvement.

Ogden JA, Alvarez R, Levitt R, Cross GL, Marlow M: Shock wave therapy for chronic proximal plantar fasciitis. *Clin Orthop* 2001;387:47-59.

The authors of this randomized, placebo-controlled study noted a success rate of 47% with high-energy shock wave therapy compared with 30% in the placebo group.

Riddle DL, Pulisic M, Pidcoe P, Johnson RE: Risk factors for plantar fasciitis: A matched case-control study. *J Bone Joint Surg Am* 2003;85:872-877.

The authors of this study used matching criteria of age and gender to analyze 50 patients with unilateral fasciitis for risk factors. They found that the risk of plantar fasciitis increases as the range of ankle dorsiflexion decreases. The risk was also increased in those who spent the majority of their work day standing as well as in those who were obese.

Watson TS, Anderson RB, Davis WH, Kiebzak GM: Distal tarsal tunnel release with partial plantar fasciotomy for chronic heel pain: An outcome analysis. *Foot Ankle Int* 2002;23:530-537.

Seventy-five patients (80 heels) who underwent distal tarsal tunnel release and partial plantar fasciotomy were retrospectively reviewed (group I). Short Form-36 (SF-36) and Foot Function Index Questionnaires were mailed to all patients, and 44 (59%) completed the questionnaires and responded

(group II). Mean follow-up was 20 months. In group I, 88% had good to excellent results. In group II, 91% of patients were somewhat to very satisfied with their outcome. Visual analog scale scores for pain were reduced by a mean of 55. SF-36 scores, matched against a control group of patients receiving just nonsurgical treatment showed a statistically significant improvement in all pain and functioning subcategories.

Midfoot

Bloome DM, Clanton TO: Treatment of Lisfranc injuries in the athlete. *Tech Foot Ankle Surg* 2002;1:94-101.

An overview of these injuries, with particular attention to current recommendations and techniques for treating these injuries in athletes.

Nunley JA, Vertullo CJ: Classification, investigation, and management of midfoot sprains. *Am J Sports Med* 2002; 30:871-878.

The authors present a new classification system, along with clinical results on 15 athletes with midfoot sprains who were treated surgically or nonsugically based on this system. The authors report an excellent outcome in 93% of the 15 athletes at an average follow-up of 27 months.

Forefoot

Anderson RB: Turf toe injuries of the hallux metatarsophalangeal joint. *Tech Foot Ankle Surg* 2002;1:102-111.

An overview of turf toe injuries, along with current recommendations for work-up and management.

Richardson EG: Hallucal sesamoid pain: Causes and surgical treatment. *J Am Acad Orthop Surg* 1999;7:270-278.

This is an excellent review of sesamoid disorders and the numerous etiologies related to the hallux MTP joint complex. The author discusses clinical and radiographic findings as well as treatment options.

Watson TS, Anderson RB, Davis WH: Periarticular injuries to the hallux metatarsophalangeal joint in athletes. *Foot Ankle Clin* 2000;5:687-713.

This is an extensive review of turf toe injuries to the hallux MTP joint in athletes. The authors describe diagnostic modalities, classification, and surgical repair and reconstruction.

Stress Fractures

Coris EE, Lombardo JA: Tarsal navicular stress fractures. *Am Fam Physician* 2003;67:85-90.

The authors of this article provide a review of the navicular stress fracture and its increasing frequency in physically active patients. They discuss prodromal symptoms, diagnostic modalities, and treatment options.

Donley BG, McCollum MJ, Murphy GA, Richardson EG: Risk of sural nerve injury with intramedullary screw fixation of fifth metatarsal fractures: A cadaver study. *Foot Ankle Int* 1999;20:182-184.

The authors of this study discuss the potential for sural nerve injury with fixation of fifth metatarsal fractures. In the 10 specimens they examined, they report that in five there was only a 2-mm distance between the sural nerve and the 4.5 mm screw head within the fifth metatarsal.

Ebraheim NA, Haman SP, Lu J, et al: Anatomical and radiological considerations of the fifth metatarsal bone. *Foot Ankle Int* 2000;21:212-215.

The authors studied the fifth metatarsal bone in cadaver specimens. They report that they found a lateral bow, with the canal being narrower in diameter in the dorsal plantar dimension than in the medial lateral dimension.

Wright RW, Fischer DA, Shively RA, Heidt RS, Nuber GW: Refracture of proximal fifth metatarsal (Jones) fracture after intramedullary screw fixation in athletes. *Am J Sports Med* 2000;28:732-736.

The authors of this article identified six refractures after intramedullary screw fixation in athletes who were permitted to return to participation in sports at 8.5 weeks after documented healing. The authors recommend using a larger diameter screw, an orthotic device with screw fixation, obtaining adequate diagnostic images to document complete healing, and management of refractures with re-reaming and larger screw fixation.

Nunley JA: Fractures of the base of the fifth metatarsal: The Jones fracture. *Orthop Clin North Am* 2001;32:171-180.

The author of this article provides an excellent review of the diagnosis and treatment of the fifth metatarsal fracture in athletes.

Rosenberg GA, Sferra JJ: Treatment strategies for acute fractures and nonunions of the proximal fifth metatarsal. *J Am Acad Orthop Surg* 2000;8:332-338.

The authors of this article provide a thorough review of the diagnosis and management of both acute fractures and nonunions of the base of the fifth metatarsal (Jones fracture).

Classic Bibliography

Anderson RB: Lisfranc's fracture-dislocation, in: Pfeffer GB, Frey CC (eds): *Current Practice in Foot and Ankle Surgery*. New York, NY, McGraw Hill, 1993, pp129-159.

Anderson RB, McBryde AM Jr: Autogenous bone grafting of hallux sesamoid nonunions. *Foot Ankle Int* 1997;18:293-296.

Bowers KD Jr, Martin RB: Turf toe: A shoe-surface related football injury. *Med Sci Sports* 1976;8:81-83.

Clanton TO, Butler JE, Eggert A: Injuries to the metatarsophalangeal joints in athletes. *Foot Ankle* 1986;7:162-176.

Eisele SA, Sammarco GJ: Fatigue fractures of the foot and ankle in the athlete. *J Bone Joint Surg Am* 1993;75:290-298.

Hardcastle PH, Reschauer R, Hutscha-Lissberg E, et al: Injuries to the tarsometatarsal joint: Incidence, classification and treatment. *J Bone Joint Surg Br* 1982;64:349-356.

Hofmeister EP, Elliott MJ, Juliano PJ: Endoscopic plantar fascia release: An anatomical study. *Foot Ankle Int* 1995;16:719-723.

Khan KM, Brukner PD, Kearney C, Fuller PJ, Bradshaw CJ, Kiss ZS: Tarsal navicular stress fractures in athletes. *Sports Med* 1994;17:65-76.

Meyer SA, Callaghan JJ, Albright JP, Crowley ET, Powell JW: Midfoot sprains in collegiate football players. *Am J Sports Med* 1994;22:392-401.

Quill GE: Fractures of the proximal fifth metatarsal. *Orthop Clin North Am* 1995;26:353-361.

Sammarco GJ: The Jones fracture. *Instr Course Lect* 1993;42:201-205.

Sellman JR: Plantar fascia rupture associated with corticosteroid injection. *Foot Ankle Int* 1994;15:376-381.

Section 4

Systemic Injuries

Section Editors:
James G. Garrick, MD
Thomas M. Best, MD, PhD, FACSM

Chapter 20

Ligamentous Injuries

Susan L. Lewis, MD

Introduction

To speak of ligament healing as a uniform orthopaedic process is a vast oversimplification of the anatomic and physiologic changes that ligaments undergo. Although there are certain similar overlying processes, ligament healing should be considered on a ligament-by-ligament basis. There are also vast differences between intra-articular and extra-articular ligament healing, as evidenced by the poor healing response of the anterior cruciate ligament (ACL) compared with the medial collateral ligament (MCL). However, the MCL has varying components, such as different insertion types proximally and distally. Therefore, how these significant variables affect ligament healing must be taken into account to understand the healing responses of ligamentous injuries.

Structure and Function

Ligaments are strong connective tissues that provide bone-to-bone connections. Collagen provides 70% of the dry weight of ligaments, and 90% of ligament collagen is type I. (Type II collagen is the primary collagen found in articular collagen.) Type III collagen constitutes the other 10%, but this amount increases when ligaments are in their healing phase. Elastin constitutes approximately 1% of ligament collagen. Although ligaments are hierarchically similar to tendons, their fibers are more variable and have a higher elastin content. The ligament hierarchy includes a series of fibrils grouped into fibers that form a subfascicular unit. These units are then surrounded by a thin layer of connective tissue. Many of these units are then bound together to form a fasciculus, which can then be oriented in the line of stress of the ligament. Although it represents only a small percentage of ligament collagen (1%), elastin is vitally important to ligament function because it allows the ligament to return to its normal length as it stores energy during loading activities. Fibroblasts, the predominant cell in ligaments, are located between rows of collagen and thus provide the extracellular matrix of the ligament. Cross-links between rows of collagen add sig-

nificant structural strength to the ligament. Cross-links are composed primarily of type VI microfibrils of collagen. Decreased cross-link density dominates ligament scarring, as do smaller diameter collagen fibrils.

There are primarily two types of ligament insertion into bone: direct and indirect (Table 1). The femoral attachment of the ACL, for example, is a direct ligament insertion. More common than indirect insertions, direct insertions have both a superficial and a deep component. The superficial fibers of a direct insertion join the periosteum, and the deep fibers attach to the bone at 90° angles and go through four distinct transition phases: (1) ligament, (2) unmineralized fibrocartilage, (3) mineralized fibrocartilage, and (4) bone. This transition spans approximately 1 mm. The tibial insertion of the MCL is an indirect ligament insertion. Indirect insertions also have both a superficial and a deep component. The superficial fibers insert at acute angles into the periosteum, and the deep fibers contain Sharpey's fibers that provide an anchor to the bone via a direct collagen connection into the bone. When avulsion injuries occur to a ligament, they typically occur between the unmineralized and mineralized fibrocartilage layers of the deep direct insertions.

Blood is supplied to ligaments primarily through the epiligamentous tissue and, contrary to what was once believed, to a lesser degree through the insertion sites into bone. The vascular supply to ligaments is critical in providing nutritional support for synthesis and repair. The nerve supply to ligaments continues to be controversial. Several studies reveal that nerve endings in ligaments and pain fibers are much less important in ligaments than proprioceptive nerves. Although not shown to be the case in the MCL, it has been well documented that lateral ankle ligaments contain proprioceptive fibers, as does the ACL.

Healing Process

Healing of the MCL has been more extensively studied than that of the ACL. In general, extra-articular ligaments undergo a healing process similar to wound heal-

TABLE 1 | Ligament Insertions Into Bone

Insertion	Superficial	Deep	Example
Direct	Periosteum	Attach to bone at 90° angles and transition in four phases (ie, ligament, unmineralized fibrocartilage, mineralized fibrocartilage, and bone) spanning 1 mm	Femoral attachment of ACL
Indirect	At acute angles into periosteum	Anchors to bone via Sharpey's fibers in a manner similar to direct collagen connection of tendon into bone	Tibial insertion of MCL

ing and scar formation that includes the four typical stages of inflammation, proliferation, remodeling, and maturation. The inflammatory process usually occurs within the first 3 days after injury. During this time, a hematoma forms that brings platelets, inflammatory cells, and erythrocytes into the area of injury. Cytokines lead to the formation of granulation tissue and further vascular stimulation. Toward the end of the inflammatory phase, fibroblast proliferation occurs, and this early scar formation is almost entirely made up of type III collagen. The proliferation phase follows, which is a period of abundant cell production. Vascular granulation tissue begins to form in any gaps, and the fibrin clot is organized. Type I collagen begins to predominate, both in the scar and in the adjacent normal ligament. During remodeling and maturation, the vascularity and the number of cells at the scar site decrease. The relative ratio of type I and type III collagen begins to approach normal, and the density of the collagen begins to increase until it plateaus at a relatively normal level. The tensile strength, although improved because of increasing cross-links, never reaches the preinjury level. The strength of the healed ligament reflects the number of cross-links as well as the concentration of large type I fibrils. Because these cross-links never reach preinjury level, the strength of the healed ligament, although good, does not reach preinjury level either.

Unlike extra-articular ligaments, intra-articular ligaments do not complete the four typical stages of inflammation, proliferation, remodeling, and maturation. Although it has been shown that the ACL does go through four phases of histologic change after injury (inflammation, epiligamentous regeneration, proliferation, and remodeling), subtle differences occur that may explain its poor healing potential. Specifically, it has been shown that alpha-smooth muscle actin forms a synovial cell layer on the surface of the ruptured ends of the ACL and may lead not only to poor healing but also retrac-

tion of the ligament. No tissue has been shown to bridge the rupture site. Although the normal human ACL is covered by synovial tissue, after tearing and during its reparative phase, epiligamentous repair leads to the formation of a synovial sheath over both ends of the ruptured ligament, which may in itself block healing. Alpha-smooth muscle actin further inhibits healing in that it may cause the ruptured ends of the ACL to retract from each other. Although the overall synovial milieu of the knee joint may also play a role, the aforementioned histologic evidence indicates that the ACL is inherently different than other extra-articular ligaments.

Numerous variables have been implicated as having positive and negative effects on ligaments and their healing potential. It has been well documented that immobilization has a particularly negative effect on ligament strength, leading to decreased load and failure. This is partly related to osteoclastic bone resorption at the insertion sites, but it has also been shown to reflect the intrasubstance of the ligament as well, specifically the collagen diameter and cross-links. Increasing age has also been implicated in leading to a decline in ligament function. Ligaments of younger patients undergo increased ultimate load and stiffness compared with those of older patients. A decline in collagen synthesis also occurs with increasing age. However, despite such theories as well as an increasingly active aging population, an increase in ligament injuries in older individuals has not occurred, calling into doubt the veracity of these theories with regard to ligament health.

Women's Ligaments and Injuries

A great deal of attention has recently been directed to ligament injury rates, specifically ACL injury rates in women. The theories explaining why ACL tears occur much more often among active young women than men include a lower center of gravity in women, poor training history, altered hormonal fluctuations during the menstrual cycle, and femoral notch anatomy. A review of the literature has yet to reveal a study that has shown any true intrinsic difference between male and female ligament structure; however, one study did reveal a significant increase in ankle ligament laxity in women compared with men. The authors examined male and female college athletes with no history of significant ankle ligament injuries to determine baseline levels. Stress radiographs revealed more laxity in women's ankles than in men's ankles. Although this study does not necessarily imply that increased laxity results in an increased incidence of ankle injuries in women, it suggests that "normal" ankle laxity should be sex-specific. Current "normal" ankle laxity levels are based on data obtained from both men and women.

It is well established that pregnancy leads to a significant increase in pelvic ligamentous laxity, and researchers have recently suggested a similar increase in laxity occurs in knee and ankle ligaments during pregnancy. One recent study investigated the effect of pregnancy on messenger RNA levels and gene expression in injured rabbit MCLs. The alterations in the behavior of MCLs in pregnant rabbits with MCL injury during adolescence were also studied to determine if pregnancy affects the previously injured MCL. Curiously, a pregnancy-associated increase in laxity was found in the MCLs of the previously uninjured group. However, no increase was observed in the previously injured rabbits during pregnancy. The injured ligament was already significantly more lax than its normal counterpart, and pregnancy did not lead to additional laxity or prevent the normal decline in laxity as the scar matured. This study suggests that the impact of pregnancy on laxity and cell activity in the MCL is dependent on whether the ligament has been previously injured. In contrast to what is generally believed, pregnancy had no significant effect on the structural (stiffness and failure load), material (stress to failure in Young's modulus), and viscoelastic (cyclic and static relaxation) properties of tissue from uninjured or injured MCL. Although these findings cannot necessarily be extrapolated to either ACLs or humans, they again call into question the role of hormones in the increased rate of ACL injuries in women.

Drugs and Ligaments

The effects of nonsteroidal anti-inflammatory drugs (NSAIDs) and cyclooxygenase (COX-)2 inhibitors on tendon and muscle healing have been studied extensively, but their effects on ligament healing have been studied to a lesser degree. One NSAID, piroxicam, has been shown to increase strength in the healing ligaments of rats when administered early (within 20 days of injury) for a short period. Piroxicam, however, had no such effect when administered late (21 days after injury). Additionally, neither doubling nor halving the standard dose altered the increased healing strength. COX-2 inhibitors have received a great deal of attention over the last few years in light of their decreased risk of gastrointestinal complications. Although their benefits have been shown to be fairly significant when used for rheumatoid arthritis or osteoarthritis, their effects on soft-tissue injuries are somewhat controversial. Recent studies demonstrated improved efficacy of using one COX-2 inhibitor (celecoxib) over ibuprofen in treating acute ankle inversion injuries. However, another study that investigated the effects of celecoxib on rat MCL healing revealed a 32% lower load to failure rate in the rats treated with celecoxib than in those that received placebos. These findings suggest that COX-2 inhibitors used to treat ligament injuries may not be beneficial. Further study is necessary to determine the effects of COX-2 inhibitors on ligament injuries.

The illicit use of anabolic steroids in body building has numerous potentially adverse effects. Many studies report severe spontaneous tendon ruptures associated with anabolic steroid intake, but very little has been published regarding such injuries occurring in ligaments. In the literature, however, there are scattered case studies and anecdotal reports of spontaneous ruptures of ACLs in body builders taking anabolic steroids. There are essentially no reports in the literature regarding the histologic changes in those taking anabolic steroids or growth hormones. There are, however, anecdotal reports of poor hamstring tendon quality in patients undergoing graft harvest who have taken anabolic steroids in the past. In light of the large number of active people improperly using anabolic steroids and growth hormones, further study is needed in this area.

Therapeutic Modalities

Ultrasound and electrical stimulation are popular physical therapy modalities used in the treatment of soft-tissue injuries. Although some orthopaedists and physical therapists question the usefulness of such treatments, some studies suggest that such treatments may actually improve ligament healing. One such study examined 87 rats that underwent transsection of their bilateral MCLs, with only one side receiving treatment with electrical stimulation. The treated side showed a statistically significant improvement in maximum rupture force, energy absorption, stiffness, and laxity, suggesting that if the correct amount of electrical stimulation is applied early, it may enhance ligament healing. A similar study using pulsed, low-intensity ultrasonography on rat MCLs revealed significantly superior mechanical properties when compared with the control side with regard to ultimate load, stiffness, and energy absorption early in the treatment protocol (12 days after injury), but the treatment did not lead to any significant advantage when the control and treated rats were tested on the 21st day. The mean diameter of the fibril, however, was significantly larger on the treatment side than on the control side. Although additional studies are needed, preliminary evidence suggests that these treatment modalities may play a role in early ligament healing.

Thermal Shrinkage

Over the past decade, the use of thermal shrinkage has gained increasing popularity, with applications expanding from the initial treatment of shoulder instability to the treatment of many other orthopaedic problems, including treatment to tighten ACLs. Nonablative thermal energy at or above 60°C appears to shrink soft-tissue collagen by inducing ultrastructural and mechanical changes in ligaments, resulting in a loss of fiber orientation and contraction of the fibrils into a shortened state. If the shrinkage is limited to less than 15%, the biome-

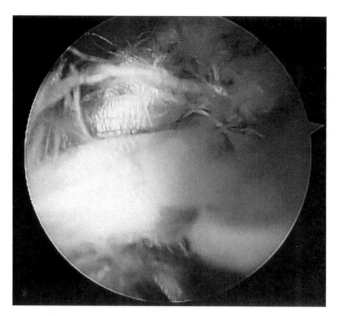

Figure 1 Arthroscopic view of a failed LAD.

chanical properties of the tissue may not be detrimentally altered. However, the true end point for the amount of thermal energy tissue can withstand with regard to optimal shrinkage is not known. In light of its technical ease of use and increased popularity, thermal shrinkage has been recommended for tightening native ACLs with intact fibers and grafts that may have stretched out over time, leading to functional laxity. Although the results of using thermal shrinkage were initially somewhat promising, long-term follow-up has shown this procedure to be ineffective. One study of patients who underwent electrothermal shrinkage for ACL laxity revealed a significant decrease in efficacy with time. Most of the patients had acceptable side-to-side differences 1 month after treatment, whereas most patients had a failed result at an average of 4 months after treatment. Although the use of thermal shrinkage continues to be quite controversial, some authors have reported good results in using thermal shrinkage to treat ACL grafts that had stretched out over time. In a recent case report, however, a 16-year-old girl who underwent ACL reconstruction using an autologous hamstring graft subsequently stretched her graft. Because continuous fibers were still present, the authors elected to perform a thermal shrinkage procedure. Several months later, the patient experienced instability. During the follow-up reconstructive procedure, the graft appeared to have been completely autodigested. Although thermal shrinkage cannot be blamed for this adverse effect, such an outcome is possible when thermal shrinkage is used. In an increasingly litigious society, not only are such complications worrisome, but the fact that this procedure has the same billing code as ACL reconstruction may also be cause for concern.

Ligament Augmentation

The use of a ligament augmentation device (LAD) is equally controversial. The first synthetic cruciate prosthesis was used in a dog model in 1960. In the 1980s, the use of an LAD to treat human ACL injuries became popular, suggesting that the need for an LAD arises from the observation that biologic grafts undergo a phase of degeneration and loss of strength before being fully incorporated and increasing strength. The LAD is intended to protect the biologic graft during ingrowth. The more popular LAD was a polypropylene braid, but other synthetic ligaments were soon widely used (eg, carbon fiber, Dacron, and Gortex grafts). Not only did these new materials fail to provide the intended added strength, but they created complications that were truly more problematic than the initial cruciate ligament injury. Well-documented adverse effects include chronic and significant synovitis, the shedding of carbon particles into the joint and lymph nodes, and extensive inflammatory reactions (Figure 1). By the early 1990s, all forms of LADs had fallen out of favor.

Recently, however, there has been a recent resurgence in the use of such devices. Although one recent study failed to document the severe complications reported in the past, it reported no positive effects of using the LAD. Whereas patients did not experience severe complications, those without the LAD fared better overall. Another similar study concurred with these results, arguing that no true need to use the LAD exists because it provided no significant advantage. One author using a polyethylene LAD in 217 patients in a recent study reported good to excellent results in 81%, but the number of complications appears unacceptably high. Three patients had infections, five underwent surgical procedures for removal of the LAD because of severe synovitis, seven reruptures occurred, and two tibial fistulas were reported. The number of complications is significantly higher than that resulting from the current standard use of an allograft or autograft.

Ligament and Tissue Engineering

As a result of the numerous problems associated with synthetic ligaments used alone or in conjunction with an augmenting device and improving cell technology and tissue engineering techniques, attention is now being directed to synthesizing or stimulating ligament healing in the laboratory. Under investigation is a biodegradable scaffold that, once implanted into the host, is subsequently invaded by native cells that populate and remodel it into a new ligament. Many of the techniques used for this investigational procedure have been based on those used for collagen scaffolds, which can be allogenic and thereby cause associated complications. Nevertheless, research into the use of biodegradable scaffolds for ligament healing has revealed some very

TABLE 2 | Summary of the Effect of Growth Factors on Tissue Regeneration Behaviors for Human ACL Cells

Growth Factor	Effect on Cell Density in the Scaffold	Effect on Cell Proliferation Rate	Effect on Cell Collagen Production Rate	Effect on Smooth Muscle Actin Expression
TGF-β1	++	NS	++	++
PDGF-AB	NS	++	++	NS
EGF	NS	NS	NS	NS
FGF-2	NS	++	NS	NS

++ = Significant increase over control values, mean at least twice the control mean. NS = No significant difference when compared with control mean. TGF-β1 = tumor growth factor-beta 1. PDGF-AB = platelet-derived growth factor–AB. EGF = epidermal growth factor. FGF-2 = fibroblast growth factor–2.

(Reproduced with permission from Meaney Murray M, Rice K, Wright RJ, Spector M: The effect of selected growth factors on human anterior cruciate ligament cell interactions with a three-dimensional collagen-GAG scaffold. J Orthop Res 2003;21:238-244.)

interesting results. One such study revealed a difference in outgrowth potential in the proximal versus distal human ACL stump, with the proximal stump having an earlier start to outgrowth as well as a potentially faster rate of outgrowth. Other studies have examined the efficacy of adding growth factors and their role in altering the capacity for growth and function of human ACL cells. Although the results of these studies have been varied, in general, there are some consistent conclusions (Table 2). For example, tumor growth factor–beta 1 has been shown to lead to a significant increase in cell density, cell collagen production, and alpha-smooth muscle actin production. It does not appear to increase cell proliferation. Platelet-derived growth factor does appear to increase cell proliferation. In addition, it has been shown to increase cell collagen production, but it has no significant effect on smooth muscle actin expression or cell density. Epidermal growth factor does not appear to have any significant effect on cell density, cell proliferation rate, cell collagen production rate, or alpha-smooth muscle actin expression. Fibroblast growth factor–2 appears only to significantly increase cell proliferation, and has no significant effect on the other parameters. Most of the studies from which these findings are derived used explants of ACLs taken during arthroplasty being performed to treat degenerative joint disease. Therefore, these findings may not be representative of outcomes involving younger patients with acute ligament injuries.

The use of other tissue-engineered ligament grafts has also recently been suggested. The authors of one recent study designed a silk fiber matrix to match the complex requirements of a native human ACL and found that the matrix supported the attachment expansion and differentiation of adult human progenitor bone marrow stromocells. They noted that if the external sericin was extracted from the silk, leaving only the core protein fibroin, the tissue was likely biocompatible and would not induce a T-cell–mediated response. Although the findings of several similar studies are quite intriguing, much more research is needed to clarify the role of tissue-engineered ligament grafts in the treatment of ligamentous injuries.

Proprioception

Technologic developments are also being made for the rehabilitation of injured ligaments. The histologic presence of mechanoreceptors in human cruciate ligaments was first demonstrated in 1984. Although such findings highlight the importance of the generation of a proprioceptive reflex arc from the cruciate ligament, the clinical relevance has been somewhat controversial over the last several decades. Some authors have suggested that once these fibers are torn, the reflex arc cannot be re-created, ligament grafts merely function as mechanical stabilizers, and no neurogenic feedback loop is created with the implantation of a graft. More recently, however, several studies have found the opposite to be true. In a 2003 study, the authors noted significant improvement in patients 6 months after ACL reconstruction in a study that matched age and gender control patients in proprioceptive testing. Moreover, decreased proprioceptive function was initially found in the uninjured side of patients with ACL tears. Bilateral deficits in knee joint proprioception were documented to be significant after unilateral ACL injury. Reconstruction of the ACL led not only to improvement in proprioception in the injured knee but the contralateral side as well. In a 2002 study, the authors found bilateral proprioceptive loss after an initial ACL injury and noted significant return with a similar time frame. In a 1996 study, it was noted that proprioception is an acquired and trainable phenomenon. Some authors have called into question the effect of muscle fatigue leading to declining joint proprioception. Others, however, have shown significant improvement with joint proprioception with a brief warm-up. Although additional study is needed regarding the effects of warm-up and muscle fatigue on proprioceptive capacities of the knee, a proprioceptive program should be included in the rehabilitation protocol of patients with cruciate ligament injuries.

The importance of a proprioceptive program after lateral ankle ligament injury is well established. In 1995, neuroanatomic data were first used to show the presence of mechanoreceptors in human ankle ligaments, which validated the long-held belief that a proprioceptive program is quite important in the rehabilitation of an ankle sprain. The importance of a proprioceptive program in recovery from an acute ankle sprain and in the prevention of a functionally unstable ankle cannot be overemphasized. Some data suggest a twofold drop in likely recurrent ankle sprains if a proprioceptive program is included in ankle rehabilitation. Other data suggest that of all patients with acute ankle sprains, even those who receive no treatment, only 10% will go on to develop chronic functionally unstable ankles. If this 10% of patients is eventually placed on a rehabilitation program that includes a proprioceptive protocol, only half will develop further functional instability. Thus, it is implied that 5% of all patients with acute ankle sprains will go on to develop chronic instability requiring surgery. Even in the setting of a chronic unstable ankle, when a proprioceptive program is instituted, it appears that there is little likelihood of continued instability requiring surgery.

Summary

The understanding of ligament repair, healing, and regeneration continues to evolve. The use of growth factors may provide an exciting frontier for the future of ligament healing. Caution should be exercised, however, with any new technology as clearly evidenced by the limitations of ligament augmentation and radiofrequency shrinkage devices. There are many questions still to be answered regarding ligament injury and repair; in particular, the role of gender and the use of anabolic steroids as they relate to ligament injury require further study.

Annotated Bibliography

Structure and Function

Fu FH, Bennett CH, Lattermann C, Ma CB: Current trends in anterior cruciate ligament reconstruction. *Am J Sports Med* 1999;27:821-830.

This review article summarizes the biology and biomechanics of ACL and reconstruction.

Murray MM, Martin SD, Martin TL, Spector M: Histological changes in the human anterior cruciate ligament after rupture. *J Bone Joint Surg Am* 2000;82:1387-1397.

This is a basic science study of the histologic changes of human ACLs. The authors suggest that a torn ACL goes through healing phases that differ from those of extra-articular ligaments.

Healing Process

Woo SL, Vogrin TM, Abramowitch SD: Healing and repair of ligament injuries in the knee. *J Am Acad Orthop Surg* 2000;8:364-372.

This review article discusses the natural stages and processes of healing and repair of knee ligament injuries.

Women's Ligaments and Injuries

Hart DA, Reno C, Frank CB, Shrive NG: Pregnancy affects cellular activity, but not tissue mechanical properties, in the healing rabbit medial collateral ligament. *J Orthop Res* 2000;18:462-471.

The authors of this prospective randomized study on the effect of pregnancy on previously injured rabbit MCLs suggest that pregnancy does not alter previously injured rat MCLs but does affect uninjured MCLs.

Wilkerson RD, Mason MA: Differences in men's and women's mean ankle ligamentous laxity. *Iowa Orthop J* 2000;20:46-48.

The authors of this prospective randomized study comparing normal values for men's and women's ankle laxity suggest that women naturally have significantly more lax ankles than men.

Drugs and Ligaments

Ekman EF, Fiechtner JJ, Levy S, Fort JG: Efficacy of celecoxib versus ibuprofen in the treatment of acute pain: A multicenter, double-blind, randomized controlled trial in acute ankle sprain. *Am J Orthop* 2002;31:445-451.

The authors of this prospective randomized double-blind study comparing the effects of a COX-2 inhibitor (celecoxib) and ibuprofen for acute ankle sprain suggest that, according to clinical parameters, the COX-2 inhibitors may benefit recovery from acute ankle sprain.

Elder CL, Dahners LE, Weinhold PS: A cyclooxygenase-2 inhibitor impairs ligament healing in the rat. *Am J Sports Med* 2001;29:801-805.

In this prospective randomized study evaluating the effects of a COX-2 inhibitor on ligament healing in rat MCLs, the authors suggest that COX-2 inhibitors may inhibit ligament healing.

Moorman CT III, Kukreti U, Fenton DC, Belkoff SM: The early effect of ibuprofen on the mechanical properties of healing medial collateral ligament. *Am J Sports Med* 1999;27:738-741.

The authors of this prospective randomized controlled study on the effect of ibuprofen on the healing properties of rabbit MCLs report no early deleterious effects of a short course of ibuprofen on the mechanical behavior of the MCLs of rabbits.

Therapeutic Modalities

Takakura Y, Matsui N, Yoshiya S, et al: Low-intensity pulsed ultrasound enhances early healing of medial collateral ligament injuries in rats. *J Ultrasound Med* 2002;21:283-288.

In this prospective randomized controlled study on the effects of ultrasound on injured MCLs in rats, the authors report that ultrasound exposure is effective for enhancing the early healing of MCL injuries in rats.

Thermal Shrinkage

Carter TR: Anterior cruciate ligament thermal shrinkage. *Clin Sports Med* 2002;21:693-700.

The author of this review article discusses the basic science and clinical applications of thermal shrinkage in the knee for ACL injuries.

Carter TR, Bailie DS, Edinger S: Radiofrequency electrothermal shrinkage of the anterior cruciate ligament. *Am J Sports Med* 2002;30:221-226.

In this prospective study of 18 patients who had continuity of the ACL but symptomatic laxity treated with arthroscopic electrothermal shrinkage of their ACL, results at 1 month revealed good function but a significant failure rate at 4 months.

Medvecky MJ, Ong BC, Rokito AS, Sherman OH: Thermal capsular shrinkage: Basic science and clinical applications. *Arthroscopy* 2001;17:624-635.

The authors of this review article discuss the basic science and clinical applications of thermal shrinkage.

Sekiya JK, Golladay GJ, Wojtys EM: Autodigestion of a hamstring anterior cruciate ligament autograft following thermal shrinkage: A case report and sentinel of concern. *J Bone Joint Surg Am* 2000;82:1454-1457.

This is a case report of a patient who underwent an ACL reconstruction and subsequently underwent thermal shrinkage for some stretching. Further investigation revealed complete autodigestion of the graft after thermal shrinkage.

Spahn G, Schindler S: Tightening elongated ACL grafts by application of bipolar electromagnetic energy (ligament shrinkage). *Knee Surg Sports Traumatol Arthrosc* 2002;10:66-72.

This is a prospective study of patients with "stretched out" ACL grafts who underwent thermal shrinkage.

Ligament Augmentation

Drogset JO, Grontvedt T: Anterior cruciate ligament reconstruction with and without a ligament augmentation device: Results at 8-year follow-up. *Am J Sports Med* 2002;30:851-856.

In this randomized controlled clinical trial on the use of ligament augmentation devices with 8-year follow-up, the authors found no positive long-term effects supporting the use of ligament augmentation devices in ACL reconstruction.

Krudwig WK: Anterior cruciate ligament reconstruction using an alloplastic ligament of polyethylene terephthalate (PET-Trevira-hochfest): A follow-up study. *Biomed Mater Eng* 2002;12:59-67.

This is a review article of 217 ACL reconstructions for which a synthetic ligament was used. Although the author reports good to excellent results, the overall complication rate is quite high.

Kumar K, Maffulli N: The ligament augmentation device: An historical perspective. *Arthroscopy* 1999;15:422-432.

This review article discusses the use of ligament augmentation devices.

Steenbrugge F, Verdonk R, Vorlat P, Mortier F, Verstraete K: Repair of chronic ruptures of the anterior cruciate ligament using allograft reconstruction and a ligament augmentation device. *Acta Orthop Belg* 2001;67:252-258.

In this clinical trial of 25 patients who underwent ligament augmentation allograft ACL reconstruction, the authors report no significant improvement using the ligament augmentation device.

Ligament and Tissue Engineering

Altman GH, Horan RL, Lu HH, et al: Silk matrix for tissue engineered anterior cruciate ligaments. *Biomaterials* 2002;23:4131-4141.

The authors of this article report on the use of silk fiber matrix as suitable material for tissue engineering of the ACL.

Koski JA, Ibarra C, Rodeo SA: Tissue-engineered ligament: Cells, matrix, and growth factors. *Orthop Clin North Am* 2000;31:437-452.

The authors of this review article discuss tissue engineering with regard to ligament and the use of growth factors.

Murray MM, Bennett R, Zhang X, Spector M: Cell outgrowth from the human ACL in vitro: Regional variation and response to TGF-beta1. *J Orthop Res* 2002;20:875-880.

In this prospective study of cell outgrowth from the human ACL, the authors report that proximal cells appear to not only express earlier outgrowth than distal but a higher rate of growth as well.

Meaney Murray M, Rice K, Wright RJ, Spector M: The effect of selected growth factors on human anterior cruciate ligament cell interactions with a three-dimensional collagen-GAG scaffold. *J Orthop Res* 2003;21:238-244.

In this article, the authors discuss the effects of a number of growth factors on human ACL growth.

Proprioception

Barlett MJ, Warren PJ: Effect of warming up on knee proprioception before sporting activity. *Br J Sports Med* 2002;36:132-134.

The results of this clinical trial reveal that proprioception within the knee benefits from a warm-up period.

Frey C: Ankle sprains. *Instr Course Lect* 2001;50:515-520.

The author of this article discusses ankle sprains and their rehabilitative treatment.

Hertel J: Functional instability following lateral ankle sprain. *Sports Med* 2000;29:361-371.

The author of this review article discusses the importance of proprioception for preventing long-term functional instability of the ankle.

Hewett TE, Paterno MV, Myer GD: Strategies for enhancing proprioception and neuromuscular control of the knee. *Clin Orthop* 2002;402:76-94.

The authors of this review article discuss strategies to improve proprioception in the therapeutic treatment after knee injuries.

Hiemstra LA, Lo IK, Fowler PJ: Effect of fatigue on knee proprioception: Implications for dynamic stabilization. *J Orthop Sports Phys Ther* 2001;31:598-605.

The authors of this review article discuss the impact of fatigue on proprioception.

Reider B, Arcand MA, Diehl LH, et al: Proprioception of the knee before and after anterior cruciate ligament reconstruction. *Arthroscopy* 2003;19:2-12.

The results of this prospective clinical trial revealed significant improvement in patients' proprioception of their lower extremity 6 months after ACL reconstruction.

Classic Bibliography

Dahners LE, Gilbert JA, Lester GE, Taft TN, Payne LZ: The effect of a nonsteroidal antiinflammatory drug on the healing of ligaments. *Am J Sports Med* 1988;16:641-646.

Frank CB: Ligament healing: Current knowledge and clinical applications. *J Am Acad Orthop Surg* 1996;4:74-83.

Freeman BJ, Rooker GD: Spontaneous rupture of the anterior cruciate ligament after anabolic steroids. *Br J Sports Med* 1995;29:274-275.

Jerosch J, Prymka M: Proprioception and joint stability. *Knee Surg Sports Traumatol Arthrosc* 1996;4:171-179.

Karlsson J, Lansinger O: Chronic lateral instability of the ankle in athletes. *Sports Med* 1993;16:355-365.

Litke DS, Dahners LE: Effects of different levels of direct current on early ligament healing in a rat model. *J Orthop Res* 1994;12:683-688.

Michelson JD, Hutchins C: Mechanoreceptors in human ankle ligaments. *J Bone Joint Surg Br* 1995;77:219-224.

Padgett LR, Dahners LE: Rigid immobilization alters matrix organization in the injured rat medial collateral ligament. *J Orthop Res* 1992;10:895-900.

Schultz RA, Miller DC, Kerr CS, Micheli L: Mechanoreceptors in human cruciate ligaments: A histological study. *J Bone Joint Surg Am* 1984;66:1072-1076.

Chapter 21

Stress Fractures and Stress Injuries in Bone

R. Dana Carpenter, MS

Gordon O. Matheson, MD, PhD

Dennis R. Carter, PhD

Introduction

The number of people participating in recreational and competitive sports has increased substantially in recent years. As a result of this and the rising volume and intensity of training, stress fractures and other overuse injuries have become an increasingly common problem. Stress fractures, which occur as a result of repetitive loading of bones during a wide variety of athletic activities, can occur in nearly every bone in the body. Because military populations participate in strictly controlled training regimens, they provide a useful model for the study of stress fracture incidence. The incidence of stress fractures in military recruits has been reported to be as high as 64% (in a group of Finnish trainees), but the incidence for US military recruits has been reported to be much lower (0.2% to 4% in men and 1% to 7% in women). The variable and individualistic training programs of athletes, however, do not lend themselves to such a standardized method of study.

Athletic training programs are specifically tailored for each particular sport, and many of these training programs put athletes at risk for stress fractures and other overuse injuries. Stress fractures may account for up to 10% of sports injuries and have been documented in virtually every sport. The severity of stress fractures varies among individual athletes and different sports, and the extent of injury also depends on skeletal site, type of bone, and local blood supply. Although a wide spectrum of stress injuries can occur, the common symptoms and basic mechanisms of injury are similar.

A stress fracture is defined as a partial or complete bone fracture resulting from repetitive application of a stress that causes damage to accumulate faster than it can be repaired. Patients typically report a gradual onset of pain that worsens during physical activity and initially subsides during rest. Injuries that have progressed further can produce pain even after sufficient rest. Because of their insidious onset and often vague symptoms, stress fractures can be challenging to diagnose, and the appropriate treatment differs on a case-to-case basis. An understanding of the underlying pathophysiol-ogy, risk factors, common symptoms, diagnostic imaging, and treatment of these injuries can aid in the diagnosis, treatment, and prevention of stress fractures.

Loading, Remodeling, and Fatigue Damage

Ground reaction forces, joint reaction forces, and muscle forces exert loads on bones during repetitive athletic activities. These forces produce an internal distribution of local force intensities called stresses (dimensions of force per unit area) within bones. The forces also cause bones to deform, and the amount of local deformation at a specific location is quantified as strain (change in length divided by length, commonly given as a percent) (Figure 1). Strain magnitude in bone is often expressed in units of microstrain ($\mu\varepsilon$), with 1 $\mu\varepsilon$ being equal to 0.0001% strain. Athletic activities that impose bending, torsional (twisting), shearing, compressive, and tensile forces create stresses and strains in bones.

Ground reaction forces are generated by the foot's contact with the ground. For example, when a runner's foot strikes a running surface, the surface exerts a reaction force in order to decelerate the foot. When the runner pushes off of the surface into the next step, the surface exerts an equal and opposite force on the runner's foot. To balance and attenuate these forces, muscles contract and produce forces of their own. Joint reaction forces and powerful muscle contractions occur at the ankle, knee, hip, sacroiliac joint, and spine. Therefore, a simple action such as taking a step produces stresses and strains throughout the entire load-bearing skeleton. Ground reaction forces can reach magnitudes of 10 to 20 times body weight during running, jumping, and weight lifting.

Muscle contractions can both increase bone stresses and attenuate the stresses caused by ground reaction forces and joint reaction forces. Muscles can produce force while shortening (concentric contraction) and while lengthening (eccentric contraction). To maintain a level posture in the stance phase of the walking gait, during which the body is balanced on one foot, the hip abductors contract concentrically with a force that is ap-

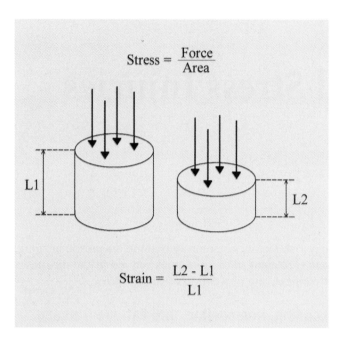

Stress = $\dfrac{\text{Force}}{\text{Area}}$

L1

L2

Strain = $\dfrac{\text{L2 - L1}}{\text{L1}}$

Figure 1 Stress and strain. The cylinder on the left, with a height of L1, is in an unloaded state. On the right, the same cylinder is loaded by a compressive stress distributed over its top surface, which causes the cylinder to shorten to a length of L2. The strain in the cylinder on the right is the amount of deformation (L2-L1) divided by the cylinder's unloaded length (L1).

proximately equal to twice the body weight. Concentric contraction of the hip abductors thus increases the force exerted on the femoral head by the acetabulum. In contrast, muscles can actually reduce forces on bones by absorbing energy through eccentric contraction. When a skier absorbs a large bump in the snow at high speed, the quadriceps muscles contract while the knee is flexing. The eccentric contraction of the quadriceps absorbs the shock of the impact and reduces the load on the skier's bones.

Cyclic stresses or strains resulting from ground reaction forces, joint reaction forces, and muscle forces elicit a remodeling response in bone. An increase in cyclic stress leads to an increase in bone mass, and a decrease in cyclic stress leads to a decrease in bone mass. These changes in bone mass occur as a result of the remodeling response of basic multicellular units (BMUs), which are made up of osteoclasts and osteoblasts. Osteoclasts resorb existing bone tissue by creating a localized acidic environment. After osteoclasts resorb bone at a given location, a cavity forms on the bone surface of cancellous bone or within the lamellar structure of cortical bone. One to 2 weeks later, osteoblasts begin to fill the cavity with type I collagen-rich matrix called osteoid. Over a period of about 3 months, hydroxyapatite crystals form within the osteoid matrix, and mineralized bone is formed. Depending on the ratio of the volume of resorbed bone to the volume of deposited bone, BMUs can effectively increase or decrease the amount of bone present at the remodeling site. Normally, when

cyclic loads on the bone are increased, bone deposition surpasses bone resorption, producing a net increase in bone mass. When the cyclic loads are decreased, a net loss in bone mass can occur.

The events that stimulate a remodeling response in bone are unclear, but substantial evidence suggests that bone remodeling repairs microdamage (microscopic cracks) that accumulate in bone as a result of cyclic loading. During rigorous activities such as running and jumping, strain levels in bone are sufficient to produce fatigue damage. When this damage is unrepaired, microdamage accumulates and eventually coalesces into a macroscopic fracture. Because bone is a metabolically active tissue that is constantly being remodeled, BMUs can resorb tissue in damaged areas and deposit new bone in its place. Evidence suggests that remodeling activity preferentially takes place in areas that have sustained microdamage. Hence, bone has the inherent ability to sense the presence of damage and may be able to direct BMUs to damaged sites for repair.

Pathophysiology

Stress fractures arise as a result of a combination of mechanical and biologic factors. The mechanical properties and geometry of a bone determine the amount of deformation that will occur when bone is subjected to a given load. For cyclic loading in both tension and compression, there appears to be a strain range in which bone's mechanical properties are relatively unaffected. Above thresholds of approximately 4,000 $\mu\varepsilon$ (0.4%) in compression and 2,500 $\mu\varepsilon$ (0.25%) in tension, severe fatigue damage occurs and bone's mechanical properties are compromised. As fatigue damage accumulates in bone under cyclic loading, more of the mechanical energy supplied by the load is dissipated because of microcrack formation (Figure 2). If the BMUs in the injured bone cannot repair this fatigue damage as fast as it occurs, a stress injury is induced. A complete stress fracture may result if the rate of damage accumulation continues to outstrip the bone's capacity for repair. In this situation, microcracks will propagate through the bone tissue and coalesce into macroscopic fractures.

Stress fractures also occur as the result of an elevated rate of remodeling in areas of bone that experience cyclic strains. The cycle begins when cyclic strains produce microdamage in bone. BMUs are activated to repair the damage, and osteoclasts resorb some of the damaged bone, leading to an increase in bone porosity. The stiffness of both cortical and compact bone is dramatically decreased by an increase in porosity. Even after osteoblasts deposit osteoid into the resorption spaces, the new bone does not have its full material properties until the osteoid is fully mineralized. Thus, an increase in bone remodeling leads to a decrease in bone stiffness that can last for weeks to months. If the high cyclic loading that produced the original damage continues to be applied, the bone with compromised stiffness will now experience even higher strains, and more damage is produced. BMUs then target the site for additional remodeling, producing even more voids in the bone tissue. This positive feedback loop can accelerate damage accumulation. When microdamage accumulates, a macroscopic stress fracture occurs.

The mechanical and physiologic components of stress fracture pathophysiology may operate independently, but they likely interact to produce the final injury. By increasing the susceptibility of bone to fatigue damage accumulation, an increased rate of remodeling can set the stage for a stress fracture. However, a stress fracture will only occur if damage accumulates faster than BMUs can repair it. Hence, these two components of stress fracture pathophysiology may lead to a downward spiral of microdamage accumulation and subsequent fracture.

Risk Factors

To prevent stress injuries and stress fractures in athletes, both the pathophysiologic processes previously described and the risk factors that can increase the chances that these mechanisms will produce clinical injuries must be understood. Risk factors for stress fractures stem from three general sources: mechanical loading, bone strength, and bone physiology.

Extrinsic loading factors such as training regimen and footwear can affect the forces applied to the skeleton. As many as 86% of athletes with stress fractures report recent changes in their training programs. Increases in training volume and changes in technique can lead to increased or altered loads on bones. Subsequent changes in damage accumulation and bone remodeling can lead to stress injuries and stress fractures. Shoes, insoles, and orthotic inserts are commonly believed to affect stress factor risk, but no conclusive scientific evidence has been obtained to explain specific effects of footwear on stress fracture incidence.

Skeletal alignment affects the transmission of forces through bones and across joints. Excessive pronation during running is often cited as a potential risk factor for stress fractures, and a recent study of military recruits found that subjects with tibial stress fractures had a higher degree of passive external rotation at the hip. Excessive pronation and external rotation are clinically useful structural measures for estimating the risk of tibial stress fractures because they can be measured without performing detailed imaging analysis. For example, external hip rotation can be measured with the patient supine on a large protractor with the hip and knee both flexed to 90°. The examiner then rotates the leg toward the midline of the trunk, using the thigh as the axis of rotation. The angle that the tibial shaft can passively ro-

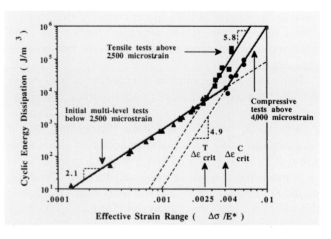

Figure 2 Effective strain range versus initial cyclic energy dissipation. As the effective strain range increases, more energy is dissipated as a result of microdamage accumulation. Above thresholds of 4,000 με (0.4%) in compression and 2,500 με (0.25%) in tension, damage accumulation increases dramatically. *(Reproduced with permission from Pattin CA, Caler WE, Carter DR: Cyclic mechanical property degradation during fatigue loading of cortical bone. J Biomech 1996;29:69-79.)*

tate is the angle of external hip rotation. External hip rotation greater than 60° indicates that the subject is at an increased risk of stress fracture.

Muscle strength and muscle fatigue also affect bone loading. Because muscles exert forces on bones and joints, stronger muscles can produce higher strains within the bone tissue. Unbalanced muscle strength may also lead to increased cyclic loading. For example, the high strength of the plantar flexors in long-distance runners can be insufficiently balanced by the relatively weaker antagonists, the ankle dorsiflexors. Evidence of muscle imbalance during clinical examination can therefore be considered a risk factor for stress fractures. Muscle fatigue is also considered a risk factor. As stated previously, many muscles absorb shock through eccentric contraction. Because fatigued muscles lose some of their ability to attenuate ground reaction forces, more of the load is transferred to the bones.

Bone strength is another important factor in determining stress fracture risk. Large, dense bones are generally stronger than small, highly porous bones. Because stronger bones are more resistant to deformation, the chance of fracture is smaller. Weaker bones, conversely, are not as resistant to deformation, resulting in a greater risk of damage accumulation and fracture.

The mechanical properties of bone tissue affect a bone's overall strength and resistance to deformation. The apparent density of bone, measured in units of grams per cubic centimeter (g/cm^3), is a valuable parameter for characterizing the mechanical behavior of bone. Because bone is a porous structure, a given volume of bone contains both bone tissue and pore spaces filled with blood, marrow, or fat. Apparent density is a measure of the amount of actual bone tissue in a given volume of bone. Bone strength is approximately proportional to the square of the apparent density. Therefore, if a bone has a relatively low apparent density, the bone can fracture when exposed to a relatively low level of local stress.

Bone size and the interior distribution of bone mass also affect a bone's resistance to deformation. The cross-sectional moment of inertia is the measure of tibial cross-sectional geometry and bone distribution, and it has been shown to be a useful indicator of stress fracture risk. A bone with a relatively large moment of inertia is more resistant to bending and torsion; therefore, strains are smaller under a given load. Bone width can also affect a bone's resistance to deformation. A study of 289 military recruits found that recruits who experienced a tibial or femoral stress fracture had significantly narrower tibial shafts than recruits without stress fractures.

Because both bone density and bone size are important in translating external forces into local bone stresses and strains, a single measurement that combines these two parameters is useful. Bone mineral density (BMD) is measured using duel-energy x-ray absorptiometry, combines both bone density and bone size parameters, and is a valuable predictor of the risk of osteoporotic fractures. For each standard deviation below the mean BMD for young, healthy women, the risk of osteoporotic fracture doubles. However, studies investigating BMD with respect to stress fractures have reported contradictory results. Some studies have determined that low BMD is associated with an increased incidence of stress fractures in male military recruits, and others have found that BMD and the risk of stress fracture are not related. Because BMD measurements are heterogeneous in both male and female athletes with stress fractures, it is probable that low BMD is not a good indicator of stress fracture risk.

Because bone physiology and overall bone health also affect bone strength, nutritional intake and hormonal factors are important in evaluating stress fracture risk. Evidence indicates that insufficient calcium intake may lead to increased risk; however, abnormal or restrictive eating habits are probably more important than specific nutritional deficiencies in determining stress fracture risk. Anorexia nervosa and bulimia nervosa commonly occur in athletes who participate in sports in which a low body weight is advantageous, such as long-distance running, ballet, and gymnastics. These eating disorders can lead to a multitude of problems, including adverse effects on bone health. Warning signs for these disorders include depression and abnormally low body weight. Early recognition of these disorders can help prevent destructive effects on the skeleton and the rest of the body. Eating disorders are also often associated with menstrual disturbances in female athletes. Amenorrhea and other menstrual irregularities are associated with abnormally low estrogen levels. Because estrogen

has an important role in regulating bone remodeling, athletes with menstrual irregularities may be at increased risk of developing stress injuries and stress fractures.

Clinical Diagnosis

Stress fractures can be difficult to diagnose because they often produce vague symptoms that develop over an extended period. Early diagnosis is important because stress fractures that go undiagnosed or are misdiagnosed can lead to complete fracture and subsequent malunion or nonunion. Recognizing the common symptoms of stress fractures and using diagnostic imaging can help to make an early and accurate diagnosis.

A review of a patient's history and a physical examination are the first steps in stress fracture diagnosis. Diffuse pain associated with stress fractures generally appears over a period of weeks. Patients typically report a dull ache that occurs with training and dissipates after a relatively short period of rest. As the injury becomes more advanced, pain occurs earlier in training and does not dissipate as quickly. Athletes with stress fractures often report a recent change in training volume or intensity, footwear, training surface, or technique. Eating disorders, previous stress injuries, leg-length discrepancy, skeletal malalignment, and muscle weakness or imbalance are also viewed as warning signs for stress fractures. When the site of an advanced stress fracture lends itself to inspection and palpation, localized tenderness and swelling are often found. Passive, active, and resisted ranges of motion are typically painless.

Stress fractures are not acute injuries. They occur over time and are part of a larger continuum of clinical responses to bone loading (Figure 3). Athletes generally will not report a stress fracture until they have reached a certain threshold of pain. Therefore, an athlete's training history, symptoms, and diagnostic imaging evidence must all be assessed to accurately diagnose the injury within the spectrum of bone's response to stress.

Diagnostic Imaging

Careful assessment of a patient's history combined with a physical examination may be sufficient for the diagnosis of a stress fracture, but diagnostic imaging is frequently needed to provide conclusive evidence. Radiography, CT, scintigraphy (bone scanning), and MRI are the most common imaging modalities used for diagnosing stress fractures. Although scintigraphy is often viewed as the current gold standard for stress fracture diagnosis, recent findings indicating that MRI provides more detailed anatomic information than scintigraphy suggest that MRI should be considered the new diagnostic gold standard.

Radiography is frequently the first imaging modality used in diagnosing stress fractures, but it is usually only

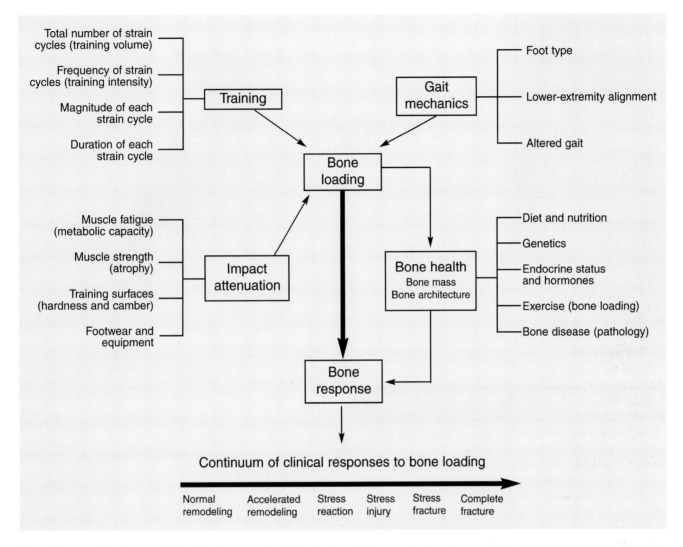

Figure 3 Summary of the factors contributing to bone's response to cyclic loading. Stress injuries occur along a continuum ranging from normal remodeling to complete stress fracture. *(Reproduced with permission from Brukner P, Bennell K, Matheson G: Stress Fractures. Carlton Victoria, Australia, Blackwell Science, 1999, p 10.)*

helpful in detecting late-stage injuries. Radiographs are not usually very effective for the early detection of stress injuries because the new periosteal bone that serves as radiologic evidence of a healing response is not visible until up to 3 months after the onset of symptoms. The sensitivity of stress injury detection using radiographs is 15% to 35% in the early stages and 30% to 70% in the later stages, but as many as 90% of all stress fractures may never be visible on radiographs. Because it is readily available, relatively inexpensive, useful for ruling out other pathologies, and can provide evidence of stress injuries some of the time, radiography can be effectively used as a first step in stress fracture detection.

The type of radiographic evidence of a stress fracture depends on the stage of injury progression at the time of imaging. The first radiographic sign of stress injury is the gray cortex, an area of low density in cortical bone that is associated with osteoclastic bone resorption. Later, thickening of the cortex can be observed on

both the periosteal and endosteal surfaces. A late-stage stress fracture can be observed in cancellous bone as a crack perpendicular to the trabeculae and in cortical bone as a radiolucent line extending partially or completely through the cortex (Figure 4).

If a radiograph provides no evidence of injury but the presence of a stress fracture is suspected, three-phase scintigraphy is often used to provide conclusive evidence of the injury. Because the sensitivity of scintigraphy is approximately 99%, it is commonly considered to be the gold standard for stress fracture detection. In three-phase scintigraphy, a bolus of a radioactive isotope tracer such as technetium Tc 99m methylene diphosphonate is injected intravenously and images are acquired at three stages. The first set of images (blood flow phase) is acquired immediately after the injection, the second set (soft-tissue phase) is acquired after approximately 5 minutes, and the third set (delayed skeletal phase) is acquired 2 to 4 hours after injection. Over

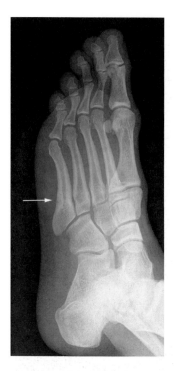

Figure 4 Radiograph showing a stress fracture (*arrow*) of the fifth metatarsal.

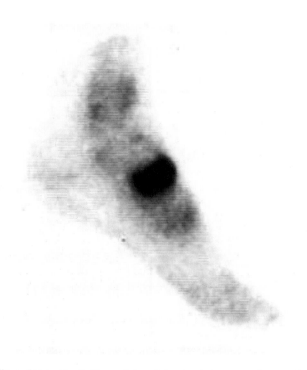

Figure 5 Technetium Tc 99m methylene diphosphonate bone scan of a stress fracture of the tarsonavicular.

TABLE 1 | Grading System for Classifying Stress Injuries Using Scintigraphy

Grade 1	Small, ill-defined foci of increased tracer uptake with mildly increased cortical activity
Grade 2	Larger lesions with a well-defined, elongated area of activity with moderately increased activity
Grade 3	Wide fusiform lesions with highly increased activity in the corticomedullary bone
Grade 4	Wide, extensive lesions with increased activity in the transcorticomedullary region

time, the tracer becomes localized in areas of high bone metabolism. These areas appear as dark "clouds" around the site of injury. Because scintigraphy is sensitive in identifying areas of increased remodeling, stress injuries can be identified at an early stage. Early injuries are seen as diffuse areas of increased tracer uptake. In more severe injuries, the tracer is much more localized and intense (Figure 5). In some cases, more detailed images must be obtained for conclusive diagnosis of stress fractures. Single-photon emission computed tomography, in which a camera is rotated 360° around the patient to produce a three-dimensional image based on radioactive tracers, can be useful for diagnosing stress fractures of the pelvis and lumbar spine.

Because stress injuries and stress fractures can vary along a continuum ranging from mild, early injury to complete fracture, a grading system has been developed to classify injury severity using scintigraphy. This system includes four grades, which are listed in Table 1. Areas

with intense tracer uptake should be the focus of further investigation. Early recognition of low-grade injuries can help increase the success of treatment and prevent injury progression and subsequent complications.

The high sensitivity of scintigraphy in identifying sites of increased bone metabolism can lead to misdiagnosis. Bone tumors, bone infections, and areas of infarction can be mistaken for stress injuries because these conditions also demonstrate increased tracer uptake. Because MRI can better differentiate between stress injuries and other highly metabolic conditions, it is becoming the method of choice for the early detection of stress fractures.

CT provides much better anatomic detail than plane radiography and is particularly useful for stress fracture diagnosis when sites of high osteoblastic activity are identified using scintigraphy. The detailed, three-dimensional images obtained using CT are useful for identifying stress fractures of the tarsal navicular, the pars interarticularis of the lumbar vertebrae, and the sacrum. As in plane radiography, stress fractures appear as radiolucent fracture lines or periosteal reactions. Longitudinal stress fractures of the tibia can also be identified using CT. These fractures appear as low-signal regions that extend through consecutive axial slices.

MRI is believed to be as sensitive as scintigraphy in detecting stress injuries, and MRI scans are more detailed and specific. Because bone does not have many free protons in solution, bone tissue itself is not represented in great detail on MRI scans. Instead, the value of MRI is in its ability to identify the soft-tissue response to stress injuries. Edema in the muscle, soft tissue, and marrow surrounding a stress injury appears as an area of high intensity on fat-suppressed, T2-weighted, and short tau inversion recovery MRI scans. In late-stage stress fractures, the fracture line appears as a band of low-signal intensity in the intermedullary space and often the cortex adjacent to the area of edema (Figure 6). Because of the high level of soft-tissue detail in these images, stress injuries can be pinpointed and distinguished from other pathologic bone conditions. A grading scale has been developed in order to classify stress injuries using fat-saturated MRI sequences. The scale has five grades, which are listed in Table 2. Using this scale to classify injuries seen on MRI scans can aid in early diagnosis and can help differentiate stress injuries and stress fractures from other conditions that cause bone marrow edema.

Radiography, CT, scintigraphy, and MRI are all valuable imaging modalities for diagnosing stress injuries and stress fractures. Although radiography and scintigraphy are usually sufficient for accurate and early diagnosis, and the cost of each is less than that of MRI, the fine detail provided by MRI leads to a more conclusive and specific diagnosis, and MRI does not require radiation exposure. MRI can also help pinpoint the location of injury and differentiate stress injuries from other pathologic conditions. As a result, MRI is replacing scintigraphy as the imaging modality of choice for detecting stress injuries and stress fractures.

Treatment

The appropriate treatment for a stress injury or stress fracture depends on the site and severity of the injury. Conservative treatment is successful for most of these injuries, but more aggressive approaches are necessary to treat severe injuries and for fractures that occur in sites that are known to commonly result in complications. Overall, modified rest and avoidance of the inciting activity are the cornerstones of stress fracture management. When rest is not sufficient to induce satisfactory healing and reduce symptoms, treatments such as bracing and internal fixation may become necessary.

After the diagnosis of a stress injury or stress fracture is made, the patient should immediately begin a period of modified rest during which the offending activity and other forms of impact loading are eliminated but normal ambulation is permitted. For lower extremity injuries, a walking boot or aircast can be used for symptomatic relief. If pain is severe, nonsteroidal anti-inflammatory drugs (NSAIDs) can be taken. There is some concern that NSAIDs may inhibit fracture healing and mask the symptoms used to gauge treatment progress, but these drugs are commonly used for man-

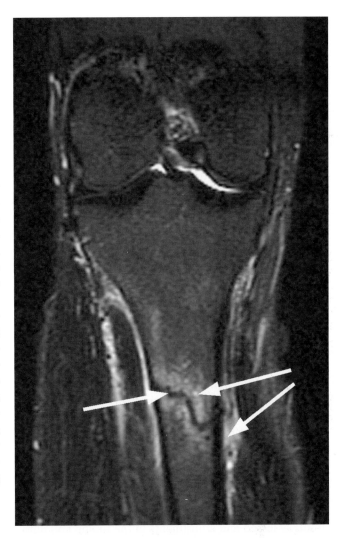

Figure 6 T2-weighted MRI scan showing marrow and periosteal edema (*right arrows*) and a low-signal stress fracture line in the proximal tibia (*left arrow*).

TABLE 2 | Grading System for Classifying Stress Injuries Using Fat-Saturated MRI Sequences	
Grade 0	Normal
Grade 1	Periosteal edema without focal marrow abnormality
Grade 2	More severe periosteal edema with bone marrow edema on T2-weighted MRI
Grade 3	Moderate to severe periosteal and marrow edema on both T1- and T2-weighted MRI
Grade 4	Low-signal fracture lines on MRIs and severe marrow edema on T1- and T2-weighted MRI

agement of very painful stress fractures. During the period of rest, the bone is able to "catch up" with the damage accumulation that has progressed, and healing can occur. During this period, consideration is also given to the modifiable contributing factors, and a program to ensure adequate muscular strength and endurance is ini-

TABLE 3	Injury Sites With a High Risk of Complication
Anterior tibial cortex
Proximal fifth metatarsal (Jones fracture)
Tarsal navicular
Femoral neck
Pars interarticularis

tiated. The length of the rest period depends on the patient's symptoms.

For stress fractures of the lower extremity, gradual resumption of activity should begin after the patient has been able to walk without experiencing pain for about 14 days. The patient should start with brisk walking for about 10 minutes per day and increase to 45 minutes per day over the course of approximately 1 week. After this time, the patient can begin to incorporate a brief period of slow jogging within the walk, starting at 5 to 10 minutes, and then increase jogging time by about 5 minutes per day. If symptoms recur during resumption of activity, 2 days of rest are recommended before continuing with the process. After the patient is able to jog without pain for 45 minutes, the pace can be gradually increased to full stride. To maintain fitness during the period of rest and resumption of activity, the patient can participate in activities such as cycling, aqua running, and resistance training in areas that avoid loading the fracture site. Although these stress fracture management guidelines can help lead to successful outcomes, they are not set in stone. Each patient's symptoms and rate of recovery should be closely assessed and adjustments in the timing and duration of rehabilitative activities made, if necessary.

When rest is not sufficient for alleviating the symptoms of a stress injury or stress fracture or when there is evidence of displacement, malunion, or nonunion of a fracture site, surgery may be warranted. Internal fixation using US Food and Drug Administration approved class II devices such as pins, plates, screws, intramedullary nails, or a combination thereof can stabilize the fracture site and promote healing. Bone autografts have also been shown to promote stress fracture healing.

Although more aggressive treatments are available, a period of rest and gradual resumption of activity is successful for most patients. The appropriate treatment depends on the site and extent of the injury as well as the personal preferences of patients and clinicians.

Higher Risk Sites

Stress fractures can occur in nearly every bone in the body, but they most frequently occur in weight-bearing bones. Common sites of injury include the tibia, fibula, tarsonavicular, fifth metatarsal, femur, pubic ramus, and pars interarticularis of the lumbar vertebrae. Several sites in particular require special attention because of

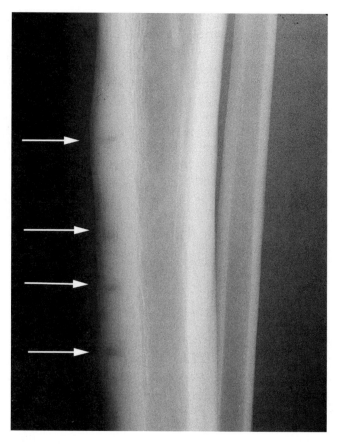

Figure 7 The "dreaded black line." Four stress fractures (*arrows*) appear in this radiograph as radiolucent lines extending into the anterior tibial cortex.

their high rates of delayed union, malunion, or nonunion. These high-risk sites are listed in Table 3.

The tibia is the most frequent site of stress fracture. Because the anterior midshaft region of the tibia typically has a relatively poor blood supply and is frequently loaded in tension, it is highly prone to nonunion. Because of its high complication rate, a fracture in the anterior tibial cortex is often called the "dreaded black line," a term derived from the appearance of this fracture as radiolucent defects on plain radiographs (Figure 7). These injuries rarely heal with conservative clinical treatment; therefore, more aggressive treatments such as intramedullary nailing are often required. A less invasive method of surgically treating the "dreaded black line" is percutaneous drilling. First described more than 40 years ago, this is the standard of treatment for this type of fracture in ballet dancers.

Stress fractures at the junction of the proximal metaphysis and diaphysis of the fifth metatarsal (Jones fracture) can also be problematic (Figure 4). The thick cortex in this location results in a relatively poor blood supply, and numerous soft-tissue connections produce a complex loading environment. Non–weight-bearing cast immobilization for 4 weeks, followed by the use of a walking cast for an additional 4 weeks, often results in

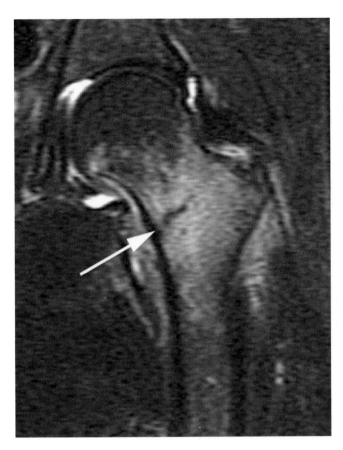

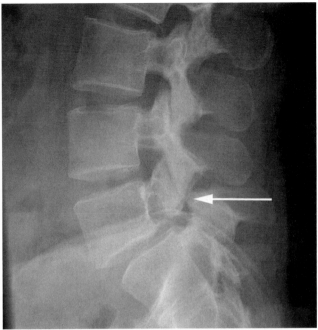

Figure 9 Radiograph showing a stress fracture *(arrow)* of the pars interarticularis of the fifth lumbar vertebra.

Figure 8 T2-weighted MRI scan showing a stress fracture of the inferior femoral neck *(arrow)*.

satisfactory healing. Internal fixation using a cannulated screw may become necessary when no evidence of healing is apparent after the period of immobilization.

Stress fractures of the tarsonavicular in the foot often result in delayed union or nonunion (Figure 5). The central portion of the tarsonavicular is relatively avascular; as a result, the healing process in this location is slow and often incomplete. Because patients with this type of fracture typically have minimal pain and swelling, accurate diagnosis via physical examination can be difficult. Although non–weight-bearing cast immobilization for 6 weeks to 3 months can often successfully treat these fractures, internal fixation and grafting are sometimes required.

Femoral neck stress injuries can cause severe, long-lasting complications if they are not recognized and treated early. There is a particularly high risk of nonunion or osteonecrosis when stress fractures of the femoral neck go untreated for a long time. Patients with femoral neck stress fractures often report pain in the groin or anterior hip region. Because radiographs often show no signs of injury, MRI and scintigraphy are more useful for early detection (Figure 8). Treatment depends on the severity of the injury and ranges from a brief period of no weight bearing for a mild stress injury to im-

mediate surgery and screw and plate fixation for a completely displaced stress fractures.

The pars interarticularis, which is the narrow portion of bone between the superior and inferior articular facets of each vertebra, is a common stress fracture site that is prone to nonunion. The pars interarticularis experiences shear stresses as a result of extension, hyperextension, and flexion of the lumbar spine, and the cyclic application of these stresses can prevent healing and union at the fracture site. Oblique radiographs can offer sufficient evidence of a pars interarticularis stress fracture, but the use of scintigraphy or MRI may be necessary when radiographs are negative (Figure 9). As a first step in the treatment of a pars interarticularis stress fracture, activities involving extension and torsion of the spine should be avoided. An antilordotic brace may be used, and exercises to strengthen the extensor muscles of the back and the abdominal muscles can help to stabilize the spine once pain has subsided.

Although they most commonly appear in weight-bearing bones, stress fractures can also occur in non–weight-bearing bones, such as the ribs, humerus, olecranon process of the ulna, and carpals. Instead of being caused by cyclic ground reaction forces, stress fractures in these bones are caused by other sources of repetitive loading such as rowing, swinging a baseball bat or tennis racquet, or even chronic coughing. Although avoidance of the initiating activity can produce satisfactory healing for most of these injuries, more aggressive treatments are sometimes warranted. Stress fractures of the olecranon, for example, may require surgery and internal fixation.

Summary

Stress injuries and stress fractures are widely variable and arise from a combination of mechanical and biologic factors. Fatigue damage accumulation and an increased rate of remodeling can produce these injuries in almost any bone in the body. Awareness of the common symptoms of stress fractures and the prudent use of available imaging modalities can help make an accurate and early diagnosis. Conservative treatment often results in satisfactory healing; however, more aggressive strategies are sometimes required, especially in fracture sites that are known to present a high risk of nonunion or other complications. A sound understanding of the pathophysiology of stress fractures, accurate and early diagnosis, and prudent treatment strategies can lead to successful stress fracture management and get athletes back on the playing field as soon as possible.

Acknowledgment

The authors wish to acknowledge Chris Beaulieu for supplying the images for this chapter.

Annotated Bibliography

General

Shaffer RA: Incidence and prevalence of stress fractures in military and athletic populations, in Burr DB, Milgrom C (eds): *Musculoskeletal Fatigue and Stress Fractures.* Boca Raton, FL, CRC Press, 2001, pp 1-33.

This review of stress fracture study designs and stress fracture incidence rates for US military and athletic populations found that study design affects reported incidence rates and that 0.2% to 4% of male military recruits and 1% to 7% of female military recruits experience at least one stress fracture during training.

Loading, Remodeling, and Fatigue Damage

Carter DR, Beaupré GS: *Mechanical Function and Form: Mechanobiology of Skeletal Development, Aging, and Regeneration.* Cambridge, England, Cambridge University Press, 2001.

This book presents current knowledge and theory of the influence of mechanics on skeletal development, remodeling, and evolution.

Pathophysiology

Milgrom C, Finestone A, Sharkey N, et al: Metatarsal strains are sufficient to cause fatigue fracture during cyclic overloading. *Foot Ankle Int* 2002;23:230-235.

In vivo metatarsal strains were measured in two subjects during walking, running, and calisthenics. The magnitude of compressive and tensile strains in these moderate activities was high enough to cause fatigue damage and failure even without an intermediate bone remodeling response.

Risk Factors

Almeida SA, Williams KM, Shaffler RA, Brodine SK: Epidemiological patterns of musculoskeletal injuries and physical training. *Med Sci Sports Exerc* 1999;31: 1176-1182.

This study of 1,296 US Marine Corps recruits indicated that the volume of rigorous physical training may be an etiologic factor in overuse injuries. Ankle sprains, iliotibial band syndrome, and stress fractures were the most common injuries.

Bennell K, Grimston S: Risk factors for developing stress fractures, in Burr DB, Milgrom C (eds): *Musculoskeletal Fatigue and Stress Fractures.* Boca Raton, FL, CRC Press, 2001, pp 35-54.

This chapter summarizes the risk factors for developing stress fractures, including measurable bone components, bone remodeling, mechanical loading, and nutritional and psychologic traits.

National Institutes of Health: Osteoporosis prevention, diagnosis, and therapy. *NIH Consens Statement* 2000;17: 1-36.

This statement from the National Institutes of Health Consensus Development Conference on Osteoporosis Prevention, Diagnosis, and Therapy summarizes the current knowledge and issues concerning osteoporosis.

Clinical Diagnosis

Perron AD, Brady WJ, Keats TA: Principles of stress fracture management: The whys and hows of an increasingly common injury. *Postgrad Med* 2001;110:115-118, 123-124.

This is a review of current knowledge of stress fracture pathogenesis, epidemiology, imaging, diagnosis, and treatment.

Diagnostic Imaging

Ishibashi Y, Okamura Y, Otsuka H, Nishizawa K, Sasaki T, Toh S: Comparison of scintigraphy and magnetic resonance imaging for stress injuries of bone. *Clin J Sport Med* 2002;12:79-84.

This prospective study of 31 patients with stress injuries to bone assessed the correlation accuracy of MRI and scintigraphy findings with clinical symptoms. The authors conclude that MRI is less invasive and provides more information than scintigraphy.

Kiuru MJ, Pihlajamaki HK, Hietanen HJ, Ahovuo JA: MR imaging, bone scintigraphy, and radiography in bone stress injuries of the pelvis and lower extremity. *Acta Radiol* 2002;43:207-212.

In this prospective study of 50 patients, the authors found 41 stress injuries to bone in 32 patients and report that MRI was more sensitive than scintigraphy in revealing stress injuries to bone.

Lassus J, Tulikoura I, Konttinen Y, Salo J, Santavirta S: Bone stress injuries of the lower extremity. *Acta Orthop Scand* 2002;73:359-368.

This is a review of the etiology, pathophysiology, diagnosis, and treatment of stress injuries in the bones of the hip, leg, and foot.

Pozderac RV: Longitudinal tibial fatigue fracture: An uncommon stress fracture with characteristic features. *Clin Nucl Med* 2002;27:475-478.

This study of three patients with longitudinal tibial stress fractures found that scintigraphs exhibiting a long area of diffusely increased activity in the distal tibia extending proximally from the tibiotalar junction are indicative of a longitudinal stress fractures.

Sijbrandij ES, van Gils APG, de Lange EE: Overuse and sports-related injuries of the ankle and hind foot: MR imaging findings. *Eur J Radiol* 2002;43:45-56.

This pictorial essay describes MRI evidence of stress injuries and other overuse injuries of the foot. Short tau inversion recovery T2-weighted MRI scans demonstrate intramedullary marrow edema adjacent to the site of a stress fracture.

Spitz DJ, Newberg AH: Imaging of stress fractures in the athlete. *Radiol Clin North Am* 2002;40:313-331.

The authors review imaging methods for the diagnosis of stress fractures including radiography, CT, scintigraphy, and MRI and report that radiographs and thorough clinical history often suffice to make the diagnosis. In patients with stress fractures that are atypical in location or clinical presentation, MRI, scintigraphy, and CT are useful.

Treatment

Brukner P: Stress fractures of the upper limb. *Sports Med* 1998;26:415-424.

This is a review of literature concerning stress fractures of the humerus, clavicle, scapula, radius, and ulna. Fractures in all patients healed with conservative management.

Ohta-Fukushima M, Mutoh Y, Takasugi S, Iwata H, Ishii S: Characteristics of stress fractures in young athletes under 20 years. *J Sports Med Phys Fitness* 2002;42:198-206.

This analysis of 222 stress fractures in 208 athletes younger than 20 years found that those athletes who visited a hospital within 3 weeks of the onset of symptoms had a significantly faster return to full activity. The tibia was the most common fracture site.

Perron AD, Brady WJ, Keats TA: Management of common stress fractures: When to apply conservative therapy, when to take an aggressive approach. *Postgrad Med* 2002;111:95-96, 99-100, 105-106.

This is a description of conservative treatment strategies for stress fractures as well as more aggressive treatments for high-risk sites, such as the fifth metatarsal and the femoral neck.

Higher Risk Sites
Brukner P, Bennell K, Matheson G: *Stress Fractures*. Carlton Victoria, Australia, Blackwell Science, 1999.

This summary of current knowledge in stress fracture pathophysiology, risk factors, diagnosis, and treatment contains treatment strategies for stress fractures in general and for specific sites.

Classic Bibliography

Bennell KL, Brukner PD: Epidemiology and site specificity of stress fractures. *Clin Sports Med* 1997;16:179-196.

Fredericson M, Bergman AG, Hoffman KL, Dillingham MS: Tibial stress reaction in runners: Correlation of clinical symptoms and scintigraphy with a new magnetic resonance imaging grading system. *Am J Sports Med* 1995;23:472-481.

Giladi M, Milgrom C, Simkin A, Danon Y: Stress fractures: Identifiable risk factors. *Am J Sports Med* 1991;19:647-652.

Matheson GO, Clement DB, McKenzie DC, Taunton JE, Lloyd-Smith DR, McIntyre JG: Stress fractures in athletes: A study of 320 cases. *Am J Sports Med* 1987;15:46-58.

Mori S, Burr DB: Increased intracortical remodeling following fatigue damage. *Bone* 1993;14:103-109.

Mulligan ME: The "gray cortex": An early sign of stress fracture. *Skeletal Radiol* 1995;24:201-203.

Pattin CA, Caler WE, Carter DR: Cyclic mechanical property degradation during fatigue loading of cortical bone. *J Biomech* 1996;29:69-79.

Reeder MT, Dick BH, Atkins JK, Pribis AB, Martinez JM: Stress fractures: Current concepts of diagnosis and treatment. *Sports Med* 1996;22:198-212.

Thomasen E: *Diseases and Injuries of Ballet Dancers*. Denmark, Universitetsforlaget/Aarhus, 1982, p 74.

Zwas ST, Elkanovitch R, Frank G: Interpretation and classification of bone scintigraphic findings in stress fractures. *J Nucl Med* 1987;28:452-457.

Chapter 22

Musculotendinous Injuries

Thomas M. Best, MD, PhD, FACSM

Hechmi Toumi, PhD

Introduction

The two main forms of trauma to skeletal muscle are indirect or strain injuries and direct or contusion injuries. Because injuries to skeletal muscle during sports are common, it is important that sports medicine physicians understand the structure and function of skeletal muscle as well as be up to date on the most recent research on musculotendinous injury and repair. It is also important to be aware of potential new treatment and rehabilitation approaches, particularly those regarding stretch injury to the myotendinous junction.

Structure and Function of Skeletal Muscle

Skeletal muscle comprises up to 45% of the average individual's total body weight. It is composed of muscle cells, nerves, blood vessels, and a connective tissue matrix. The primary function of skeletal muscle is to contract, resulting in the generation of force and torque about a joint that brings about movement. A second function of skeletal muscle is energy absorption, which plays a much more significant role in injury and injury mechanisms than first recognized.

Skeletal muscle consists of four major myofibrillar proteins: myosin, actin, tropomyosin, and troponin. These four proteins and their enzymes (myosin ATPase) interact with intermediate filament proteins such as desmin and dystrophin to regulate the speed and intensity of muscle contraction. It is increasingly recognized that collectively these proteins also play a role in injury and repair and the ability of skeletal muscle to adapt to altered patterns of mechanical loading. The plasticity of skeletal muscle can also be attributed to satellite cells, which are primordial cells that trigger new muscle growth, lie dormant within the basal lamina, and can be activated by a variety of conditions, intrinsic growth factors, and cytokines (Tables 1 and 2).

Skeletal muscle function is largely influenced by the nerve entering the muscle at its motor point. Each muscle fiber is contacted by one nerve terminal at its neuromuscular junction. Collectively, the nerve and all of the muscle fibers it innervates are known as a motor unit. Each motor unit contains a specific number of fibers that is largely dictated by the accuracy and speed of movement necessary.

Muscle Injury and Repair

Muscle injury can occur through a variety of mechanisms such as mechanical injury, muscular dystrophies, infectious diseases, and biochemical toxicities. Regardless of the type of insult to muscle, a key event in the early stages of repair is the inflammatory response resulting in both polymorphonuclear and mononucleated cellular infiltration of the injury site. The process begins with cytokine and growth factor release from injured muscle fibers that produce chemotactic signals to invading inflammatory cells. The neutrophil is the first cell to appear following all forms of muscle injury. Neutrophils, produced in the bone marrow, circulate in the bloodstream and represent 50% to 60% of the total circulating leukocytes. Neutrophil invasion of damaged muscle occurs as early as 1 hour after injury, but recent reports suggest that it may occur within minutes. A primary function of neutrophils following injury is phagocytosis of necrotic muscle fibers and cellular debris. In addition, invading neutrophils signal for the arrival of proinflammatory cytokines such as interleukin (IL)-1, IL-8, and tumor necrosis factor–alpha (TNF-α). These cytokines may play a role in the upregulation of inflammation and provide a signal for further invasion by both neutrophils and monocytes.

The initial damage that occurs with stretch injury to the myotendinous junction is likely a combination of the initial mechanical damage and the loss in calcium homeostasis through stretch-activated channels and ruptures in the sarcoplasmic reticulum or sarcolemma. Release of proteolytic enzymes such as calpain from the injured myofibers may also contribute to the initial damage. Immediate functional and structural deficits are followed by evidence of further damage within the first 24 hours. Recent observations have suggested that neutrophils may be responsible, in part at least, for the secondary damage that occurs with a stretch injury. Neutrophils contain several enzymes such as myeloperoxidase and

TABLE 1 | Proinflammatory Cytokines and Their Role in the Pathogenesis of Arthritis

Cytokine	Major Cellular Source	Major Targets and Biologic Effects
TNF-α	Monocytes Macrophages T lymphocytes	Monocytes, synovial macrophages, fibroblasts, chondrocytes, endothelial cells Stimulation of proinflammatory cytokine and chemokine synthesis Activation of granulocytes Increase MHC class II expression Secretion of MMPs leading to cartilage matrix degradation
IL-1	Monocytes Macrophages Many cell types	Monocytes, synovial macrophages, fibroblasts, chondrocytes, endothelial cells Inhibition of matrix synthesis in chondrocytes Secretion of MMPs leading to matrix degradation Stimulation of proinflammatory cytokine and chemokine synthesis Fibroblast proliferation T cell proliferation
IL-6	Activated T cells (Th2) Many cell types (induced by IL-1 or TNF-α)	Stimulation of acute phase protein synthesis in liver B cell proliferation and differentiation T cell proliferation Differentiation of hematopoietic precursor cells Differentiation and maturation of osteoclasts (induction of MMP-inhibitor, TIMP-1)

TGF-β	Many cell types	Immune suppression (inhibition of B and T cell proliferation)
		Monocyte chemotaxis
		Differentiation of mesenchymal and epithelial cells (chondrogenesis)
		Anabolic for cartilage
		  Stimulation of matrix synthesis
		  Reduced production of MMPs
		  Increased production of proteinase inhibitors

MHC = major histocompatibility complex, MMP = matrix metalloproteinase, TIMP = tissue inhibitors of matrix metalloproteinases

(Reproduced from Recklies AD, Poole AR, Banerjee S, et al: Pathophysiologic aspects of inflammation in diarthrodial joints, in Buckwalter JA, Einhorn TA, Simon SR (eds): Orthopaedic Basic Science: Biology and Biomechanics of the Musculoskeletal System, ed 2. Rosemont, IL, American Academy of Orthopaedic Surgeons, 2000, pp 489-530.)

nicotinamide adenine dinucleotide phosphate oxidase that are capable of generating free radicals such as superoxide, hydrogen peroxide, nitric oxide, and hydroxyl radicals. It is possible that these highly reactive molecules cause direct cell damage, including modification of nucleic acids, proteins, and lipids that would therefore suggest a negative effect on the repair process. The presence of neutrophils has been correlated with structural damage and tissue injury in other models of muscle damage. Peak neutrophil infiltration of stretch-injured muscle occurs within 24 hours. This peak correlates with peak free radical production as well as maximum myofiber damage. An attractive hypothesis suggests that neutrophils invade the damaged muscle and produce free radicals that lead to further damage. Conversely, it is possible that free radicals act to amplify the host's inflammatory response by the upregulation of proinflammatory cytokines such as nuclear factor κB.

In addition to neutrophil invasion of the injury site, monocytes appear that eventually mature and differentiate into macrophages. Adhesion molecules such as E-selectin and P-selectin appear critical for the influx of leukocytes (neutrophils and monocytes) to the injured tissue. Neutrophils can stimulate the proliferation of res-

ident macrophages, of which two subtypes are now recognized to play a role in muscle injury and repair. The first subpopulation expresses the ED1[+] antigen and is capable of invading damaged muscle fiber to phagocytose cellular debris and damaged myofibrillar material. The ED2[+] macrophages are resident macrophages present throughout the regenerative process, but their exact role remains unknown. ED2[+] macrophages do not appear to invade damaged tissue; rather, their primary function may be to serve as sources of growth factors and cytokines such as insulin-like growth factor (IGF)-I, IL-6, and platelet-derived growth factor that may regulate myoblast proliferation and/or differentiation.

Following removal of damaged cellular products by infiltrating inflammatory cells, a series of events occurs that involves two competing events: muscle fiber regeneration and collagen synthesis. The satellite cells that reside in the periphery of the muscle fiber between the basal lamina and the sarcolemma are the primitive cells for muscle regeneration. An intact basal lamina appears to be essential to satellite cell activation and is capable of expressing various extracellular matrix components necessary for regeneration. If the basal lamina of the damaged fiber remains intact following injury, satellite

TABLE 2 | Major Cytokines Involved in Immune Regulation

Cytokine	Cellular Source	Biologic Effects
IL-2	Activated T cells (Th1)	Clonal proliferation of T cells Proliferation of B cells
IFN-γ	Activated T cells (Th1)	Induction of MHC class II expression on monocytes, connective tissue cells (fibroblasts, chondrocytes) and endothelial cells Increased expression of MHC class I molecules
IL-4	Activated T cells (Th2)	B cell proliferation and class switching of immunoglobulin synthesis Inhibition of production of proinflammatory cytokines by monocytes
IL-5	Activated T cells (Th2)	Growth and differentiation of eosinophils
IL-12	Activated macrophages	Development of the Th1 response
IL-10	Activated T cells (Th2) Macrophages	Inhibition of synthesis of proinflammatory cytokines by T cells and macrophages
IL-15	Activated macrophages Connective tissue cells?	T cell proliferation (similar to IL-2)
IL-17	Activated memory T cells	Proinflammatory; stimulation of cytokine secretion (IL- 6, IL-8, MCP1, granulocyte-stimulating factor) and prostaglandin E_2 in epithelial, endothelial, and fibroblastic cells

IFN-γ = interferon-γ, MHC = major histocompatibility complex, MCP1 = monocyte chemotactic protein 1

(Reproduced from Recklies AD, Poole AR, Banerjee S, et al: Pathophysiologic aspects of inflammation in diarthrodial joints, in Buckwalter JA, Einhorn TA, Simon SR (eds): Orthopaedic Basic Science: Biology and Biomechanics of the Musculoskeletal System, ed 2. Rosemont, IL, American Academy of Orthopaedic Surgeons, 2000, pp 489-530.)

cells form myogenic cells that fuse with existing fibers or with each other to form myotubules. In vitro experiments have shown satellite cell proliferation can occur within hours of injury. It has been previously shown that there are two populations of satellite cells. Committed satellite cells can directly enter the differentiation pathway and begin to produce myogenic transcription factors and muscle-specific proteins. Stem satellite cells first divide, most probably so that one of the offspring replenishes the pool of reserve cells and the other may enter the differentiation pathway.

A delicate balance of several factors exists that determines both the speed and the extent of myofiber regeneration following injury. Growth factors such as basic fibroblast growth factor (bFGF), IGF-I, and transforming growth factor (TGF)-β have received the most attention to date. These growth factors are made available to the injured tissue via local availability, disruption of the extracellular matrix, local synthesis, and blood-borne arrival. Studies have shown an increased expression of IGF-I in satellite cells, myoblasts, and myotubules during skeletal muscle regeneration. IGF-I levels increase significantly under the influence of growth hormone after muscle injury. Furthermore, an acute bout of eccentric exercise increases IGF-I levels in muscle tissue sections for up to 4 days; however, the exact significance of this increase is not known.

Satellite cells proliferate, differentiate into myoblasts, and fuse to form myotubules, which fill the old basal lamina cylinder and become closely apposed to the surviving parts of the torn and/or transected myofibers. Newly formed myotubules are reported to fuse with the surviving parts of damaged myofibers by the fourth day after injury. If an intervening scar is formed at the site of injury, however, the transected myofibers do not fuse with each other. Regenerating myofibers are unable to penetrate through the scar and instead become attached to the scar by the formation of new myotendinous junctions. Adequate connective tissue production is necessary at the same time for normal force transmission to occur and for the muscle's resistance to tensile loading to be preserved. Excessive collagen synthesis can lead to fibrosis that can potentially alter muscle stiffness and joint range of motion and performance.

Collagen types I and III constitute the major types of collagen within skeletal muscle. Type I collagen, present primarily in the muscle fiber's epimysium and perimysium, possesses relatively high tensile strength and stiffness and is therefore suitable for transmission of musculotendinous forces. Type III collagen is located primarily within the perimysium and endomysium. Its structure is similar to that of type I collagen, but it forms thinner and more elastic fibers. In response to skeletal muscle injury, collagen types I and III are produced. Type III collagen synthesis increases before mature fibroblasts can be detected, with primitive, multipotent cells as the presumed source. Later in the repair process, there is marked production of type I collagen and restoration of the normal ratio of collagen types I and III. Clinicians and therapists face an ongoing dilemma of requiring some new collagen formation for the musculotendinous unit to carry load and generate torque about a joint while at the same time seeking minimal scar formation to minimize stiffness and loss of coordinated motion patterns. Recent studies have suggested that collagen types IV and V may also be involved in the repair of damaged skeletal muscle.

Role of Growth Factors and Cytokines in Muscle Injury

Cytokines are a diverse family of intercellular signaling proteins that influence the movement, proliferation, differentiation, and metabolism of target cells. These actions can occur by direct interaction of the cytokine with its particular receptor or by the ability of one cytokine to induce synthesis of other cytokines and hormones. Stimuli such as mechanical damage, oxidants, and stress hormones may modulate or induce cytokine activity. Some generalizations about their role in soft-tissue injury and repair appear possible. First, IL-1β and TNF-α are proinflammatory cytokines that upregulate inflammation. On the other hand, TGF-β, IL-4, and IL-10 assist in downregulation of the host inflammatory response. Cytokines also appear to play an important role in muscle repair through satellite cell chemotaxis. For example, FGF-2 and TGF-β promote the migration of muscle precursor cells in vitro.

Modulation of Inflammation

Skeletal muscle injury, induced by eccentric contractions, direct muscle trauma, or overstretch is associated with increased neutrophil concentrations within the muscle. Traditionally, the primary roles of neutrophils were thought to be phagocytosis and removal of cellular debris; however, studies suggest that neutrophils may play a role in secondary injury to the muscle. Because of the temporal relationship between muscle neutrophil concentrations and secondary injury, it is plausible to think that these cells play a role in injury. Animal models have shown that peak neutrophil concentrations are present at the same time as peak myofiber damage occurs. Neutrophils release potentially damaging reactive oxygen and nitrogen intermediates that conceivably could result in damage. Experiments with blocking antibodies have demonstrated that limiting neutrophil invasion and blocking oxygen-free radical generation can limit muscle damage following stretch injury. Moreover, tissue culture experiments have confirmed that neutrophils can injure healthy skeletal myotubules; however, the exact significance of these findings in vivo is uncertain at this point.

It is therefore conceivable that one way of limiting muscle damage would be to attenuate certain aspects of neutrophil function. Rest, cold, compression, and elevation are early treatments traditionally implemented to limit bleeding, whereas nonsteroidal anti-inflammatory medications are prescribed to suppress the response of the inflammatory cells. Despite the frequent use of nonsteroidal anti-inflammatory medications to treat sports-related trauma, the scientific basis for this application based on animal models and clinical trials is rather limited. The use of corticosteroid injections after acute muscle injury is controversial because experimental models have shown that direct corticosteroid injection can briefly weaken the musculotendinous unit. However, a recent study of professional football players with hamstring strains and palpable defects demonstrated that a corticosteroid injection reduced the time for rehabilitation and return to sport without an increase in the rerupture rate. Although the results were dramatic, the study was retrospective and without a control group. As more is learned about the role of inflammatory cells and the modulation of inflammation, treatment methods may become more effective when specific functions of these cells are targeted. Perspectives for rational approaches to handle the development of tissue injury during neutrophil invasion and activation show some promise.

Despite the fact that corticosteroids appear to be catabolic and inhibit the healing process, there is tremendous interest and some findings in the literature to suggest their efficacy in the treatment of muscle injuries. On the other hand, anabolic steroids have been shown to promote muscle growth and regeneration in some circumstances. They have also been shown to speed the recovery of force-generating capacity after certain injuries. Their use in the treatment of muscle injury may warrant further research.

Use of Growth Factors To Improve Muscle Healing

Over the past 5 years, there have been major advances in understanding the mechanisms of scar formation and muscle healing. An exciting new approach to improve muscle healing and limit scarring and fibrosis involves the use of certain growth factors. Although limited to in vivo animal studies and in vitro assays at this point, it appears that growth factors such as bFGF, IGF-I, and nerve growth factor are capable of enhancing muscle regeneration and accelerating recovery of muscle force in strain-injured tissues. These three growth factors in particular appear to positively influence satellite cell proliferation and formation of new myotubules, an early step in myofiber regeneration.

Another exciting development is the synthesis of antifibrotic agents. TGF-β has been implicated in the development of fibrosis in various tissues including skeletal muscle and is expressed at high levels. It is also associated with fibrosis in the skeletal muscle of patients with Duchenne muscular dystrophy. The use of antifibrosis agents that inactivate TGF-β have been shown to reduce muscle fibrosis and improve muscle healing following laceration injury in an animal model.

The use of human recombinant growth factors also invites the intriguing possibility of using gene therapy to transport satisfactory concentrations of growth factor to injured muscle. Both viral and nonviral vectors have been studied. Each method offers distinct advantages and disadvantages and is the subject of ongoing investigations to develop safe and rational delivery methods.

Rehabilitation Strategies and Injury Prevention

Sports-related muscular trauma can result in significant morbidity and time loss from competition. For example, hamstring injuries, which are the most common muscle injury in running and sprinting athletes, result in significant pain, disability, and time lost from sports competition. Despite the frequency of muscle injuries, the current understanding of risk factors and prevention of injury is far from complete. Although both intrinsic and extrinsic risk factors have been proposed, it is difficult from epidemiologic studies to determine the role of factors such as strength and flexibility in predicting injury and recovery from injury. It appears clear that the main risk factor for a stretch-related injury is a previous similar injury. Although a fair proportion of muscle strains recur during the first week of return to competition, there appears to be a persistent significant risk of recurrence for many weeks after return to play. Imaging studies have shown that the injury can be much more extensive than initially appreciated by clinical examination. Therefore, primary prevention of muscle strain injury is a topic of great interest and debate. Recent studies suggest that a preseason strengthening program involving the hamstrings and quadriceps can reduce the incidence of hamstring strains in elite athletes. Additional studies are needed before these results are applicable to other populations and muscle groups.

The role of stretching in injury treatment and prevention has recently been questioned. Although stretching can alter the short-term viscoelastic properties of the muscle, the extrapolation of these findings to humans has not provided conclusive evidence that stretching can prevent or even reduce the incidence of sports-related muscle injury. Few prospective randomized studies have been done that critically evaluate whether stretching can prevent injury or reduce the severity of sports-related muscular injury. An important concern may be whether a stretch-injured muscle should be placed in a lengthened or shortened position of immobilization for a short period after injury. Recent studies have shown that immobilization of a muscle in a lengthened position for a short period after a contusion injury appears to result in a faster return to sports participa-

tion without posing an increased risk for reinjury. Most studies showing any protective benefit of stretching have included a cointervention such as a warm-up, making it impossible to identify the potential benefit of stretching alone. If stretching is to be implemented, body position may be important. For example, stretching the hamstring muscle with an anterior pelvic tilt may be more effective because it minimizes compensation from the cervical, thoracic, and lumbar spine. Recent studies point to the possibility that trunk stabilization and neuromuscular control exercises may be advantageous in the treatment of patients with acute hamstring strains. Other studies have demonstrated that a similar approach implementing motions in the frontal plane together with core stability exercises is advantageous over passive stretching and strengthening in the treatment of rugby players with chronic groin pain. The current understanding of the role of strengthening after muscle injury is based largely on basic physiologic principles. Because the majority of tears involve muscles with type II fibers, it is thought that activities of high velocity are optimal for muscle training. Whether this is correct has not been assessed in any prospective studies comparing different strategies of muscle strengthening.

There is no consensus as to when an athlete can safely return to athletic activity following a muscle strain. It now appears that a recent history of strain to one muscle group actually increases the risk of injury to surrounding muscle groups. This observation suggests that biomechanical and perhaps neurologic alteration in muscle and joint function subsequent to injury are important in the rehabilitation phase. Obviously, this is dependent on the functional demands of the sport and position played by the individual. No single test or clinical observation is regarded as the gold standard despite the common approach for full range of motion and strength. An analogous situation may be the decision making that occurs following an injury and repair of the anterior cruciate ligament. Many practitioners will allow an athlete to return to sports participation within 6 to 8 months, even though basic science studies report that the anterior cruciate ligament graft is still maturing between 12 and 24 months after reconstruction.

The indications for surgical treatment of sports-related musculotendinous trauma are not clear or evidence-based at this time; however, many studies suggest that surgical repair is advantageous for total or near-total muscle rupture and should be considered in cases of bony avulsion with more than 2 cm of displacement. Nonetheless, no prospective clinical studies are available to support these assertions.

Summary

Musculotendinous injuries continue to be a challenge for athletes and physicians. Recent studies suggest the possibility for new treatment strategies to limit fibrosis and scarring and improve healing. Prospective studies are needed to address optimal treatment and prevention strategies.

Annotated Bibliography

Muscle Injury and Repair

Belcastro AN, Shewchuk LD, Raj DA: Exercise-induced muscle injury: A calpain hypothesis. *Mol Cell Biochem* 1998;179:135-145.

The sequestration of calcium and release of proteases such as calpain after injury are hypothesized to contribute to the secondary damage seen with repetitive eccentric contractions.

Brickson S, Corr DT, Hollander J, Ji L, Best TM: Oxidant production and immune response after stretch injury in skeletal muscle. *Med Sci Sports Exerc* 2001;33: 2010-2015.

Oxygen-free radicals derived from neutrophils may mediate damage following stretch injury to skeletal muscle.

Cannon JG, St. Pierre BA: Cytokines in exercise-induced skeletal muscle injury. *Mol Cell Biochem* 1998; 179:159-167.

The authors of this article describe the biologic actions and potential adaptive values of cytokines through the course of muscle necrosis and degeneration.

Pizza FX, McLoughlin TJ, McGregor SJ, Calomeni EP, Gunning WT: Neutrophils injure cultured skeletal myotubes. *Am J Physiol Cell Physiol* 2001;281:C335-C341.

Neutrophils can damage skeletal myotubules and prevent new muscle growth in vitro.

St. Pierre Schneider B, Brickson S, Corr DT, Best TM: CD11b$^+$ neutrophils predominate over ram11$^+$ macrophages in stretch-injured muscle. *Muscle Nerve* 2002; 25:837-844.

Neutrophils are reported to be the predominant leukocyte invading skeletal muscle within minutes of a controlled stretch injury, which has implications for control and treatment of inflammation.

Modulation of Inflammation

Levine WN, Bergfelf JA, Tessendorf W, Moorman CT: Intramuscular corticosteroid injection for hamstring injuries. *Am J Sports Med* 2000;28:297-299.

This is a case series of 53 athletes with near-complete hamstring tears treated with corticosteroid injections to provide earlier return to sport without an increased risk of rerupture.

Use of Growth Factors to Improve Muscle Healing

Best TM, Shehadeh SE, Leverson G, Corr DT, Michel JT, Aeschlimann D: Analysis of changes in mRNA levels of myoblast- and fibroblast-derived gene products in healing skeletal muscle using quantitative reverse transcription-polymerase chain reaction. *J Orthop Res* 2001;19:565-572.

Early signal for types I and III collagen along with protein deposition occur with little signal for new myosin expression, suggesting the formation of scar at the expense of myofiber regeneration.

Fukushima K, Badlan N, Usas A, Fiane F, Fu F, Huard J: The use of an antifibrosis agent to improve muscle recovery after laceration. *Am J Sports Med* 2001;29:394-402.

Decorin, an inhibitor of TGF, can decrease fibrosis and improve recovery of function (strength) after a laceration injury in rabbit skeletal muscle.

Kasemkijwattana C, Menetrey J, Bosch P, et al: Use of growth factors to improve muscle healing after strain injury. *Clin Orthop* 2000;370:272-285.

This article summarizes the use of growth factors to improve healing and decrease fibrosis in an animal model.

Rehabilitation Strategies and Injury Prevention

Beiner JM, Jokl P, Cholewicki J, Panjabi MM: The effects of anabolic steroids on healing of muscle contusion injury. *Am J Sports Med* 1999;27:2-9.

The authors report that anabolic steroids may speed the recovery of muscle force-generating capacity after contusion injury.

Herbert RD, Gabriel M: Effects of stretching before and after exercise on muscle soreness and risk of injury: Systematic review. *BMJ* 2002;325:468-470.

This meta-analysis suggests that there is little prospective evidence supporting a link between stretching and the prevention of sports-related muscle injuries.

Orchard J: Intrinsic and extrinsic risk factors for muscle strains in Australian football. *Am J Sports Med* 2001;29: 300-303.

The author identifies intrinsic and extrinsic risk factors for hamstring and quadriceps strains in Australian athletes.

Classic Bibliography

Burke RE: Motor unit properties and selective involvement in movement. *Exerc Sport Sci Rev* 1975;3:31-81.

Close RI: Dynamic properties of mammalian skeletal muscles. *Physiol Rev* 1972;52:129-197.

Kibble MW, Ross MB: Adverse effects of anabolic steroids in athletes. *Clin Pharm* 1987;6:686-692.

Ryan JB, Wheeler JH, Hopkinson WJ, Arciero RA, Kolakowski KR: Quadriceps contusions: West Point update. *Am J Sports Med* 1991;19:299-304.

Tidball JG: Inflammatory cell response to acute muscle injury. *Med Sci Sports Exerc* 1995;27:1022-1032.

Section 5

Medical Disorders in Athletes

Section Editor:
Thomas M. Best, MD, PhD, FACSM

Chapter 23

Infectious Diseases

David T. Bernhardt, MD

Introduction

Infectious diseases occur among recreational, competitive, and elite athletes at a rate comparable to that of the general population. The training and competitive demands of sports can affect the immune system. In addition, infectious diseases may negatively impact the athlete's performance and put athletes at risk for injury. Therefore, it is important for sports medicine physicians to understand the effects of exercise on the immune system and the unique aspects of infectious diseases as they relate to athletic participation.

Exercise and the Immune System

Many elite athletes and their coaches believe that intense exertion decreases resistance to infections, especially viral respiratory infections. Others believe that daily exercise protects against frequent infections. Who is correct? One study suggests that both theories are correct, with moderate exercise being associated with fewer upper respiratory infections and overtraining associated with an increased risk of more frequent upper respiratory infections when compared with baseline.

Exercise raises the levels of all types of white blood cells, including polymorphonuclear neutrophils, lymphocytes, and monocytes. This occurs in response to any stressful activity because of the hormonal influences of norepinephrine and cortisol. In athletes, decreased fitness or higher intensity workouts will therefore likely result in a greater effect. This effect has also been reported recently in a group of adolescent tennis players, with more mild changes noted after less intense, shorter workouts and more prolonged effects noted after more stressful, intense conditioning. A study of elite swimmers showed an acute decrease in salivary immunoglobulin A and immunoglobulin M levels immediately after exercise along with a decline in natural killer cell numbers. However, no association among upper respiratory tract infection, changes in the immune system, and the stressful exercise regimen used in this study was reported.

Recovery after exercise results in a suppression of the immune system. With prolonged strenuous exercise, such as that used by athletes who participate in ultra-marathons, decreased lymphocyte counts and a drop in mucociliary clearance and T cell function have been noted.

Respiratory Infections

Viral Upper Respiratory Tract Infections

Viral upper respiratory tract infections (common colds), the most commonly occurring infections among athletes and nonathletes, are often caused by the rhinovirus and other viruses. Symptoms include mild fever, rhinorrhea, sore throat, fatigue, malaise, and possibly cough. The classic viral upper respiratory tract infection is a self-limiting illness that lasts approximately 3 to 14 days and is usually spread via respiratory droplets. Although viral upper respiratory tract infections are usually benign, self-limiting, and rarely require a visit to a primary care provider, athletes and physicians should be aware of how these infections impact athletics. Some viruses that cause the common cold can also cause myocarditis; sudden death in athletes has been triggered by arrhythmias related to myocarditis.

Exercise and performance can be affected by viral upper respiratory tract infections. Pulmonary manifestations may include a drop in peak flow, gas exchange, and respiratory muscle strength. Cardiac output and stroke volume may also be diminished. Constitutional symptoms include myalgias, weakness, and fatigue that may result in a decrease in strength. Associated fever and malaise along with the illness itself may result in psychologic effects that directly affect an athlete's ability to train and perform.

Treatment of athletes with viral upper respiratory tract infections is usually supportive. Rest and fluids are recommended. Symptomatic treatment of fever and myalgias may involve the use of antipyretics and analgesics. Because of the increasing threat of drug-resistant organisms, antibiotics should not be prescribed for viral upper respiratory tract infections. Antibiotics should only be prescribed for possible secondary bacterial infections.

Supportive treatment may also include the judicial use of over-the-counter cold medications. Athletes and physicians must be aware of rules regarding the use of these medications because several have been banned by different sport-governing bodies. In addition, many of these medications have adverse effects (for example, drowsiness, dizziness, and effects on temperature regulation, heart rate, and blood pressure) that may be detrimental to athletic performance.

Athletes and physicians must also be aware of the dangers of using herbal remedies to treat viral upper respiratory tract infections and other ailments. Not only can some of the substances contained in herbal remedies be outright dangerous, but they may also be contaminated with substances not listed in the ingredients. For example, *Ephedra sinica*, also known as ma huang, is an herbal supplement that is often used as a dietary supplement; its alkaloid derivative, ephedrine, is commonly used as a nasal decongestant, and some athletes will use this herbal supplement to treat viral upper respiratory tract infections and for weight control. Other unapproved products containing ephedra or ephedrine include *Sida cordifolia* and epitonin. Recent studies report that although ephedra and ephedrine may promote modest short-term weight loss, there is no sufficient evidence to support the use of these compounds to improve athletic performance. In addition, a two to three times increased risk of psychiatric, autonomic, and upper gastrointestinal symptoms and heart palpitations has been reported with its use. Ephedra has also been linked to an increased risk of hemorrhagic stroke and to at least two recent cases of sudden death during sports participation.

Contamination of herbal substances occurs on a regular basis. A study of performance-enhancing herbal supplements found that 11 of 12 brands tested did not meet the labeling requirements set out in the 1994 Dietary Supplement Health and Education Act.

Other supportive measures may include the use of beta-agonists (such as albuterol and salmeterol), but the evidence supporting their use to treat viral upper respiratory tract infections is controversial. Limited evidence suggests that the beneficial effects of beta-agonists may occur only in patients with bronchial hyperresponsiveness, wheezing, or airflow limitation (such as with viral-induced asthma).

Competition and practice limitations are usually based on the severity of the illness. Because of the possible association of viral upper respiratory tract infections and myocarditis, physicians should limit the athletic activities of patients with high fever, myalgias, chills, and significant fatigue. Athletes with more mild symptoms of viral upper respiratory tract infection should modify activity based on energy level. Because

of increased cardiopulmonary effort, reduced maximum exercise capacity, increased likelihood of heat illness, and increased orthostatic hypertension during exercise, the American Academy of Pediatrics recommends that athletes with illnesses associated with fever do not participate in competitive athletic activities. What defines a high fever in these guidelines, however, and the evidence supporting the risk of playability can be questioned.

Athletes could be at increased risk for viral upper respiratory tract infections for several reasons, including sharing locker room facilities and water bottles, prolonged intense training, frequent travel, and the stress of competition. Coaches should consider altering practice duration and intensity when a viral upper respiratory tract infection outbreak occurs on a team. Prohibiting athletes from sharing water bottles and towels and frequent cleaning of equipment is recommended. Getting adequate rest from practice and other nightlife activities can also lead to a more rapid recovery.

Pharyngitis

Pharyngitis can be caused by a variety of different viruses including the adenovirus, Coxsackie virus, influenza, respiratory syncytial virus, and herpesvirus. Symptoms consist of a sore, scratchy throat, malaise, and headache; with many of the viral causes, symptoms may also include rhinorrhea and possibly cough. Signs of a viral pharyngitis include a variable, low-grade fever and mild erythema of the pharynx with or without exudate. Herpesvirus (type 1 or 2) results in vesicles with more serious erythema, fever, and tender anterior cervical adenopathy. The Coxsackie virus causes herpangina in younger athletes; patients typically have small vesicles on the soft palate, low-grade fever, and possibly associated lesions on the palms and soles (classic hand-foot-mouth disease). Because the Coxsackie virus has been associated with myocarditis in the past, it is important to recognize this condition in athletes.

Decisions regarding treatment and playability for patients with viral pharyngitis are made in a manner similar to those for patients with viral upper respiratory tract infections; supportive treatment is the mainstay. Maintaining adequate hydration may be difficult, however, because patients with viral pharyngitis often have pain with swallowing.

Bacterial causes of pharyngitis include group A β-hemolytic and other types of *Streptococcus*, *Arcanobacterium*, and possibly anaerobic infections. A patient with group A β-hemolytic streptococcal pharyngitis classically presents with a sore throat of variable severity and possibly headache and abdominal pain. Rhinorrhea, cough, or other gastrointestinal symptoms are rarely present. Examination classically reveals swollen, erythematous tonsils with tender anterior cervical adenopathy. Group A β-hemolytic streptococcus can be diagnosed with a streptococcal rapid antigen test or traditional culture. For over 50 years, an orally administered 250-mg dose of potassium phenoxymethyl penicillin (penicillin VK) two to three times daily for 10 days has remained the standard of care. In patients with penicillin allergy, treatment options include macrolide antibiotics (erythromycin) and cephalosporins. Treatment with antibiotics is recommended to prevent possible complications, including rheumatic fever or peritonsillar abscess formation. Because other types of streptococcus are not associated with rheumatic fever and do not usually result in additional complications, they do not need to be treated with antibiotics unless symptoms warrant. Most athletes with classic bacterial streptococcal pharyngitis will not feel well enough to practice or compete. Supportive care with analgesics and hydration should be recommended.

Arcanobacterium is a less common cause of pharyngitis. Presentation includes a severe sore throat, exudative pharyngitis, and anterior cervical adenopathy. Although diagnosis is made via throat culture, the throat culture should be screened for all organisms and not just for *Streptococcus*. Erythromycin is the treatment of choice.

Influenza

Influenza is a respiratory illness that begins with a scratchy throat and cold symptoms and progresses within 2 to 3 days to a more severe illness with constitutional symptoms, including high fever, malaise, myalgias, and persistent cough. Athletes infected with influenza will have a difficult time participating in athletic activities because of the severity of the symptoms. Complications such as secondary bacterial pneumonia should be suspected when influenza persists for longer than 1 week. Other rare complications include encephalitis and myocarditis.

Treatment for influenza consists of supportive treatment with rest, hydration, antipyretics, and, if necessary, cough suppressants to aid with sleep. Amantidine, rimantadine, oseltamivir, and zanamivir can shorten the course of the illness if started within 48 hours after the onset of symptoms. Amantadine and rimantadine are effective only in treating influenza A; oseltamivir and zanamivir can be used to treat either influenza A or B, but some drug-resistant strains may exist. These medications can also be used prophylactically when an outbreak occurs.

The influenza vaccine is effective and is recommended for all athletes who compete during the winter months and individuals with chronic cardiovascular or respiratory diseases, including asthma. An allergy to eggs is the main contraindication to receiving this vaccine.

TABLE 1 | Clinical Presentation of Infectious Mononucleosis

Feature	Frequency %
Lymphadenopathy	100
Splenomegaly*	> 90
Malaise and fatigue	> 90
Fever	> 80
Sore throat	> 80
Pharyngitis	> 70
Anorexia	> 50
Periorbital edema (Hoagland's sign)	20 to 40
Rash	10 to 40

*Only palpable in 50% of patients

Infectious Mononucleosis

Infectious mononucleosis is a viral syndrome that is caused by Epstein-Barr virus. Other viruses such as cytomegalovirus can cause similar symptoms. Athletes with infectious mononucleosis classically present with a 3- to 5-day prodrome consisting of nonspecific fatigue, malaise, headache, and possibly cold-like symptoms, which gradually progresses to fatigue, sore throat with signs of severe exudative pharyngitis, anterior and posterior tender cervical adenopathy, and splenomegaly. Symptoms may last for up to 2 weeks, after which a convalescent phase with fatigue can affect patients for up to 6 additional weeks (Table 1).

Laboratory findings include a lymphocytosis with greater than 10% of lymphocytes classified as atypical. Mild neutropenia and thrombocytopenia may be noted in the first 2 weeks of the illness. During the second week, 90% of patients have mild elevations of liver function.

Diagnosis is confirmed via a positive heterophile antibody test. Although usually negative in the first week of the illness, 90% of patients will have positive results by the end of the third week. False-positive test results can be caused by a variety of different infections including cytomegalovirus, adenovirus, and toxoplasmosis. Confirmatory serologic testing specific for Epstein-Barr virus can be performed when the reliability of the heterophile antibody test result is questionable.

Complications may include a concurrent group A β-hemolytic streptococcal infection in approximately 15% of patients. Because treatment with ampicillin or amoxicillin usually results in an antibody-mediated rash in these patients, penicillin or erythromycin is preferable.

Upper airway obstruction secondary to severe tonsillar enlargement may result in dehydration caused by the inability to swallow or severe respiratory compromise.

Treatment with corticosteroids can dramatically reduce tonsillar size and is indicated for patients with upper airway obstruction complications.

Although splenomegaly is almost universally seen in patients with infectious mononucleosis, an enlarged spleen is palpable in only 50% of patients. Although rupture of the spleen is a rare complication, it is certainly a concern for any athlete participating in contact sports. Most ruptures occur spontaneously and are not related to athletic competition or any collision.

Almost all complications occur within the first 3 weeks of the illness. Other rare complications associated with Epstein-Barr virus infections include hematologic disorders such as autoimmune hemolytic anemia and thrombocytopenia. Rare neurologic complications include encephalitis, Bell's palsy, and Guillain-Barré syndrome. Infectious complications may include a secondary bacterial infection resulting in a peritonsillar abscess.

Treatment recommendations usually consist of rest, fluids, and analgesic management of pharyngitis. The pharyngitis may be severe enough to warrant the use of viscous lidocaine or narcotic medication. Stool softeners to decrease straining with bowel movements can help prevent splenic rupture associated with Valsalva maneuvers. Concomitant strep throat must be treated with appropriate antibiotics.

Treatment with corticosteroids is indicated for patients with impending respiratory compromise or dehydration related to severe tonsillar hypertrophy. Other indications for treatment with corticosteroids include neurologic complications and immune-mediated abnormalities related to anemia or thrombocytopenia (depending on severity). Treatment with corticosteroids has no proven benefit in the prevention of splenomegaly and splenic rupture and should not be used to allow athletes with infectious mononucleosis to return to play more quickly.

Return to play recommendations for athletes with infectious mononucleosis are based on risk for splenic rupture and the patient's overall recovery. No strict return-to-play criteria or guidelines currently exist. Because the risk of splenic rupture is greatest during the first 3 weeks, most sports medicine practitioners prohibit athletic activity for a minimum of 3 weeks after onset, after which athletes are allowed to return to athletic activity gradually based on their general energy levels and how they respond to more stressful conditioning sessions.

Diarrhea Illnesses

Viral Gastroenteritis

Viral gastroenteritis, usually caused by the rotavirus or Norwalk virus, is spread via fecal-oral transmission. The classic patient presentation includes diarrhea, crampy abdominal pain, malaise, and possibly vomiting. Physical examination typically reveals nonlocalized abdominal tenderness and a mild fever. Signs of dehydration may also be present. Although viral gastroenteritis is a self-limited illness and no treatment is indicated, hydration should be maintained with an oral electrolyte solution or, if necessary, intravenous hydration. Because of the increased risk for heat-related injury secondary to dehydration and fever, athletes with viral gastroenteritis who have subjective symptoms of significant malaise or objective findings of fever or dehydration should be restricted from athletic activity.

Blood-Borne Pathogens

Human Immunodeficiency Virus

Human immunodeficiency virus (HIV) is caused by human retrovirus and directly affects immune function by attacking CD-4 helper T cells. The progressive immune suppression leads to opportunistic infections and malignancy. The overall incidence of infection in the United States is approximately 1:250. Transmission can occur via sexual contact, parenteral exposure, wound contamination, and mother-fetus transmission. The two major issues regarding athletes with HIV are the possibility of transmission through possible wound contamination and guidelines for exercise.

The number of athletes infected with HIV is unknown. The risk of transmission is similar to that for nonathletes and is directly attributable to high-risk behavior such as intravenous drug use, multiple sexual contacts, and unprotected sex. Although it is possible to transmit HIV to another competitor through an open wound or blood spill, the risk of this happening is quite low for three reasons. First, the organism is quite fastidious and does not tolerate drying or exposure to air. Second, the concentration of viral particles in the blood is actually quite small compared with other blood-borne pathogens such as hepatitis B. Third, given that the risk of infection or transmission via direct needle-stick exposure with infected blood is 1 in 300, the risk of infection or transmission via an open wound or blood spill during athletic competition is likely comparable or lower. Thus far, there has been no evidence documenting transmission of HIV during athletic competition. Although the risk of transmission is remote, it is very important for those treating a wound or blood spill of an athlete with HIV to be familiar with universal precautions to reduce the risk of transmission to themselves.

In terms of exercise recommendations for athletes with HIV, as with other athletes with chronic disease, exercise can improve the quality of life, maintain fitness, and improve psychologic well-being. Mild to moderate exercise is recommended, and any exercise program should be guided by a physician who specializes in the care of patients with HIV. Theoretically, exhaustive, stressful exercise can further stress an already threatened immune system and is therefore discouraged; however, a single bout of exercise does not increase HIV-RNA levels, and exercise is thought to be safe in individuals with HIV. Specific exercise guidelines for athletes with HIV are listed in Table 2. Strength training can increase lean mass and reduce fat mass in patients with HIV if adequate energy balance is provided. As with the general population, aerobic exercise can help maintain weight in patients with HIV.

The mandatory testing of athletes for HIV is controversial and not recommended at this time. Before such testing can be instituted, several issues must be resolved, including who to test, how often to test, what to do about false-positive and false-negative results, and whether test results change any recommendations regarding sports participation or make a sport safer than it is currently.

Voluntary testing of at-risk athletes is no different than that of the nonathletic population. The results of testing provide a window of opportunity to educate and counsel at-risk athletes in terms of decreasing high-risk behavior. In addition, if diagnosed early, a positive test for HIV allows the infected individual to start therapy, which is generally promising. All voluntary testing should involve counseling in which the meaning of the test is explained to the patient and additional information regarding prevention, decreasing risk, and possible referral resources are provided for those with a positive test result.

Whether to disclose the results of HIV testing is currently the right of the individual patient. As the risk of HIV transmission during athletic activity is low, physicians are not obligated to inform other team members, opponents, coaches, or even athletic trainers when they are caring for an athlete with HIV.

Hepatitis B Virus

The transmission of the hepatitis B virus is a much more serious concern for athletes and those who provide their medical care. Of all people infected with hepatitis B, 1% will die from fulminant liver failure, and up to 10% will become chronic carriers of the hepatitis B virus.

As with HIV, transmission of the hepatitis B virus can occur via parental exposure. Hepatitis C can also be transmitted via parenteral exposure, but because it is not seen as frequently as hepatitis B, it is less of a health risk, especially as it pertains to athletics. Transmission of the hepatitis B virus to other athletes and those who provide their medical care is of much greater concern. The hepatitis B virus is the most sustainable of the blood-borne pathogens; fomites can serve as agents of transmission for several days. Transmission of the hepatitis B virus has been reported among household contacts from shared razors and toothbrushes. Approximately one of every three needle sticks with infected

TABLE 2 | Empirical Guidelines for Athletes With HIV

A complete physical examination should be conducted before initiating any new exercise program.

Healthy, asymptomatic athletes should avoid overtraining but can otherwise continue to train and compete without restriction.

Athletes with acquired immunodeficiency syndrome–related complex should avoid exhaustive training and competition but can train as their energy levels allow.

Athletes with frank acquired immunodeficiency syndrome may remain physically active depending on their energy levels and should avoid strenuous exercise; athletes with acute illness should avoid exercise entirely.

(Adapted with permission from Calabrese L, LaPierre D: HIV infections: Exercise in athletes. Sports Med 1993;15:1-3.)

blood will result in transmission. In addition to being able to live outside of the body for a long period, the concentration of the hepatitis B virus in the blood is quite high. Most importantly, the risk of transmission in athletics is not theoretical because it has been reported to occur among Sumo wrestlers in Japan.

Symptoms and signs of hepatitis B include anorexia, fatigue, and possibly low-grade fever. Although the disease may be mild in many patients, in others it may progress to fulminant hepatitis and death. Chronic carriers remain contagious. Specific exercise guidelines have not yet been developed for patients with hepatitis B.

Treatment consists of hepatitis B immunoglobulin and vaccine. Baseline laboratory cultures need to be obtained along with serology to monitor the patient's infectious state. Hepatitis B virus antigen is the best marker for infectivity; patients with the hepatitis B virus e antigen remain infective and should avoid participation in contact or collision sports to avoid infecting others.

All individuals at risk for acquiring hepatitis B, including health care workers and athletes, should be immunized. Most children born in the United States receive a series of three vaccines at birth to immunize them from contracting hepatitis B.

Immunizations

Many infectious diseases can be easily prevented with immunization. Therefore, team physicians and athletic training staff must have an up-to-date record of an athlete's immunization status. The most practical immunizations for athletes are the tetanus primary series and booster, a meningococcus vaccine for athletes living in dormitories during college, and an influenza vaccine on an annual basis if participating in athletic activities during the winter months. The other vaccine of importance is the tetanus vaccine because of the risk of exposure to contaminated wounds in many sports.

Summary

Infectious diseases can affect the recreational and elite athlete in many different ways. Although many basic science research studies have investigated the role of exercise and immune function, how this affects the athlete's performance or clinical status is still under investigation. Common infections such as viral respiratory infections, strep throat, and infectious mononucleosis all affect the athlete's ability to perform, train, and compete. Recognition and management of these infections is essential for the sports medicine physician to allow safe return of the athlete to athletic activity. Blood-borne pathogens such as HIV and hepatitis B play a unique role in possibly affecting both infected athletes and their competitors in contact sports.

Annotated Bibliography

Exercise and the Immune System

Gleeson M, McDonald WA, Pyne DB, et al: Immune status and respiratory illness for elite swimmers during a 12-week training cycle. *Int J Sports Med* 2000;21:302-307.

This is a prospective study of systemic and mucosal immunity in elite swimmers. The authors found that despite changes in some immune parameters during a 12-week training program prior to competition there were no associations detected with upper respiratory tract infections for this cohort of elite swimmers.

Mackinnon LT: Chronic exercise training effects on immune function. *Med Sci Sports Exerc* 2000;32(suppl 7): S369-S376.

This article reviews the literature on the chronic training effects on immune function.

MacKinnon LT: Overtraining effects on immunity and performance in athletes. *Immunol Cell Biol* 2000;78:502-509.

This review article summarizes neuroendocrine and immune changes related to overtraining or prolonged periods of intense training.

Nieman DC: Is infection risk linked to exercise workload? *Med Sci Sports Exerc* 2000;32:S406-S411.

This article reviews the immune response to acute bouts of exercise and points out that there is a need for further research in this area.

Nieman DC, Kernodle DA, Sonnenfeld G, Morton DS: The acute response to the immune system to tennis drills in adolescent athletes. *Res Q Exerc Sport* 2000;71: 403-408.

This study examined the acute immune response to tennis training in 20 elite adolescent tennis players. The authors report that 2-hour sessions of tennis performed by these athletes resulted in mild changes in cell counts and immune function.

Respiratory Infections

Committee on Sports Medicine and Fitness: Medical conditions affecting sport. *Pediatrics* 2001;107:1205-1209.

This policy statement reviews medical conditions such as fever, diarrhea, and mononucleosis and makes recommendations as they pertain to sports participation.

Del Mar CB, Glasziou P: Upper respiratory tract infection. *Clin Evid* 2002;7:1391-1399.

This brief review critically examines the efficacy of various common treatments for upper respiratory tract infections, including antibiotics, over-the-counter medications, and herbal remedies.

Green GA, Catlin DH, Starcevic B: Analysis of over-the-counter dietary supplements. *Clin J Sport Med* 2001; 11:254-259.

This study assessed the purity of over-the-counter steroid supplements and demonstrated that 11 of 12 brands did not meet the requirements outlined in the 1994 Dietary Supplement Health and Education Act.

Blood-Borne Pathogens

Roubenoff R, McDermott A, Weiss L, et al: Short-term progressive resistance training increases strength and lean body mass in adults infected with human immunodeficiency virus. *AIDS* 1999;13:231-239.

The authors of this article studied 25 adults with human immunodeficiency virus who were trained using a progressive resistance training program. They report that the subjects had improvements in strength, lean body mass, and body fat at the end of 8 weeks of training.

Roubenoff R, Skolnik PR, Shevitz A, et al: Effect of a single bout of acute exercise on plasma human immunodeficiency virus RNA levels. *J Appl Physiol* 1999;86: 1197-1201.

This study of 25 patients with human immunodeficiency virus showed that no increased viral load was associated with acute exercise.

Immunizations

Boozer CN, Nasser JA, Heymsfield SB, Wang V, Chen G, Solomon JL: An herbal supplement containing Ma Huang-Guarana for weight loss: A randomized, double-blind trial. *Int J Obes Relat Metab Disord* 2001;25:316-324.

The authors studied 67 overweight subjects who were given placebo or an herbal supplement for weight loss. They report that the Ma Huang-Guarana group had greater weight loss and body fat decrease over an 8-week period.

Classic Bibliography

American Medical Society for Sports Medicine (AMSSM), American Orthopedic Society for Sports Medicine (AOSSM): Human immunodeficiency virus (HIV) and other blood borne pathogens in sports. Joint Position Statement, 1995.

Calabrese L, LaPierre D: HIV infections: Exercise in athletes. *Sports Med* 1993;15:1-3.

Eichner ER, Calabrese LH: Immunology and exercise: Physiology, pathophysiology and implications for HIV infection. *Med Clin North Am* 1994;78:377-388.

Farley DR, Zietlow SP, Bannon MP, Farnell MB: Spontaneous rupture of the spleen due to infectious mononucleosis. *Mayo Clin Proc* 1992;67:846-853.

Henderson DK, Fahey BJ, Willy M, et al: Risk for occupational transmission of human immunodeficiency virus type 1 (HIV:1) associated with clinical exposure. *Ann Intern Med* 1990;113:740-746.

Kashiwagi S: Outbreak of hepatitis B in members of a high school wrestling club. *JAMA* 1982;248:213-214.

Nieman DC: Immune response to heavy exertion. *J Appl Physiol* 1997;82:1385-1394.

Chapter 24

Dermatologic Problems

William W. Dexter, MD, FACSM

Laurie D. Donaldson, MD

Introduction

Dermatologic disorders can affect athletes on multiple levels. Pain, irritation, and pruritus are aggravating factors that can adversely affect athletic performance. Although some dermatologic conditions such as skin disorders caused by trauma, environment, and infectious agents may pose harm to athletes, they are rarely life threatening; however, these conditions may affect return to play. Disqualification from competition and team disruption may also be of concern. When treating athletes with dermatologic conditions, the psychologic impact of the disease should be taken into account as well as the etiology of the disease, diagnostic clues, and prevention.

Traumatic Disorders

Corns and calluses are the most common dermatologic problem encountered in athletes. Repetitive injury and overuse leads to a buildup in the skin of protective layers of keratin that can be problematic. Corns are small, hard, conical lesions that can be quite painful. Most commonly they are located on the little toe. Soft corns may be present between the toes; these are known as a "kissing lesion." Calluses are broad, thick lesions that occur over pressure points and are commonly located on the plantar surface of the foot, on the great toe, and over the metatarsal heads. Foot anatomy, biomechanics, and footwear all may be causative factors in the development of corns and calluses. When symptomatic, the treatment of corns and calluses includes evaluating and correcting any of the contributing factors. Eliminating pressure points, padding the corn or callus, and using shoe inserts are often sufficient treatment. Judicious use of paring, after soaking the foot for several minutes, can be performed with a pumice stone or emery board. For recalcitrant lesions, radiographs can help identify underlying bony deformities that may be correctable.

Abrasions received as a result of trauma caused by sudden impact with the ground ("road rash") can be quite painful and are typically seen in cyclists. Infections and permanent "tattooing" of the skin may occur if foreign material is not removed. Treatment consists of thorough cleansing and scrubbing with soap to remove debris and grease. Dish detergent can be an effective cleansing agent. Sedation and/or anesthesia should be considered when the lesion is extensive because this procedure can be very painful. Topical lidocaine gel for small or moderate lesions will provide sufficient anesthesia. Cleansing should be followed with the application of an antibacterial agent and dressing changes to prevent infection.

Shearing forces from repetitive rubbing or from rapid starts and stops can lead to the formation of blisters. These are common in almost all athletes and can occur on both the hands and feet. Treatment consists of making a small incision at the periphery of the blister to allow for drainage of the underlying fluid while preserving the protective roof of skin. Antibiotic ointment is rarely required. A simple bandage, tape, or second skin may be placed over the blister after drainage. Commercial products such as Moleskin (Schering-Plough, Kenilworth, NJ) may help prevent blister formation. Blisters occurring deep to calluses are treated by débridement of the overlying callus, drainage, and a protective covering. Blisters can be prevented by gradually increasing activity to toughen the skin. Well-fitting footwear, moisture-wicking socks, and appropriate gloves (such as those used in cycling) are also useful preventive measures.

Poorly fitting footwear also can be responsible for lesions known as runner's toenail, tennis toe, skier's toe, or jogger's nails (Figure 1). A subungual hematoma forms from repetitive contact of the distal end of the nail with the shoe. This can be a painful condition that can progress to onycholysis and dystrophy of the nail. With atypical or unresolving lesions, a high degree of suspicion for melanoma should be maintained, a biopsy of the lesion should be performed, and the patient should be referred for further consultation, if necessary. Rest and soaking of the foot in warm water is usually adequate treatment. For more immediate relief from acute bleeding, however, a large (18-gauge) needle can be used to drill through the nail by gently rolling the needle between the fingers while applying downward

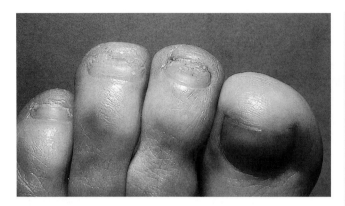

Figure 1 Jogger's nails. *(Reproduced with permission from the American Academy of Dermatology, Schaumburg, IL.)*

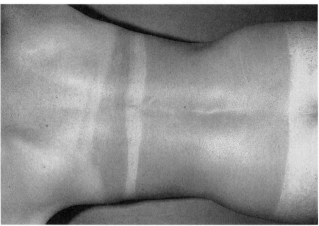

Figure 2 Sunburn reaction. *(Reproduced with permission from the American Academy of Dermatology, Schaumburg, IL.)*

pressure. This drains blood and relieves pressure. Keeping the toenails trimmed, short, and straight and wearing shoes with an adequate toe box may help prevent subungual hematoma.

Talon noir (black heel) and tache noir (black palms) are lesions caused by shearing forces on the epidermis that result in intraepidermal bleeding and blue-black macular lesions. Talon noir is common in basketball players and is associated with the frequent stop and start nature of the sport. Tache noir is often seen on the palms of skiers as a result of repetitive pole planting in downhill skiing. Tache noir is also occasionally caused by repetitive shearing trauma in weight lifters, tennis players, golfers, and mountain climbers. These lesions are asymptomatic, completely innocuous, and do not require treatment. However, the level of suspicion for melanoma should remain high; thus, follow-up is important. Once the causative trauma is eliminated, these lesions should spontaneously resolve.

Repetitive friction in runners can result in a condition known as jogger's nipples, which occurs more commonly in males than females. This is because most female runners wear supportive brassieres during running that add a protective layer. Especially common in long-distance runners in cold weather, bleeding erosions on the nipples after a long run can be exquisitely painful. Treatment includes the application of petroleum jelly or antibiotic ointment. Wearing soft-fiber running bras for women or cotton or silk shirts for men can prevent this type of trauma. Petroleum jelly can be applied before long runs or protective tape or a bandage can be applied to the size and shape of the areola.

Runner's rump and rower's rump are two additional traumatic skin conditions seen in the gluteal cleft area. In the former, small ecchymoses occur on the superior portion of the gluteal cleft. These often occur in long-distance runners as a result of the repetitive contact between the cheeks of the buttocks with each running stride. Rower's rump, a form of lichen simplex chronicus, is caused by repetitive friction from the seat of a

rowing machine. Surfer's nodules are fibrous nodules that occur on the anterior tibial prominence of the leg or mid dorsum of the foot as a result of repetitive blunt trauma from the surfboard. Modifying or eliminating the responsible source of contact can treat all of these conditions.

Traumatic skin lesions should always be evaluated using universal precautions. Return to play will be guided by the nature and healing of the wound and by the player's desire to return. There should be no active bleeding from healing wounds; healing wounds should be covered if athletes will be participating in contact sports.

Environmental Disorders

Contact dermatitis in athletes can be caused by outdoor plant exposure (for example, poison ivy) or by allergens in athletic equipment (such as rubber swim caps or goggles, diving equipment, or helmets). Contact dermatitis usually presents as a localized, erythematous, urticarial or vesicular rash. It may take 7 days for symptoms to appear after initial exposure. Repeated outbreaks usually occur within a day of contact with the allergen. Identifying the cause of contact dermatitis can be difficult. Once identified, optimal treatment includes avoidance of the offending material, and mild over-the-counter steroids can usually treat the rash effectively. Nonallergenic athletic equipment should be used by athletes with contact dermatitis.

Athletes who participate extensively in outdoor activities are at high risk for sun damage. The acute effects of sun exposure are manifested as sunburn (Figure 2). Within hours after exposure, tender, red, raised areas with sharply demarcated borders may appear. Patients with first-degree sunburn, the mildest form of sunburn, typically have erythema and mild discomfort. Patients with second-degree sunburn typically have erythema and blisters, and those with third-degree sunburn typically have erythema, blisters, and ulcers. Treatment of sunburn should consist of cooling the skin with cold water compresses and emollients. Compresses placed over a low- or moderate-potency topical corticosteroid cream applied for 1 hour three times a day can provide pain relief, and anti-inflammatory agents can be used for the first 1 to 2 days. Analgesics and anti-inflammatory agents can also be used to decrease pain and inflammation. Rarely, a short course of oral steroids may be necessary.

Excessive sun exposure is also linked to premature aging, photosensitivity, immunosuppression, and skin cancer. Prevention of harmful exposure is the best treatment. Broad UV-A/UV-B spectrum, sweat-proof, water-resistant sunblock with a sun-protection factor of 15 or higher should be applied liberally and frequently when athletes are outdoors. Sun-protective clothing, wide-brimmed hats, and UV-A/UV-B–screening sunglasses also should be worn when possible. Finally, the sun should be avoided when possible, particularly between 10 AM and 2 PM when UV rays are most intense. These protective measures are especially important at higher altitudes because the intensity of the sun increases 20% for every 5,000-foot increase in elevation.

Insect bites and stings also present another outdoor exposure risk for the athlete. Because of the risk of anaphylaxis, it is important to be able to recognize the signs and symptoms of insect bites and stings. Team medical records should also include any allergies players may have (such as an allergic reaction to bee stings). This information should be included on the preseason history and the trainer and/or physician should be aware of it in advance of preparation. Minutes after such a bite or sting, athletes can manifest any number of symptoms, such as apprehension, generalized urticaria, edema, wheezing, cough, or cyanosis.

Exercise-induced urticaria and anaphylaxis are other entities to consider. These are pruritic conditions that produce skin wheals and intense itching, which usually occur within 5 minutes of beginning exercise. Flushing, headache, abdominal cramping, and diarrhea may also be present. These attacks may last from 30 minutes to 4 hours. If untreated, it may progress to angioedema, respiratory distress, hypotension, and, rarely, vascular collapse. Initial treatment involves immediate cessation of exercise followed by a dose of 25 to 50 mg of diphenhydramine. Progressive symptoms should be treated with injectable epinephrine; 0.5 mL of epinephrine (in a concentration of 1:1,000) can be subcutaneously injected into a nonoccluded limb every 5 to 30 minutes as required. Patients with exercise-induced urticaria and anaphylaxis should always carry an autoinjector that administers epinephrine (EpiPen, Dey, Napa, CA) and never exercise alone. Taking a long-acting, nonsedating antihistamine 1 hour before exercise may prevent the

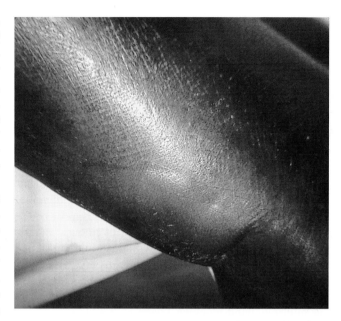

Figure 3 Frostbite. *(Reproduced with permission from the American Academy of Dermatology, Schaumburg, IL.)*

milder form of exercise-induced urticaria. Not eating before working out and not exercising in hot weather may also prevent outbreaks. Because of the potential for these more serious outcomes, epinephrine and diphenhydramine should be a mainstay in the team physician's sideline bag.

Dry (xerotic) skin is a common finding in athletes with frequent exposure to cold or wet environments. There is often a genetic atopic predisposition for this condition. Athletes with dry skin typically have dry, red, scaly skin that may or may not be pruritic. Itching often increases when undressing at bedtime and is less evident in skin folds and moist areas such as the groin and axilla. Because bathing removes the natural protective oils of the skin, athletes with dry skin should limit bathing to only one brief, lukewarm shower per day and avoid drying soaps and astringents. Long, hot baths or showers, bubble baths, whirlpools, and hot tubs should be avoided. Mild, unscented soaps should be used without excessive scrubbing and should be rinsed off completely. Immediately following the shower, a light, hypoallergenic, unscented moisturizer should be applied. Eczematous patches can be treated with a moderate-potency corticosteroid.

Frostbite and frostnip are environmental risks for winter sports enthusiasts such as skiers, mountain climbers, ice fishers, and long-distance runners. Frostbite refers to cold-induced trauma that can damage skin, subcutaneous tissue, muscle, and bone (Figure 3). In contrast, frostnip refers to the more common milder injury involving only the skin and superficial subcutaneous tissue. Temperatures below 32°F (0°C) combined with windy, wet weather increase the risk for frostbite and frostnip. Altitude also increases the risk. The face is the most common area where frostnip occurs because of increased exposure. Local frostbite reactions may occur with direct contact of exposed skin with cold metal objects such as ski poles, sleds, or chair lifts. Penile frostnip may be seen in joggers and cross-country skiers who are inadequately protected from the cold. With frostnip, the skin will take on a white, waxy appearance following the initial symptoms of numbness, stiffness, or pain. Frostbitten areas progress to blisters and necrosis. The fingers, nose, toes, and ears are most commonly involved. Partial rewarming and refreezing can increase tissue damage; therefore, the affected area should only be fully rewarmed when the patient is ensured of no risk for refreezing. Warming by an open fire and rubbing of the injured skin should be avoided. Treatment involves rapid rewarming in a circulating water bath of 38°C to 44°C for 20 minutes. This can be a very painful process. Wearing multiple, wind-blocking layers of clothing that trap air to provide an insulating effect can help prevent frostbite. Because the face is the most common site of frostnip, the protective effect of natural sebum should be maximized; therefore, exposed skin should not be washed or shaven before cold-weather activities. Petroleum jelly can be applied as a protective layer, if needed. All skin should be covered if at all possible to prevent frostnip of exposed skin.

Infectious Disorders

Data from the National Collegiate Athletic Association (NCAA) Injury Surveillance System show that skin infections result in a 10% loss of time from participation in the sport of wrestling. Because of the close contact of participants in this sport, NCAA guidelines have been developed with regard to the management of skin infections and return to play. Under NCAA rules, thorough skin checks by certified athletic trainers and/or physicians should be conducted before all wrestling competitions. Open wounds and infectious skin lesions that cannot be adequately covered should be considered cause for disqualification from both practice and competition. If the athlete is undergoing treatment of a communicable skin disease at the time of competition, written documentation of diagnosis, culture results (if possible), specific therapy, and dates of treatment should be provided. The team physician may also find this information useful when making clinical decisions in other sports in which equipment is shared or contact occurs.

Bacterial Infections

The NCAA wrestling guidelines provide general management and return-to-play instructions for all bacterial skin infections, including furuncles, carbuncles, folliculitis, impetigo, cellulitis or erysipelas, and staphylococcal disease. The guidelines recommend that athletes be without any new skin lesions for 48 hours before a wrestling event. Athletes also must have completed 72 hours of antibiotic therapy and have no moist, exudative, or draining lesions. When lesions are questionable, a Gram stain of the exudate should be obtained. Sites of active bacterial infection should not be covered to allow athletic participation.

Impetigo contagiosa is a common bacterial infection spread by direct contact to skin. *Staphylococcus* or *Streptococcus* is usually the infecting organism. Impetigo is common among athletes who participate in sports with close contact, such as football, rugby, and wrestling. Diagnostically, impetigo initially appears as vesicles on an erythematous base that coalesce and are present on the extremities or head and neck. Yellowish drainage and honey-colored crusting are characteristic. Occasionally, there may be a bullous appearance that is more characteristic of a staphylococcal infection. Although usually self-limited, these lesions may persist from weeks to months and are quite contagious. Treatment involves removing the crust, cleansing the lesion with antibacterial soap, and then using a drying agent, such as Burow's solution. Topical antibiotics, such as mupirocin, can be used to treat very small areas. Otherwise, oral antibiotics such as cephalexin (500 mg three times daily) or dicloxacillin (500 mg three times daily) should be used. Erythromycin is a good alternative for patients who are allergic to penicillin. Athletes may be able to prevent spreading this infection by not sharing equipment or towels.

Furunculosis is another skin infection often caused by *Streptococcus* or *Staphylococcus*. Patients with this type of infection typically present with acute, deep-seated, red, hot, and exquisitely tender lesions that are frequently located on the upper extremities. Furuncles or boils can be seen in other areas of the body, especially in areas of friction. These can be recurrent and chronic. One study showed that up to 25% of football players develop furunculosis. For larger lesions, treatment initially includes frequent warm compresses, incision, drainage, and packing. Oral antibiotics with *Staphylococcus* coverage should be instituted promptly to help treat this condition. Treatment failure or recurrence suggests that there may be possible nasal carriage of *Staphylococcus*, in which instance mupirocin can be applied to the anterior nares twice daily for 1 week to clear carriage.

Folliculitis, which is often the initial lesion that leads to the more severe furuncle, is the inflammation of hair follicles as a result of infection, chemical, or mechanical factors (Figure 4). Shaving with the grain if using a blade or using electric razors may also prevent this type of infection. Again, *Staphylococcus* is the most common infecting organism. Small pustules may be present in any hair-bearing area of the body. Treatment with topical antibiotics is often ineffective. For wide distribution,

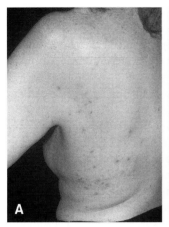
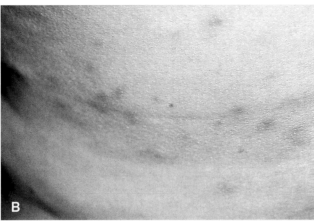

Figure 4 A, Hot tub folliculitis. **B**, Close-up of the same patient. *(Reproduced with permission from the American Academy of Dermatology, Schaumburg, IL.)*

oral antistaphylococcal antibiotics should be used.

Pseudomonas folliculitis or "hot tub folliculitis" often occurs in athletes using whirlpools or hot tubs for rehabilitation. Follicular, pruritic lesions are seen 2 to 3 days after exposure, are distributed diffusely on the exposed area, and may only be seen on the area of the body covered by a bathing suit. Treatment is usually not necessary; however, the contaminated water source should be drained and cleaned.

Fungal Infections

Fungal infections often occur in epidemic proportions in wrestlers. Close skin-to-skin contact allows for transfer of fungal species. These organisms infect and dwell on dead keratin, especially in warm, moist areas, and are not ordinarily present on mucosal surfaces. Tinea corporis among wrestlers is called tinea corporis gladiatorum and is most commonly caused by the fungus *Trichophyton tonsurans*. Macerated skin from sweating, abrasions, occlusion by equipment, and carriers with asymptomatic tinea capitis (Figure 5) may play a role in transmission. Wrestling mats are an unlikely medium for transmission. Tinea corporis gladiatorum characteristically appears as a scaly, red, pruritic plaque with a well-defined raised border and central clearing. These lesions do not exhibit the ring-shaped appearance seen with other forms of tinea. Lesions are present most commonly on the head, neck, and upper extremities. Clinical confirmation may be performed with application of potassium hydroxide to skin scrapings that under the microscope will demonstrate branching hyphae.

Treatment includes both topical and oral antifungal agents. Traditionally, griseofulvin has been the oral drug of choice, with treatment usually lasting 4 to 8 weeks. This, however, may not always be effective because of organism resistance. Systemic ketoconazole, fluconazole, and itraconazole have been used more recently with excellent results; however, extended use of these medications may cause liver toxicity. One study demonstrated that treatment with 100 mg of fluconazole weekly for

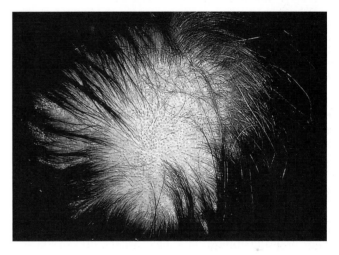

Figure 5 Tinea capitis. *(Reproduced with permission from the American Academy of Dermatology, Schaumburg, IL.)*

3 weeks resulted in negative cultures in 100% of the athletes treated.

Athletes with tinea corporis gladiatorum should not share equipment or towels. The NCAA wrestling guidelines require a minimum of 72 hours of topical therapy with medications such as terbinafine or naftifine for tinea infections before athletes with tinea corporis gladiatorum will be permitted to wrestle. For scalp lesions, a minimum of 2 weeks of systemic therapy is required. When documentation of adequate treatment is provided, athletes may participate with the lesion covered. The recommended covering regimen includes washing the lesion with selenium sulfide or ketoconazole shampoo, followed by application of a topical antifungal medication. A gas-permeable dressing such as OpSite (Smith & Nephew, Memphis, TN) or Bioclusive (Johnson & Johnson Medical Ltd, Somerville, NJ) should be placed over the lesion and then wrapped with ProWrap (Fabrifoam, Exton, PA) and stretch tape. Dressing changes are required after each wrestling match to allow the lesion to air dry.

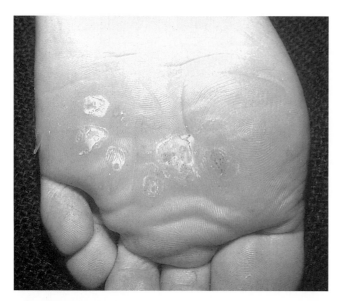

Figure 6 Plantar warts. *(Reproduced with permission from the American Academy of Dermatology, Schaumburg, IL.)*

Tinea pedis (athlete's foot) is another fungal infection that commonly occurs in athletes. Patients with tinea pedis will typically have dry, peeling, or flaking skin between the toes or on the plantar surfaces of the feet. The skin may become macerated and blistered. Over-the-counter topical antifungal powder can be used to treat mild cases. Moderate tinea pedis can be treated with antifungal cream. More severe cases may require both oral and topical antifungal agents. Prevention includes keeping the feet clean and dry; the use of synthetic socks with frequent changing should be encouraged. Wearing sandals in the locker room and shower may help prevent transmission.

Viral Infections

Herpes simplex virus (HSV), also called herpes gladiatorum, can cause epidemic outbreaks on athletic teams, especially in wrestling and rugby. Herpes gladiatorum may occur in up to one third of wrestlers. HSV type 1 and type 2 can produce lesions anywhere on the body. Both are highly contagious agents, secreted from active blisters, saliva, and mucous membranes. Infection usually presents on the head, neck, or upper extremities of athletes. These lesions consist of painful, small-grouped vesicles on an erythematous base that may eventually ulcerate. Usually self-limited, HSV infection lasts 1 to 2 weeks. Diagnosis is clinical; however, Tzanck preparation and cultures can be used to definitively distinguish the signs and symptoms of HSV infection from those of similar rashes. Treatment may begin as soon as the prodrome is noted, which is when the patient reports local pain and/or tingling, fever, malaise, and other systemic symptoms. Lesions may be prevented if antiviral treatment is initiated with the onset of prodromal symptoms.

For active lesions, antiviral agents such as valacyclovir (1 g twice daily) or famciclovir (250 mg three times daily) are effective. However, the duration of treatment before athletes are allowed to return to competition is controversial.

For wrestlers, the NCAA states that the athlete must be free of systemic symptoms and any new blisters for 72 hours before being allowed to participate in athletic activity. Additionally, the wrestler must have no moist lesions, all lesions must be dry and crusted, and at least 120 hours of appropriate antiviral therapy should have been instituted before the meet or tournament. Finally, no active herpetic lesion should be covered to allow participation. Unfortunately, despite therapy, herpes tends to recur, often at the site of the initial lesion. Recurrent lesions should be managed similar to that above; however, athletes with recurrent herpes should be considered for season-long prophylaxis.

Warts and plantar warts are caused by the human papilloma virus (HPV) (Figure 6). This DNA virus usually penetrates small wounds either on the hands or feet. There may be an incubation period of several months, and most will resolve spontaneously and without treatment within 2 years. Plantar warts appear as thick, round callosities that are painful with weight bearing. Confusion with a simple callus can be addressed by paring the hyperkeratotic material of the wart; this will reveal many punctate black spots. Treatment should only be initiated if warts are painful, enlarging, or spreading. Single warts respond well to surgical removal by blunt dissection. Multiple warts are more difficult to treat, and surgical excision is not recommended.

There are numerous methods of treatment of the symptomatic wart or plantar wart. Liquid nitrogen, salicylic acid, silver nitrate, and paring are a few treatment options; however, these may prevent athletes from returning to athletic activity immediately because of discomfort. Treatment with duct tape has not been shown to work reliably. A newer immunomodulating agent, imiquimod, which is available as a 5% cream, is approved for treating genital and nongenital warts. It is applied and left on the skin for 6 to 10 hours and then washed off. This regimen should be repeated three times a week; a typical course of treatment lasts from 4 to 16 weeks. Return to play for athletes with HPV is allowed if the lesion is adequately covered. Again, wearing sandals in the locker room can help prevent the spread of HPV and should be encouraged.

Infestation

Scabies is caused by the mite *Sarcoptes scabiei* that burrows into the epidermis of infected skin (Figure 7). Symptoms may not occur until 3 to 4 weeks after exposure. Athletes will typically present with red burrows or papules, usually in the areas of the palms, wrists, genita-

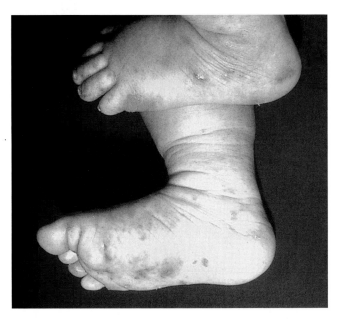

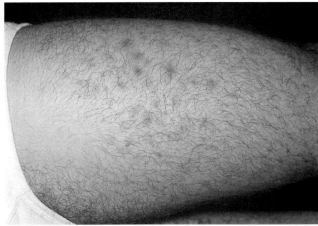

lia, ankles, or umbilicus. Pruritus is often out of proportion to clinical findings and is usually worse at night. Secondary infection may present in areas of excoriation. Treatment includes washing all bed linens and clothing in hot water; items that are not washable should be isolated for 3 days. Application of a scabicide topical agent such as permethrin (5%) or lindane (1%) should be applied to the whole body from the neck down and left on overnight. The scabicide should be reapplied in 7 days. Given the highly contagious nature of scabies infection, athletes involved in contact sports or activities in which athletic equipment is shared should be restricted from play until the infection is cleared, which is usually within 1 week of treatment. NCAA wrestlers are required to have a negative scabies prep at the time of a meet or tournament.

Pediculosis (lice infestation) may occur on the genitalia (pediculosis pubis), head (pediculosis capitis), or body (pediculosis corporis). Patients with pediculosis typically report severe itching in the area of infestation. Moving lice and clusters of louse eggs (nits) usually can be visualized on shafts of hair. There may be localized lymphadenopathy associated with both head and pubic lice. Although pubic lice are commonly acquired through sexual contact, other types of pediculosis infestation can be easily transmitted among athletes involved in contact sports.

Treatment is with permethrin (1%), lindane (1%), or pyrethrins applied for 10 minutes followed by bathing. Clothing and bed linens should be washed in hot water. Topical treatment also should be repeated in 1 week. Before returning to play, the athlete should be nit free. NCAA wrestling guidelines require documentation of

treatment and reexamination for completeness of response before allowing athletes to return to wrestling.

Acne

Acne is a general concern that many athletes are hesitant to discuss. Despite this reluctance, acne can be a psychologically debilitating and physically disfiguring skin condition that can be treated effectively. Puberty and hormonal status play a large part in the development of acne. Other more sport-specific factors may also be responsible. Acne mechanica is a superficial folliculitis caused by the mechanical irritation of equipment, such as tight synthetic clothing, helmets, headgear, tape, or padding (Figure 8). Heat, pressure, friction, occlusion, and moisture of the skin all contribute to development of acne mechanica. Football players are especially affected as the bulk of their uniform is in contact with areas of the body with the highest concentration of sebaceous glands. Acne mechanica can also occur in dancers wearing occlusive leotards, hockey players, weight lifters in contact with weight benches, and golfers who carry golf bags over the shoulder.

In athletes with acne mechanica, well-defined erythematous papules and pustules usually occur in areas such as the shoulders, back, and head that are in contact with protective equipment. Adjusting or minimizing physical factors and improving basic hygiene can improve the condition of the skin. A clean, cotton T-shirt should be worn underneath uniforms and equipment. Immediately after exercise, athletes should wash thoroughly with a mildly abrasive soap, scrubbing the affected area with a washcloth or bath brush. This scrubbing may be followed by application of a keratolytic solution such as 3% salicylic acid and 8% resorcinol in 70% alcohol. Systemic antibiotics are less beneficial in the treatment of acne mechanica than they are in the treatment of acne vulgaris.

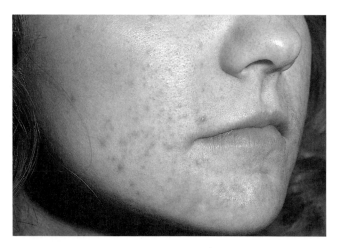

Figure 9 Steroid-induced acne. *(Reproduced with permission from the American Academy of Dermatology, Schaumburg, IL.)*

The use of anabolic steroids can also affect the development of acne in athletes (Figure 9). The sports medicine physician should maintain a high index of suspicion for steroid use in the athlete who has acne that presents suddenly or whose acne is highly resistant to treatment. If the acne is steroid-induced, moderate to severe lesions will be seen on the upper arms and shoulders. For female athletes who are hirsute and have irregular menses, steroid use should also be suspected, but a hormonal abnormality such as polycystic ovarian disease should be considered when anabolic steroid use is ruled out.

Summary

A wide variety of dermatologic conditions can affect athletes at any level of competition. Traumatic skin lesions are often easily preventable. Environmental injury can be reduced by proper preparation for exposure to sun, heat, and cold. The infectious etiologies of dermatologic diseases in athletes pose a special dilemma when determinations need to be made regarding return to play. Although guidelines exist that restrict athletes from competition to prevent the spread of infectious diseases, they often give rise to controversy. Team physicians should be aware of the current return-to-play guidelines that affect athletes under their care. Finally, physicians taking care of athletes should be aware that certain dermatologic conditions may affect athletic performance and that timely diagnosis, treatment, and preventive measures can help athletes succeed in their sport.

Annotated Bibliography

Traumatic Disorders

Adams BB: Dermatologic disorders of the athlete. *Sports Med* 2002;32:309-321.

In addition to a discussion of cutaneous reactions to the environment, infections, and neoplasm, traumatic skin disorders unique to athletes, such as mogul's palm, jogger's nipples, and talon noire are discussed in this all-inclusive review article on dermatology and the athlete.

Basler RS: Cutaneous injuries in women athletes. *Dermatol Nurs* 1998;10:9-18.

This article focuses on the female athlete and skin conditions that may occur as a result of athletic activities.

Fisher AA: Sports-related cutaneous reactions: Part III. Sports identification marks. *Cutis* 1999;63:256-258.

In the final article in a three-part series regarding dermatologic problems in sports medicine, the author focuses on specific skin injuries and "marks" of various sports such as baseball, bowling, fishing, tennis, and wrestling.

Kanerva L: Knuckle pads from boxing. *Eur J Dermatol* 1998;8:359-361.

This is a case report of a 21-year-old male boxer who developed painful callosities on his knuckles (knuckle pads) after frequent boxing. The author also briefly reviews other traumatic entities unique to particular sports, including jogger's toe, athlete's nodule, jogger's nipple, runner's rump, runner's bump, rower's rump, tennis toe, skier's shin, surfer's nodule, black heel, black palm, jazz ballet bottom, and stria distensae.

Environmental Disorders

Castells MC, Horan RF, Sheffer AL: Exercise-induced anaphylaxis. *Curr Allergy Asthma Rep* 2003;3:15-21.

Exercise-induced anaphylaxis has been recognized as a life-threatening problem in athletes, and studies have shown that food may play a role in this syndrome through a mast cell reaction. This article discusses the clinical findings in exercise-induced anaphylaxis, the role of foods, prevention, and treatment of this problem.

Davis JL: Sun and active patients: Preventing acute and cumulative skin damage. *Phys Sportsmed* 2000;28:79-85.

This review article discusses the both the acute and cumulative effects of the sun on the athlete. The treatment of sunburn is also discussed and prevention is stressed.

Fisher AA: Sports-related cutaneous reactions: Part II, Allergic contact dermatitis to sports equipment. *Cutis* 1999;63:202-204.

In the second article in a three-part series regarding dermatologic problems in sports medicine, the author reports that many contact allergens in sports are rubber (For example, swim goggles). The identification of allergy through testing, avoidance of particular products, and recommended alternative equipment are also discussed.

Kanzenbach TL, Dexter WW: Cold injuries: Protecting your patients from the dangers of hypothermia and frostbite. *Postgrad Med* 1999;105:72-78.

Hypothermia is an especially important concern among people who enjoy cold weather sports. This review article discusses proper recognition and treatment of frostbite, frostnip, and hypothermia.

Infectious Disorders

Edwards L: Imiquimod in clinical practice. *J Am Acad Dermatol* 2000;43:12-17.

Topical imiquimod (aldara) has been shown to be effective in the treatment of genital warts. With the antiviral and antiproliferative effects of imiquimod, as well as data from early reports, there is an indication that this medication may prove useful in the treatment of other dermatologic problems such as nongenital warts and molluscum contagiosum. The author reports that imiquimod is a good alternative for athletes who need to return to play quickly.

Green JJ: Localized whirlpool folliculitis in a football player. *Cutis* 2000;65:359-362.

Hot tub folliculitis is seen commonly from exposure to water contaminated with *Pseudomonas aeruginosa.* This article discusses the case of a football player with hot tub folliculitis who was being treated for an ankle injury with whirlpool therapy.

Halpin T: *NCAA 2001 Wrestling Championship Handbook.* Indianapolis, IN, National Collegiate Athletic Association, 2002. Available at http:www.ncaa.org/library/handbooks/wrestling/2003/d1_wrestling.pdf. Accessed: March 1, 2004.

This handbook provides the NCAA wrestling championship guidelines regarding the appropriate identification and treatment of skin infections in wrestlers, and return to play guidelines are specified.

Kohl TD, Lisney M: Tinea gladiatorum. *Sports Med* 2000;29:439-447.

This review article discusses tinea gladiatorum and its epidemic outbreak among wrestlers as well as distinguishing factors, diagnosis, treatment, and prevention.

Kohl TD, Martin DC, Nemeth R, Hill T, Evans D: Fluconazole for the prevention and treatment of tinea gladiatorum. *Pediatr Infect Dis J* 2000;19:717-722.

This double-blind, placebo-controlled trial assessed the effectiveness of fluconazole for the prevention of tinea gladiatorum in wrestlers. A significant reduction in the total number of tinea infections was seen in the fluconazole group, and the authors concluded that this drug is effective and safe for primary prevention of the disease in this population.

Acne

Bender TW III: Cutaneous manifestations of disease in athletes. *Skinmed* 2003;2:34-40.

In this review article on skin disorders that occur in athletes, the author concludes with a discussion of performance-enhancing drugs and their effects on the skin of athletes. The author also discusses how the team physician can identify and perhaps prevent the long-term sequelae of dietary supplement abuse.

Fisher AA: Sports-related cutaneous reactions: Part I. Dermatoses due to physical agents. *Cutis* 1999;63:134-136.

In the first article in a three-part series regarding dermatologic problems in sports medicine, the author briefly reviews traumatic and environmental skin findings in athletes. This article contains a good discussion on acne mechanica and its treatment. In addition, the author cautions against the use of isotretinoin in athletes because of adverse effects on athletic performance.

Lee DJ, Van Dyke GS, Kim J: Update on pathogenesis and treatment of acne. *Curr Opin Pediatr* 2003;15:405-410.

This is a recent review article on the pathogenesis, identification, and treatment of acne in the general population.

Classic Bibliography

Bergfeld WF: Dermatologic problems in athletes. *Clin Sports Med* 1982;1:419-430.

Bergfeld WF, Taylor JS: Trauma, sports, and the skin. *Am J Ind Med* 1985;8:403-413.

Leshaw WL, Dightman L: Pinning down skin infections: Diagnosis, treatment, and prevention in wrestlers. *Phys Sportsmed* 1997;25:45-56.

Leshaw SM: Itching in active patients. *Phys Sportsmed* 1997;26:47-53.

McKeag DB, Hough DO, Zemper ED: *Primary Care Sports Medicine.* New York, NY, WCB/McGraw-Hill, 1993.

Reichel M, Laib D: From acne to black heel: Common skin injuries in sports. *Phys Sportsmed* 1992;20:2.

Sosin DM, Gunn RA, Ford WL, Skaggs JW: An outbreak of furunculosis among high school athletes. *Am J Sports Med* 1989;17:828-832.

Chapter 25

Cardiopulmonary Disease

Rebecca A. Demorest, MD

Gregory L. Landry, MD

Introduction

Cardiopulmonary disease in athletes can be responsible for significant morbidity and mortality. This chapter will cover the most important issues related to the heart and lungs in the athlete and is in no way meant to be a complete discussion of all of the issues.

The Athlete's Heart

An athlete's heart undergoes normal physiologic changes from repetitive dynamic and static exercise secondary to chronic pressure and volume overload on the heart. An alteration in the normal autonomic feedback system, where sympathetic tone dominates, creates an increased resting vagal tone in many elite athletes during extensive training. Increased vagal tone along with physiologic cardiac hypertrophy creates athletically advantageous changes in the athlete's heart by making the heart more efficient. Athletes with an increased resting vagal tone may experience increased episodes of vasovagal syncope. The athlete's heart is seen more frequently in men than women and may occur within the first week of training.

There are many manifestations attributable to the athlete's heart. A combination of these findings may be seen in over 50% of athletes. Common rhythm findings include sinus bradycardia, sinus arrhythmias, and first-degree arteriovenous block. Electrocardiogram (ECG) changes are seen, including ST-segment elevation with peaked T waves, ST-segment depression, T-wave inversion in the lateral precordium, increased P-wave amplitude, increased QRS voltage, and criteria for left and right ventricular hypertrophy. Many of these ECG changes are present at rest when vagal tone is high and then normalize during activity. On echocardiogram, athletes participating in dynamic and aerobic activities may have an increased left ventricular end diastolic diameter secondary to chronic volume overload, with a compensatory increase in ventricular wall thickness. Athletes participating in primarily static or isometric activities may show an increase in left ventricular wall thickness secondary to chronic pressure overload without a change in left ventricular end diastolic diameter. As most athletic activities involve both static and dynamic components, combinations of these changes are present in many athletes.

Increases in posterior and septal wall ventricular thickness that occur in the athlete's heart may mimic hypertrophic cardiomyopathy (HCM), a common cause of sudden cardiac death (SCD) in athletes. Left ventricular hypertrophy in an athlete's heart is typically a concentric hypertrophy between 13 and 16 mm, whereas heterogeneous hypertrophy greater than 16 mm is suspicious for HCM. Diastolic left ventricular cavity size is usually normal or increased (> 55 mm) in the athlete's heart and decreased (< 45 mm) in the hearts of patients with HCM. An athlete's heart maintains normal left ventricular compliance and filling, whereas the hearts of patients with HCM do not. Many of the echocardiographic changes seen in an athlete's heart will regress after 3 months of no training, whereas those that occur in the hearts of patients with HCM are permanent. Any athlete with ECG changes found in an athlete's heart along with cardiac symptoms of syncope, chest pain, shortness of breath, palpitations, or exercise fatigue should be evaluated for HCM.

Sudden Cardiac Death

SCD is the most frequent cause of sports-related deaths in young athletes. Defined as witnessed or unwitnessed natural death resulting from sudden cardiac arrest occurring unexpectedly within 6 hours of a previously normal state of health, SCD occurs in 1 in every 200,000 young athletes annually. The SCDs of sports legends such as Reggie Lewis, Hank Gathers, and Sergi Grinkov have brought this entity to public attention.

SCDs are most often caused by rare congenital cardiac diseases, which affect less than 0.3% of the population. The authors of one study reviewed instances of SCD in 134 high school and college athletes between 1985 and 1995 and found HCM and coronary artery anomalies to be the leading causes of SCD (Figure 1). In addition, SCD was reported to affect males more

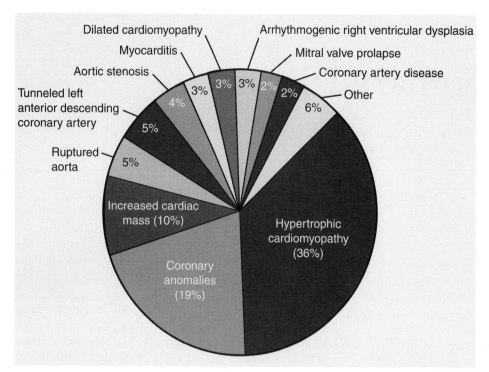

Figure 1 The causes of sudden cardiac death in 134 high-school and college athletes.

commonly than females (a ratio of 5:1). Ninety percent of the instances of SCD occurred between the hours of 3 PM and 9 PM, either during or immediately following afternoon sports practice; 18% had prodromal cardiac symptoms within the preceding 36 months. Although athletes who eventually die as a result of SCD may report initial symptoms of syncope, dyspnea, fatigue, or chest pain, most die suddenly.

HCM, a familial cardiac malformation with heterogeneous expression from mutations in proteins encoding cardiac sarcomere genes, causes a hypertrophied but not dilated left ventricle. HCM is the most common genetic cardiovascular disease and affects 1 in every 500 persons. Obstruction secondary to a hypertrophied subaortic septum occurs in 20% to 25% of patients with HCM and is responsible for a soft systolic murmur at the second right intercostal space and along the left sternal border that increases with standing or Valsalva maneuver. Most patients with HCM do not have this classic murmur because the unobstructive form of HCM is more prevalent. Risk factors for SCD from HCM include a family history of premature SCD, prior cardiac arrest, ventricular tachycardia, hypotension with exercise, young age at onset of symptoms, and extreme left ventricular hypertrophy (> 30 mm). Sudden death occurs secondary to obstruction or, more commonly, a fatal arrhythmia (ventricular fibrillation) from hypertrophied and scarred myocardium. Although not diagnostic, 75% to 95% of athletes with HCM will have abnormalities on ECG. With HCM, the echocardiogram shows asymmetric left ventricular wall hypertrophy

(> 16 mm), a diminished left ventricular cavity (< 45 mm), and diastolic dysfunction.

Other causes of SCD include coronary artery anomalies; most commonly, an aberrant left main coronary artery from the right sinus causes ischemia from compression of the artery between the aorta and right ventricular outflow tract. Difficult to diagnose by echocardiogram, coronary artery anomalies are usually diagnosed by cardiac arteriography. Ten percent of the instances of SCD are caused by idiopathic left ventricular hypertrophy, which is hypertrophy that does not meet strict criteria for HCM. Athletes with Marfan syndrome, a connective tissue disorder responsible for arachnodactyly, arm span greater than height, pectus excavatum, ligamentous laxity, ectopia lentis, and vertebral column deformities can experience aortic root dilatation and rupture resulting in SCD.

Arrhythmogenic right ventricular dysplasia (ARVD) is caused by patchy fibrofatty replacement of the right ventricle, which predisposes the athlete to aneurysms and fatal ventricular arrhythmias. Cardiac MRI can usually diagnose ARVD. Responsible for approximately 3% of all SCDs in the United States, ARVD is the most common cause of SCD in Venito, Italy, where there is mandatory cardiac screening of athletes with an ECG and echocardiogram. This cardiac screening may disqualify participants with structural lesions detected on ECG and echocardiogram, such as HCM, before athletic participation. Wolf-Parkinson-White syndrome and long QT syndrome can also cause life-threatening cardiac arrhythmias in athletes. In athletes older than 35 years, atherosclerotic coronary artery disease accounts for 80% of SCDs.

The biggest issue relating to SCD is whether it is preventable. Although preparticipation physical examination (PPE) screening is recommended by the American Heart Association (AHA) every 2 years (with an interim history) for high school athletes and during the entry athletic year (with interim history and follow-up examinations as needed) for college athletes, debate exists as to how effective history and PPE screening really are. In the retrospective analysis of 134 cases of SCD discussed previously, of those athletes who had undergone a PPE, only 3% were suspected to have cardiac disease and less than 1% received a correct cardiac diagnosis. Because of the inadequacy, variability, and lack of core uniformity in PPE questionnaires, examination forms, and medical examiners at both the high school and college levels, the PPE may have limited potential as a screening tool for cardiac disease causing SCD. The components of cardiac screening as proposed at the 26th Bethesda Conference and recommended by the AHA are listed in Table 1.

It has been proposed that in addition to the PPE, ECG and echocardiogram screening may help detect those at risk for SCD. Current recommendations by the AHA, however, do not advocate using ECG or echocardiogram as a screening tool. The athlete's heart causes many false-positive results on both ECGs and echocardiograms. In one study of 1,005 predominantly male athletes screened with ECG, 40% had abnormal ECGs, but only 5% had structural cardiovascular abnormalities. Conversely, normal ECG and echocardiogram studies do not always signify an absolute zero risk for cardiovascular disease responsible for SCD. False-negative results from echocardiogram testing can occur because phenotypic expression of HCM may not be complete during the adolescent years.

The AHA estimates that it would cost $250,000 to detect one undiagnosed case of HCM using echocardiogram as a screening tool. Echocardiograms would need to be done for 200,000 athletes to diagnosis that one instance of HCM. One study, however, examined the costs for screening athletes with an ECG and echocardiogram and found that ECG was the most cost-effective modality for diagnosing cardiac abnormalities when compared with the cost of cardiac history and physical examination or two-dimensional echocardiogram. In athletes older than 35 years with ischemic symptoms, coronary risk factors, or with a strong family history of premature cardiac disease, it is prudent to perform an exercise stress test before allowing athletic participation. In younger athletes, routine screening with ECG and echocardiogram is not recommended by any group. The PPE should focus on obtaining a good cardiac history and conducting a physical examination as recommended by the AHA.

TABLE 1 | Components of the Cardiac Screening Examination as Recommended by the AHA

Family History

Premature sudden death

Heart disease in surviving relatives younger than 50 years

Specific conditions: hypertrophic cardiomyopathy, dilated cardiomyopathy, long QT, Marfan syndrome, clinically significant arrhythmias

Personal Medical History

Heart murmur

Systemic hypertension

Excessive fatigue with exercise

Exertional syncope

Exertional chest pain

Excessive exertional shortness of breath

Physical Examination

Heart murmur: precordial auscultation in supine and seated position

Femoral pulses to rule out coarctation of the aorta

Stigmata of Marfan syndrome

Brachial blood pressure in seated position

(Adapted with permission from Maron BJ, Thompson PD, Puffer JC, et al: Cardiovascular preparticipation screening of competitive athletes: A statement for health professionals from the Sudden Death Committee (clinical cardiology) and Congenital Cardiac Defects Committee (cardiovascular disease in the young), American Heart Association. Circulation 1996;94:850-856.)

Commotio Cordis

Commotio cordis, usually seen in young males, is sudden death caused by ventricular arrhythmias from a sudden, blunt, low-impact force to the chest without apparent heart injury. According to the US Consumer Products Safety Commission, between 1973 and 1995, 88 baseball-related deaths from commotio cordis were reported. Approximately two to four incidents of commotio cordis are reported annually. The majority of incidents were ball-related chest impacts, with some incidents occurring after being struck by the bat. Commotio cordis has also been reported in softball, ice hockey, football, lacrosse, basketball, and the martial arts. Young athletes are particularly susceptible because of a narrow AP chest diameter and an increased chest wall compliance that allows delivery of transmitted forces directly to the heart.

A blow to the precordial area is usually followed by ventricular fibrillation, with immediate death or a brief period of consciousness occurring before collapse. Impacts during the vulnerable portion of the cardiac cycle, 15 to 30 milliseconds before the T-wave peak, are thought to pose the most significant risk for a fatal arrhythmia. Survival is low despite cardiopulmonary resuscitation attempts. The effectiveness of safety baseballs in reducing the risk of commotio cordis is still being studied. Current results are mixed regarding their

TABLE 2 | 1997 Classification of Hypertension by Age in Children and Adolescents

Age (years)	High Normal[*]	Significant Hypertension[†]	Severe Hypertension[‡]
6 to 9			
Systolic	111-121	122-129	> 129 (129)[§]
Diastolic	70-77	70-85	> 85 (84)
10 to 12			
Systolic	117-125	126-133	> 133 (134)
Diastolic	75-81	82-89	> 89 (89)
13 to 15			
Systolic	124-135	136-143	> 143 (149)
Diastolic	77-85	86-91	> 91 (94)
16 to 18			
Systolic	127-141	142-149	> 149 (159)
Diastolic	80-91	92-97	> 97 (99)

Highest reading (systolic or diastolic) tabulates hypertension severity.

[*]90th to 94th percentile for age, boys and girls combined.

[†]95th to 98th percentile for age, boys and girls combined.

[‡]99th percentile for age, boys and girls combined.

§ Values in parentheses are those used for classification of severe hypertension by the 26th Bethesda Conference.

(Reproduced with permission from Risser WL, Anderson SJ, Boldec SP, et al: Committee on Sports Medicine and Fitness: Athletic participation by children and adolescents who have systemic hypertension. Pediatrics 1997;99:637-638.)

TABLE 3 | 2003 Joint National Committee 7 Classification of Adult Hypertension

	Prehypertension	Stage I Hypertension	Stage II Hypertension
Adults > 18 years			
Systolic	120-139	140-159	≥ 160
Diastolic	80-89	90-99	≥ 100

(Reproduced with permission from Chobanian AV, Bakins GL, Black HR, et al: The Seventh Report of the Joint National Committee on Prevention, Detection, Evaluation, and Treatment of High Blood Pressure: The JNC 7 Report. JAMA 2003;289:2560-2572.)

protective effect. Batting chest protectors have not been shown to decrease the risk of commotio cordis and are not currently recommended. Other protective measures include elimination of the on-deck circle, helmets with protective facemasks, and eyewear for batters, base runners, and fielders.

Hypertension

According to the 26th Bethesda Conference Task Force, systemic hypertension is the most common cardiovascular condition observed in athletes. Ninety-five percent of systemic hypertension is primary essential hypertension. Although not a direct cause of SCD, hypertension is thought to be a risk factor for cardiac disease that can lead to SCD.

Systemic hypertension is defined as elevated systolic or diastolic pressures (> 95th percentile for age) re-

corded on at least three separate occasions. The most recent guidelines for hypertension in children and adults are listed in Tables 2 and 3. Discrepancies exist between the classification of adult and child hypertension and may be a result of the guidelines of the Joint Committee on Prevention, Detection, Evaluation and Treatment of High Blood Pressure released in May 2003 that introduce new categories of hypertension. If high readings exist for both systolic and diastolic measurements, the higher category should be used to define the athlete's hypertension. Blood pressure should be taken with an appropriate sized cuff (bladder diameter at least two thirds the length of the upper arm) with the athlete in a seated position and the arm supported at the level of the heart after resting quietly for 5 minutes. If an inappropriately small cuff is used, patients can have falsely elevated readings. Children with hypertension should always be evaluated for significant medical causes of hypertension (for example, kidney disease and coarctation of the aorta). If blood pressure readings are consistently elevated, it is appropriate to evaluate patients for target end organ damage by assessing electrolytes, blood urea nitrogen, creatinine, glucose, cholesterol, and urinalysis.

Stage I hypertension or significant hypertension in the absence of end organ damage does not preclude physical activity because exercise is thought to help decrease mild hypertension. Severe or stage II hypertension in the absence of end organ damage requires activity restriction (especially from competitive sports and highly static activities) until blood pressure is controlled with a low-fat and low-salt diet, lifestyle modifications (avoiding use of tobacco, alcohol, anabolic steroids, and street drugs), or antihypertensive medications. Although a variety of antihypertensive medications exist to decrease blood pressure, most athletes should avoid taking beta-blockers and diuretics. Beta-blockers may decrease exercise tolerance and are not recommended in patients with asthma, and diuretics can cause an increased risk of dehydration. Certain governing athletic committees have banned the use of both of these medications. Angiotensin-converting enzyme inhibitors are used to treat most athletes with hypertension. If cardiovascular disease does exist concomitantly with hypertension, activity restrictions should be based on the severity of cardiovascular disease. Regardless of the stage of hypertension, blood pressure should be monitored regularly every 2 to 3 months.

For most young athletes, additional cardiovascular testing is not essential when primary hypertension is diagnosed. For athletes with hypertension who are older than 35 years, an echocardiogram and exercise stress test are recommended before proceeding with athletic participation.

Syncope

Syncope is defined as sudden loss of consciousness with loss of postural tone. There are numerous etiologies that may cause syncope in athletes (Table 4). Most commonly, syncopal episodes result from vasovagal autonomic instability caused by decreased cerebral blood flow. Increased vagal tone, a physiologic adaptation to vigorous exercise in elite athletes, may also contribute to syncopal episodes. A classic prodrome of lightheadedness, dizziness, tunnel vision, abrupt fainting, recall of the episode, and complete recovery within minutes usually signals vasovagal syncope; however, this should be a diagnosis of exclusion. Other symptoms such as chest pain, palpitations, diaphoresis, nausea, seizure activity, dyspnea, headache, extreme fatigue, exercise intolerance, syncope during exercise, or recurrent syncope over a short duration may suggest a more serious etiology. Syncope is the most common symptom before SCD.

TABLE 4 | Causes and Common Symptoms of Syncope

Causes	Common Symptoms
Vasovagal	Prodrome (lightheadedness, dizziness, nausea)
Orthostatic hypotension	Prodrome, dehydration
Arrhythmias	Palpitations, dizziness, chest pain, dyspnea, fatigue
Long QT syndrome	
Wolf-Parkinson-White syndrome	
Sick sinus syndrome	
Mitral valve prolapse	
Atrial flutter	
Atrial fibrillation	
Junctional rhythm	
Supraventricular tachycardia	
Ventricular tachycardia	
Ventricular fibrillation	
Arteriovenous block	Fatigue, heart irregularity
Cardiac anomalies	Fatigue, decreased exercise tolerance, dyspnea
Hypertrophic cardiomyopathy	
Coronary artery anomaly	
Aortic stenosis	
Pulmonary stenosis	
Exercise associated collapse (heat illness)	Prodrome, exercise in extremes of temperature or high humidity
Myocardial infarction	Chest pain, fatigue, diaphoresis
Seizure	Loss of consciousness, seizure-like activity
Anemia	Fatigue, blood loss
Hypertension	Headaches, vision changes
Hypoglycemia	Prodrome, history of diabetes, lack of calories
Severe anxiety	Palpitations, situation specific symptoms

Diagnosing the correct etiology for syncope can be challenging. Approximately 50% of patients with syncope will have a cause for their syncopal episodes identified. A careful history and thorough physical examination are imperative to making the diagnosis. The history should distinguish when, where, and how syncopal episodes occur in relationship to exercise (maximal versus submaximal exercise, static versus dynamic activity, syncope during exercise versus syncope after exercise completion), prodromal symptoms, previous syncope, precipitants to the episodes (visual cues), cardiac symptomatology, and seizure activity. Diet and fluid intake history can be helpful in identifying hypoglycemia or orthostatic episodes. Obtaining a family history regarding cardiac disease (especially sudden death), arrhythmias, hypertension, and hypercholesterolemia can be helpful. If syncope occurs during exercise or if there is a

TABLE 5 | Causes of Chest Pain

Traumatic
    Pneumothorax
    Rib fracture
    Sternoclavicular separation
    Clavicular fracture
    Sternal fracture
    Cardiac contusion
    Pulmonary contusion
    Abdominal trauma
Nontraumatic
    Asthma
    Spontaneous pneumothorax
    Costochondritis
    Viral or bacterial pneumonia
    Tuberculosis
    Herpes zoster
    Prolonged cough
    Pulmonary embolus
    Arrhythmia
    Coronary artery disease/myocardial infarction
    Myocarditis/pericarditis
    Dissecting aneurysm
    Sickle cell disease
    Gastroesophageal reflux
    Breast tenderness
    Anaphylaxis/allergic reaction
    Anxiety
    Cocaine use

family history of SCD, a cardiac workup must be done. Tests including an ECG and possibly an echocardiogram, Holter monitor, or exercise stress test are warranted to rule out cardiac arrhythmias or structural heart disease. If an arrhythmia is suspected, invasive electrophysiologic testing may be done. Cardiac MRI will diagnose ARVD, and cardiac catheterization is usually necessary to diagnose coronary anomalies. Neurologic testing including an electroencephalogram and occasionally head MRI are done if seizures are suspected. Tilt-table testing is occasionally done to establish a diagnosis of autonomic instability; however, a high rate of false-positive and false-negative results makes this test unreliable in many situations.

Return to athletic activity after syncopal episodes depends on the etiology. Vasovagal episodes may be lessened with proper hydration, an increase in dietary salt intake, and a decrease in caffeine. Most athletes with vasovagal syncope are not restricted from athletic participation. Athletes experiencing syncope from heat illness should be hydrated, and immediate measures should be taken to decrease core body temperature. If an arrhythmia or cardiac disease is diagnosed, return to play is based on guidelines set forth in the 26th Bethesda Conference Recommendations for Determining Eligibility for Competition in Athletes with Cardiovascular Abnormalities. Uncontrolled seizure activity usually prohibits return to play. Diving, water sports, archery, riflery, power lifting, and sports involving heights should be avoided. Athletes with controlled seizures may return to participation in most sports with no restrictions.

Chest Pain

There are numerous etiologies for chest pain in athletes (Table 5). The most common nontraumatic cause of chest pain in young athletes is asthma. Chest pain in most children and adolescents will not have a cardiac origin; however, individuals older than 35 years are at an increased risk for cardiovascular disease, myocardial infarction, pulmonary embolism, and aortic aneurysms. Athletes participating in contact sports, sports using high-velocity equipment (baseball, softball, lacrosse, hockey, bicycle racing, and motor sports), or sports involving heights are at increased risk for chest pain caused by trauma.

A thorough history for an athlete presenting with chest pain should include the identification of the frequency, severity, and other characteristics of the pain (sharp, dull, stabbing, or radiating); associated symptoms (fever, cough, cold symptoms, dyspnea, allergic response, reflux, or pain with deep breathing or position changes); what relieves and exacerbates the pain; history of trauma; and medical history (asthma, allergies, sickle cell disease, cystic fibrosis, cardiovascular disease, myocardial infarction). Physical examination should include a complete cardiac, pulmonary, abdominal, and related musculoskeletal examination. The examination should determine whether there is any chest wall tenderness suggesting costochondritis. A chest radiograph, ECG, pulse oximetry, spirometry, and blood work including complete blood count and cardiac enzyme levels can be helpful when the history and examination suggest a cardiac or pulmonary etiology. Any athlete with suspected trauma, cardiovascular disease, myocardial infarction, or pulmonary embolism should be referred for additional evaluation immediately. Return to play is based on the etiology of the chest pain.

Syncopal episodes associated with chest pain occurring during maximal exercise suggest a cardiac origin such as arrhythmia, HCM, coronary artery anomaly, and aortic or pulmonic stenosis. Rib fracture complications include pneumothorax, hemothorax, and splenic and liver lacerations. Although sternoclavicular dislocation is rare, it can cause mediastinal hemorrhage, tracheal rupture, or esophageal perforation if the dislocation is posterior. Cardiac contusions can lead to life-threatening arrhythmias, hemopericardium, and cardiac rupture.

Automatic External Defibrillators

Used with increasing frequency over the past 10 to 20 years, automatic external defibrillators (AEDs) can reverse life-threatening arrhythmias by analyzing cardiac rhythm and administering an electric countershock. Studies have suggested that early defibrillation is the most important intervention in saving the lives of those with cardiovascular collapse. Immediate defibrillation may result in a survival rate greater than 90%, with each minute of ventricular fibrillation reducing the survival rate by 10%. Several studies have documented the effectiveness and usefulness of AED use by first responders in public areas such as airports and at sporting events.

Most AEDs are compact, and minimal training is required for their use because instructions are mounted on the device and voice prompts tell the operator what to do. Biphasic waveform countershocks are administered by pushing a button when an appropriate rhythm (ventricular fibrillation) is present. Most AEDs cost between $3,000 and $4,500 and have a 5-year nonrechargeable lithium battery that automatically self-tests its power on a daily or weekly basis. Study results are mixed regarding the rate of survival with AED use. Although most studies suggest that decreased time to defibrillation and an increased survival rate do occur with the use of AEDs, some evidence suggests that defibrillation alone without other lifesaving measures such as cardiopulmonary resuscitation or emergency medical service support may not increase the number of lives saved. The 2000 AHA Guidelines for Cardiopulmonary Resuscitation and Emergency Cardiovascular Care suggest placement of AEDs in areas where reliable emergency medical services cannot be guaranteed to arrive within 5 minutes from call to arrival and where AEDs would likely be used at least once within 5 years.

Future studies need to assess the use of AEDs on young athletes during sporting events to determine their effectiveness for saving the lives of those who collapse on the court or field. Although many colleges, universities, and high schools have AEDs on hand at athletic events, the cost of these devices may be prohibitive for some sports programs.

Exercise-Induced Asthma

Exercise-induced asthma (EIA) is reversible airway hyperreactivity consisting of bronchial smooth muscle constriction, airway inflammation, cytokine release, and increased mucus production. Depending on the sport, approximately 10% to 35% of athletes have EIA. Of individuals with asthma, 50% to 90% have bronchial reactivity to exercise. Controversy exists as to whether there is a difference between exercise-induced bronchospasm

(EIB), which is seen predominantly in cold-weather athletes, and EIA. Some researchers propose that EIB is a related but separate entity consisting of transient airway narrowing from cold or dry air causing inflammation and permanent airway remodeling that is unresponsive to typical asthma prophylaxis. Others suggest that EIB is associated with the airway inflammation seen in EIA and that EIA is a better term for describing exercise-related bronchoconstriction.

Although the pathogenesis of EIA is not completely understood, two hypotheses exist. The osmotic hypothesis suggests that airway cooling from rapid breathing of cold, dry air creates an increased bronchial osmolarity that subsequently increases mast cell degradation and the release of inflammatory markers. Alternatively, the thermal theory suggests that rapid airway rewarming after exercising (which causes airway drying and cooling) causes increased bronchial permeability and edema leading to airway obstruction. The pathogenesis is probably a combination of the two mechanisms.

Symptoms of EIA include difficulty breathing, shortness of breath, chest tightness or pain, cough, wheezing, decreased endurance performance, and postexercise cough. The most sensitive symptom is cough; occasionally, cough is the only symptom. Asthma triggers for athletes include high ventilation rates in cold, dry air; allergens; and indoor air pollutants. At least 3 to 8 minutes of maximal exercise ($\geq$ 80% of the maximal heart rate) is usually necessary to produce symptoms of EIA. Symptoms usually begin with cessation of exercise and peak at 8 to 15 minutes after exercise; however, some athletes experience symptoms during exercise. Spontaneous recovery occurs in approximately 30 to 60 minutes. About 50% of athletes with EIA will experience a refractory period of 40 minutes to 3 hours after an initial asthma exacerbation during which further symptoms are absent or reduced if exercise continues. The differential diagnosis for athletes with EIA symptoms includes performance anxiety, vocal cord dysfunction, gastroesophageal reflux, poor conditioning, anemia, cardiac disorders, and other pulmonary diseases.

Although most primary care physicians diagnose and treat EIA in accordance with athlete-reported symptoms, some studies suggest that this may not be a reliable method for accurate diagnosis. One recent study of elite athletes showed that self-reported symptoms did not predict the presence of EIA because 41% of athletes reporting asthma-like symptoms had normal spirometry values. Spirometry is the standard test for reversible airway constriction. A 10% to 15% decrease in forced expiratory volume over 1 second (FEV_1) with improvement after use of a beta-agonist is diagnostic for asthma. If results are equivocal, a methacholine- or histamine-challenge test can provoke airway constriction. Osmotic challenges with dry powdered mannitol and nebulized hypertonic saline may also be used to confirm an EIA diagnosis. Eucapnic voluntary hyperventilation, which may cause bronchoconstriction in some patients, is done by having the athlete breathe a dry test gas composed of 5% carbon dioxide, 21% oxygen, and nitrogen at 60% to 85% of maximal ventilation rate, which simulates competitive conditions when bronchospasm occurs better than traditional methacholine- or histamine-challenge tests. Many athletes, however, will not respond to spirometry or a bronchial-inhalation challenge test if their bronchoconstriction occurs only during a specific athletic activity. An exercise-challenge test, usually performed on a treadmill or stationary bicycle, simulates the specific athletic activity in which symptoms are experienced. After 6 to 10 minutes of an exercise challenge at 80% to 85% of the maximal predicted heart rate, FEV_1 is measured with the athlete sitting at 5, 10, 15, 20, and 30 minutes after exercise; a 10% to 15% decline in FEV_1 is diagnostic for EIA. Since 2001, the International Olympic Committee now requires all athletes involved in international competition who are using inhaled beta-agonists to have clinical and laboratory confirmation of asthma or EIA.

Treatment of EIA consists of a combination of preventive and "rescue" medications and asthma education. Educating athletes, coaches, and parents about EIA, the proper management of EIA symptoms, and the acute treatment of asthma exacerbations is imperative. A proper warm-up period of 10 to 30 minutes is recommended to help induce a refractory period for competition. Avoiding exercise in cold weather, avoiding triggering allergens, and covering the nose and mouth to warm the air that is inhaled during exercise in colder temperatures may help prevent EIA.

When athletes have asthma symptoms, a beta-agonist (albuterol) is the drug of choice for immediately decreasing bronchoconstriction. For athletes with EIA, a beta-agonist given 15 to 20 minutes before exercise is recommended to prevent symptoms. Prevention of EIA is much more effective than using a beta-agonist for rescue. The onset of action for beta-agonists is approximately 15 to 30 minutes, with peak effect at 60 minutes and maximal effects lasting up to 3 to 4 hours. Frequent use of beta-agonists can cause tachyphylaxis and may worsen symptoms. Nedocromil and cromolyn, mast cell stabilizers, can also be used 15 to 20 minutes before exercise to prevent EIA, but these are not usually as effective as beta-agonists; a combination of the two may be more effective than either medication alone.

Long-acting beta-agonists (salmeterol) can be useful when exercise is unpredictable. Although the effects of long-acting beta-agonists last for 8 to 12 hours, tachyphylaxis and tolerance can occur with regular use for longer than 1 month. Athletes having symptoms more than twice weekly or symptoms outside of exercise require a daily anti-inflammatory medication, such as an inhaled corticosteroid to control airway inflammation. A combination medication consisting of both a long-acting beta-agonist and an inhaled corticosteroid is available for prevention. For athletes with more severe asthma, leukotriene antagonists (montelukast) help control symptoms when used as a preventive medication. Some studies suggest that leukotriene antagonists may be more effective for controlling symptoms when compared with long-acting beta-agonists.

The International Olympic Committee rules allow the use of albuterol, salmeterol, leukotriene antagonists, cromolyn, and inhaled corticosteroids by athletes during competition; however, because of possible ergogenic effects, the use of certain inhaled beta-agonists, all oral and injectable beta-agonists, and all systemic corticosteroids are banned for competition at the Olympic level.

Vocal Cord Dysfunction

Vocal cord dysfunction (VCD) is an underrecognized and underdiagnosed entity in athletes. Occurring more frequently in adolescent female athletes, the true prevalence of VCD in athletes is unknown. A recent study estimated that 5% of elite athletes might experience VCD. Most athletes in this study competed in winter sports, and a significantly higher incidence of VCD occurred among outdoor athletes.

VCD is categorized by the paradoxical closure of the vocal cords during inspiration and occasionally during expiration. The anterior portion of the vocal cords is predominantly affected, creating a diamond-shaped passage for airflow. This adduction causes airflow obstruction and stridor. In many cases, this airway dysfunction leads to a diagnosis of asthma, without much consideration of the presence of VCD until typical asthma medications are proven to be nonbeneficial to the athlete. Asthma, gastroesophageal reflux disease, depression, and anxiety may be comorbid conditions in athletes with VCD.

Unlike EIA in which chest symptoms peak after exercise, VCD usually causes throat symptoms at the beginning of exercise. The classic symptom of VCD is abrupt onset of inspiratory stridor with exercise. The onset of EIA symptoms is typically more gradual and is primarily expiratory. Dyspnea, throat tightness, shortness of breath, difficulty inhaling, and a change in voice may also occur. Expiratory wheezing is not a typical symptom of VCD, although athletes may mistake inspiratory stridor for wheezing. VCD symptoms usually resolve within a few minutes after stopping activity, whereas EIA symptoms may take 30 minutes to 1 hour to resolve.

Flow-volume spirometry can be useful in differentiating VCD from asthma. In many but not all athletes with VCD, the inspiratory loop of the flow curve is blunted as opposed to the decline in FEV_1 seen with asthmatics. Flow-volume loops are not done in standard pulmonary function tests and must be requested specifically. Although a methacholine-challenge test is used to predict asthma, a recent study suggests that this test may not be specific for diagnosing asthma because acute episodes of VCD occurred after methacholine administration in some patients without suggesting airway reactivity. Definitive diagnosis is made with direct observation of the vocal cords via endoscopy during a VCD episode. This is not always possible, however, because some symptoms are only present during intense exercise.

Treatment of VCD focuses on speech therapy to teach respiratory control and diaphragmatic breathing. One study showed that athletes with VCD were able to control symptoms for up to 6 months after speech pathology intervention. Biofeedback and psychotherapy are also used. Occasionally, antidepressants or anxiolytics may be helpful in reducing attacks. Because VCD is highly associated with gastroesophageal reflux, treatment with histamine H_2 receptor antagonists or proton-pump inhibitors can be helpful.

Anaphylaxis

True anaphylaxis is rare in athletes. Anaphylaxis is the culminating event of an allergic reaction in which the systemic release of histamine and cytokines occurs in response to an allergen. Anaphylaxis is a life-threatening emergency consisting of airway constriction, angioedema, and hypotension. Common allergens that can cause anaphylaxis include bee or wasp stings, insect bites, food, latex, medicine, or exercise.

Symptoms include diffuse pruritic hives; skin flushing; local swelling; chest tightness; difficulty breathing; lip, tongue, and oral mucosa swelling; a change in voice; anxiety; nausea; and abdominal pain. Athletes with a history of anaphylaxis from exposure to known allergens should carry an epinephrine pen at all times in case of an unavoidable exposure. If an allergic reaction does occur that proceeds to anaphylaxis, immediate intramuscular administration of an epinephrine pen (0.3 mg of epinephrine into the anterolateral thigh through clothing if the area is unexposed) is recommended, followed by immediate transport to an emergency medical facility.

Anaphylactic reactions encompass a broad spectrum of histamine-related disorders in athletes, including cholinergic urticaria, classic exercise-induced anaphylaxis, food-dependent exercise-induced anaphylaxis, and variant exercise-induced anaphylaxis. Cholinergic urticaria, thought to be caused by an augmented cholinergic response to warming, occurs in response to exercise, fever, or stress. It is characterized by the appearance of localized 2- to 4-mm punctate pruritic erythematous papules and macules on the neck that spread distally without systemic symptoms. Occasional bronchospasm can also occur.

Classic exercise-induced anaphylaxis is triggered by systemic mast cell release of histamine and other cyto-kines in response to exercise or cold air inhalation but not to passive warming. A generalized urticarial reaction is typically characterized by the appearance of hives (10 to 15 mm), flushing, airway obstruction, and cardiovascular collapse. Symptoms include shortness of breath, chest tightness, wheezing, headache, nausea and vomiting, cyanosis, mental status changes, angioedema, hypotension, and brief loss of consciousness. Symptoms last for up to 4 hours after cessation of activity. One study looking at the natural history of exercise-induced anaphylaxis found that endurance activities such as jogging, walking, racquetball, and dance were most commonly associated with this disorder. Exercising in humid, hotter climates triggered reactions, whereas stopping exercise early decreased symptoms. Up to 50% of the athletes in this study had allergic rhinitis, allergies, or a family history of atopy in a first-degree relative. Over a period of 10 years, the frequency of episodes of exercise-induced anaphylaxis either decreased or remained the same.

Foods or medications are also precipitants for anaphylaxis; raw celery, shellfish, tomatoes, alcohol, and nuts are the most common precipitants when eaten 2 to 4 hours before exercise. Aspirin, nonsteroidal anti-inflammatory drugs, certain antibiotics, and cold medications may also cause a similar reaction. Variant type exercise-induced anaphylaxis, precipitated by exercise only, typically causes the appearance of 2- to 4-mm punctate urticarial lesions and eventual cardiovascular collapse.

Although diagnosis is usually made by medical history, an exercise challenge test can be done, provided emergency airway equipment and personnel are readily available. Avoiding activity in hot, humid weather may decrease risk. For those with food or medication-induced anaphylaxis, avoiding specific foods or medications for at least 4 hours before exercise may decrease symptoms. Pretreatment with an antihistamine (H_1 receptor antagonist) may prevent or decrease symptoms in patients with cholinergic urticaria or exercise-induced anaphylaxis. Antihistamines and epinephrine must be used on an emergent basis when symptoms arise. Runners with a history of exercise-induced anaphylaxis should always carry an epinephrine pen with them during activity and should never run alone. Immediate treatment with epinephrine and transport to an emergency medical facility is recommended for patients with acute symptoms.

Summary

Several cardiopulmonary diseases can result in significant morbidity and mortality in athletes. The athlete's heart occurs in elite athletes secondary to adaptive physiologic cardiac changes from repetitive dynamic and static exercise. SCD, a rare event in athletes, is difficult to prevent. The use of protective baseballs and chest protectors are being studied for their ability to decrease the risk of commotio cordis (sudden death from a blunt chest impact causing fatal arrhythmias in young athletes). Most athletes with mild hypertension can still participate in sports; however, athletes with severe hypertension will require further evaluation and treatment before participation. Syncope that occurs during exercise or is associated with a family history of early sudden death warrants a complete cardiac evaluation. Chest pain in young athletes is usually caused by asthma or costochondritis. Cardiac causes of chest pain should be strongly considered in athletes with chest pain who are older than 35 years. AEDs should be available at any sporting venue that cannot be reached by emergency medical personnel within 5 minutes. The most sensitive symptom of EIA is cough. Athletes with EIA must be taught how to prevent symptoms. VCD produces breathing difficulty that has an abrupt onset and is associated with difficulty inhaling and speaking. Exercise-induced anaphylaxis can be controlled by avoiding precipitant foods or medications for at least 4 hours before exercise and by using antihistamines before exercising.

Annotated Bibliography

The Athlete's Heart

Pelliccia A, Maron BJ, Culasso F, et al: Clinical significance of abnormal electrocardiographic patterns in trained athletes. *Circulation* 2000;102:278-284.

Of the 1,005 athletes examined in this study, 40% had abnormal ECGs but only 5% had structurally abnormal cardiac disease. Most abnormal ECGs represented physiologic remodeling of the athlete's heart as a result of intense training and exercise.

Sudden Cardiac Death

Basillico FC: Cardiovascular disease in athletes. *Am J Sports Med* 1999;27:108-121.

This review article describes the epidemiology and etiology of various causes of SCD, changes that occur in the physiologically conditioned athlete's heart, and current recommendations for cardiac screening tools and implementations.

Fuller CM: Cost effectiveness analysis of screening of high school athletes for risk of sudden cardiac death. *Med Sci Sports Exerc* 2000;32:887-889.

When assessing the cost-effectiveness of various screening tools for SCD, the author found the 12-lead ECG to be the most cost-effective screening device for distinguishing athletes at risk for SCD when compared with history and physical examination and two-dimensional echocardiogram.

Glover DW, Maron BJ: Profile of preparticipation cardiovascular screening for high school athletes. *JAMA* 1998;279:1817-1819.

Because of the inadequacy, variability, and lack of core uniformity in cardiac questionnaires, examination forms, and medical examiners at the high-school level, the PPE may have limited potential for screening for cardiac disease responsible for SCD.

Pfister GC, Puffer JC, Maron BJ: Preparticipation cardiovascular screening for US collegiate student-athletes. *JAMA* 2000;283:1597-1599.

The authors of this study report that the inadequacy, variability, and lack of core uniformity in cardiac questionnaires, examination forms, and medical examiners at the college level may result in the PPE having limited potential for screening for cardiac disease responsible for SCD.

Commotio Cordis

Vincent GM, McPeak H: Commotio cordis: A deadly consequence of chest trauma. *Phys Sportsmed* 2000;28: 31-39.

This article summarizes the incidence, clinical profile, proposed pathophysiology of commotio cordis and discusses current studies and protective measures.

Hypertension

Chobanian AV, Bakins GL, Black HR, et al: The Seventh Report of the Joint National Committee on Prevention, Detection, Evaluation, and Treatment of High Blood Pressure: The JNC 7 Report. *JAMA* 2003;289: 2560-2572.

This article provides the most recent adult hypertension guidelines regarding prevention, detection, evaluation, and treatment; prehypertension is presented as a new blood pressure classification for adults.

Syncope

Mounsey JP, Fergusin JD: The assessment and management of arrhythmias and syncope in the athlete. *Clin Sports Med* 2003;22:67-79.

This article reviews the presentation and management of arrhythmias and syncope in athletes.

Chest Pain

Perron AD: Chest pain in athletes. *Clin Sports Med* 2003;22:37-50.

This review article outlines the presentation, management, and return-to-play guidelines regarding the various causes of chest pain in athletes.

Automatic External Defibrillators

Marenco JP, Wang PJ, Link MS, Homoud MK, Estes NA III: Improving survival from sudden cardiac arrest: The role of the automated external defibrillator. *JAMA* 2002;285:1193-1200.

This article reviews recent studies assessing the use, effectiveness, and cost of AEDs to treat out-of-hospital cardiovascular collapse.

Exercise-Induced Asthma

Anderson SA, Holzer KH: Exercise-induced asthma: Is it the right diagnosis in elite athletes? *J Allergy Clin Immunol* 2000;106:419-428.

This article suggests that in elite athletes EIB is a separate entity from EIA. The authors also suggest that a milder form of airway narrowing in elite athletes, bronchial hyperresponsiveness, may be the result of pathophysiologic changes in the airway resulting from dehydration injury during exercise.

McKenzie DC, Stewart IB, Fitch KD: The asthmatic athlete, inhaled beta agonists, and performance. *Clin J Sport Med* 2002;12:225-228.

This article examines the International Olympic Committee requirement of medical justification for EIA, the use of beta-agonists in Olympic athletes, and the lack of ergogenic properties of inhaled beta-agonists when used at therapeutic doses.

Rundell KW, Jenkinson DM: Exercise induced bronchospasm in the elite athlete. *Sports Med* 2002;32:583-600.

This article describes the prevalence, pathophysiology, diagnosis, and treatment of EIB in elite athletes.

Rundell KW, Johee LB, Wilber RL, et al: Self-reported symptoms and exercise-induced asthma in the elite athlete. *Med Sci Sports Exerc* 2001;33:208-213.

Self-reported asthma symptoms in 158 elite athletes were compared with the results of preexercise and postexercise spirometry testing. The reported symptoms did not effectively predict positive or negative spirometry results.

Rundell KW, Spiering BA: Inspiratory stridor in elite athletes. *Chest* 2003;123:468-474.

The authors of this study examined 374 elite athletes and identified inspiratory stridor in 5% with comorbid EIB in 53%. Lack of beta-agonist response and spirometry testing helped distinguish inspiratory stridor from EIB.

Tan RA, Spector SLA: Exercise-induced asthma: Diagnosis and management. *Ann Allergy Asthma Immunol* 2002;89:226-236.

This article discusses the pathogenesis, clinical features, diagnosis, testing for, and management of EIA.

Vocal Cord Dysfunction

Perkins PJ, Morris MJ: Vocal cord dysfunction induced by methacholine challenge testing. *Chest* 2002;122:1988-1993.

Although the methacholine-challenge test is used to predict asthma, this study suggests that this test may not be specific for diagnosing asthma because acute episodes of VCD occurred after methacholine administration in some patients without suggesting airway reactivity.

Sullivan MD, Heywood BM, Beukelman DR: A treatment for vocal cord dysfunction in female athletes: An outcome study. *Laryngoscope* 2001;111:1751-1755.

In this study, 20 adolescent female athletes with VCD were successfully treated with speech pathology that focused on breathing control. Most patients were still able to control VCD symptoms for up to 6 months after treatment.

Anaphylaxis

Shadick NA, Liang MH, Partridge AJ, et al: The natural history of exercise-induced anaphylaxis: Survey results from a 10-year follow-up study. *J Allergy Clin Immunol* 1999;104:123-127.

This 10-year follow-up study of 671 people with exercise-induced anaphylaxis attempts to determine the natural history of exercise-induced anaphylaxis. Although the number of episodes decreased or remained the same over time, activity modification helped to improve symptoms in most patients.

Classic Bibliography

Huston TP, Puffer JC, Rodney WM: The athletic heart syndrome. *N Engl J Med* 1985;313:24-32.

Maron BJ, Mitchell JH: 26th Bethesda Conference: Recommendations for determining eligibility for competition in athletes with cardiovascular abnormalities. *J Am Coll Cardiol* 1994;24:845-899.

Maron BJ, Shirani J, Poliac LC, Mathenge R, Roberts WC, Mueller FO: Sudden death in young competitive athletes: Clinical, demographic, and pathologic profiles. *JAMA* 1996;276:199-204.

Maron BJ, Thompson PD, Puffer JC, et al: Cardiovascular preparticipation screening of competitive athletes: A statement for health professionals from the Sudden Death Committee (clinical cardiology) and Congenital Cardiac Defects Committee (cardiovascular disease in the young), American Heart Association. *Circulation* 1996;94:850-856.

Maron BJ, Thompson PD, Puffer JC, et al: Cardiovascular preparticipation screening of competitive athletes: Addendum, An addendum to a statement for health professionals from the Sudden Death Committee (Council on Clinical Cardiology) and the Congenital Cardiac Defects Committee (Council on Cardiovascular Disease in the Young), American Heart Association. *Circulation* 1998;97:2294.

Risser WL, Anderson SJ, Boldec SP, et al: Committee on Sports Medicine and Fitness: Athletic participation by children and adolescents who have systemic hypertension. *Pediatrics* 1997;99:637-638.

Volcheck GW, Li JT: Exercise-induced urticaria and anaphylaxis. *Mayo Clin Proc* 1997;72:140-147.

Chapter 26

Nutrition and Eating Disorders

Albert C. Hergenroeder, MD

Introduction

Nutritional problems are ubiquitous in orthopaedic sports medicine practice. The field of sports nutrition includes diverse topics such as the use of performance enhancers, dietary supplements, fluids and electrolytes, and body weight. The issue of body weight presents formidable clinical challenges.

Eleven percent of US adolescents are overweight and another 16% are at risk for being overweight. Sixty-four percent of US adults are either overweight or obese. Obesity causes or complicates the treatment of many musculoskeletal problems, including low back pain and degenerative joint disease. Conversely, malnutrition can result in amenorrhea, which is a risk factor for stress fractures and osteopenia. Five percent of female adolescents in the United States have anorexia nervosa or bulimia nervosa. A comparable percentage of young female athletes who have weight loss and some features of an eating disorder but lack sufficient criteria for the diagnosis of anorexia nervosa or bulimia nervosa could possibly have an eating disorder not otherwise specified (EDNOS).

The drive to maintain a low body weight is intensified in sports that are governed by weight class or appearance. In all sports, excessive exercise coupled with inadequate caloric intake can result in what is known as the female athlete triad, which refers to the interrelatedness of disordered eating, amenorrhea, and osteoporosis. In a culture that promotes thinness for young females and urges athletes to win at all costs, patients can be vulnerable to unsubstantiated claims about dietary supplements, ergogenic aids, definitions of healthy eating, and weight loss and gain strategies. Physicians sometimes can contribute to this vulnerability by not recognizing harmful weight loss or gain or, if recognized, offering no practical advice. The dietary supplement industry is often affiliated with health care providers who lack the training in physiology, biochemistry, and medicine needed to provide dietary and exercise guidance. (For example, a dietitian requires a bachelor's degree in nutrition, whereas a nutritionist can be any-

one who chooses that title and has little or no formal training; much of the public is unaware of this distinction and its implications.)

Forty percent of the US population older than 2 months has taken a mineral, vitamin, or dietary supplement in the past month. A well-balanced diet obviates the need for most of these dietary supplements. Additionally, athletes with high caloric needs who eat highly fortified foods are at risk of exceeding the upper tolerable limit for vitamins and minerals. Healthy weight gain and loss can be achieved incrementally with a measured, common sense approach to caloric intake and caloric expenditure. To the extent that orthopaedic problems are made worse if weight problems are ignored, orthopaedic surgeons may be inclined to incorporate basic dietary advice and exercise guidelines into their practice. Orthopaedic surgeons should gain a better understanding of basic clinical nutrition and be able to categorize a patient's body weight as normal, malnourished, or obese; categorize the degree of malnutrition; provide a baseline of accurate advice regarding appropriate weight loss and gain strategies using the concept of caloric balance; and recognize and manage the eating disorders of female athletes.

Body Weight

The first step in attempting to address a patient's questions or concerns about body weight and the desire for weight loss or gain is to estimate the patient's ideal body weight (IBW). IBW is not to be used as the target weight, but rather as a reference point to recommend a weight range goal. Weight is a function of age, gender, and height. It can be estimated for 12- to 17-year-old patients using the data provided in Tables 1 and 2.

Body weight equal to 90% to 110% of IBW is normal. Body weight greater than 120% of IBW is the definition of obesity; 80% to 85% of IBW indicates mild malnutrition (although the body weight of some healthy, well-conditioned athletes may be approximately 85% of IBW); 70% to 80% of IBW indicates moderate malnutrition; and less than 70% is consistent with severe mal-

TABLE 1 | IBW (50th Percentile) by Height Group for Females 12 to 17 Years of Age

Height (cm)	IBW (kg) by Age (years)					
	12	13	14	15	16	17
135.0-139.9	28.9					
140.0-144.9	36.8	36.7				
145.0-149.9	38.5	40.5	42.3	45.4	51.0	45.1
150.0-154.9	42.8	42.9	47.9	48.1	48.9	48.9
155.0-159.9	46.8	48.4	49.6	50.8	51.6	53.2
160.0-164.9	51.1	52.2	53.0	55.0	55.5	55.4
165.0-169.9	53.1	58.1	56.8	58.4	59.1	59.3
170.0-174.9	56.7	52.9	59.8	61.2	62.1	60.2
175.0-179.9			59.8	62.4	65.9	61.7

(Adapted with permission from US Department of Health, Education, and Welfare Public Health Service: Plan and Operation of a Health Examination Survey of US Youths 12-17 Years of Age: A Description of the Health Examination Survey's Third Cycle-Examinations of a Probability Sample of United States Youths 12-17 Years of Age. Rockville, MD, Health Resources Administration, National Center for Health Statistics, 1974. DHEW Publication No. (HRA) 75-1018.)

TABLE 2 | IBW (50th Percentile) by Height Group for Males 12 to 17 Years of Age

Height (cm)	IBW (kg) by Age (years)					
	12	13	14	15	16	17
135.0-139.9	31.6	31.0				
140.0-144.9	34.1	36.1				
145.0-149.9	38.2	37.9	40.6			
150.0-154.9	42.1	41.0	41.4	44.7		
155.0-159.9	46.2	45.8	46.1	49.2	46.8	49.7
160.0-164.9	48.4	50.4	52.1	51.5	51.4	56.9
165.0-169.9	54.4	53.6	55.4	56.4	58.0	61.5
170.0-174.9	61.0	60.1	59.4	61.9	61.6	64.6
175.0-179.9		63.3	64.7	64.3	65.4	66.5
180.0-184.9			69.4	70.2	68.9	71.2
185.0-189.9				70.7	78.4	75.3
190.0-194.9				73.8		87.3

(Adapted with permission from US Department of Health, Education, and Welfare Public Health Service: Plan and Operation of a Health Examination Survey of US Youths 12-17 Years of Age: A Description of the Health Examination Survey's Third Cycle-Examinations of a Probability Sample of United States Youths 12-17 Years of Age. Rockville, MD, Health Resources Administration, National Center for Health Statistics, 1974. DHEW Publication No. (HRA) 75-1018.)

Using the table, the estimated IBW of a 15-year-old female who is 162 cm tall and weighs 58.0 kg is 55 kg; the percent of IBW, calculated as (body weight/IBW) × 100 is 105%. For patients younger than 12 years, the use of standard height and weight graphs is recommended. For patients older than 17 years, IBW is estimated as follows: IBW (lb) = 100 + 5 lb per inch over 60 inches of height (for women) and IBW (lb) = 106 + 6 lb per inch over 60 inches of height (for men).

nutrition. Superobesity, or morbid obesity, is a term used to indicate those with a body weight greater than 200% of IBW. Alternatively, body mass index, which is calcu-

lated as body weight in kilograms divided by height in meters squared, can be used as a screening assessment tool for body weight.

Caloric Balance

In the absence of a disease process characterized by fluid shifts, such as congestive heart failure, renal disease, malabsorption, or dehydration as can occur in athletes with eating disorders, weight changes in otherwise healthy people can be interpreted in the context of caloric balance, which is defined as caloric intake minus caloric expenditure. Negative caloric balance occurs when caloric expenditure exceeds caloric intake.

Estimated Caloric Intake

Management of a patient's weight begins with estimating typical daily caloric intake, which can be done using a 3-day food record. Overweight patients tend to underestimate their caloric intake, whereas malnourished patients with eating disorders may overestimate their caloric intake. Patients need guidance in estimating portion sizes for any dietary recall method, and this is where consultation with a dietitian is invaluable. Ideally, the dietitian should work in the same clinic as the treating physician. Alternatively, someone in the office can be trained by a dietitian to instruct patients in the completion of the food record. Insurance companies tend to not reimburse for assessments and care provided by dietitians in this setting. Advocacy efforts seeking to improve insurance reimbursement for medical nutritional therapy by dietitians is an important part of making this model of integrated physician-dietitian practice a fiscal reality.

Estimated Caloric Expenditure

For most patients, a precise estimate of caloric expenditure is unnecessary. In adolescent females, the average daily caloric need is approximately 14 kilocalories per centimeter of height; in adolescent males, the average daily caloric need is approximately 16.5 kilocalories per centimeter of height. For adults with normal weight, the daily resting energy (calorie) expenditure (REE) can be estimated as follows: 1 kilocalorie/body weight in kilograms/hour × 24 hours (for males) and 0.9 kilocalorie/body weight in kilograms/hour × 24 hours (for females). For obese adults, rather than using body weight, which would overestimate the REE, the estimated IBW plus 25% of the estimated IBW should be used. For sedentary individuals, total daily caloric expenditure can be estimated by adding 20% to 30% to the REE; for moderately active individuals, 50% should be added; and for active individuals, 80% to 100% should be added.

Knowing the caloric expenditure of common activities can be useful in the clinical setting. For example, running or walking 1 mile for a healthy older adolescent/adult consumes approximately 100 kilocalories. Obese patients who lose approximately 20% or more of their original weight should be advised that walking a certain distance will use less calories, even after adjusting for the reduced body weight. Therefore, for weight loss maintenance, they may need to increase the time of exercise.

In practice, estimates of caloric expenditure may be used to monitor patients who are not gaining weight in spite of reporting a positive caloric balance, which is caloric intake in excess of caloric expenditure. For patients with eating disorders characterized by malnutrition, patients may underestimate energy expenditure by exercise and overestimate caloric intake. In this context, the direct measure of REE, using a metabolic cart, may be considered. The Harris-Benedict equation has correction factors for malnutrition, indicating the malnourished patient may have a reduction in REE of 10% to 40%.

Nutrition and Exercise

Losing 10% of the presenting body weight is a reasonable initial goal for obese patients. When a sedentary individual starts an exercise program, exercise volume rather than intensity should be emphasized because carbohydrates tend to be the preferred energy source in high-intensity, short-duration activity, whereas fat tends to be the preferred energy source in low- to medium-intensity exercise of a longer duration. Sedentary patients should also be advised to increase the amount of exercise slowly (for example, 10% to 15% per week). They should also be advised that 1 lb of mixed tissue (fat and fat-free mass) weight loss represents approximately 3,500 kilocalories. If patients achieve a daily caloric deficit of 500 kilocalories, then in 1 week they can be expected to lose 1 lb (ie, caloric deficit of 500 kilocalories per day × 7 days = 3,500 kilocalories).

Simple suggestions to promote weight loss include avoiding consumption of sugared drinks, soft drinks, juice drinks, lemonade, and sweetened tea; building a healthy plate at mealtime, in which one half of the portion consists of fruits and vegetables, one fourth consists of starch foods, and one fourth is meat or other sources of protein; limiting the addition of fat by avoiding the consumption of mayonnaise, margarine, sour cream, and salad dressing; and limiting television viewing.

Patients may report being refractory to weight loss even though they follow prescribed menu and exercise plans. In one study, a group of obese adults that was refractory to weight loss on a 1,200-kilocalorie per day diet overestimated caloric expenditure from physical activity by a mean of 51% and underestimated caloric intake by 47%. Therefore, when treating obese patients for weight management, it is important to be aware that

obese patients may overestimate caloric expenditure and underestimate caloric intake.

Eating Disorders and Female Athletes

Although the female athlete triad is defined as the constellation of disordered eating, amenorrhea, and osteoporosis, oligomenorrhea with amenorrhea and osteopenia with osteoporosis may be included in this definition. Amenorrhea in this context is hypothalamic amenorrhea, which reflects the loss of normal pulsatile release of gonadotropin luteinizing hormone (LH) and follicle-stimulating hormone (FSH). It is not exercise per se that causes the loss of normal LH and FSH secretion; rather, it is the inability to match caloric intake with caloric expenditure (negative caloric balance) that is etiologic in hypothalamic amenorrhea.

Female athletes with amenorrhea or oligomenorrhea have lower bone mineral density (BMD) and a higher rate of stress fractures than athletes with eumenorrhea. A long-term consequence of amenorrhea and osteopenia during the second decade of life is an increased risk of postmenopausal osteoporosis.

Clinical Presentation

Patients with eating disorders may present to the orthopaedic surgeon with a stress fracture. The *Diagnostic and Statistical Manual of Mental Disorders, Fourth Edition* criteria for anorexia, bulimia nervosa, and EDNOS are listed in Table 3. A teen or young adult with a stress fracture should have the percentage of IBW calculated and a menstrual history recorded. Those with oligomenorrhea or amenorrhea and/or malnutrition should be referred for evaluation and treatment of the cause of these conditions while the stress fracture is being treated. Failure to recognize and treat an eating disorder and/or malnutrition may result in a chronic stress fracture that does not respond to treatment as expected.

Patients with the female athlete triad can also report cold intolerance and orthostatic instability. The cold intolerance, in part, is secondary to a reduced REE. The most important predictor of REE is lean body mass. Because lean body mass is reduced during prolonged starvation, REE and, therefore, endogenous heat production, are reduced. Peripheral fat stores are also reduced, leading to easier heat loss across the skin. The patient will typically report being cold and will have progressively lower body temperature as the starvation progresses. Another manifestation of reduced REE is a low resting pulse (eg, 30 to 45 beats per minute [bpm]).

Orthostatic instability is manifested as presyncope or syncope when going from the lying to standing position and as orthostatic tachycardia with or without orthostatic hypotension. Orthostatic tachycardia is defined as a pulse increase of 35 bpm or greater at 5 minutes of standing after rising directly from the lying position.

TABLE 3 | Definitions of Eating Disorders

Anorexia nervosa

Refusal to maintain body weight at or above a minimally normal weight for one's age and height (eg, weight loss leading to maintenance of body weight less than 85% of that expected or failure to make expected weight gain during a period of growth that results in body weight less than 85% of that expected).

Intense fear of gaining weight or becoming fat, even though underweight.

Disturbance in the way in which one's body weight or shape is experienced, undue influence of body weight or shape on self-evaluation, or denial of the seriousness of the current low body weight.

In postmenarchal females, amenorrhea (ie, the absence of at least three consecutive menstrual cycles); a woman is considered to have amenorrhea if her periods occur only following hormone (eg, estrogen) administration.

Bulimia nervosa

Recurrent episodes of binge eating. (An episode of binge eating is characterized by eating, in a discrete period of time [eg, within any 2-hour period], an amount of food that is definitely larger than most people would eat during a similar period of time and under the same circumstances and a sense of lack of control over eating during the episode [eg, a feeling that one cannot stop eating or control what or how much one is eating]).

Recurrent inappropriate compensatory behavior to prevent weight gain, such as self-induced vomiting; misuse of laxatives, diuretics, enemas, or other medications; fasting; or excessive exercise.

The binge eating and inappropriate compensatory behaviors both occur, on average, at least twice a week for 3 months.

Self-evaluation is unduly influenced by body shape and weight.

The disturbance does not occur exclusively during episodes of anorexia nervosa.

EDNOS

For females, all of the criteria for anorexia nervosa are met except the individual has normal menses.

All of the criteria for anorexia nervosa are met except that, despite significant weight loss, the individual's weight is still within the normal range.

All the criteria for bulimia nervosa are met except that the binge eating and inappropriate compensatory mechanisms occur at a frequency of less than twice per week or for a duration of less than 3 months.

The regular use of inappropriate compensatory behavior by an individual of normal body weight after eating small amounts of food (eg, self-induced vomiting after the consumption of two cookies).

Repeatedly chewing and spitting out (not swallowing) large amounts of food.

Binge-eating disorder (recurrent episodes of binge eating in the absence of the regular use of inappropriate compensatory behaviors characteristic of bulimia nervosa).

tion, including decreased cardiac output and decreased peripheral vascular tone. (The treatment implications of hypothermia and cardiovascular dysfunction are discussed later.) Appropriate treatment and follow-up should be planned for patients who meet the criteria for an eating disorder (Table 3) or the female athlete triad.

Patients or their families may ask whether growth can be compromised by excessive participation in sports and exercise in the prepubertal and/or pubertal years. One study compared a group of adolescent gymnasts with a mean bone age of 12.3 ± 0.2 years that exercised a mean of 22 hours per week with a group of swimmers that exercised a mean of 8 hours per week; the authors reported evidence of reduction in growth potential in the group of adolescent gymnasts. Another study reported a negative impact of gymnastics training (10 to 20 hours per week) on statural growth. The consensus is that short stature in gymnastics is related to selection bias and not intense training. Nonetheless, patients with eating disorders characterized by chronic malnutrition can have short stature as a result of nutritional deficiencies. Therefore, adult stature can be compromised by excessive participation in sports and exercise when the athlete develops malnutrition. The inability to match high caloric expenditure with caloric intake and the resultant malnutrition affects growth, not the exercise per se in nearly all instances.

Evaluation

History

When evaluating a young female athlete with weight loss, it is useful to ask the patient what she would like to weigh. A dietary history is also useful and should be evaluated by a dietitian. The first step in addressing primary or secondary amenorrhea is to make a correct diagnosis. Hypothalamic amenorrhea associated with exercise and inadequate caloric intake is a diagnosis of exclusion. The diagnosis is made on the basis of the exercise history, a 3-day food record, a physical examination, and a medical history that suggests no evidence of chronic disease, such as chronic diarrhea in inflammatory bowel disease, peripheral edema in malabsorptive conditions, or nephrotic syndrome. Patients with bulimia nervosa commonly present with a body weight that is normal. Therefore, inquiry about vomiting and other purging behavior should be made. Academic pressure with stress for any reason with or without excessive exercise training can be associated with amenorrhea; therefore, not all patients with amenorrhea have undiagnosed eating disorders.

Physical Examination

During the physical examination, the patient's percentage of IBW should be calculated. Lying pulse and blood pressure should also be taken and repeated at 5 minutes

Orthostatic hypotension is defined as a systolic blood pressure decrease of 20 mm Hg or a diastolic decrease of 10 mm Hg from baseline after 5 minutes of standing. These are manifestations of altered cardiovascular func-

after going from the lying to the standing position. Although the following items are not typically part of the orthopaedic surgeon's routine physical examination of athletes with weight loss, they can provide data that are key in establishing the correct diagnosis. The presence of severe acne or hirsutism noted during skin examination may be consistent with a hyperandrogenic state, such as occurs in patients with polycystic ovarian syndrome or an androgen-secreting tumor. A history of blurry vision and bulging optic disks with galactorrhea noted during funduscopic examination suggest the presence of a hypothalamic or pituitary mass. An enlarged thyroid gland on palpation can be consistent with hyperthyroidism or hypothyroidism, depending on the primary process. The presence of nipple discharge during physical examination is consistent with hyperprolactinemia. An elevated prolactin level is consistent with galactorrhea, which occurs in patients with a pituitary microadenoma or other pituitary masses or primary hypothyroidism. Therefore, serum thyroid stimulating hormone concentration should be measured if the prolactin level is elevated.

A patient with hypothalamic amenorrhea secondary to excessive exercise and inadequate caloric intake is likely to have normal breast and pubic hair development; however, breast size may be reduced. A pelvic examination is necessary. Amenorrhea without breast and/or uterine and vaginal development may be the manifestation of a chromosomal, gonadal, or anatomic abnormality. Common conditions that need to be ruled out in the evaluation of primary amenorrhea include chromosomal abnormalities, such as Turner syndrome; vaginal agenesis, such as that which occurs in patients with androgen insensitivity; pregnancy; hyperprolactinemia associated with a prolactin-secreting pituitary adenoma or primary hypothyroidism; polycystic ovarian syndrome; and primary ovarian failure, such as that which can occur in patients after pelvic radiation or use of alkylating chemotherapeutic agents for the treatment of cancer and hypothyroidism. Any additional diagnostic testing to evaluate amenorrhea should be done by specialists.

Dual-Energy X-ray Absorptiometry

Measuring the BMD of the lumbar spine and hip using dual-energy x-ray absorptiometry (DEXA) should be considered when the patient has been amenorrheic for longer than 6 months. If the patient has been amenorrheic for more than 1 year and is malnourished, then DEXA is recommended. DEXA should not be repeated more often than 12 months apart. The World Health Organization has established criteria for the diagnosis of osteopenia (T-score, –1.0 or less) and osteoporosis (T-score, –2.5 or less). The T-score, similar to one standard deviation above or below ideal bone mass (normal T-score, +1 to –1), is based on a comparison of a pa-

tient's bone density and the peak bone density of the healthy, young adult population. Its significance as a predictor of subsequent stress fractures or clinical osteoporosis (manifest as a fracture in young athletes with amenorrhea) is not known. Caution should be exercised in interpreting T-scores and Z-scores (based on age-matched bone mass) in patients with short stature because DEXA tends to underestimate BMD in these patients and overestimate BMD in patients with tall stature. This could lead to overdiagnosis of osteoporosis in short patients.

Treatment

When the diagnosis of hypothalamic amenorrhea or oligomenorrhea is made, reduction in training volume and increased caloric intake are indicated. Specific recommendations should be made on a case-by-case basis, depending on the patient's clinical assessment, percentage of IBW, body temperature, pulse, and blood pressure. In general, the physician should propose a plan in which energy intake exceeds energy expenditure. This, however, depends on patient report, and often female athletes with eating disorders overestimate their energy intake. There is no universal set of guidelines regarding the amount of energy reduction and increased energy intake. A general statement regarding the patient with mild malnutrition and amenorrhea would be that the energy intake should be increased by 5% to 10% and the energy expenditure reduced by 5% to 10%. In general, a resting pulse below 40 bpm and a body temperature less than 36°C could be considered contraindications to exercise in a patient with a suspected eating disorder, regardless of a patient's percentage of IBW. For an athlete with a suspected eating disorder and 90% to 100% of IBW, normal pulse, normal temperature, and no evidence of orthostatic instability, another approach is to reduce the exercise volume by one third. For example, if the athlete is participating in similar amounts of exercise 6 days per week, exercise volume should be reduced to 4 days per week, with no increased training on the remaining days. Daily caloric intake could be increased by a adding a 250-kilocalorie supplement to this athlete's diet. For an athlete with 85% to 90% of IBW, exercise volume could be reduced by half. For example, if the athlete exercises daily, exercise should be reduced to 3 days a week and one or two 250-kilocalorie dietary drinks or snacks per day should be added to the athlete's diet. For patients with less than 80% of IBW, exercise is not recommended.

In general, no exercise is recommended for athletes with less than 85% of IBW who also have hypothalamic amenorrhea and an eating disorder. Exceptions include the female athlete with eumenorrhea and 80% to 85% of IBW. The reason why some women with a weight equal to 80% to 85% of IBW have eumenorrhea but the typical patient with anorexia nervosa resumes menses at 90% of IBW is not known. Patients with an EDNOS may be allowed to participate in limited exercise with the contingency that weight should gradually increase as they increase their volume of exercise. This weight increase can be as little as 0.1 kg per week. Patients with 80% to 85% of IBW who are recovering from an eating disorder and who can be monitored during exercise may also be allowed to participate in limited exercise (such as stretching for 5 to 10 minutes and 5 minutes of walking per day) with the understanding that the exercise is contingent on consistent weight gain.

Reduced training assumes the participation of a supportive coach. A written plan should be given to the athlete and she should be encouraged to show it to her coach and ask the coach to call the physician or dietitian with questions.

Follow-up Care

Athletes should be observed weekly until weight increases consistently. Weight should be measured after the patient urinates and while wearing a gown and underclothes; the same scale should be used each time. This protocol addresses weight fluctuations caused by clothing variations, water intake, and variations in different scales. Urine-specific gravity should be assessed to help evaluate the degree of dehydration or water overload. Once the patient's weight increases to 90% of IBW, visits can be reduced to every 2 weeks.

If osteopenia is present, even in the face of normal menses, then increased emphasis is placed on weight gain. Amenorrheic athletes who gain weight as a result of reduced training and improved diet can resume menses spontaneously and increase their BMD. Exercise may attenuate bone loss in patients with bulimia nervosa and anorexia nervosa. Strain placed on bone through exercise and adequate serum estrogen levels appear to have additive effects on improving bone strength. The effectiveness of bone modeling through exercise may be limited, however, when serum estrogen levels are below normal.

Exercise in patients with bulimia nervosa is appropriate if their weight is greater than or equal to 90% of IBW; if their pulse, blood pressure, and temperature are normal; if they are menstruating; and if a recent set of serum electrolytes measurements is normal.

Female athletes who increase body weight in response to dietary and exercise recommendations are patients who are able to regulate exercise and caloric intake in a manner consistent with good health. However, these athletes are probably at risk for developing the female athlete triad and must be observed regularly (ie, every 3 months over the course of 1 year) to ensure that weight and menstrual function are normal. Patients who experience weight loss, alteration in vital signs, or oligomenorrhea or amenorrhea require closer monitoring

and reinstitution of exercise and calorie guidelines. Some patients will be able to improve clinically with dietary and medical management alone. The female athlete triad can be prevented in some patients if relatively simple exercise prescriptions and dietary management are implemented before pathologic eating disorder behavior becomes entrenched and significant malnutrition develops. Some patients are not diagnosed early or, if diagnosed, are observed for too long before referral to an eating disorder program. This implies an important role for the preseason examination. The team physician should work with an interdisciplinary team and with coaches and administrators to address eating disorders before they become refractory to care. Some programs welcome this approach, whereas others do not.

Referral to a Psychologist or Psychiatrist

If patients meet the criteria for anorexia nervosa, bulimia nervosa, or an EDNOS, they should be referred to a mental health professional with expertise in managing eating disorders. In the context of the clinical scenarios discussed previously in which an eating disorder is suspected but not diagnosed, if weight gain does not ensue after a few weeks of medical and nutritional therapy, or if weight loss occurs after an initial period of progress, then referral to a mental health professional is indicated. If the patient refuses to see the mental health provider or is noncompliant with follow-up psychotherapy, then the physician should consider advising the patient and family that optimal care includes psychotherapy. If the noncompliance persists and the clinical condition does not improve, then the physician should consider advising the patient and family to seek the consultation of another physician. Although some may interpret this is an abrogation of the physician's responsibility, to the contrary, the physician's responsibility is to provide optimal care, which for patients with eating disorders is complex and interdisciplinary by necessity. A physician cannot care for these patients alone. Because the criteria for anorexia nervosa includes denial of the seriousness of the current low body weight, part of the pathology is manifested as the patient and/or family understating the seriousness of the condition, which can result in noncompliance with counseling or medical and nutritional recommendations. To treat the patient without the necessary counseling is to reinforce denial, which is ultimately counterproductive.

Hormone Replacement Therapy

It has never been demonstrated that the use of estrogen-progestin prevents stress fractures in young women with hypothalamic amenorrhea. Controversy also exists whether the use of estrogen-progestin (in the form of oral contraceptive pills) or estrogen replacement therapy (0.3 to 0.625 mg of conjugated estrogen) increases BMD. Some research suggests that the use of oral contraceptive pills by premenopausal women is associated with a reduced risk of postmenopausal osteoporosis. Another study supports the use of estrogen-progestin replacement therapy for severely malnourished patients (those with body weight ≤ 70% of IBW and eating disorders, but not those with body weight > 70% of IBW). One recent trial of women (mean age, 25 years) with anorexia nervosa who received oral contraceptive pill therapy with or without insulin-like growth factor (IGF)-I or placebo reported no improvement in BMD after 9 and 12 months of treatment, respectively. Oral contraceptive pill therapy did appear to have a synergistic effect on spine BMD in those treated with recombinant IGF-I in the study on older women. A nonrandomized trial of females (two groups; mean age, 16 to 17 years) with anorexia nervosa showed no difference in BMD after 12 months of treatment. A randomized controlled trial showed an improvement in BMD in women with hypothalamic amenorrhea (mean age, 19 years) who received either oral contraceptive pill therapy or placebo over 12 months.

A problem with many of these studies is that BMD (measured in g/cm^2) is an areal bone mineral measurement, which is subject to interpretation in estimating the two-dimensional area measured using DEXA. This is the outcome measure for bone mineralization in many research studies. Absolute bone mineral content (BMC) in grams is not subject to interpretation of the vertebral and femoral neck surface area, as is BMD; therefore, BMC is a more direct measure of bone mineral and should be used in experimental studies. Most studies, however, do not report BMC. The randomized controlled study of women with hypothalamic amenorrhea (mean age, 19 years) showed improvement in total body BMC and lumbar spine BMC.

Other investigators have stressed the importance of focusing on bone size and BMC instead of BMD. Bone fragility is a function of bone size and volumetric BMD (the latter being an estimate of volume, not area). One cross-sectional, nonrandomized retrospective cohort study reported that women with anorexia nervosa treated with estrogen replacement over 2 years had greater lumbar vertebral body size and BMC compared with those who were not treated with estrogen replacement.

The decision to treat with estrogen-progestin should be individualized. If the amenorrhea persists for 6 months or longer and the athlete is malnourished, then estrogen-progestin therapy in oral contraceptive pill form should be considered. Of concern is the perception of weight gain in patients with eating disorders. There is evidence that oral contraceptive use is associated with weight gain as an independent factor in teenagers with eating disorders. Some oral contraceptive pill users have reported the perception of weight gain despite having gained no weight at all. In patients with eating disorders, there is also a concern that oral contraceptive pill ther-

apy could interfere with psychologic function. A patient with an eating disorder who takes oral contraceptive pills may ascribe mood changes and depressed feelings to the treatment, whereas, in most cases, the mood changes and depressed feelings are better correlated to the stressors in the patient's life. Occasionally, oral contraceptive pill therapy will be changed if the discussion about the effect of treatment on mood becomes a focal point of therapy.

There is a gap in the literature with respect to whether oral contraceptive pill therapy improves bone mineralization in athletes with hypothalamic amenorrhea. A prospective, longitudinal, randomized trial is needed to answer this question. However, the dropout rate in studies with amenorrheic subjects treated with hormonal therapy is 25% to 50%, making longitudinal studies difficult to complete.

In the absence of an established standard for the use of estrogen to prevent osteopenia in adolescent and young adult females with secondary or primary amenorrhea caused by overtraining and caloric restriction, the following factors should be noted: (1) young women with anorexia nervosa and secondary amenorrhea have serum estradiol levels that approximate those of postmenopausal women; (2) osteopenia and osteoporosis are two of the more serious, long-term consequences of anorexia nervosa, with 92% and 38% of patients with anorexia nervosa having osteopenia and osteoporosis, respectively; (3) most published studies use BMD and not BMC and bone size as the outcome measures of interventions with estrogen therapy; and (4) hypoandrogenemia, reduced IGF-I serum levels, and hypercortisolemia in patients with anorexia nervosa contribute to bone mineral loss. These factors will improve with weight gain, may be unaffected by estrogen-progestin therapy, and unless improved, the therapeutic effect of estrogen-progestin supplementation alone is probably limited. Weight gain is the priority. Given these issues, treatment of amenorrheic patients with oral contraceptive pills for more than 6 months still should be considered in addition to the lifestyle changes previously discussed.

Regarding the use of estrogen-progestin in adolescent females with hypothalamic amenorrhea and the potential effects of estrogen on hastening epiphyseal plate growth, bone age is important. A 15-year-old girl, for example, has achieved 96.4% of her adult height with a bone age of 13 years, 98.3% of her adult height with a bone age of 14 years, and 99% of her adult height with a bone age of 15 years. The mean height of females in North America at 19 years is 163 cm. If estrogen replacement completely arrested height gain at the onset of therapy, then a female patient with a bone age of 15 years could potentially lose 1.6 cm of height if her potential adult height was 163 cm. More likely, height attainment would not be arrested, and some height would still be achieved.

Alternatively, the loss of height could be immeasurable. Significant arrest of bone mineral acquisition could occur before menarche as the result of malnutrition caused by an eating disorder. The onset of bone loss relative to bone development is important in that the onset of anorexia nervosa in girls younger than 15 years will affect bone size and volumetric BMD more than it will in those 15 years of age and older. Bone fragility is a function of bone size and volumetric BMD, both of which increase during pubertal growth. There is a risk to BMD acquisition from chronic hypoestrogenemia when epiphyseal growth is occurring. Estrogen-progesterone replacement for females with amenorrhea at 15 years of age and a bone age of 15 years and for those with a bone age of 14 years, depending on the degree of osteopenia and malnutrition, should be considered. This is an area that requires further investigation.

Other Pharmacologic Treatments

Other pharmacologic treatments are available to help prevent osteoporosis. Selective estrogen receptor modulators have been developed to maximize the effect of estrogen on bone while minimizing the effect of estrogen on the breasts and endometrium. Raloxifene is a selective estrogen receptor modulator that has been approved by the US Food and Drug Administration for the prevention and treatment of osteoporosis in postmenopausal women, but its effect on the skeletons of adolescent and young adult females is not known and is currently being investigated.

Recombinant IGF has been shown to increase markers of bone turnover in women with anorexia nervosa and to improve spinal BMD alone or in combination with oral contraceptive pill therapy. Animal studies suggest that leptin may help regulate bone remodeling via the sympathetic nervous system. Further research is needed, however, to determine the role of these agents in improving BMD status in young women with hypothalamic amenorrhea.

Calcium Intake

It is recommended that amenorrheic athletes have an elemental calcium intake of 1,500 mg/day. Calcium sources from dairy or juice products containing the calcium salt calcium-citrate-maleate are preferred. For example, an 8-ounce serving of milk or yogurt can provide 300 mg of calcium. Calcium supplements in the form of calcium salts such as calcium carbonate can be used if patients have difficulty consuming 1,500 mg of calcium daily from food sources. Calcium supplementation alone, however, with or without supplemental vitamin D intake, will not improve BMD in young women with hypothalamic amenorrhea.

Summary

Weight-related issues commonly arise in orthopaedic sports medicine. The initial goal for weight loss in obese patients is 10% of the presenting weight. Patients with stress fractures should have their percentage of IBW calculated and a menstrual history recorded. The management of weight gain or loss should start with estimating the patient's caloric balance. Females with hypothalamic amenorrhea can continue with prescribed exercise as long as increases in caloric intake result in weight gain. The degree of exercise restriction and increased caloric intake recommended depends on the percentage of IBW and other vital signs. Patients with the female athlete triad should be cared for by an interdisciplinary team and observed weekly until there is evidence of consistent, slow weight gain. Dietary management should be done by a dietitian. Mental health care is necessary when the patient is unable to gain weight despite appropriate medical care, dietary management, and exercise guidelines. DEXA should be considered for patients who have had hypothalamic amenorrhea longer than 6 months. Estrogen replacement therapy with oral contraceptive pills should be considered for these patients.

Annotated Bibliography

Nutrition and Exercise

Bass S, Bradney M, Pearce G, et al: Short stature and delayed puberty in gymnasts: Influence of selection bias on leg length and the duration of training on trunk length. *J Pediatr* 2000;136:149-155.

In this study, which included cross-sectional and longitudinal study design components, the only predictor of height velocity in elite gymnasts was caloric intake. The upper body growth velocity was delayed in gymnasts until they stopped competing; then there was an acceleration in upper body (sitting height) velocity. There is an important selection bias in studying elite gymnasts for short stature.

Damsgaard R, Bencke J, Matthiesen G, Petersen JH, Muller J: Is prepubertal growth adversely affected by sport? *Med Sci Sports Exerc* 2000;32:1698-1703.

This retrospective cohort study supports the conclusions that there is no effect of exercise and sports participation on prepubertal growth and constitutional factors play an important role in sports selection; therefore, these selection biases need to be considered in growth issues across sports in the prepubertal years.

Department of Health and Human Services: *National Health and Nutrition Examination Survey: Use of Dietary Supplements.* Atlanta, GA, Centers for Disease Control and Prevention, National Center for Health Statistics. Available at www.cdc.gov/nchs/data/nhanes/databriefs/dietary.pdf. Accessed: December 8, 2003.

This publication discusses use of dietary supplements in the United States.

Eating Disorders and Female Athletes

American Academy of Pediatrics: Committee on Adolescence Policy Statement: Identifying and treating eating disorders. *Pediatrics* 2003;111:204-210.

This is a review of the standard of care for adolescents with eating disorders.

Golden NH, Lanzkowsky L, Schebendach J, Palestro CJ, Jacobson MS, Shenker IR: The effect of estrogen-progestin treatment on bone mineral density in anorexia nervosa. *J Pediatr Adolesc Gynecol* 2002;15:135-143.

This nonrandomized intervention trial compared patients treated with various estrogen-progestin combinations and those receiving no hormonal therapy. Although the group that chose the estrogen-progestin replacement was older and had a longer duration of illness, the authors did not control for this in the analysis.

Grinspoon S, Thomas L, Miller K, Herzog D, Klibanski A: Effects of recombinant human IGF-I and oral contraceptive administration on bone density in anorexia nervosa. *J Clin Endocrinol Metab* 2002;87:2883-2891.

This is a randomized controlled trial for women with anorexia nervosa who received estrogen-progestin (oral contraceptive pill) versus no estrogen-progestin with or without IGF-I over 9 months. The IGF-I group showed a significant increase in bone density when compared with the group that was not treated with IGF-I; the estrogen-progestin had a synergistic effect in the IGF-I group. The estrogen-progestin group showed no significant improvement in bone density compared with the group treated without estrogen-progestin.

Karlsson MK, Weigall SJ, Duan Y, Seeman E: Bone size and volumetric density in women with anorexia nervosa receiving estrogen replacement therapy and in women recovered from anorexia nervosa. *J Clin Endocrinol Metab* 2000;85:3177-3182.

Using a cross-sectional, nonrandomized, retrospective study design, the authors of this study report that women with anorexia nervosa who received estrogen replacement therapy over 2 years had greater lumbar vertebral bone size and BMC compared with those who did not receive estrogen replacement therapy.

Michalsson K, Baron JA, Farahmand BY, Persson I, Ljunghall S: Oral-contraceptive use and hip fracture: A case-control study. *Lancet* 1999;353:1481-1484.

Using a case-control study design, the authors report that those who used oral contraceptive pills after age 40 years had a significantly lower odds ratio (95% confidence interval, 0.5 to 0.9) than those who had never used oral contraceptive pills.

Takeda S, Elefteriou F, Lecasseur R, et al: Leptin regulates bone formation via the sympathetic nervous system. *Cell* 2002;111:305-317.

This study demonstrated that central control of the sympathetic nervous system is important in bone regulation. Treatment with a beta-adrenergic antagonist medication (leptin) improved bone mass in ovariectomized, wild-type mice.

Yanovski SZ, Yanovski JA: Obesity. *N Engl J Med* 2002; 346:591-602.

This is a review of pharmacologic and nonpharmacologic treatment strategies for obesity.

Classic Bibliography

American Psychiatric Association: *Diagnostic and Statistical Manual of Mental Disorders, ed 4*. Washington, DC, American Psychiatric Association, 1994.

Drinkwater BL, Nelson K, Chestnut CH, Bremner WJ, Shainholtz S, Southworth MD: Bone mineral content of amenorrheic and eumenorrheic athletes. *N Engl J Med* 1984;311:277-281.

Dueck CA, Matt KS, Manore MM, Skinner JS: Treatment of athletic amenorrhea with a diet and training intervention program. *Int J Sport Nutr* 1996;6:24-40.

Gruelich WW, Pyle SI: *Radiographic Atlas of Skeletal Development of the Hand and Wrist*, ed 2. Stanford, CA, Stanford University Press, 1959.

Kleerekoper M, Brienza RS, Schultz LR, Johnson CC: Oral contraceptive use may protect against low bone mass. *Arch Intern Med* 1991;151:1971-1976.

Klibanski A, Biller B, Schoenfeld D, Herzog D, Saxe V: The effect of estrogen administration on trabecular bone loss in young women with anorexia nervosa. *J Clin Endocrinol Metab* 1995;80:898-904.

Lightman SW, Pisarska K, Berman ER: Discrepancy between self-reported and actual caloric intake and exercise in obese subjects. *N Engl J Med* 1992;327:1893-1898.

Lindholm C, Hagenfeldt K, Ringertz BM: Pubertal development in elite juvenile gymnasts: Effects of physical training. *Acta Obstet Gynecol Scand* 1994;73:269-273.

Theintz GE, Howald H, Weiss U, Sizonenko PC: Evidence for a reduction of growth potential in adolescent female gymnasts. *J Pediatr* 1993;122:306-313.

Subcommittee on the Tenth Edition of the RDAs, Food and Nutrition Board, Commission on Life Sciences, National Research Council: *Recommended Dietary Allowances*, ed 10. Washington, DC, National Academy Press, 1989.

US Department of Health, Education, and Welfare, Public Health Service: *Plan and Operation of a Health Examination Survey of US Youths 12-17 Years of Age: A Description of the Health Examination Survey's Third Cycle-Examinations of a Probability Sample of United States Youths 12-17 Years of Age*. Rockville, MD, Health Resources Administration, National Center for Health Statistics, 1974. DHEW Publication No. (HRA) 75-1018.

Section 6

Selected Sports-Related Issues

Section Editors:
Marlene DeMaio, MD, CAPT, MC, USN
Thomas M. Best, MD, PhD, FACSM

Chapter 27

Performance-Enhancing Supplements

Robert Sallis, MD, FACSM

Introduction

Competitive athletes often feel compelled to try anything that may give them an advantage on the playing field. Dietary supplements are commonly seen as a way to gain that advantage, and their use is encouraged by heavy marketing, increased availability of these products through the Internet and mail order, and recent reports of famous athletes using them. The dietary supplement market is largely unregulated; the US Food and Drug Administration (FDA) has little jurisdiction over these supplements because they are not considered drugs. This has given dietary supplement manufacturers the opportunity to make claims about the effectiveness and safety of their products, sometimes without good scientific evidence. In what has been estimated to be a $12 billion industry, approximately 89 brands of dietary supplements exist that offer more than 300 products. Of these, at least 235 claim to enhance muscle growth and/or performance. Because of the widespread use of dietary supplements, team physicians should have a working knowledge of the most common supplements used by competitive athletes.

Prevalence of Dietary Supplement Use

The biomedical literature contains little information regarding the prevalence of dietary supplement use among competitive athletes, and patterns of use are constantly changing. A 1994 meta-analysis of supplement use involving 10,274 athletes from 15 sports at all levels revealed a prevalence of 46%. Dietary supplement use was more common among elite athletes, followed by college athletes, and then by high school athletes. This study also showed that the use of such supplements by women was greater than among men, and use by athletes was greater than among the general population.

Each year the National Collegiate Athletic Association (NCAA) surveys athletes on substance use. The 2001 survey included questions regarding dietary supplements. Fifty-three percent of all athletes surveyed (from multiple sports) had used dietary supplements, with the most common among them being creatine and protein products.

A group of 263 NCAA Division III college football players was surveyed in 1998 to determine the prevalence and type of supplements used to enhance athletic performance. Of the 263 athletes surveyed, 230 (87%) admitted to previous use of dietary supplements to enhance athletic performance. A total of 24 substances were identified as having been used by these players. The most common dietary supplements used were creatine (78%), protein supplements (44%), antioxidant vitamins (37%), amino acids (32%), caffeine (19%), β-hydroxy-β-methylbutyrate (HMB) (16%), chromium (15%), androstenedione (13%), ephedrine (13%), dehydroepiandrosterone (DHEA) (8%), carnitine (7%), and pyruvate (4%).

Common Dietary Supplements Used by Athletes

Sports medicine physicians should be familiar with the dietary supplements that are commonly used by athletes to enhance athletic performance as well as have a working knowledge of the theories behind their use, dosing, adverse effects, and the scientific evidence that either supports or refutes the benefits of these supplements. A summary of the theories behind the use of less commonly used dietary supplements as well as their adverse effects, legal status, and the scientific evidence supporting or refuting their benefits is provided in Table 1. A list of NCAA banned-drug classes appears in Table 2.

Creatine

Creatine is an amino acid that is synthesized in the liver, pancreas, and kidneys. It is also available in meats and fish. Creatine can act as an energy bank by serving as a substrate for adenosine triphosphate (ATP) formation in skeletal muscles. In theory, higher creatine levels may accelerate regeneration of ATP (from adenosine diphosphate) and thus improve athletic power, strength, and speed. Creatine is also purported to decrease fatigue by buffering and delaying the buildup of lactic acid in skeletal muscle (Figure 1).

TABLE 1 | Summary of Less Commonly Used Nutritional Supplements

Supplement	Theory	Adverse Effects	Legality	Science
Arginine, ornithine, lysine	Stimulate growth hormone release	None at doses used	Legal	No benefit
Aspartate	Increase free fatty acid use, sparing muscle glycogen	Mild at high doses	Legal	Mixed, some positive benefits
Bee pollen	Increases strength and endurance	Allergic reaction	Legal	Refutes, no benefits
Boron	Increases endogenous steroid production	Mild at high doses	Legal	Refutes, no benefit
Calcium	Increases muscle contractility, enhances glycogen metabolism	Mild at high doses	Legal	Refutes, no benefit
Carbohydrates	Increase endurance, decrease fatigue	Mild at high doses	Legal	Supports
Carnitine	Increases fat metabolism	None	Legal	Refutes
Chrysin	Inhibits aromatase, increases endogenous steroids	None	Legal	Limited, refutes
Coenzyme Q10 (ubiquinone)	Delays fatigue, acts as antioxidant	None	Legal	Refutes, no benefit
Coenzyme Q12	Increases aerobic capacity, speeds muscle repair	None	Legal	Refutes, no benefit
Fat supplements	Increase endurance	Mild	Legal	Refutes
Folic acid	Increases aerobic capacity	None	Legal	Refutes
Gamma-hydroxybutyrate	Stimulates growth hormone release and muscle growth	Significant, dose-related; abuse potential	Illegal	Limited, refutes
Ginseng	Increases endurance, enhances muscle recovery	Mild, abuse syndrome reported	Legal	Limited, refutes, no benefit
Glucosamine	Serves as a nonsteroidal anti-inflammatory drug alternative, enhances recovery	None	Legal	Limited, may have limited nonsteroidal anti-inflammatory drug abilities
Glutamine	Boosts immunity and growth hormone levels	None	Legal	May boost immunity, no other benefits
Glycerol	Improves hydration and endurance	Mild	Legal (oral)	Limited, supports
Guarana (herbal caffeine)	Increases muscle contractility and aerobic endurance, enhances fat metabolism	Mild	Legal to urine level 12-15 µg/mL	Supports
Inosine	Enhances energy production, improves aerobic capacity	Mild	Legal	Refutes, no benefit
Iron	Increases aerobic capacity	Mild, toxic at high doses	Legal	No benefit unless preexisting deficiency
Leucine	Decreases muscle breakdown and spare muscle glycogen stores	None	Legal	Limited, no ergogenic effect
Magnesium	Enhances muscle growth	Mild at high doses	Legal	No benefit unless preexisting deficiency
Multivitamins	Increase energy, endurance and aerobic capacity, enhance recovery	None at recommended daily allowances, some toxicities at high doses	Legal	No benefit unless preexisting deficiency
Niacin	Increases energy and endurance	Mild at high doses	Legal	No benefit unless a preexisting deficiency
Phosphates	Increase adenosine triphosphate production, energy and muscle endurance	Mild at high doses	Legal	Mixed, negative
Phytosterol	Stimulates release of endogenous steroids and growth hormone	Little data, allergic reaction possible	Legal	Refutes, no benefit
Pycnogenol	Boosts antioxidant levels, enhances recovery	None	Legal	Supports, dietary sources offer same benefit

The body normally uses 2 grams of creatine daily. The liver, kidneys, and pancreas produce about 1 gram, whereas the remainder is derived from dietary sources, especially beef and fish. Synthetic creatine is manufactured as powders, pills, and chewable tablets. Manufacturers recommend using a loading dose of 20 g/day for

TABLE 1 | Summary of Less Commonly Used Nutritional Supplements (*continued*)

Supplement	Theory	Adverse Effects	Legality	Science
Pyruvate	Increases lean body mass	None	Legal	Limited research, benefit only in specific cases
D-Ribose	Increases cellular adenosine triphosphate and muscle power	None known	Legal	No human research
Selenium	Enhances antioxidant functions	Mild at high doses	Legal	Limited, no benefit
Sodium bicarbonate	Buffers lactic acid production, delays fatigue	Mild, dangerous at high doses	Legal	Supports
Strychnine	Unknown	Significant, dangerous	Legal	No research on ergogenic benefits
Tribulus terrestris	Increases endogenous steroid production	Potentially dangerous at high doses	Legal	Refutes
Tryptophan	Decreases pain perception, increases endurance	Mild, potentially dangerous	Legal	Mixed, no benefit in trained athletes
Vanadyl sulfate	Increases glycogen synthesis, enhances muscle recovery	Mild	Legal	Refutes, no benefit in healthy individuals
Vitamin B1 (thiamin)	Enhances energy production, increases aerobic capacity, improves concentration	None	Legal	No benefit unless preexisting deficiency
Vitamin B2 (riboflavin)	Increases aerobic endurance	None	Legal	No benefit unless preexisting deficiency
Vitamin B6 (pyridoxine)	Enhances muscle growth, decreases anxiety	Mild at high doses	Legal	No benefit unless preexisting deficiency
Vitamin B12 (cyanocobalamin)	Enhances muscle growth	None	Legal	No benefit unless preexisting deficiency
Vitamin B15 (dimethylglycine)	Increases muscle energy production	None proven, but concerns raised	Legal	Mixed, negative
Yohimbine	Increases endogenous steroid production	Mild	Legal	Refutes, no benefit
Zinc	Enhances muscle growth, increases aerobic capacity	Mild	Legal	Limited, negative

(Adapted with permission from Ahrendt DM: Ergogenic aids: Counseling the athlete. Am Fam Physician 2001;63:913-922.)

5 to 7 days, followed by a 2- to 5-gram daily dose. Alternatively, a "slow load" of 3 g/day for 28 days can be used. Both methods of supplementation have been shown to increase intracellular levels of creatine in muscle by about 20%.

Few clinically significant adverse effects have been reported for creatine, and short-term supplementation appears to be safe. However, the adverse effects of weight gain, nausea, bloating, diarrhea, and abdominal cramping may deter some from using this substance. Because of the increased protein load from creatine use (it may increase urinary creatinine 90-fold and serum creatinine by 20%), it is recommended that users of this dietary supplement stay well hydrated.

Numerous studies have demonstrated that creatine supplementation has ergogenic potential. Although not all studies are in agreement, there is a consensus that creatine use can improve the effects of short-duration (under 30 seconds), repetitive, high-intensity exercise. This may be beneficial in power sports such as football and sprinting. It has no effect on aerobic training or per-

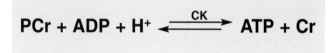

Figure 1 Reversible equilibrium of creatine (Cr) and phosphocreatine (PCr). ADP = adenosine diphosphate, H = hydrogen, CK = creatine kinase, ATP = adenosine triphosphate.

formance. Its value appears limited in those who have saturated baseline creatine stores (it may work better in vegetarians).

Protein Supplements

Protein supplements are manufactured in the form of powders, tablets, or liquids and have not shown any higher muscle absorption than natural sources of protein (beef, chicken, fish, legumes, or nuts). Protein supplementation beyond American Dietary Association recommendations is purported to aid in the synthesis of

Table 2 | NCAA Banned-Drug Classes (2002-2003)

Stimulants
Amiphenazole
Amphetamine
Bemigride
Benzphetamine
Bromantan
Caffeine (guarana)
Chlorphentermine
Cocaine
Cropropamide
Crothetamide
Diethylpropion
Dimethylamphetamine
Doxapram
Ephedrine (ephedra, ma huang)
Ethamivan
Ethylamphetamine
Fencamfamine
Meclofenoxate
Methamphetamine
Methylene-dioxymethamphetamine (Ecstasy)
Methylphenidate
Nikethamide
Pemoline
Pentetrazol
Phendimetrazine
Phenmetrazine
Phentermine
Phenylpropanolamine (effective August 2003)
Picrotoxine
Pipradol
Prolintane
Strychnine
  and related compounds*

Anabolic Agents
Anabolic steroids
Androstenediol
Androstenedione
Boldenone
Clostebol
Dehydrochlormethyl-testosterone
Dehydroepiandrosterone
Dihydrotestosterone
Dromostanolone
Fluoxymesterone
Mesterolone
Methandienone
Methenolone
Methyltestosterone
Nandrolone

Anabolic Agents (*continued*)
Norandrostenediol
Norandrostenedione
Norethandrolone
Oxandrolone
Oxymesterone
Oxymetholone
Stanozolol
Testosterone
  and related compounds*

Other Anabolic Agents
Clenbuterol

Substances Banned for Specific Sports (Riflery)
Alcohol
Atenolol
Metoprolol
Nadolol
Pindolol
Propranolol
Timolol
  and related compounds*

Diuretics
Acetazolamide
Bendroflumethiazide
Benzthiazide
Bumetanide
Chlorothiazide
Chlorthalidone
Ethacrynic acid
Flumethiazide
Furosemide
Hydrochlorothiazide
Hydroflumethiazide
Methyclothiazide
Metolazone
Polythiazide
Quinethazone
Spironolactone
Triamterene
Trichlormethiazide
  and related compounds*

Street Drugs
Heroin
Marijuana
Tetrahydrocannabinol

Peptide Hormones and Analogs
Chorionic gonadotrophin (human chorionic gonadotrophin)
Corticotrophin (adrenocorticotrophic hormone)
Growth hormone (human growth hormone, somatotrophin)

*The term "related compounds" comprises substances that are included in the class by their pharmacologic action and/or chemical structure. No substance belonging to the prohibited class may be used, regardless of whether it is specifically listed as an example. Nutritional supplements are not strictly regulated and may contain substances banned by the NCAA. All the respective releasing factors of the above-mentioned substances also are banned (erythropoietin and sermorelin). Definitions of positive test results depend on the following: (1) if the concentration in urine exceeds 15 µg/mL for caffeine; (2) if the administration of testosterone or the use of any other manipulation has the result of increasing the ratio of the total concentration of testosterone to that of epitestosterone in the urine to greater than 6:1, unless there is evidence that this ratio is the result of a physiologic or pathologic condition; and (3) if the concentration of tetrahydrocannabinol metabolite in the urine exceeds 15 ng/mL for marijuana and tetrahydrocannabinol. (Available at: http://www1.ncaa.org/membership/ed_outreach/health-safety/drug_testing/index.html.)

new muscle proteins and thus enhance strength.

The recommended daily allowance (RDA) for protein is 0.8 mg/kg/day. For athletes training in strength and endurance sports, an intake of 1.2 to 2.0 g/kg/day of protein has been recommended. The average American diet supplies 1.4 g/kg/day (about 119 grams) of protein. The extra protein needs of athletes can be easily met by increasing the amount of protein derived from food sources. Excess protein is not converted to additional muscle; instead, it is converted to energy stores in the form of fat. No serious adverse effects have been shown at doses up to 2 g/kg/day, and the most commonly reported adverse effects are stomach cramps and diarrhea. Its use in high doses may be a concern in athletes with renal insufficiency.

Athletes engaging in regular strength and endurance training appear to need more protein than when not training. However, the scientific literature does not show that protein supplementation beyond recommended levels has an ergogenic effect. Protein supplements may be helpful for female athletes consuming low-protein diets because of concern over body weight.

Antioxidant Vitamins

Vitamin C

Vitamin C (ascorbic acid) is a water-soluble substance commonly found in citrus fruits, tomatoes, strawberries, and other fresh fruits and vegetables. Vitamin C is required for a variety of biochemical functions (ie, synthesis of collagen, adrenaline, and the stress hormone cortisol). It is also important for connective tissue stability, wound healing, and energy production in muscle cells. A powerful antioxidant, vitamin C scavenges free radicals produced during exercise that can cause tissue damage. Based on these effects, a high dose of vitamin C has been purported to improve physical and aerobic power, speed recovery from injury, and enhance immunity.

The RDA for vitamin C is 60 mg/day, but doses up to 1,000 mg/day are commonly used. Doses of 1 to 3 g/day have been described for treatment of the common cold. The primary risk is the formation of kidney stones, but this is controversial.

Current research suggests that inadequate vitamin C intake can decrease athletic performance. However, high-dose dietary supplementation with vitamin C has not been shown to have ergogenic effects in humans. An interesting finding is that high-dose vitamin C supplementation has shown evidence of improved muscle endurance in animals. Although dietary supplementation with vitamin C is not clearly ergogenic in humans, athletic performance may be impaired if vitamin C stores are low. Also, vitamin C may provide immunologic benefits to endurance athletes. Daily supplementation with vitamin C 1 to 3 weeks before participating in a marathon or ultra-

marathon has been shown to decrease the incidence of postrace upper respiratory tract infection by as much as 33%.

Vitamin E

Vitamin E (α-tocopherol) is a fat-soluble vitamin that can scavenge free radicals. It is widely available in food, primarily vegetable oils, whole grains, and nuts. The theory behind the beneficial effect of vitamin E supplementation is that by scavenging free radicals formed during exercise, it may decrease delayed onset muscle soreness and improve anaerobic capacity.

The RDA for vitamin E is 10 to 30 IU/day, but supplementation can be as high as 800 to 1,200 IU/day. A typical dose is 400 IU/day. Vitamin E is generally safe, even at high doses. Reported adverse effects include gastrointestinal upset, weakness, fatigue, and rash.

Studies suggest that vitamin E supplementation may increase the anaerobic threshold and time to exhaustion at high altitudes via antioxidant protection. No proven benefit has been found for low-level exercise or in the prevention of delayed onset muscle soreness.

Amino Acids

Amino acids are the building blocks of protein and are available in tablet or powder form. Two formulations are commonly used: amino acids (essential and nonessential) and branched-chain amino acids (BCAAs). Because amino acids are the structural building blocks of protein, increasing the bioavailability of amino acids in the body is believed to cause a subsequent rise in protein synthesis. This rise is particularly important to athletes because of the catabolic effect exercise can have on protein metabolism through amino acid oxidation. BCAAs (leucine, isoleucine, and valine) have been advertised as being an important source of energy during endurance-type athletic activities. The theory behind the use of BCAAs is known as the central fatigue hypothesis. It is a complex theory that proposes the levels of BCAAs decrease with exercise and that more tryptophan therefore crosses the blood-brain barrier and leads to increased serotonin levels and fatigue. BCAAs in supplements are thought to compete with tryptophan and thus ward off fatigue.

BCAAs are available in tablet or powder form and are often mixed with other amino acids. Typical doses range from 5 to 10 g/day before exercise and are often added to carbohydrate solutions. Although minimal harm comes from short-term supplementation with small quantities of amino acids, increased dosages can cause gastrointestinal adverse effects such as stomach upset and diarrhea; the long-term adverse effects, however, have not been determined.

Numerous studies have shown that athletes undertaking strength and endurance training have a higher protein requirement than other people. In addition, it is known that particular amino acids are essential for human functioning. Despite these findings, the ergogenic benefit of dietary supplementation with amino acids for athletes remains unproven.

The central fatigue hypothesis has been researched in numerous ways: by measuring the rate of perceived exertion, by cognitive testing, and by measuring the time to exhaustion. Increases in plasma BCAA levels have been observed, but results showing ergogenic benefits of BCAA supplementation have been equivocal at best.

Athletes should be educated about the limited evidence that currently exists for using amino acid supplements, and less expensive options for increasing protein intake (through dietary modification) should be recommended.

Caffeine

Caffeine is a xanthine derivative and is the most widely consumed drug in the world. Caffeine is purported to increase the metabolic rate and mental awareness and decrease the perception of fatigue. By doing so, the time to exhaustion in middle-distance aerobic activity is increased. The beneficial effects of caffeine may be central or peripheral.

Most studies have used a single dose of 3 to 15 mg/kg (equivalent to 210 to 1,050 mg in a 70-kg man) taken before exercise. Caffeine concentrations in beverages include 60 to 150 mg per cup of brewed coffee (40 to 110 mg for instant coffee) and 40 to 50 mg per 12-ounce cola beverage. Vivarin (GlaxoSmithKline, Brentford, UK) tablets contain 200 mg of caffeine. Higher doses of caffeine (8 to 10 cups of coffee) can cause headache, palpitations, heartburn, stomach upset, the urge to defecate, and dizziness. The diuretic effect of caffeine may hinder athletic performance in hot weather.

The International Olympic Committee has set a threshold for caffeine in Olympic athletes at 12 µg/mL in urine (the NCAA threshold is 15 µg/mL for NCAA athletes). This limit can be achieved with 5 to 6 cups of coffee (urinary excretion of caffeine is decreased with exercise). Caffeine is the only dietary supplement with a threshold, rather than an absolute ban.

Low to moderate doses of caffeine may be ergogenic for endurance activities. At least one study of endurance cyclists and runners has shown that caffeine increases time to exhaustion by as much as 50%. It seems that caffeine's main benefit is for intense exercise of longer than 5 minutes occurring at the end of a prolonged bout of exercise (for example, the final stretch of a 10-kilometer race). The benefits seem to be less significant in untrained or recreational athletes. Additionally, benefits may depend on caffeine abstinence for several days before caffeine administration.

β-hydroxy-β-methylbutyrate

HMB is an amino acid metabolite of leucine that is not considered an essential nutrient. It is also found in citrus fruits, catfish, and breast milk. HMB is one of the newest supplements reported to have ergogenic properties. Although the function of HMB in the body is not fully known, it has been hypothesized to inhibit protein breakdown. Promoters of HMB suggest that an increase in HMB levels decrease protein catabolism and thus creates an anabolic effect, leading to increased muscle mass and strength. Body builders often use it.

HMB is available as an over-the-counter supplement, with a suggested dosage of 1 gram three times per day. The mean cost for a 10-day supply of over-the-counter HMB is $25. Although preliminary information on HMB is encouraging, little information exists as to potential adverse effects or consequences of long-term use. Several studies in animals and a peer-reviewed, randomized, double-blind, placebo-controlled study in humans suggest that HMB enables muscle mass and strength to increase in a dose-dependent fashion. Because information about HMB is limited, however, any recommendation favoring HMB as a safe ergogenic supplement would be premature.

Chromium

Chromium is an essential trace mineral that is found in various foods such as mushrooms, prunes, nuts, whole grains, breads, cereals, and American cheese. It is sold predominantly in the form of chromium picolinate (because picolinic acid is thought to aid chromium absorption). Chromium is a known cofactor of insulin that enhances its action at the cellular level. Chromium initially gained popularity as a dietary supplement because of claims that it could enhance weight loss and decrease body fat. Its use became popular among athletes after an increase in chromium excretion was observed following exercise. This conclusion led to a still unproved belief that athletes could easily become chromium-deficient. More recently, aggressive promotion of chromium as a "safe alternative" to anabolic steroids—both for increasing muscle mass and for decreasing body fat—caused a surge of chromium use among bodybuilders and weightlifters.

No RDA for chromium has been set, but the current Estimated Safe and Adequate Daily Dietary Intake is 50 to 200 µg/day. In doses of 50 to 200 µg/day taken for less than 1 month, few adverse effects other than gastrointestinal intolerance are reported. More serious adverse effects (anemia, interstitial nephritis, cognitive impairment, and chromosomal damage) have been shown to occur with prolonged use or excessive dosages of chromium.

Chromium has been shown to increase muscle mass in animals, but results of human studies are less convincing. Early studies did show an increase in lean body mass after chromium use; however, the results of these studies have since come into question because of the body fat measurement techniques used. More recent studies using better measurement techniques showed no benefit of chromium supplementation on lean body mass. In addition, no known study has shown a clinically significant increase in strength after chromium supplementation, and the ineffectiveness of chromium as an ergogenic aid is becoming increasingly obvious with each new study. In a 1996 attempt to regulate misleading advertisements, the US Federal Trade Commission ordered chromium manufacturers to cease making unsubstantiated claims that their product promoted weight loss and health benefits. Considering the potential risks of chromium supplementation and the lack of proof for its ergogenic benefits, health care practitioners should strongly discourage the use of chromium supplements.

Androstenedione

Androstenedione has been called a steroid "prohormone" that is converted to testosterone in the body (Figure 2). It is produced in small quantities by the gonads and adrenal glands. Although androstenedione is advertised as a dietary supplement, it is not part of a normal diet. It is popular among weightlifters and became world famous after home-run hero Mark McGwire admitted to using it during his record-breaking 1998 season. Androstenedione has little intrinsic activity, but it is a direct precursor of both testosterone and estrogen. The basis for use of androstenedione is evidence that supraphysiologic doses of testosterone increase muscle mass and strength. Manufacturers of commercial androstenedione characterize it as a "prohormone" and claim that it can raise the testosterone level and thus increase strength and athletic performance. The recommended dose is 50 mg orally twice a day in pill form. Concerns exist that athletes are exceeding this dose in the belief that more is better.

There are currently no known studies that accurately assess the adverse effects of androstenedione. If androstenedione does in fact increase testosterone levels, it potentially has adverse effects similar to those of anabolic steroids. Additionally, there may be potential adverse effects related to increased estrogen levels. Athletes should also be advised that the use of androstenedione is banned by many athletic organizations, including the International Olympic Committee, the NCAA, and the National Football League, and its use can cause a positive steroid drug test result.

A recent study showed that neither short- nor long-term administration of androstenedione increased serum concentrations of free or total testosterone. It did, however, increase serum concentrations of estradiol and estrone. In addition, no difference in either strength or

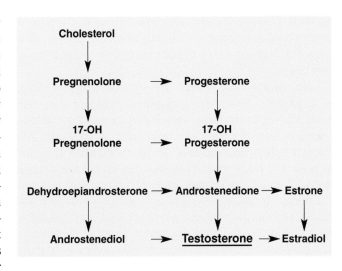

Figure 2 Pathway for testosterone synthesis.

lean body mass in response to training was shown when comparing androstenedione and placebo groups. Because androstenedione has questionable efficacy and the potential for adverse effects, its use should be strongly discouraged.

Ephedrine

Ephedrine is a sympathomimetic drug and central nervous system stimulant that has a structure and action similar to amphetamine. It is available as commercial ephedrine and in the herbs ma huang and *Ephedra sinica*. Although the FDA issued a ban on the sale of dietary supplements containing ephedrine in 2004, many athletes continue to use stockpiled stores of the drug. In addition, the FDA ban does not apply to traditional Chinese herbal remedies or teas that contain ephedrine. Ephedrine is listed as an ingredient in decongestants and in weight-loss products, and it is commonly added to creatine or protein powders when marketed to athletes. It is also commonly taken in combination with caffeine. Ephedrine is marketed as an energy booster that can aid workouts and enhance speed, strength, and performance. More recently, ephedrine has been touted as a fat burner and used by athletes to maintain or improve leanness.

Ephedrine is usually taken 45 minutes before a workout in doses of 25 mg per 100 lb, and it is often used 3 to 6 days per week for a 10- to 12-week period and combined with caffeine and aspirin (the ephedrine-caffeine-aspirin stack). Ephedrine users have been shown to have increased resting and exercise heart rates as well as longer cardiac recovery periods after exercise. Ephedrine can have a stimulatory effect on the central nervous system and can result in nervousness, insomnia, irritability, elevated blood pressure, and psychosis. Studies have also shown tolerance and dependence effects similar to those of alcohol or amphetamines. The Centers for Disease Control and Prevention has reported multiple adverse effects, including death, in people who ingested high doses of ephedrine before weight-lifting workouts.

No studies have proved that ephedrine taken alone is ergogenic. Ephedrine combined with caffeine has been shown to decrease run time, increase time to exhaustion, and decrease rate of perceived exertion. Although ephedrine has been shown to increase thermogenesis and body weight loss in obese individuals, there are no known studies that show ephedrine will act as a fat burner to promote leanness in athletes who are not obese. Despite its potential adverse effects and evidence that ephedrine does not enhance athletic performance, the stimulatory effect of this substance may continue to attract athletes.

Dehydroepiandrosterone

DHEA is an androgen produced by the adrenal glands and is a precursor in the formation of estrogen and testosterone (Figure 2). It can also be found in wild yams. Touting that DHEA has anabolic effects similar to those of testosterone, manufacturers have in recent years intensified their marketing efforts to encourage bodybuilders to use DHEA. Some advising bodybuilders claim that anabolic effects may be achieved by taking higher doses than manufacturers suggest. DHEA is also touted to enhance physical and psychologic well being in men older than 50 years.

DHEA is consumed orally in 50-mg and 100-mg tablet form and is widely available in pharmacies and grocery stores. Potential adverse effects of DHEA are similar to those of anabolic steroids and include acne, hair loss, increased levels of low-density lipoprotein, decreased levels of high-density lipoprotein cholesterol, gynecomastia in men, and hirsutism in women. Use can also alter the T:E ratio (the ratio of the concentration of testosterone to the concentration of epitestosterone), resulting in a positive steroids drug test result.

No evidence clearly shows that DHEA or similar testosterone precursors are anabolic, increase strength, or improve athletic performance when used at the recommended over-the-counter doses. Although several studies have shown DHEA can increase serum androstenedione concentrations, serum levels of testosterone were not affected.

Summary

Physicians who care for athletes should be aware of the dietary supplements commonly used today, as well as the efficacy and potential adverse effects of these products as described in the medical literature. Clinicians must be vigilant in asking patients about their use of dietary supplements because many patients fail to mention usage of these products unless specifically asked.

Current evidence suggests that creatine, HMB, caffeine, and ephedrine (when combined with caffeine) may provide some ergogenic or anabolic effects. In certain settings, the use of vitamin C and vitamin E may have some benefit for athletes participating in endurance sports and high-altitude exercise, respectively. No benefits have been proven for protein supplements, amino acids, chromium, androstenedione, ephedrine, and DHEA. Ephedrine and chromium have been associated with serious adverse effects. Athletes should understand that most studies on these substances have not examined their long-term effects. Dietary supplement use must not be viewed as the key to athletic success and cannot be a substitute for hard work and proper training.

Annotated Bibliography

Prevalence of Dietary Supplement Use
Green GA, Uryasz FD, Petr TA, Bray CD: NCAA study of substance use and abuse habits of college student-athletes. *Clin J Sport Med* 2001;11:51-56.

The authors of this study report that most student athletes engage in substance use, including dietary supplements to enhance athletic performance.

Common Dietary Supplements Used by Athletes
Ahrendt DM: Ergogenic aids: Counseling the athlete. *Am Fam Physician* 2001;63:913-922.

This article provides an in-depth review of some of the more popular dietary supplements used by athletes and provides basic information on many others.

Becque MD, Lochmann JD, Melrose DR: Effects of oral creatine supplementation on muscular strength and body composition. *Med Sci Sports Exerc* 2000;32:654-658.

The authors of this study report that creatine supplementation during arm flexor strength training improved strength compared with training alone.

Congeni J, Miller S: Supplements and drugs used to enhance athletic performance. *Pediatr Clin North Am* 2002;49:435-461.

This article provides a review of the literature for studies involving four common performance enhancing substances: anabolic steroids, prohormones, creatine, and Ephedra.

Greydanus DE, Patel DR: Sports doping in the adolescent athlete: The hope, hype and hyperbole. *Pediatr Clin North Am* 2002;49:829-855.

The authors of this study review the literature for studies on sports doping, including those that assess supplements, anabolic steroids, and blood doping.

Johnson WA, Landry GL: Nutritional supplements: Fact vs. fiction. *Adolesc Med* 1998;9:501-513.

The authors of this article summarize the facts and fiction surrounding the use of popular products that may be found at the pharmacy and health food store that are being used by high school and college athletes in the United States. They urge clinicians to stress the value of a well-balanced diet to their active adolescent patients and discourage nutritional supplement use.

Juhn MS, Tarnopolsky M: Oral creatine supplementation and athletic performance: A critical review. *Clin J Sport Med* 1998;8:286-297.

This study was conducted to review current data on oral creatine supplementation regarding its potential efficacy in athletic performance, mechanism of action, and metabolism.

King DS, Sharp RL, Vukovich MD, et al: Effect of oral androstenedione on serum testosterone and adaptations to resistance training in young men: A randomized controlled trial. *JAMA* 1999;281:2020-2028.

This study was conducted to determine whether short- and long-term oral androstenedione supplementation in men increases serum testosterone levels and skeletal muscle fiber size and strength and to examine its effect on blood lipids and markers of liver function. The authors conclude that androstenedione supplementation does not increase serum testosterone concentrations or enhance skeletal muscle adaptations to resistance training in normotestosterogenic young men and may result in adverse health consequences.

Powers SK, Hamilton K: Antioxidants and exercise. *Clin Sports Med* 1999;18:525-536.

The authors of this article review the basic science underlying the use of antioxidants to improve muscular performance and conclude that there is little evidence to support their use in this manner.

Schwenk TL, Costley CD: When food becomes a drug: Anabolic nutritional supplement use in athletes. *Am J Sports Med* 2002;30:907-916.

The authors of this article review the most commonly used nonanabolic nutritional supplements and offer suggestions for counseling athletes regarding their usage.

Sturmi JE, Diorio DJ: Anabolic agents. *Clin Sports Med* 1998;17:261-282.

The authors of this article provide a comprehensive assessment of four anabolic agents used by athletes: anabolic-androgenic steroids, DHEA, human growth hormone, and insulin-like growth factor.

Williams MH: Facts and fallacies of purported ergogenic amino acid supplements. *Clin Sports Med* 1999;18:633-649.

This article reviews data on the use of amino acid supplements to enhance athletic performance and concludes that the necessary amino acids are best obtained from natural high-quality protein foods.

Classic Bibliography

Armsey TD Jr, Green GA: Nutrition supplements: Science vs hype. *Phys Sportsmed* 1997;25:77-90.

Clarkson PM, Thomas HS: Drugs and sport: Research findings and limitations. *Sports Med* 1997;24:366-384.

Dekkers JC, van Doornen LJ, Kemper HC: The role of antioxidant vitamins and enzymes in the prevention of exercise-induced muscle damage. *Sports Med* 1996;21:213-238.

Nissen S, Sharp R, Ray M, et al: Effect of leucine metabolite beta-hydroxy-beta-methylbutyrate on muscle metabolism during resistance-exercise training. *J Appl Physiol* 1996;81:2095-2104.

Peters EM, Goetzsche JM, Grobbelaar B, Noakes TD: Vitamin C supplementation reduces the incidence of postrace symptoms of upper-respiratory-tract infection in ultramarathon runners. *Am J Clin Nutr* 1993;57:170-174.

Chapter 28

The Female Athlete Triad

Darryl B. Thomas, MD, MAJ, MC, USA

Dean C. Taylor, MD, COL, MC, USA

Introduction

When women first participated at the Olympic Games in 1928, fewer than two dozen competed in athletic events. At the 2000 Olympic Games held in Sydney, Australia, 38% of the approximately 10,000 athletes were women. In the United States, the prime impetus for increased participation by girls and women in sports occurred in 1972, when Title IX of the Education Amendment Act was passed. This law mandated that all schools receiving federal funding must provide equal opportunities for women's sports, and as a result, the number of girls participating in high school and collegiate sports has increased dramatically. In the 1971-1972 academic year, 294,015 girls participated in high school sports in the United States. By the 1998-1999 school year, this number had increased to over 2,652,000. Along with this surge in female athletic participation has come the awareness that female athletes may develop a unique set of medical and orthopaedic issues.

The term "female athlete triad" was coined in 1992 by the American College of Sports Medicine to describe three interrelated conditions that often occur together in female athletes: amenorrhea, disordered eating, and osteoporosis. The female athlete triad is being diagnosed with increasing frequency, particularly in young female athletes. It is caused by an imbalance between energy intake and energy expenditure. Athletes sometimes resort to disordered eating patterns for a variety of reasons, including weight requirements and a desire to achieve a specific physical image. Inadequate nutrition combined with excessive athletic training may lead to menstrual dysfunction and premature osteoporosis. The results not only impair health and athletic performance, but also can have negative effects on future well being.

Amenorrhea

Amenorrhea is the absence of menses. Typically, amenorrhea is classified as either primary or secondary. Primary amenorrhea, or delayed menarche, is defined as the absence of the onset of menstruation by the age of 16 years. Secondary amenorrhea is defined as the absence of menstrual bleeding for 6 months or the absence of three to six consecutive menstrual cycles after normal menses has begun. The mean age for menarche in the United States is 12.7 years, but menarche has been shown to be delayed in athletes who begin training before menarche. One study of 75 ballet dancers found the mean age of menarche to be 14.5 years, whereas another study of 201 gymnasts found the mean age to be 15.6 years.

Although approximately 2% to 5% of nonathletic women of reproductive age who are not pregnant or lactating experience some form of secondary amenorrhea, an increased incidence of amenorrhea has been found among female athletes. Amenorrhea coincident with heavy physical activity has long been recognized, and although the exact prevalence of amenorrhea is unknown, studies estimate the observed prevalence to be 10% to 20% in women who exercise vigorously and as high as 40% to 66% in elite runners and professional ballet dancers. The prevalence of secondary amenorrhea depends on the intensity of training. For example, it is 20% in women who run 20 miles per week, but it jumps dramatically to 43% in women who run more than 60 miles per week. Amenorrhea associated with exercise, or athletic amenorrhea, is a diagnosis of exclusion, and all other causes of amenorrhea must first be evaluated. Pregnancy is by far the most common cause of amenorrhea, and all sexually active amenorrheic women should be tested for pregnancy as part of their standard medical evaluation. Other important causes of amenorrhea include thyroid disease, polycystic ovary syndrome, premature ovarian failure, pituitary dysfunction, and anatomic or developmental disorders of the genital tract.

Amenorrhea is caused by a reduction in the frequency of luteinizing hormone (LH) and follicle-stimulating hormone pulses from the anterior pituitary gland. This suppresses estradiol from the ovaries and results in the loss or absence of menses. An interference in the frequency of gonadotropin releasing hormone secretion from the hypothalamus is thought to decrease LH pulses. The disruption of the hypothalamic-pituitary axis is the focus of current research on amenorrhea. In the 1970s, low body weight and low body fat were thought

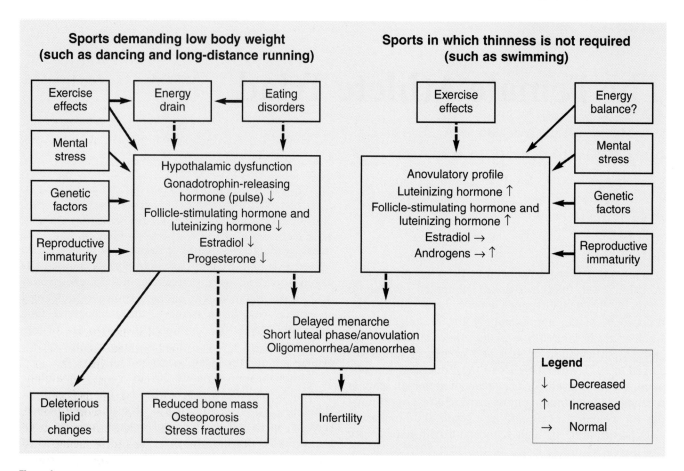

Figure 1 Two proposed mechanisms that can lead to menstrual dysfunction in female athletes. *(Reproduced with permission from Warren MP, Shantha S: The female athlete. Baillieres Best Pract Res Clin Endocrinol Metab 2000;14:37-53.)*

to be the primary causes of amenorrhea, but subsequent research has refuted these hypotheses and suggests other causes, including excessive amounts of physical training, skeletal immaturity or early age at which intense training starts, the stress or anxiety of training and competition, and poor nutrition. Although the etiology of athletic amenorrhea is most likely multifactorial, there are two main theories regarding its mechanism (Figure 1). One hypothesis involves hypothalamic dysfunction and prolonged periods of hypoestrogenism, which can occur in female athletes who participate in sports that demand low body weight. The other hypothesis involves mild hyperandrogenism, which is associated with participation in sports that do not require thinness.

Once thought to be a benign, reversible condition, amenorrhea is becoming recognized as a serious medical problem. Athletic amenorrhea can result in hypoestrogenemia similar to menopause and is associated with decreased bone mineral density (BMD) and increased risk for injury. Athletes particularly at risk are those who participate in endurance sports, such as long-distance running, rowing, cycling, and ballet. In the past, many serious athletes have mistakenly viewed amenor-

rhea as an indicator of adequate training intensity. Ballet dancers have been silently aware of this problem for at least the past decade, and some even consider amenorrhea to be a blessing in disguise. It must be emphasized that amenorrhea is not a desirable or even a "normal" result of heavy physical training.

The association between amenorrhea and cardiovascular disease is a focus of current research. The increased risk of cardiovascular disease in postmenopausal women led one center to undertake a study of 21 amenorrheic female runners. One of the associated precursors of cardiovascular disease is thought to be a loss of blood vessel dilation. Ultrasound was used to measure the ability of the blood vessels to dilate under various training conditions. Impaired vessel dilating capacity was identified in all 10 women with secondary amenorrhea and was similar to that found in 50-year-old postmenopausal women. No impairment was found in the 11 eumenorrheic control subjects.

Amenorrhea is the most recognizable symptom of the female athlete triad, and it may have serious long-term consequences. The loss of normal menses is a symptom of a serious condition that requires prompt medical assessment within the first 3 months of occurrence.

Disordered Eating

Adolescent male athletes are encouraged to gain weight to increase muscle mass and improve physical performance, whereas their female counterparts are often encouraged to lose weight to improve performance and/or physical appearance. High societal standards along with pressure from peers, coaches, and judges cause many young women to have unrealistic goals and perceptions regarding ideal body weight. Although competitive sports often require athletes to maintain daily caloric intake commensurate with the demands of an intense training regimen, many young female athletes choose to restrict their caloric intake (particularly protein) in an attempt to lose weight or body fat. This caloric restriction results in a failure to balance energy expenditures with energy intake and can cause multiple adverse changes throughout the musculoskeletal, cardiovascular, thermoregulatory, and endocrine systems.

Disordered eating refers to a continuum of abnormal eating patterns with poor nutritional habits at one end and anorexia and bulimia at the other. Anorexia nervosa is a severe restrictive eating disorder in which the individual views herself as overweight even though she is at least 15% below ideal body weight. Its prevalence is approximately 1% among young women. Amenorrhea is listed as one of the diagnostic criteria for anorexia nervosa in the *Diagnostic and Statistical Manual of Mental Disorders,* Fourth Edition (see chapter 26). Bulimia nervosa involves a cycle of food restriction leading to overeating or binging followed by purging. Its prevalence ranges from 1% to 4% among young women. This purging commonly involves self-induced vomiting, but it can also include the use of laxatives, diuretics, enemas, and excessive exercise. Acutely, these eating habits can cause fluid and electrolyte imbalances. Short-term morbidity including dehydration, acid-base imbalances, and cardiac arrhythmia has been reported. If not treated, these habits can also lead to more chronic medical problems including erosion of tooth enamel, gray-appearing teeth, halitosis, parotid gland enlargement, and gastrointestinal disorders.

Although most female athletes do not meet the criteria for anorexia nervosa or bulimia, many may be considered to have disordered eating habits. Disordered eating occurs in 5% of the general population, and female athletes often display various disordered eating practices. Vomiting, food restriction, prolonged fasting, low calorie diets (< 1,200 kcal/day), as well as diet pill, laxative, and supplement abuse should all be recognized as characteristics of disordered eating patterns requiring evaluation and treatment.

Disordered eating is often difficult to detect and treat. Because of the secretive nature of disordered eating patterns, it is difficult to establish their prevalence. Self-report questionnaires suggest a prevalence of 22% to 34%, whereas published studies report that between 32% and 64% of female athletes display some type of disordered eating. In another study, disordered eating was reported in 74% of gymnasts, 47% of long-distance runners, and 15% of elite swimmers.

In an attempt to lose weight, many female athletes practice unhealthy weight-control methods, have suboptimal caloric (energy) intake, and are at risk of compromised nutritional status. Coaching techniques that use strict weight standards, such as frequent weigh-ins, as well as pressure from peers and overly controlling parents, may all contribute to the development of eating disorders. This problem is not unique to female athletes; male wrestlers experience it as well. One study involving female US gymnasts demonstrates the dramatic results that coaching weigh-ins have had on young female participants. The results reveal a sharp reduction in mean height (4.9 inches), weight (28 lb), and age (2.3 years) over the past 40 years.

Any female athlete is at risk for the development of eating disorders and the female athlete triad. Athletes particularly at risk are those who participate in sports emphasizing leanness (long-distance running, cycling, and cross-country skiing), those who participate in activities in which performance is subjectively scored (dance, figure skating, diving, and gymnastics), those who compete in sports with weight categories (horse racing, wrestling, and rowing), and those who are involved in sports that require body contour-revealing clothing (swimming, diving, figure skating, ballet, cheerleading, and track). Many factors contribute to the development of disordered eating behaviors, including pressure to be thin, chronic dieting, low self-esteem and depression, familial dysfunction, physical or sexual abuse, and biologic factors.

Because disordered eating patterns are more likely to occur in women with a family history of disordered eating, familial patterns of disordered eating should be closely evaluated during the physical examinations of female athletes. Additional factors affecting the female athlete include perfectionism, lack of nutritional knowledge, the impact of injury and lost training time, and the drive to excel or win at any cost. In reality, despite the intention of the athlete, inadequate caloric intake and disordered eating ultimately impairs health and physical performance. Serious problems can result from the depletion of muscle glycogen stores, dehydration, loss of muscle mass, hypoglycemia, and anemia.

The effects of chronic poor nutritional health on the immune system are currently being studied. Exercise, competition, and training have all been shown to affect various components of the immune system, including lymphocyte subsets, immunoglobulin levels, the mononuclear phagocytic system, polymorphonuclear leukocytes, and cytokines (Figure 2). Changes in metabolism and hormone secretion are proportional to the degree

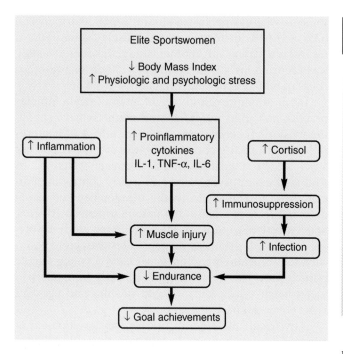

Figure 2 Severe consequences of low-caloric intake together with physiologic and psychologic stress on muscle, endurance, and goal achievements in women who participate in sports. IL = Interleukin, TNF-α = Tumor necrosis factor-alpha. *(Reproduced with permission from Montero A, Lopez-Varela S, Nova E, Marcos A: The implication of the binomial nutrition-immunity on sportswomen's health. Eur J Clin Nut 2002;56(suppl 3):S38-S41.)*

TABLE 1 | World Health Organization Guidelines for Interpretation of Bone Densitometry Results*

Normal	A value for BMD or BMC not more than 1 standard deviation below the average value of young adults
Low bone mass or osteopenia	A value for BMD or BMC more than 1 standard deviation below the young adult average, but not more than 2.5 standard deviations below
Osteoporosis	A value for BMD or BMC more than 2.5 standard deviations below the young adult average
Severe osteoporosis	A value for BMD or BMC more than 2.5 standard deviations below the young adult average value and the presence of one or more fragility fractures

*1 standard deviation change in BMD equals a 10% to 12% change in bone density; for every standard deviation of decrease in BMD in the elderly, the relative risk of fracture increases by a factor of 1.5 to 1.8. BMC = bone mineral content

(Adapted from Genant HK, van Kuijk, C: Bone densitometry, in Buckwalter J, Einhorn T, Simon S (eds): Orthopaedic Basic Science: Biology and Biomechanics of the Musculoskeletal System. Rosemont, IL, American Academy of Orthopaedic Surgeons, 2000, p 285.)

of physiologic stress encountered. Exercise-induced elevations in plasma catecholamines and corticosteroids are of particular interest because of their immunoregulatory effects. Although exercise is known to stimulate many immune functions, more rigorous training and the stress of competition can suppress various immune responses. According to one study, there is an increased risk of subclinical and clinical infection during these periods, most frequently upper respiratory tract infections.

There is also some evidence that immunocompetent cells are less effective in signaling defense mechanisms against infection after rigorous exercise. Intense training coupled with low caloric intake seems to be responsible for the altered immunocompetence, particularly cell-mediated immunity. Another study of elite gymnasts demonstrated decreased T-lymphocyte counts and increased production of inflammatory cytokines. Severely impaired nutritional intake may be partially responsible. It is imperative that those taking care of athletes are aware of the importance of good nutrition, not only to avoid medical problems, but also to improve their overall athletic performance.

Osteopenia and Osteoporosis

Osteopenia (reduced bone mass) is a frequent associated finding in patients with amenorrhea and low estrogen levels. The World Health Organization has defined osteopenia as BMD that is 1.0 to 2.5 standard deviation

points below the young adult reference mean (Table 1). Osteoporosis is defined as BMD that is more than 2.5 standard deviation points below the mean and is associated with pathological fractures, pain, and disability. The bone loss seen in young amenorrheic athletes is comparable to the bone loss seen in postmenopausal women or in women with a pathologic hypoestrogenic condition, such as premature ovarian failure, a pituitary tumor, or anorexia nervosa. Concern for athletes with low BMD caused by hypoestrogenemia revolves around the risk of the development of stress fractures and other injuries during their competitive years. Several published studies report a higher incidence of injuries and stress fractures among amenorrheic and oligomenorrheic athletes when compared with eumenorrheic athletes.

Risk factors for the development of stress fractures in young athletes include female sex, low bone density, delayed menarche, menstrual irregularities, lower dietary calcium, lower dietary fat, decreased calf girth, reduced lower extremity bone mass, limb-length discrepancy, increased training intensity, and a prior history of stress fracture. One survey of 71 young ballet dancers found that 61% had sustained stress fractures. Other prospective studies of female track and field athletes found the stress fracture incidence rate to be between 11% and 27%. Although these stress fractures commonly occur at the tibia, fibula, metatarsal, and navicular, fractures of the femoral neck and vertebral bodies can be particularly problematic and often career ending. Furthermore, if unrecognized and untreated, athletes with these types of stress fractures are also at future risk for the development of premature osteoporotic fractures, such as thoracolumbar compression fractures most commonly seen in the postmenopausal elderly.

Studies of postmenopausal women have shown that the degree of osteopenia is directly related to the age of onset and duration of amenorrhea. The degree of osteopenia also depends not only of the rate of bone loss, but on peak bone mass (PBM), which is the maximum amount of bone present at skeletal maturity. A person's PBM is one of the most important protective factors against osteoporosis, and the adolescent years are critical for PBM acquisition. PBM is typically achieved between the age of 24 and 34 years, and between 60% and 70% of PBM is accrued during adolescence. Any condition negatively impacting the accumulation of PBM can have long-lasting morbidity. If a young female athlete is amenorrheic and does not have a normal amount of bone during adolescence, she may always have decreased bone mass. Therefore, it is important to stress to these young women and their coaches and trainers that poor nutrition and the hypoestrogenemic state secondary to amenorrhea can have serious, life-long implications.

Researchers report that prior menstrual history is the best predictor of current BMD, and it has been shown that women with a history of amenorrhea have a lower BMD than those who have always been cyclic. Young amenorrheic athletes have been found to lose as much as 2% to 6% of bone mass per year. For example, an amenorrheic athlete in her 20s may lose as much as 25% of her bone density over time, leaving her with a bone mass comparable to that of a 60-year-old woman. Because the rate of bone loss is greatest within the first 5 to 6 years after the initial decrease in levels of endogenous estrogen, there may only be a brief window of opportunity to prevent irreversible bone loss.

Although higher body weight and exercise are associated with increased BMD, once the athlete becomes amenorrheic, the protective effect of weight-bearing exercise is lost. Amenorrheic runners have lower vertebral BMD than eumenorrheic runners. Although resumption of menses is usually associated with an increase in bone mass, the transient loss may not be reversible. It is important to know whether the hypoestrogenic low BMD condition can be treated or reversed to allow the accretion of normal bone mass. Several studies report an increase in BMD in amenorrheic athletes resuming their normal menses, but the gains in BMD appear to be limited. Furthermore, amenorrheic athletes using hormone replacement therapy (HRT) in doses typically reserved for menopausal women have shown maintenance of BMD, but no gains. Overall, the current literature suggests that restoration of normal menses may retard the rate of further bone loss, but that bone already lost may not be fully replaced.

The association of low BMD with increased injury rates has been well established. One recent study questions the association of osteoporosis with the female athlete triad. The authors scrutinized previous research examining BMD data for athletes at risk of the female athlete triad and found that although osteopenia has a significant prevalence, osteoporosis is relatively uncommon. One large review of athletes at risk found only a 10.3% lower lumbar spine BMD (as measured by dual energy x-ray absorptiometry), which falls within the lower limit of normal BMD or very early osteopenia. By definition, osteoporosis causes microarchitectural deterioration, increases skeletal fragility, and increases risk for fractures of the hip, wrist, and vertebral bodies. These fractures commonly occur in the elderly as a result of extremely low bone mass. The authors argue that bone disease that occurs in athletes with the female athlete triad places those athletes at increased risk for stress fractures, but not osteoporotic fractures. Therefore, osteopenia is the more appropriate term to use for most of these athletes. Osteoporosis can and does occur in athletes; however, authors are concerned that requiring this condition to be present in the female athlete triad relegates this syndrome to relative obscurity. They suggest that if either osteopenia or osteoporosis were accepted as criteria for impaired bone health, the female athlete triad would have greater prevalence and clinical relevance. Any female athlete with osteopenia would benefit from optimizing her lifestyle to maintain bone mass and increase bone strength.

Prevention and Treatment

The most effective treatment of the female athlete triad is prevention. Physicians must educate athletes, parents, coaches, and trainers about the dangers of the female athlete triad, with emphasis on proper nutritional requirements for normal growth and development during adolescence as well as increased energy requirements during intensive training. Early diagnosis is critical, and early signs may be subtle. An ideal time to screen for those athletes at risk is during the preparticipation physical examination. The history and physical form recommended by the American College of Sports Medicine contains questions about menstrual history, including age at menarche, last menstrual period, frequency and duration of periods, and the use of birth control pills or HRT (Table 2). Amenorrhea should be seen as a red flag that necessitates a more detailed history and physical examination.

A thorough nutritional history is another important part of the preparticipation physical examination. Questions should include the number of daily meals and snacks, a list of forbidden foods, the amount of satisfaction with current body weight, the highest and lowest weights since menarche, recent weight loss, and the use of vomiting, laxatives, diet pills, or diuretics to control weight. It is imperative that young athletes consume enough daily calories to meet their increased energy requirements. Despite running an average of 10 miles per

TABLE 2 | Screening History for the Female Athlete Triad

Menstrual History

Age at menarche

Frequency and duration of menstrual cycles

Longest period of time without menstruation

Last menstrual period

Physical signs of ovulation, such as cervical mucus change or menstrual cramps

Hormonal replacement therapy taken previously and currently

Diet History

What was eaten in the past 24 hours?

List of any forbidden foods

Highest/lowest weight since menarche

Satisfaction with current weight

Ideal weight according to the patient

Disordered eating practices (bingeing and purging)

Use of laxatives, diuretics, or pills

Exercise History

Exercise patterns and training intensity for the sport (hours per day and days per week)

Additional exercise outside of required training

History of previous fractures

History of overuse injuries

(Reproduced with permission from Hobart JA, Smucker DS: The female athlete triad. Am Fam Physician 2000;61:3357-3367.)

TABLE 3 | Guidelines for Calcium Requirements

Group	Daily Elemental Calcium Requirements (mg)*
Children	500 to 700
Growth spurt to young adult (10 to 25 years of age)	1,300
Adult male (25 to 65 years of age)	750
Adult female (25 to 65 years of age)	
Postmenopausal	1,500
Elderly	1,200
Pregnant	1,500
Lactating	2,000
Healing long bone fracture (women and men)	1,500

*One daily equivalent of calcium is equal to 250 mg of elemental calcium; one equivalent is equal to an 8-ounce glass of milk

(Adapted from Broström MPG, Boskey A, Kaufman J, Einhorn TA: Form and function of bone, in Buckwalter J, Einhorn T, Simon S (eds): Orthopaedic Basic Science: Biology and Biomechanics of the Musculoskeletal System. Rosemont, IL, American Academy of Orthopaedic Surgeons, 2000, p 356.)

day, the mean daily caloric intake of one group of amenorrheic runners was reported to be only 1,600 calories. The recommended daily caloric intake for female runners to preserve proper menstrual function and prevent BMD loss is 2,500 calories per day.

Physical signs of disordered eating should be identified during the physical examination. These athletes may not necessarily be very thin. Presenting signs include bradycardia and/or hypotension, lanugo hair, parotid gland swelling, erosion of tooth enamel, and skin trauma to the hand (from persistent gastric secretion during induced vomiting).

Athletes should be questioned about the history of stress fractures because such fractures are not only a major indicator of low BMD, but also a strong predictive factor for the future development of stress fractures. A summary of typical weekly training and competition regimens can help identify those athletes who should be observed closely throughout the season. Weight-bearing exercise and resistance training have been shown to be important in maintaining adequate BMD. A recent study also identified lean body mass and leg power to be predictors of BMD, suggesting a role for muscle mass development during growth to maximize peak bone density. Other researchers have found similar relationships between BMD and muscle strength in fe-

male college athletes when compared with nonathletic young women. Plyometric training has also been shown to increase BMD, but many athletes find that these routines exacerbate stress injuries of the lower extremities. Data are still lacking regarding the optimal exercise program that would minimize injury while effectively stimulating bone mass accretion in those who have not yet reached their PBM.

Calcium is one of the most important interventions in optimizing bone health. Several controlled trials in prepubescent and adolescent girls found that calcium supplementation resulted in an increase in BMD as high as 14%. Proper therapy should follow the National Institutes of Health guidelines for calcium intake by age group, with the added recommendation of 1,500 mg per day in the female athlete with oligomenorrhea or amenorrhea (Table 3). Vitamin D, which stimulates osteoblasts and increases calcium absorption must be supplemented in the range of 400 to 800 IU per day.

Nasal calcitonin used to increase BMD has been approved by the US Food and Drug Administration (FDA) for the treatment of osteoporotic stress fractures in postmenopausal women and elderly men, but its role in the treatment of young female athletes has not yet been elucidated. Although bisphosphonates have been used to treat postmenopausal women, they are not recommended nor are they approved by the FDA for the treatment of women of child-bearing age because of the teratogenic effects seen in animal studies. In addition, the selective estrogen receptor modulators approved for the prevention and treatment of postmenopausal osteoporosis have been shown to cause bone loss in premenopausal women in several studies and should therefore not be used to treat women of child-bearing age.

Although many physicians use HRT to treat athletic amenorrhea, no published longitudinal studies exist evaluating the long-term benefits of HRT to slow or reverse the loss of BMD or decrease the risk of stress fractures. Most of the evidence is extrapolated from data supporting the use of HRT to treat postmenopausal women. Some short-term controlled studies have found an increase in BMD in those receiving HRT compared with placebo. Other retrospective studies of athletes have shown that birth control pill use may result in a decreased risk of stress fracture. Despite the lack of direct evidence on the appropriate timing for initiation of HRT, most physicians will consider HRT after 6 months of amenorrhea. Those athletes already exhibiting decreased BMD should also be strongly encouraged to start HRT. Currently, estrogen therapy is favored over progesterone therapy.

Summary

The female athlete triad, a syndrome of amenorrhea, disordered eating, and impaired bone health (osteoporosis versus osteopenia), is now a clearly recognizable condition in competitive female athletes. The components of this triad are linked pathophysiologically and can result in significant immediate and life-long morbidity. Principles of treatment include reducing the intensity of training until menses resumes, increasing caloric intake, ensuring adequate calcium and vitamin D supplementation, encouraging weight-bearing exercise when appropriate, and considering HRT. Although HRT can be used to treat athletic amenorrhea, the ultimate goal is the return of normal menses. Adequate, long-standing intervention often requires a multidisciplinary approach, involving parents, athletic trainers, physicians, coaches, and frequently sports psychologists. Prevention of the female athlete triad through education, recognition of those at risk, and early diagnosis is paramount to the health and safety of female athletes.

Annotated Bibliography

General

Golden NH: A review of the female athlete triad (amenorrhea, osteoporosis and disordered eating). *Int J Adolesc Med Health* 2002;14:9-17.

This article outlines the principles of treatment for the female athlete triad, including prevention, reducing the intensity of training until menses resumes, increasing caloric intake, ensuring adequate calcium and vitamin D intake, and considering HRT.

Amenorrhea

Donaldson ML: The female athlete triad: A growing health concern. *Orthop Nurs* 2003;22:322-324.

The female athlete triad is a significant health concern. As more young women participate in sports, the population at risk is increasing. The authors conclude, therefore, that it is imperative that orthopaedic surgeons are educated about its detection and treatment.

Sabatini S: The female athlete triad. *Am J Med Sci* 2001; 322:193-195.

This article reports that the female athlete triad is often seen in athletes who participate in sports that place an emphasis on "thinness," including gymnastics, figure skating, and ballet. The author concludes that the female athlete triad is difficult to treat and requires a multidisciplinary approach with intense psychologic counseling.

Warren M, Shantha S: The female athlete. *Baillieres Best Pract Res Clin Endocrinol Metab* 2000;14:37-53.

This article reports that reduced nutritional intake and negative caloric balance lead to reproductive system dysfunction in female athletes. The authors conclude that a hypoestrogenemic state results from hypothalamic dysfunction and leads to decreased BMD, decreased PBM, and stress fractures.

Wilson S: An ignored epidemic. *Training & Conditioning* 2002;12.8:12-19. [serial online] Available at http://www.momentummedia.com/articles/tc/tc1208/epidemic.htm. Accessed February 19, 2004.

The author of this article reports that athletic amenorrhea is a growing problem among female student athletes. The author concludes that because current studies estimate that 28% of collegiate female athletes experience amenorrhea, education, recognition, and early treatment are essential to maintaining life-long health.

Disordered Eating

Bass M, Turner L, Hunt S: Counseling female athletes: Application of the stages of change model to avoid disordered eating, amenorrhea, and osteoporosis. *Psychol Rep* 2001;88:1153-1160.

Because health professionals can play an important role in the prevention and treatment of the female athlete triad, the authors of this article examine the stages of change model and provide theoretical applications of this model for reducing harmful behaviors in female athletes.

Beals KA, Manore MM: Disorders of the female athlete triad among collegiate athletes. *Int J Sport Nutr Exerc Metab* 2002;12:281-293.

The authors report that athletes at risk for eating disorders more frequently have menstrual irregularity and bone injuries. They conclude that although the prevalence of clinical eating disorders is low in female college athletes, many are at risk for an eating disorder and its associated problems.

Montero A, Lopez-Varela S, Nova E, Marcos A: The implication of the binomial nutrition-immunity on sportswomen's health. *Eur J Clin Nut* 2002;56(suppl 3):S38-S41.

Because the combination of poor nutrition and stress faced by the female athlete is linked to damaged immunocompetence and increases susceptibility to infections, the authors of this article suggest that it is important to take care of nutritional status in this population to improve performance and avoid medical complications.

Osteopenia and Osteoporosis

Khan KM, Liu-Ambrose T, Sran MM, Ashe MC, Donaldson MG, Wark JD: New criteria for female athlete triad syndrome? As osteoporosis is rare, should osteopenia be among the criteria for defining the female athlete triad syndrome? *Br J Sports Med* 2002;36:10-13.

Osteoporosis does occur in female athletes, but osteopenia is far more prevalent. The authors argue that requiring osteoporosis to be present to diagnose the female athlete triad may miss a large number of athletes with suboptimal bone mass who are at risk for injury.

Nattiv A: Stress fractures and bone health in track and field athletes. *J Sci Med Sport* 2000;3:268-279.

The authors report that the incidence of stress fractures in female track athletes is 11% to 21% and that the tibia is the common site of such fractures. They also report that the risk factors for stress fractures include delayed menarche, menstrual dysfunction, low BMD, low calcium intake, and a prior history of stress fractures.

Prevention and Treatment

Hobart JA, Smucker DR: The female athlete triad. *Am Fam Physician* 2000;61:3357-3364, 3367.

Because the consequences of lost BMD can be devastating for the female athlete and result in premature osteoporotic fractures, the authors of this article suggest that early recognition of the female athlete triad can be accomplished via risk factor assessment and screening questions.

Witzke KA, Snow CM: Lean body mass and leg power best predict bone mineral density in adolescent girls. *Med Sci Sports Exerc* 1999;31:1558-1563.

The authors of this study found that lean body mass and leg power best predicted bone mineral content and BMD of the whole body, lumbar spine, femoral shaft, and hip in young female athletes. They also report that plyometric jump training improved bone mass.

Classic Bibliography

Calabrese LH: Nutritional and medical aspects of gymnastics. *Clin Sports Med* 1985;4:23-37.

Classens AL, Malina RM, Lefevre J, et al: Growth and menarcheal status of elite female gymnasts. *Med Sci Sports Exerc* 1992;24:755-763.

Drinkwater BL, Bruemner B, Chesnut CH: Menstrual history as a determinant of current bone density in young athletes. *JAMA* 1990;263:545-548.

Marcus R, Cann C, Madvig P, et al: Menstrual function and bone mass in elite women distance runners: Endocrine and metabolic features. *Ann Intern Med* 1985;102:158-163.

Marshall LA: Clinical evaluation of amenorrhea, in Agostini R, Titus S (eds): *Medical and Orthopaedic Issues of Active and Athletic Women*. Philadelphia, PA, Hanley & Belfus, 1994, pp 152-163.

Myburgh KH, Bachrach LK, Lewis B, et al: Low bone mineral density at axial and appendicular sites in amenorrheic athletes. *Med Sci Sports Exerc* 1993;25:1197-1202.

Nattiv A, Agostini R, Drinkwater B, Yeager KK: The female athlete triad: The inter-relatedness of disordered eating, amenorrhea, and osteoporosis. *Clin Sports Med* 1994;13:405-417.

Otis CL, Drinkwater B, Johnson M, Loucks A, Wilmore J: ACSM position stand: The female athlete triad. *Med Sci Sports Exerc* 1997;29:i-ix.

Renckens ML, Chesnut CH III, Drinkwater BL: Bone density at multiple sites in amenorrheic athletes. *JAMA* 1996;276:238-240.

Teitz C, Hu S, Arendt E: The female athlete: Evaluation and treatment of sports-related problems. *J Am Acad Orthop Surg* 1997;5:87-96.

Theintz GE, Howard H, Weiss U, et al: Evidence for a reduction of growth potential in adolescent female gymnasts. *J Pediatr* 1993;122:306-313.

Warren MP, Brooks-Gunn J, Hamilton LH, Warren LF, Hamilton WG: Scoliosis and fractures in young ballet dancers: Relations to delayed menarche and secondary amenorrhea. *N Engl J Med* 1986;314:1348-1353.

Yeager KK, Agostini R, Nattiv A, et al: The female athlete triad: Disordered eating, amenorrhea, osteoporosis. *Med Sci Sports Exerc* 1993;25:775-777.

Chapter 29

Ultrasound and Radiofrequency in Sports Surgery

George A. Corbett, MD

Marc T. Galloway, MD

Introduction

Ultrasound and radiofrequency energy devices are becoming increasingly popular as therapeutic modalities in the treatment of sports-related injuries. Each has inherent advantages as well as potential adverse effects that warrant further investigation. Although their use is becoming more widespread, the science supporting them is still developing.

Ultrasound

Ultrasound refers to energy above the audibly perceptible range of frequencies (20 Hz to 20 kHz). The frequency used for therapeutic ultrasound is usually 0.5 MHz, whereas the frequency for diagnostic ultrasound ranges from 2 to 10 MHz. Ultrasound is a form of mechanical energy that is transmitted through and into biologic tissues as acoustic pressure waves.

Musculoskeletal ultrasound is increasingly being used in the evaluation and treatment of sports-related injuries. The technique is widely available, rapid, noninvasive, and has a high rate of patient acceptance. Sonography has several inherent diagnostic advantages, including accessibility, quick scan time, multiplanar capability, and the ability to perform dynamic real-time imaging that can be correlated to clinical symptoms and compared with contralateral structures. In experienced hands, ultrasound is sensitive and specific in the diagnosis of a variety of musculoskeletal pathologies.

In addition to its many diagnostic advantages, ultrasound has become a popular nonsurgical treatment modality for a variety of sports-related injuries. Physical therapists often use ultrasound acutely to decrease joint stiffness, reduce pain and muscle spasms, and improve muscle mobility. In the clinical setting, ultrasound is being investigated in the treatment of fractures and ligament, tendon, muscle, cartilage, and chronic inflammatory injuries.

Fractures

Ultrasound affects the three phases of fracture healing (inflammation, repair, and remodeling) by enhancing angiogenic, chondrogenic, and osteogenic activity. Angiogenesis is enhanced by increasing blood flow to the fracture site, which increases the delivery of components necessary for fracture healing. Ultrasound may induce conformational changes in cell membranes and alter their ionic permeability and second messenger expression. This could lead to downstream alterations in gene expression, resulting in accelerated fracture repair via the upregulation of cartilage- and bone-specific genes. Reports suggest that ultrasound stimulates chondrogenesis and cartilage hypertrophy, resulting in an earlier onset of enchondral formation and leading to increased stiffness and strength of the fracture site.

The US Food and Drug Administration approved the use of low-intensity ultrasound for the accelerated healing of fresh fractures in October 1994 and for the treatment of established nonunions in February 2000. Clinical studies have demonstrated that ultrasound can accelerate fracture healing. One article reported the results of a meta-analysis of studies published from 1966 through December 2000 that assessed the effects of pulsed ultrasound therapy on time to fracture healing. Inclusion criteria for the studies were as follows: randomization, skeletally mature patients of either sex with one or more fractures, double-blinded as to fracture healing, administration of pulsed low-intensity ultrasound to at least one treatment group, and assessment of fracture healing as determined radiographically by the bridging of three of four cortices. Based on analysis of these randomized trials, the authors reported that low-intensity ultrasound treatment may significantly reduce the time to fracture healing for fractures treated nonsurgically.

Recent studies have also evaluated the effectiveness of ultrasound in treating established nonunions and stress fractures. In a study of nonunions in rats treated with ultrasound, the authors reported an 86% union rate for fractures treated with ultrasound alone. Another study evaluated the use of ultrasound to treat stress fractures of the tibia in athletes and reported that ultrasound treatment was effective in pain relief and early return to vigorous activity without bracing.

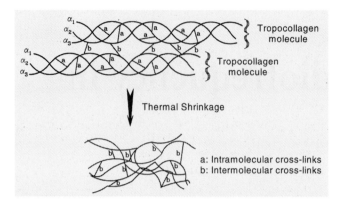

Figure 1 Molecular mechanism of collagen shrinkage. The intramolecular cross-links within the tropocollagen molecules are denatured, but the intermolecular cross-links between the tropocollagen molecules are maintained. *(Reproduced from Arnoczky SP, Aksan A: Thermal modification of connective tissue: Basic science considerations and clinical implications.* J Am Acad Orthop Surg 2000;8:305-313.)

Cartilage Repair

Ultrasound has a direct stimulatory effect on cartilage formation, maturation, and extracellular matrix production. Animal studies have demonstrated that treatment with low-intensity ultrasound has a significant positive effect on the healing of osteochondral defects. An in vivo study of full-thickness osteochondral defects in New Zealand rabbits showed that the treated group had repaired cartilage with improved morphologic features and histologic characteristics. The authors reported that not only did the repair occur earlier but also fewer degenerative changes at later times were observed in defects treated with ultrasound. Therapeutic ultrasound has also been shown to improve the quality of investigational chondrocyte implants for transplantation into articular cartilage defects.

Ligament and Tendon Injuries

The use of pulsed low-intensity ultrasound to treat ligament and tendon injuries has been reported in several animal studies. In a study of dogs with surgically tenotomized Achilles tendons followed by surgical repair, ultrasound therapy resulted in earlier improvement in the ultrasound echotexture, histologically better union with less inflammatory reaction, and earlier and more organized collagen bundle formation. Another study reported that the medial collateral ligaments of rats when treated with ultrasound demonstrated superior mechanical properties in regard to ultimate load, stiffness, and energy absorption compared with controls in the early phases of healing. Ultrasound treatment has also been shown to decrease the adhesions surrounding healing ligaments, leading to improved range of motion.

Muscle Injuries

Although clinical studies assessing its efficacy are rare, therapeutic ultrasound has been used to treat muscle in-

juries. Ultrasound has been shown to increase the number of muscle precursor cells at the site of injury, but it has no effect on the amount of actual muscle cell regeneration. Nonetheless, recent animal studies have shown that ultrasound can improve force production after contraction-induced muscle injuries.

Inflammatory Lesions

Ultrasound has also been reported to have a beneficial effect in the short-term treatment of calcific rotator cuff tendinitis. In one study, patients with symptomatic calcific rotator cuff tendinitis who were treated with pulsed ultrasound had better resolution of calcifications and improved short-term clinical outcomes. The results at longer follow-up (9 months), however, were not significant.

Radiofrequency

Radiofrequency energy devices work by generating a high-frequency alternating electromagnetic current that flows from the tip of a probe to the adjacent tissues. Intracellular and extracellular ions are moved by the alternating current, and this molecular agitation causes frictional heating within the tissue.

In monopolar radiofrequency, current flows from the active electrode in the probe tip to the return electrode (a grounding pad). The current flows through the interposed tissue, which is the path of least resistance. The amount of heat developed by the high-frequency alternation current increases by the square of the current density. A high-current density develops at the small active electrode, and a low-current density develops at the large grounding electrode. The tissue just beneath the tip of the active electrode is heated, but little or no heat is generated at the grounding pad because of its large surface area and low-current density.

Bipolar radiofrequency uses two electrodes at the tip of the probe. Current passes between the two electrodes, and heating occurs only at the tissue adjacent to the active electrode. The amount of frictional heating is determined by many factors. The heat generated is inversely proportional to the distance from the probe, and this relationship is exponential. Heat production is directly proportional to the duration of the application of heat and probe tip size.

The effect of heat on collagen has a predictable course that is affected by temperature, exposure time, and tissue (or the quality of the collagen) (Figures 1 and 2). It is highly dependent on the collagen cross-linking of the tissue, which in turn is dependent on the age of the patient. When sufficient heat is applied, the heat-sensitive bonds of the collagen are broken, and its triple-helix structure is unwound (denatured) and takes on a shorter configuration. Because collagen is at its longest configuration in the triple-helix, loss of this tertiary structure can reduce the length of collagen by as much as 50%.

The critical temperature range to achieve shrinkage in capsular and ligamentous tissue is 65°C to 75°C. Little or no shrinkage will occur at temperatures below 65°C. With increasing age, collagen cross-links begin to fail, which will further influence the effect of heat. In tissues that have low impedance (joint capsule and ligaments), sufficient heat penetrates the tissue to cause cell death to a depth of approximately 3 to 4 mm. Articular cartilage has much higher impedance, so the energy path actually flows through the irrigation solution and results in a more limited depth of penetration (approximately 0.4 mm to 0.9 mm). The depth of penetration depends on the temperature setting of the probe, the electrical conduction path, and the thermal conductivity of the tissue.

The thermal effect on treated tissue is significant. Capsular tissue shows an immediate drop in stiffness, which peaks 2 weeks after surgery. Thereafter, a gradual improvement in the mechanical properties of the tissue occurs, and by 12 weeks, the tissue has regained its normal mechanical properties. Histologically, large hyalinized regions with pyknotic nuclei and denatured tissue are seen after thermal treatment. Two weeks later, the beginnings of a fibroblastic and vascular invasion are observed. There is almost no inflammatory response at this point. By 6 weeks after thermal application, the angiogenic and fibroblastic response is dramatic. By 12 weeks, the hyalinized collagen has been completely replaced, although the tissue remains hypercellular. This cellular and vascular reaction may persist for months and has been reported to persist as long as 1 year.

Because the fibroblasts involved in the healing process arise from tissue adjacent to the affected area, it was hypothesized that if a grid pattern instead of a paintbrush type pattern were used, then the healing process could be shortened. This hypothesis has been tested, and results demonstrate that the time for the mechanical properties to return to normal was reduced to 6 weeks.

In contrast to capsular tissue, the effects of the thermal treatment of articular cartilage are permanent. Cell death begins at 45°C; at 55°C to 60°C cells within articular cartilage die. It is believed, however, that thermal chondroplasty can result in a more accurate débridement without damaging adjacent unaffected tissue as much as mechanical débridement. The therapeutic benefit of thermal chondroplasty may be achieved from annealing the surface of the cartilage. Fibrillated cartilage releases collagen and proteoglycan epitopes that travel to the synovial membrane. The synovium then releases various substances including metalloproteinases that cause further degradation of the articular cartilage. This creates more inflammation, leading to swelling and pain.

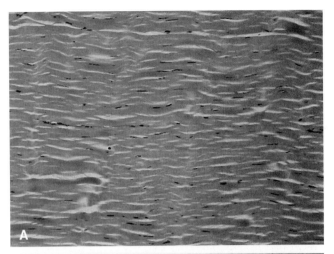

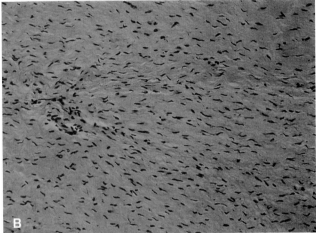

Figure 2 Photomicrographs of a longitudinal section of a normal rabbit patellar tendon before **(A)** and 8 weeks after **(B)** thermal modification (hematoxylin-eosin, original magnification x100). Note the marked fibroblastic response still present within the tissue at 8 weeks. *(Reproduced from Arnoczky SP, Aksan A: Thermal modification of connective tissue: Basic science considerations and clinical implications. J Am Acad Orthop Surg 2000;8:305-313.)*

Annealing the surface may reduce or eliminate the release of these epitopes.

Clinical Use
Shoulder
The primary use of thermal energy in the treatment of shoulder injuries is capsular shrinkage for glenohumeral instability. Although it has been used extensively, the exact indications, technique, amount of delivered energy, and postoperative therapy regimens have not been established or controlled. There are also scant reports in the literature regarding the clinical effect of thermal energy on capsular tissue over time.

Thermal energy has been used as a stand-alone treatment or as an adjunct to other arthroscopic procedures. Success rates using pure thermal treatment have been reported to range from 70% to almost 100%; however, prospective randomized studies with adequate follow-up are lacking. One study reported on 54 patients with a minimum follow-up of 2 years. The patients were treated with thermal capsulorrhaphy alone or with supplemental fixation. The author reported a success rate that exceeded 90%, with only 6 patients having poor results. Another study reported on 30 patients with capsular laxity who were treated with thermal capsulorrhaphy or arthroscopic plication of the rotator interval. Patient satisfaction was reported as satisfactory in 93% of the patients. Another study reported favorable results in throwing athletes with internal impingement who underwent treatment with thermal shrinkage compared with similar athletes who did not have the procedure.

Despite the lack of controlled studies and long-term follow-up, thermal capsulorrhaphy remains an attractive treatment option because it is technically easier to use than other treatment options. Thermal capsulorrhaphy can result in complications, however, including instability, recurrence, stiffness, axillary nerve injury, and capsular necrosis. The most frequently reported complication after arthroscopic stabilization is recurrence. Recurrence after thermal procedures has been reported to range from 0% to 47%. Stiffness can occur after thermal procedures, but the true rates are unknown. It has been reported to be as high as 10%. Axillary nerve injury associated with thermal procedures has been reported to be approximately 8%. Most reports involved temporary axillary nerve injury, but permanent injuries have also been reported. Thermal necrosis of the capsule has been reported, but again the true complication rates are unknown. Applying the treatment using a grid pattern has been proposed to correct this problem.

Knee

When treating knee injuries, radiofrequency can be used to cut tissue, remove tissue, and prepare the anterior and/or posterior cruciate ligament site by exposing bony landmarks in the knee. Radiofrequency can also facilitate the removal of soft tissue during notchplasty and lateral releases, access difficult to reach areas of the meniscus, and shrink the medial retinaculum.

Recurrent patellofemoral instability can be treated using medial capsular plication and lateral retinacular release. For patients who undergo this procedure, the resulting tissue is weak, and activities are restricted for 3 months. Although early reports demonstrate results comparable to those using traditional open methods, outcome data are limited.

The treatment of articular cartilage with radiofrequency is controversial, and conflicting results with thermal chondroplasty have been reported. Early reports demonstrated beneficial effects of using bipolar radiofrequency when compared with mechanical shaving for treating chondromalacia. Recent studies using confocal laser microscopy, however, have demonstrated that significant chondrocyte death occurs after the use of ra-

diofrequency, some to the level of the subchondral bone. To date, there are no known human clinical studies on the use of radiofrequency devices to treat articular cartilage lesions.

Ankle

For ankle injuries, radiofrequency can be used to tighten the lateral ligaments in a manner similar to that achieved using a Broström procedure. After this procedure, the ankle should be protected for 3 months. Other applications of radiofrequency in the treatment of ankle injuries include lysis of arthrofibrosis and removal of meniscoid lesions.

Summary

Therapeutic ultrasound has been shown to be an effective modality in the treatment of acute fractures and, more importantly, in the treatment of nonunions and stress fractures. Its use in other areas is widespread, but objective data documenting its clinical effectiveness are still lacking. Radiofrequency devices have become popular among many orthopaedic surgeons. The reasons for this may vary, but ease of use when compared with traditional arthroscopic treatment modalities is consistently cited. Despite the popularity of radiofrequency devices, the science behind most applications is lacking (or conflicting at best), and care should be exercised with their use.

Annotated Bibliography

Ultrasound

Azuma Y, Ito M, Harada Y, Ohta T, Jingushi S: Low-intensity pulsed ultrasound accelerates rat femoral fracture healing by acting on the various cellular reactions in the fracture callus. *J Bone Miner Res* 2001;16:671-680.

In this in vivo animal study of 69 male rats with bilateral closed femur fractures, the right femur was the treatment group and the left femur served as the control group. Rats were divided into four groups based on timing and duration of treatment. Results indicated that ultrasound accelerated fracture healing, and longer treatments were more effective.

Brand JC, Brindle T, Nyland J, Caborn DN, Johnson DL: Does pulsed low-intensity ultrasound allow early return to normal activities when treating stress fractures? A review of one tarsal navicular and eight tibial stress fractures. *Iowa Orthop J* 1999;19:26-30.

This study evaluated the efficacy of daily pulsed low-intensity ultrasound with early return to activities for the treatment of tibial stress fractures. Although no controls were used, results showed that treatment of tibial stress fractures with daily pulsed low-intensity ultrasound was effective in pain relief and allowed early return to vigorous activity.

Busse JW, Mohit B, Kulkarni AV, Tyunks E: The effect of low-intensity pulsed ultrasound therapy on time to fracture healing: A meta-analysis. *CMAJ* 2002;166: 437-441.

Five electronic databases were searched to identify reports on the use of ultrasound for fracture healing published from 1966 to 2000. The criteria for pooling included random allocation of treatments, inclusion of skeletally mature patients of either sex with one or more fractures, blinding of both the patient and the assessor(s) as to fracture healing, administration of low-intensity pulsed ultrasound treatments to at least one of the treatment groups, and assessment of time to fracture healing as determined radiographically by bridging of three or four cortices. Pooled results showed that the time to fracture healing was significantly shorter in the treatment groups receiving ultrasound therapy.

Cook SD, Salkeld SL, Popich-Patron LS, Ryaby JP, Jones DG, Barrack RL: Improved cartilage repair after treatment with low-intensity pulsed ultrasound. *Clin Orthop* 2001;391(suppl):S231-S243.

The authors of this study evaluated the effectiveness of low-intensity pulsed ultrasound on the repair of full-thickness osteochondral defects in the patellar grooves of rabbits. They report that ultrasound treatment significantly improved the morphologic features and histologic characteristics of the repair cartilage compared with untreated control subjects.

Da Cunha A, Parizotto NA, Vidal BC: The effect of therapeutic ultrasound on repair of the Achilles tendon of the rat. *Ultrasound Med Biol* 2001;27:1691-1696.

In this study of the effect of ultrasound on the healing of 15 tenotomized Wistar rat Achilles tendons, the authors reported that histologic findings using pulsed ultrasound showed a high birefringence and better organization and aggregation of collagen fibrils.

Ebenbichler GR, Erdogmus CB, Resch KL, et al: Ultrasound therapy for calcific tendinitis of the shoulder. *N Engl J Med* 1999;340:1533-1538.

In this randomized, double-blinded study of the use of ultrasound to treat patients with symptomatic calcific tendonitis of the shoulder, 63 patients (70 shoulders) were enrolled in the study, and 54 patients (61 shoulders) completed the study. Results showed that patients who received ultrasound had greater decreases in pain and greater improvements in the quality of life. At 9 months, however, the results were no longer significant.

Karnes JL, Burton HW: Continuous therapeutic ultrasound accelerates repair of contraction induced skeletal muscle damage in rats. *Arch Phys Med Rehabil* 2002;83: 1-4.

The authors of this randomized, case-controlled study assessed the effect of ultrasonography on the repair of muscle injured through repeated eccentric contractions. They report

that 7 days of continuous therapeutic ultrasound improved force production after contraction-induced muscle injury.

Mayr E, Mockl C, Lenich A, Ecker M, Ruter A: Is low-intensity ultrasound effective in treatment of disorders of fracture healing? *Unfallchirurg* 2002;105:108-115.

In this prospective study of 100 nonunions treated with low-intensity ultrasound, 86 of the fractures healed with no surgical intervention.

Nishikori T, Ochi M, Maniwa S, et al: Effects of low-intensity pulsed ultrasound on proliferation and chondroitin-sulfate synthesis of cultured chondrocytes embedded in Atelocollagen gel. *J Biomed Mater Res* 2002;59:201-206.

In this in vitro study of the proliferation and chondroitin synthesis in articular chondrocytes harvested from the hip, knee, and shoulder joint of Japanese white rabbits and exposed to low-intensity pulsed ultrasound, the authors report that exposure promoted the synthesis of chondroitin sulfate but not cell number or stiffness.

Nolte PA, van der Krans A, Patka P, Janssen IM, Ryaby JP, Albers GH: Low-intensity pulsed ultrasound in the treatment of nonunions. *J Trauma* 2001;51:693-702.

This study assessed the use of low-intensity pulsed ultrasound in the treatment of 29 established nonunions in the tibia, femur, radius/ulna, scaphoid, humerus, metatarsal, or clavicle. The average postfracture duration from time of injury to time of treatment was 61 weeks; 25 of the 29 nonunions (86%) healed in an average treatment time of 22 weeks.

Rantanen J, Thorsson O, Wollmer P, Kalimo H: Effects of therapeutic ultrasound on the regeneration of skeletal myofibers after experimental muscle injury. *Am J Sports Med* 1999;27:54-59.

This descriptive study assessed the regeneration of skeletal myofibers of the gastrocnemius muscle using pulsed ultrasound. Immunohistochemical, morphometric, and scintigraphic analysis were performed. The authors report that treatment promoted satellite cell proliferation phase of myoregeneration, but it did not have significant effects on the overall morphologic manifestations of muscle regeneration.

Rubin C, Bolander M, Ryaby JP, Hadjiargyrou M: The use of low-intensity ultrasound to accelerate the healing of fractures. *J Bone Joint Surg Am* 2001;83:259-270.

This is a review of the biomedical applications and basic science of using ultrasound for fracture treatment. Clinical studies are also discussed.

Saini NS, Roy KS, Bansal PS, Singh B, Simran PS: A preliminary study on the effect of ultrasound therapy on the healing of surgically severed Achilles tendons in five dogs. *J Vet Med A Physiol Pathol Clin Med* 2002;49:321-328.

The authors of this study used ultrasound to treat the surgically repaired Achilles tendons of five dogs that were previously surgically tenotomized. Ultrasound treatment resulted in better ultrasound echotexture, grossly fewer adhesions, and a better union as determined using histologic analysis.

Takakura Y, Matsui N, Yoshiya S, et al: Low-intensity pulsed ultrasound enhances early healing of medial collateral ligament injuries in rats. *J Ultrasound Med* 2002; 21:283-288.

Ultrasound was used to treat 13 male Sprague Dawley rats after surgical transection of the medial collateral ligament. The contralateral limbs were the controls. After 12 days, ligaments treated with ultrasound exhibited significantly superior mechanical properties.

Zhang ZJ, Huckle J, Francomano CA, Spencer RG: The influence of pulsed low-intensity ultrasound on matrix production of chondrocytes at different stages of differentiation: An explant study. *Ultrasound Med Biol* 2002; 28:1547-1553.

Cartilage explants from chicken embryos were exposed to low-intensity pulsed ultrasound. The authors report that exposure to ultrasound resulted in increased matrix synthesis, indicating a potential role for this treatment modality in cartilage repair.

Radiofrequency

Anderson K, Warren RF, Alchek DW, Craig EV, O'Brien SJ: Risk factors for early failure after thermal capsulorrhaphy. *Am J Sports Med* 2002;30:103-107.

In this retrospective review of 106 patients who underwent thermal shrinkage, 15 patients were identified as treatment failures, and previous surgeries and multiple recurrent dislocations were associated with poor outcome.

Andrews JR, Dugas JR: Diagnosis and treatment of shoulder injuries in the throwing athlete: The role of thermal-assisted capsular shrinkage. *Instr Course Lect* 2001;50:17-21.

The authors of this article believe that addressing capsular laxity arthroscopically at the same time that the intra-articular pathology is addressed is the best form of treatment for athletes with overuse-type injuries and affords them the best chance of returning to competition at the same or higher level.

Arnoczky SP, Aksan A: Thermal modification of connective tissue: Basic science considerations and clinical implications. *J Am Acad Orthop Surg* 2000;8:305-313.

This is a review of the mechanism of thermal shrinkage, experimental studies, and clinical implications of using thermal energy therapy.

Barber FA, Uribe JW, Weber SC: Current application for arthroscopic thermal surgery. *Arthroscopy* 2002; 18(suppl 1):40-50.

The authors of this article provide a review of the basic science and clinical applications of using thermal energy during arthroscopic surgery.

Fanton GS: Arthroscopic electrothermal surgery of the shoulder. *Oper Tech Sports Med* 1998;6:139-146.

In this study, 54 patients were treated with thermal capsulorrhaphy; two thirds of the patients were treated with thermal capsulorrhaphy alone and the remainder with supplemental fixation. The author reports a success rate of 90%, with only six patients having fair or poor results.

Grylar EC, Greis P, Burks RT, West J: Axillary nerve temperatures during radiofrequency capsulorrhaphy of the shoulder. *Arthroscopy* 2001;17:567-572.

This cadaveric study was conducted to determine the temperature along the course of the axillary nerve during radiofrequency application. The authors report that heating of the axillary nerve can occur during radiofrequency capsular shrinkage of the shoulder and may reach levels that can damage neural tissue.

Hecht P, Hayashi K, Lu Y, et al: Monopolar radiofrequency energy effects on joint capsular tissue: Potential treatment for joint instability. *Am J Sports Med* 1999;27: 761-771.

This animal study was conducted to evaluate the thermal effect of monopolar radiofrequency energy on the mechanical, morphologic, and biochemical properties of joint capsular tissue. Monopolar radiofrequency energy was arthroscopically applied to the synovial surface of the femoropatellar joint of 24 sheep; sheep were sacrificed at 0, 2, 6, and 12 weeks after surgery and synovial surfaces analyzed. The authors report that this treatment initially caused a significantly deleterious effect on the mechanical properties of the joint capsule, but it was followed by gradual improvement of the mechanical, morphologic, and biochemical properties of the tissue over time.

Hecht P, Hayashi K, Cooley J, et al: The thermal effect of monopolar radiofrequency energy on the properties of joint capsule. *Am J Sports Med* 1998;26:808-814.

This in vivo study of 12 mature sheep was conducted to analyze the short-term tissue response to treatment with monopolar radiofrequency energy. Five different power settings at 65°C were studied. Thermal damage at all power settings was noted at 7 days postoperatively.

Kaplan L, Uribe JW, Sasken H, Marmarian G: The acute effects of radiofrequency energy in articular cartilage: An in vitro study. *Arthroscopy* 2000;16:2-5.

The purpose of this study was to determine the effect of radiofrequency energy on six fresh human articular cartilage specimens obtained from patients undergoing total knee arthroplasty for unicompartmental osteoarthritis. Radiofrequency energy was applied to normal and diseased areas at three voltage settings. At the treated site, chondrocytes remained viable, no collagen abnormalities were identified, and diseased areas were smoothed.

Lopez MJ, Hayashi K, Fanton GS, Thabit G III, Markel MD: The effect of radiofrequency energy on the ultrastructure of joint capsular collagen. *Arthroscopy* 1998; 14:495-501.

The authors of this study evaluated the effect of radiofrequency energy on the histologic and ultrastructural appearance of joint capsular collagen. They report that thermally induced ultrastructural collagen fibril alteration is likely the predominant mechanism of tissue shrinkage caused by the application of radiofrequency energy.

Lu Y, Edwards RB III, Cole BJ, Markel MD: Thermal chondroplasty with radiofrequency energy. *Am J Sports Med* 2001;29:42-49.

This in vitro study was conducted to examine the effects of three radiofrequency energy devices on bovine cartilage during thermal chondroplasty. The authors report that significant chondrocyte death as determined by confocal laser microscopy occurred with each device and that bipolar radiofrequency energy penetrated to the level of subchondral bone.

Lu Y, Edwards RB III, Klscheur VL, Nho S, Cole BJ, Markel MD: Effect of bipolar radiofrequency energy on human articular cartilage: Comparison of confocal laser microscopy and light microscopy. *Arthroscopy* 2001;17: 117-123.

The authors of this study evaluated chondrocyte viability with confocal light microscopy following exposure to bipolar radiofrequency energy. Confocal light microscopy showed that bipolar radiofrequency energy delivered through the probe created significant chondrocyte death. These changes were not apparent using standard light microscopy.

Lu Y, Hayashi K, Edwards RB III, Fanton GS, Thabit G, Markel MD: The effect of monopolar radiofrequency treatment pattern on joint capsular healing. *Am J Sports Med* 2000;28:711-719.

This study compared two delivery patterns of monopolar radiofrequency energy: uniform (paintbrush) pattern and multiple single line passes (grid pattern). The authors report that the grid pattern allowed faster healing than tissue treated with a paintbrush pattern.

Obrzut SL, Hecht P, Hayashi K, Fanton GS, Thabit G III, Markel MD: The effect of radiofrequency energy on the length and temperature properties of the glenohumeral joint capsule. *Arthroscopy* 1998;14:395-400.

In this in vitro study of the effect of radiofrequency energy on the glenohumeral joint capsules of sheep, the authors

found that tissue shrinkage was less than 4% for treatment temperatures below 65°C and increased to 14% for treatment temperatures at 80°C. The length of tissue after treatment was significantly shorter for treatment temperatures of 65°C, 70°C, 75°C, and 80°C.

Savoie FH III, Field LD: Thermal versus suture treatment of symptomatic capsular laxity. *Clin Sports Med* 2000;19:63-75.

This is a report on 30 patients who were treated with thermal capsulorrhaphy and arthroscopic suture plication of the rotator interval. Findings suggested that thermal capsulorrhaphy with rotator interval plication is an effective treatment for managing multidirectional instability of the shoulder, with results comparable to previous open and arthroscopic procedures.

Shellock FG, Shields CL: Radiofrequency energy-induced heating of bovine articular cartilage using a bipolar radiofrequency electrode. *Am J Sports Med* 2000; 28:720-724.

This in vitro study of the effects of different radiofrequency energy settings on bovine cartilage was conducted to determine the temperature changes associated with the use of radiofrequency energy. The authors performed the procedures in a temperature-controlled saline bath and report that there were significant increases in temperatures associated with all settings tested.

Turner AS, Tippett JW, Powers BE, Dewell R, Mallinckrodt CH: Radiofrequency ablation of articular cartilage: A study in sheep. *Arthroscopy* 1998;14:585-591.

The knee articular cartilage of two groups of sheep were treated with either mechanical shaving or bipolar radiofrequency energy. For all variables tested, the joints treated with bipolar radiofrequency energy had more favorable responses. Cartilage treated with bipolar radiofrequency energy also demonstrated less severe histologic changes.

Classic Bibliography

Hayashi K, Thabit G III, Massa KL, et al: The effect of thermal heating on the length and histological properties of the glenohumeral joint capsule. *Am J Sports Med* 1997;25:107-112.

Kristiansen TK, Ryaby JP, McCabe J, Frey JJ, Roe LR: Accelerated healing of distal radial fractures with the use of specific, low-intensity ultrasound: A multicenter, prospective, randomized, double blind, placebo-controlled study. *J Bone Joint Surg Am* 1997;79:961-973.

Chapter 30

Total Joint Arthroplasty in Sports

Brett Miller, MD

Michael H. Huo, MD

Eugene G. Galvin, MD

Introduction

Total joint arthroplasties of the hip, knee, and shoulder have successfully alleviated pain and improved function in older patients with advanced arthritis. Predictable efficacy has led orthopaedic surgeons to extend the indications for arthroplasty to younger and more active patients. Available data have shown, however, that activity rather than age or body weight is the main factor in predicting implant survival. Close follow-up is important in younger and more active patients. Of particular importance is awareness that radiographic detection of wear and related periprosthetic osteolysis is a slow process, often taking 5 years or longer to become evident.

Young Patients With Total Joint Arthroplasties

Total Hip Arthroplasty

Total hip arthroplasty (THA) has become one of the most successful joint replacement operations. The success of this operation has led surgeons to offer this procedure to younger patients with rheumatoid arthritis and other inflammatory arthropathies, osteonecrosis, posttraumatic arthritis, developmental dysplasia of the hip, Legg-Calvé-Perthes disease, and previous septic arthritis. Functional capacity is more relevant for younger patients because many of these patients must remain employed. Moreover, many younger patients participate in recreational sports. The failure rates resulting from aseptic loosening have been greater in younger patients, a factor that is primarily attributable to participation in athletic activities.

The indications for THA in younger patients are the same as those in older patients. Every effort should be made to offer alternative treatments to younger patients before THA. Because multiple joint involvement is more likely to be one of the principal indications for total joint arthroplasties at a young age, however, younger patients are less likely to have a satisfactory result with alternative treatment methods.

Fixation durability of both the implant stem and cup has been improved greatly with the development of newer designs, materials, and surgical techniques. Two recent prospective studies evaluated the results of THAs done with cemented and cementless stems in patients younger than 50 years. A cementless cup was inserted. The cemented stem group was observed for an average of 9.4 years. There were no revisions because of aseptic loosening, but one patient required revision surgery because of infection. The rate of implant survival was 99% at 10 years. There was a significant relationship between polyethylene wear in patients younger than 40 years, male gender, and higher abduction angle of the cup. The authors concluded that good outcomes were principally the result of using improved cementing techniques and a smaller diameter femoral head with a thicker polyethylene liner. The other prospective study evaluated cementless femoral stems in a comparable patient population and reported no aseptic loosening at a mean follow-up of 9.8 years. One patient, however, underwent revision surgery because of recurrent dislocation.

The high incidence of polyethylene wear and osteolysis in younger patients has led orthopaedic surgeons to seek alternative bearing surfaces for THAs. One group reported on the result of alumina-on-alumina THA in patients younger than 40 years. With revision for mechanical failure considered as the end point, the survival rates at 10 and 15 years were 84.6% and 80%, respectively. The overall survival rates for the stem were 94.8% at 10 years and 84.8% at 15 years. Another group reported the results of using ceramic THAs in patients younger than 50 years. The survival rate at 14 years was 80% for those patients receiving cemented stems and cups. For cemented prostheses with threaded cups, the survival rate was only 45%. Newer designs with improved fixation and ceramic-on-ceramic articulation may further reduce the incidence of osteolysis over the long term.

Young patients seeking THA should be counseled on the importance of health and weight maintenance and moderation in activity level. Regardless of the type of prosthesis used, early failure and wear are unavoidable. Close monitoring, therefore, is crucial in this population.

Total Knee Arthroplasty

With middle-aged adults (particularly women) who participate in exercise and sporting activities, there has been a concomitant increase in injuries about the knee. Injury of the ligaments, menisci, and osteochondral surfaces can lead to accelerated degenerative joint disease, for which total knee arthroplasty (TKA) can successfully alleviate pain and disability. TKA has also been shown to be effective in patients younger than 55 years with osteoarthritis and rheumatoid arthritis. As with THA, the main concern with younger patients undergoing TKA is that revision surgery may be required because of loosening and wear.

One study recently reported on the use of cementless TKA in patients younger than 50 years. No revision surgeries were required to treat implant loosening. Five of 75 patients underwent polyethylene exchange for wear. The mean knee score improved from 67 (preoperatively) to 97 (at final follow-up). Radiography revealed that all implants were stable. The authors contended that the principal advantage of cementless fixation was preservation of bone stock in anticipation of future revisions. Another study reported the results of using cemented TKAs in patients with osteoarthritis who were younger than 40 years; 82% of patients had good or excellent results at a mean follow-up of 7.9 years. The aseptic failure rate was 12.5% at 8 years. The mean knee score for this group of patients was lower than that for older patients. Another study reviewed 1,301 revision TKAs. The lowest implant failure rate was found in patients with rheumatoid arthritis. Young age (< 55 years) was associated with the shortest implant survival time.

Meticulous surgical techniques emphasizing limb alignment, component orientation, soft-tissue balance, and preservation of bone stock are crucial to ensure long-term implant survival in younger patients. Improving durability in younger patients also relies on appropriate implant selection and counseling about the importance of limiting activity levels. As with THA, early wear, loosening, and ultimately failure are seen in younger patients without rheumatoid arthritis who undergo TKA.

Unicompartmental Knee Arthroplasty

Unicompartmental knee arthroplasty (UKA) has been controversial since its introduction in the early 1970s. Initial results of first generation designs resulted in unsatisfactory results. By the 1980s, improved results were reported, and enthusiasm for the procedure increased. Refinements in patient selection, surgical technique, and prosthetic design led to acceptable results. Ten-year follow-up studies have reported a rate of UKA implant survival that is only slightly less than that for TKA implants. One study recently reported the results of 511 UKAs. The 10-year survival rate was 88.3% compared with 95.0% for TKAs.

Indications for UKA include noninflammatory osteoarthritis or osteonecrosis of one femoral condyle, less than 10° varus or 15° valgus deformity, intact cruciate ligaments, and a flexion contracture less than 10°. The patellofemoral joint can have up to grade 3 changes if this compartment is not symptomatic. In general, UKA is most appropriate for older, more sedentary patients (generally those older than 60 years) with unicompartmental tibiofemoral arthritis. Optimal results are obtained in nonobese patients without patellofemoral symptoms who have functioning cruciate ligaments and range of motion greater than 90°. UKA is contraindicated in patients with an active lifestyle (because of concerns regarding accelerated component wear), significant deformity, neuropathic arthropathy, or patellofemoral symptoms. Unfortunately, these contraindications apply to most patients who participate in athletic activities. Metallic spacers have been available for over 50 years with studies reporting good short-term results in 85% of patients. Although the UniSpacer Knee System (Zimmer, Warsaw, IN) is being used more commonly, there are no long-term published reports of its effectiveness.

Total Shoulder Arthroplasty

Of all patients who undergo major total joint arthroplasty, those who undergo total shoulder arthroplasty (TSA) have the lowest mean age. Osteoarthritis of the glenohumeral joint in the young patient is rare and is usually secondary to prior instability surgery, trauma, inflammatory arthropathy, rotator cuff tear arthropathy, or osteonecrosis. Other treatment alternatives such as arthroscopic débridement, subacromial decompression, and synovectomy have limited efficacy in patients with advanced disease.

The indication for shoulder arthroplasty in young patients is pain after failure of conservative or other less definitive surgical treatments. The decision to treat patients with hemiarthroplasty or TSA is based on several factors. Humeral head replacement is reserved for patients with functioning deltoid and rotator cuff muscles and concentric glenoids. For patients with eccentric glenoid wear, glenoid replacement should be considered. The contraindications for TSA include nerve or muscle damage causing muscle imbalance and subluxation of the glenohumeral joint. Severe rotator cuff deficiency can cause eccentric loading of the glenoid component and lead to early loosening. The loss of sensation and potential muscle weakness associated with neuropathic arthropathy is a relative contraindication to TSA because it can lead to early loosening and failure of the prosthesis.

Preoperative planning is crucial in the younger patient undergoing TSA. MRI can help determine the status of the rotator cuff. If bony anatomy is in question in the case of eccentric glenoid wear, CT is helpful. In patients with neuropathic arthropathy, electromyography and nerve conduction velocity studies should be included in the preoperative workup. For patients suspected of having an infection, appropriate laboratory studies and nuclear medicine scanning are warranted.

The results of TSA in young patients are mixed. TSA has been shown to be reliable in producing excellent pain relief and improved range of motion. One study reported the results of TSA in patients younger than 50 years. The survival rates for hemiarthroplasties were 92% at 5 years, 83% at 10 years, and 73% at 15 years. The survival rate for TSA was 97% at both 5 and 10 years and 84% at 15 years. Radiographic evidence of loosening of the humeral component was seen in 24% of the hemiarthroplasties and 53% of the TSAs. Radiographic evidence of loosening of the glenoid component was 59%. Increased risk for revision was attributed to a deficient rotator cuff. The authors concluded that although TSA provided effective relief of pain and improvement in motion, nearly half of the patients had an unsatisfactory result according to the shoulder rating system. Therefore, caution should be exercised when making recommendations for either hemiarthroplasty or TSA for a young patient.

Exercise Prescription for the Total Joint Arthroplasty Patient

As the average life expectancy in the United States continues to increase, the number of patients seeking total joint arthroplasty is also increasing. After successful total joint arthroplasty, most patients increase their physical activity. One study demonstrated improvements in exercise duration, maximum workload, peak oxygen consumption, and percentage of predicted maximum oxygen intake in patients who had undergone total joint arthroplasty. Resumption and increase in physical activity after total joint arthroplasty is associated with an improvement in cardiovascular fitness.

There are many considerations and potential risks in resuming athletic activity after undergoing total joint arthroplasty. Joint-bearing surface wear, traumatic complications, and implant failure caused by loosening should all be considered when making activity recommendations for patients who have undergone total joint arthroplasty. The preoperative level of athletic activity should be taken into consideration along with postoperative limitations. Patients who were active before surgery are generally the best candidates for safely resuming high-demand activities after surgery.

Patient activity was always assumed to be the variable that accounted for most of the effect of age on the durability of implants used for THA. This supposed relationship between patient activity and implant survival has been further supported by the fact that implant sur-

vival length can vary widely among patients within the same age range. It is difficult to quantify patient activity level. It is even more difficult to define a heterogeneity of activity levels among patients. Moreover, the activity level in the same patient is a dynamic process that is a function of many factors including overall health status, mental status, degenerative conditions of other joints or the spine, employment, and changing lifestyle selections over a decade or longer.

Strong data exist that support a correlation between articulation surface wear and physical activity as a function of the number of steps in gait measured by pedometers or other instruments. In a recent study, however, the authors were unable to correlate pedometer measurements with polyethylene wear at 5- to 6-year follow-up in a group of young patients who underwent THA. Despite the controversies, most surgeons believe that some objective measurement of activity level is critical in clinical studies of the implants used in THA.

Any attempt to assess patient activity must be dynamic enough to allow for multiple measurements over time. It is clear that precise and standardized methodologies of activity evaluation must be used to make fair comparisons between the results of procedures done with different designs and at different medical centers for patients with different diagnoses. Validated patient questionnaires must be developed with the collection of relevant data regarding all aspects of patient activity (nature of the activity, frequency, duration, and intensity). A summary numerical score can then be calculated to reflect the relative weight of all different aspects of activity. Sporting activities must be taken into consideration in the development of such a questionnaire. The importance of sporting activities was clearly reported in one study in which patients rated the resumption of sports as their highest priority after the elimination of pain and the return to normal activities of daily living. It is hoped that the development and implementation of any patient activity questionnaire can be facilitated by the use of the Internet. It is believed that Internet access to patient activity questionnaires will provide patients with the ability to answer questions in the privacy of their own homes rather than in the physician's office, thereby resulting in patients providing more complete and accurate information.

Catastrophic implant and bearing surface fractures are uncommon with contemporary designs and biomaterials. Dislocation and periprosthetic fractures are potentially serious complications in patients who have undergone total joint arthroplasty and continue to participate in athletics. Athletic activity has been shown to adversely contribute to implant loosening rates. Durability of implant fixation has been improved with newer designs, surface texture, adjuncts to fixation (such as hydroxyapatite coating), and surgical techniques. Newer bearing surface alternatives may improve the risks of ar-

TABLE 1 | Activity After THA: 1999 Hip Society Survey

Recommended/Allowed	Allowed With Experience	Not Recommend	No Conclusion
Stationary bicycling	Low-impact aerobics	High-impact aerobics	Jazz dancing
Croquet	Road bicycling	Baseball/softball	Square dancing
Ballroom dancing	Bowling	Basketball	Fencing
Golf	Canoeing	Football	Ice skating
Horseshoes	Hiking	Gymnastics	Roller/inline skating
Shooting	Horseback riding	Handball	Rowing
Shuffleboard	Cross-country skiing	Hockey	Speed walking
Swimming		Jogging	Downhill skiing
Doubles tennis		Lacrosse	Stationary skiing
Walking		Racquetball	Weight lifting
		Squash	Weight machines
		Rock climbing	
		Soccer	
		Singles tennis	
		Volleyball	

(Reproduced with permission from Healy WL, Iorio R, Lemos MJ: Athletic activity after joint replacement. Am J Sports Med 2001;29:377-388.)

ticulated wear debris generation and the adverse biologic consequences. Only a few known reports have been published with regard to sporting and athletic activity guidelines after undergoing total joint arthroplasty.

Total Hip Arthroplasty

Active, high-demand patients with THA implants are at risk for implant loosening and wear. During walking, forces 2.5 to 3.5 times body weight can be placed across the hip joint. These forces can increase as much as 50% during jogging. The decision for participation in athletic activity after undergoing THA should be individualized. Patients should be educated about the risks associated with sporting activities. The most significant risk is wear at the joint surface; secondary risks include implant loosening and traumatic complications. A Hip Society survey was conducted to develop guidelines for athletic participation for patients after undergoing THA. The recommendations are listed in Table 1.

Total Knee Arthroplasty

One study examined the athletic participation of 160 patients (208 implants) who had undergone TKA. Seventy-nine patients participated in sports at least once a week before undergoing TKA, and 51 patients participated in sports at least once a week after undergoing TKA. Twenty percent returned to high-impact athletic activities, whereas 91% returned to low-impact athletic activities. In general, most surgeons discourage participation in high-impact activities after undergoing TKA. A Knee

Society survey was conducted to develop guidelines for athletic participation after undergoing TKA. The results are listed in Table 2.

Total Shoulder Arthroplasty

Many athletic activities place demand and stress on the upper extremity and the shoulder. Some athletic activities that are acceptable for patients who have undergone THA or TKA create unacceptable levels of stress for patients who have undergone TSA. One study evaluated the influence of glenohumeral implant geometry and position on shoulder muscle forces and found that changes in the geometric center of the humeral head can cause up to a 300% increase in joint-reaction forces, depending on retroversion angle. Moreover, the forces generated during translation and rotation of the humeral head may contribute to glenohumeral loosening. Less constrained and less conforming implant designs are, therefore, recommended, particularly those that reduce mechanical loosening of the glenoid component.

The incidence of revision TSAs varies from 4.6% for proximal humeral hemiarthroplasty to 30% to 40% for constrained TSAs. One evaluation of 419 unconstrained TSAs demonstrated a survival rate of 96% at 2 years, 92% at 5 years, and 88% at 10 years. The durability of cementless fixation of the humeral component of TSA implants has been reported to be good. A meta-analysis of 11 studies demonstrated a loosening rate of < 1% in cementless humeral implant stems. In younger and active patients, a cementless humeral implant component may be more suitable. Another study retrospectively re-

TABLE 2 | Activity After TKA: 1999 Knee Society Survey

Recommended/Allowed	Allowed With Experience	Not Recommend	No Conclusion
Stationary bicycling	Road bicycling	Basketball	Fencing
Croquet	Canoeing	Football	Roller/inline skating
Golf	Hiking	Gymnastics	Downhill skiing
Horseshoes	Rowing	Handball	Weight lifting
Shooting	Cross-country skiing	Hockey	
Shuffleboard	Stationary skiing	Jogging	
Swimming	Speed walking	Lacrosse	
Walking	Tennis	Racquetball	
Low-impact aerobics	Weight machines	Squash	
Bowling	Ice skating	Rock climbing	
Dancing		Soccer	
Horseback riding		Singles tennis	
		Volleyball	

(Reproduced with permission from Healy WL, Iorio R, Lemos MJ: Athletic activity after joint replacement. Am J Sports Med 2001;29:377-388.)

TABLE 3 | Activity After TSA: 1999 American Shoulder and Elbow Surgeons Survey

Recommended/Allowed	Allowed With Experience	Not Recommend	No Conclusion
Cross-country skiing	Golf	Football	High-impact aerobics
Stationary skiing	Ice skating	Gymnastics	Baseball/softball
Speed walking and jogging	Shooting	Hockey	Fencing
Swimming	Downhill skiing	Rock climbing	Handball
Double tennis			Horseback riding
Low-impact aerobics			Lacrosse
Bicycling, road and stationary			Racquetball/squash
Bowling			Skating, roller/inline
Canoeing			Rowing
Croquet			Soccer
Shuffleboard			Tennis, singles
Horseshoes			Volleyball
Dancing			Weight training

(Reproduced with permission from Healy WL, Iorio R, Lemos MJ: Athletic activity after joint replacement. Am J Sports Med 2001;29:377-388.)

viewed 24 golfers who underwent TSA and reported that 96% of the patients were able to resume playing golf. The average length of time to return to play was 4.5 months. The authors noted that playing golf did not result in increased radiographic evidence of component loosening, and no increase occurred in radiographic evidence of lucent lines when the golfers were compared with a control group of 76 patients with osteoarthritis who had 103 shoulder arthroplasties ($P < 0.05$). An American Shoulder and Elbow Surgeons survey was conducted to develop guidelines for athletic participation after undergoing TSA. The results are listed in Table 3.

Summary

When considering total joint arthroplasty for younger and more active patients, preoperative discussions must convey the importance of appropriate postoperative activity and sports participation and the need for close clinical and radiographic follow-up. In general, lower impact activities (with decreased joint loading) are recommended after undergoing total joint arthroplasty. Preoperative athletic participation is another important factor in recommending activities after undergoing total joint arthroplasty. Early implant failure can be expected in young patients without rheumatoid arthritis who undergo THA and TKA.

Annotated Bibliography

Young Patients With Total Joint Arthroplasties

Bizot P, Banallec L, Sedel L, Nizard R: Alumina-on-alumina total hip prosthesis in patients 40 years of age or younger. *Clin Orthop* 2000;379:68-76.

This study assessed 128 alumina-on-alumina THAs in 104 consecutive patients with a maximum age of 40 years. The main diagnoses were osteonecrosis and congenital hip dislocation. The implant survival rates after 7 years were 94.1% for the cemented cup, 88.8% for the screw-in ring, 95.1% for the cementless press-fit socket, and 94.3% for the metal-back press-fit component. The 10-year survival rate was 90.4% for the cemented socket and 88.4% for the screw-in ring component. The 15-year survival rate was 78.9% for the cemented socket implant.

Coyte PC, Hawker G, Croxford R, Wright JG: Rates of revision knee replacement in Ontario, Canada. *J Bone Joint Surg Am* 1999;81:773-782.

This study of 18,530 TKAs was conducted to assess the longevity of knee replacements; 1,301 of the TKAs were classified as revisions and the revision rate ranged from 4.3% to 8%.

Duffy GP, Trousdale RT, Stuart MJ: Total knee arthroplasty in patients 55 years old or younger: 10- to 17-year results. *Clin Orthop* 1998;356:22-27.

At an average 13-year (minimum 10-year) follow-up, the authors of this study reported 99% implant survival at 10 years and 95% at 15 years. No radiographic evidence of loose implants was detected at the latest follow-up. The average knee score at latest follow-up was 84.

Gioe TJ, Killeen KK, Hoeffel DP, et al: Abstract: Analysis of unicompartmental knee arthroplasty in a community-based implant registry, in *Annual Meeting Proceedings of the American Academy of Orthopaedic Surgeons, February 5-9, 2003, New Orleans, LA.* Rosemont, IL, American Academy of Orthopaedic Surgeons, 2003, p 561. Abstract 069.

This prospective study reviewed the outcomes of 511 UKAs done by 23 surgeons over 10 years. The implants of nine different manufacturers were used. Implant survival was 93.6% at 5 years and 88.3% at 10 years compared with 95.0% at 10 years for primary cemented TKAs. The major reason for revision UKA was progression of arthritis to the uninvolved compartments.

Harris WH: Wear and periprosthetic osteolysis: The problem. *Clin Orthop* 2001;393:66-70.

The author of this article presents several key features of periprosthetic osteolysis and focuses on its general progressive nature and consequences as well as the current understanding of the diverse radiographic evidence of this disease.

Hayes PR, Flatow EL: Total shoulder arthroplasty in the young patient. *Instr Course Lect* 2001;50:73-88.

The authors present a comprehensive review of the indications for hemiarthroplasty versus TSA in young patients.

Hofmann AA, Heithoff SM, Camargo M: Cementless total knee arthroplasty in patients 50 years or younger. *Clin Orthop* 2002;404:102-107.

The authors of this study report that at a mean follow-up of 111 months the knee scores of patients undergoing cementless TKA improved from 67 to 97 on average. Fifty-seven percent of the patients had a diagnosis of posttraumatic arthritis, which indicates that most were young and active. No revision surgeries were required for implant loosening or failure.

Huo MH, Brown BS: What's new in hip arthroplasty. *J Bone Joint Surg Am* 2003;85:1852-1864.

The authors of this review article discuss fixation with cement, fixation without cement, revision surgery, complications, surgical techniques, articulation and wear, growth factors and biology, and outcome analysis and practice management.

Kim YH, Kook HK, Kim JS: Total hip replacement with a cementless acetabular components and a cemented femoral component in patients younger than fifty years of age. *J Bone Joint Surg Am* 2002;84:770-774.

In this study, the authors used a 22-mm femoral head with a smooth femoral stem (Ra, 0.6). At a mean follow-up of 9.4 years, the average linear and volumetric wear was 0.96 mm and 364.7 mm, respectively. Nine percent of patients had an osteolytic lesion in the calcar (zone 7). Although the average hip score improved from 44 to 95 at final follow-up, the authors conclude that the high rates of volumetric and linear wear are concerning.

Kim YH, Oh SH, Kim JS: Primary total hip arthroplasty with a second-generation cementless total hip prosthesis in patients younger than fifty years of age. *J Bone Joint Surg Am* 2003;85:109-114.

In this prospective study at a mean 9.8-year follow-up (range, 8 to 11 years), the average hip score improved from 48.8 to 92.0 at final follow-up. No aseptic loosening was reported, and the average amount of linear wear was 1.18 mm (0.12 mm/yr). Twelve percent of patients had femoral osteolysis and 9% had acetabular osteolysis.

Lonner JH, Hershman S, Mont M, Lotke PA: Total knee arthroplasty in patients 40 years of age and younger with osteoarthritis. *Clin Orthop* 2002;380:85-90.

In this study, the authors review the outcomes of 32 TKAs in 32 patients who had osteoarthritis and were 40 years of age or younger. At a mean 7.9-year follow-up, good or excellent results were reported in 82% of patients. Three revision surgeries were done to treat aseptic loosening, representing a failure rate of 12.5% at 8 years.

Mont MA, Lee CW, Sheldon M, Lennon WC, Hungerford DS: Total knee arthroplasty in patients younger or equal than 50 years old. *J Arthroplasty* 2002;17:538-543.

In this study, 30 patients (30 TKAs) were evaluated with an average follow-up of 7 years. One patient underwent revision surgery because of unexplained pain. In the other patients, there was no radiographic evidence of implant loosening. Ninety-seven percent of the patients rated their TKA outcomes as good or excellent at latest follow-up.

Sperling JW, Cofield RH, Rowland CM: Neer hemiarthroplasty and Neer total shoulder arthroplasty in patients fifty years older or less: Long-term results. *J Bone Joint Surg Am* 1998;80:464-473.

The authors of this study report on 74 hemiarthroplasties (34 shoulders) at a mean 12.3-year follow-up. They report that both the Neer hemiarthroplasty and the Neer TSA procedures resulted in significant long-term pain relief and improvement in abduction and external rotation; no significant difference between the two procedures was reported. The estimated survival of the Neer hemiarthroplasty was 92% at 5 years, 83% at 10 years, and 73% at 15 years. The estimated survival of the Neer TSA was 97% at 5 and 10 years and 84% at 15 years.

Exercise Prescription for the Total Joint Arthroplasty Patient

Bradbury N, Borton D, Spoo G, Cross MJ: Participation in sports after total knee replacement. *Am J Sports Med* 1998;26:530-535.

In this review of 160 patients who underwent TKA, the authors report that patients were more likely to return to low-impact activities than to high-impact activities after surgery. Seventy-seven percent of patients who participated in regular exercise in the year before surgery returned to athletic activity, whereas only 5% of patients who were not involved in athletic activities in the year before surgery participated in sports after surgery.

Healy WL, Iorio R, Lemos MJ: Athletic activity after joint replacement. *Am J Sports Med* 2001;29:377-388.

This comprehensive article provides recommendations for specific athletic activities for patients who have undergone THA, TKA, or TSA. Included in this article are tables from the surveys of the Hip Society, the Knee Society, and the American Shoulder and Elbow Surgeons Society for appropriate athletic activity for patients who have had joint replacement operations.

Healy WL, Iorio R, Lemos MJ: Athletic activity after total knee arthroplasty. *Clin Orthop* 2000;380:65-71.

The authors of this article outline activity recommendations for patients who have undergone TKA. In general, these patients are encouraged to participate in low-impact, low-demand athletic activities and to avoid high-impact, high-demand athletic activities.

Jensen KL, Rockwood CA Jr: Shoulder arthroplasty in recreational golfers. *J Shoulder Elbow Surg* 1998;7:362-367.

In this retrospective review, the authors report that of 24 patients who had shoulder arthroplasty 23 were able to resume playing golf.

McClung CD, Zahiri CA, Higa JK, Amstutz HC, Schmalzreid TP: Relationship between body mass index and activity in hip or knee arthroplasty patients. *J Orthop Res* 2000;18:35-39.

The authors of this study report that a higher body mass index (greater obesity) was associated with a lower activity level. With regard to the rate of polyethylene wear in patients with hip or knee implants, decreased ambulatory activity may counterbalance weight, which may explain why weight has not been shown to have a consistent effect on polyethylene wear in clinical studies.

Schmalzried TP, Szuszczewicz ES, Northfield MR, et al: Quantitative assessment of walking activity after total hip or knee replacement. *J Bone Joint Surg Am* 1998;80:54-59.

In this study, a pedometer was used to record the number of steps taken by 111 patients who underwent either TKA or THA. The authors report that age was significantly associated with activity. Patients who were younger than 60 years walked 30% more on average than those who were older than 60 years. Men who were younger than 60 years walked 40% more on average than the rest of the patients.

Classic Bibliography

Cirincione RJ: Sports after total joint replacement. *Md Med J* 1996;45:644-647.

Gill GS, Chan KC, Mills DM: 5- to 18-year followup study of cemented total knee arthroplasty for patients 55 years old or younger. *J Arthroplasty* 1997;12:49-54.

Mallon WJ, Callaghan JJ: Total joint replacement in active golfers. *J South Orthop Assoc* 1994;3:295-298.

Chapter 31

Epidemiology and Prevention of Sports Injuries

Anthony I. Beutler, MD

Stephen W. Marshall, PhD

Introduction

As is true for many aspects of medical knowledge, many things that are "known" about preventing sports injuries are not understood; for example, why female soccer players are more likely to tear their anterior cruciate ligaments than male soccer players. In short, even though scientific knowledge is incomplete, measures can still be taken to prevent injuries. Studies of injury epidemiology provide both factual knowledge; very few studies provide factual knowledge and conceptual understanding. Building effective prevention strategies for sports injury requires a differentiation between what is and what is not known; what is proven effective, proven ineffective, or simply unproven; and what has been confirmed as "cost-effective," either in financial or injury prevention terms. By exploring the overall significance of sports injuries, the sport-specific patterns of injury, and the contribution of specific intrinsic and extrinsic factors to injury risk, all that is known can be distinguished from the little that is truly understood.

The Significance of Sports Injuries

The burden on society from sports-related injuries is considerable (Table 1). It has been estimated that the medical costs alone for sports injuries exceed $282 million in the United States each year. In 1972, it was suggested that recreational and sports injuries account for more productive time lost than industrial injuries. The Centers for Disease Control and Prevention estimates that sports injuries account for 16% of all unintentional injuries treated in hospital-based emergency departments. Among children 10 to 14 years old, sports injuries are the most common cause of emergency department visits for unintentional injury (52% for boys and 38% for girls). In deployed US military forces, far more duty days are lost because of injuries from sports and recreation than combat casualties or illnesses. Based on data from the National Health Interview Survey, a federal survey of over 37,000 US households, the rate of sports and recreational injury was calculated to be 26 episodes per 1,000 persons per year or 1 out of every 5 medically attended injury episodes (2 out of every 5 injury episodes for patients 5 to 24 years old). These data suggest that the injury rate for sports participation exceeds the injury rate for motor vehicle accidents. Data from this same survey also indicate that 20% of school children miss school at least 1 day each year because of sports injuries and 28% of working adults miss at least 1 day of work per year because of sports injuries.

Sport-Specific Injury Patterns

Sports and recreational injuries arise in a wide variety of activities and affect individuals at all levels of fitness and conditioning. By far the biggest determinant of injury risk in sports and recreational injury is the nature of the activity itself, with contact sports carrying the greatest risk of injury. Yet even in full-contact sports, up to 40% of injuries are the results of overuse mechanisms. Overuse injuries have been estimated to account for more than 50% of all sports-related injuries. Numerous descriptive studies have documented the specific epidemiology of injuries in individual athletic activities ranging from bobsledding to Australian Rules football. Although these studies are helpful in identifying injuries common to a particular sport, they often provide limited insight into the mechanism by which injuries occur, which in turn limits their utility from a preventive perspective. Age, gender, level of competition, and level of fitness influence injury incidence. Age is an important risk factor, especially in patients with patellofemoral dysfunction, stress fractures, and apophyseal injuries. Older athletes more commonly experience metatarsal pain syndromes, plantar fasciitis, and degenerative tendinopathies. It is commonly accepted that gender predisposes athletes to certain overuse injuries (for example, female athletes may experience more patellofemoral pain and stress fractures than their male counterparts). Recent data, however, demonstrate that overuse injuries to female athletes are more sport-specific than gender-specific. With respect to fitness, unfit military recruits experience substantially more injuries during training than more fit individuals. The most dramatic data on fit-

TABLE 1 | Estimated Annual Injury Episodes in the United States by Age Group and Activity (National Health Interview Survey, 1997-1999)

| | Activity | | | |
| | No. of Injuries in 1000s (%) | | | |
Rank	5 to 14 years of age	15 to 24 years of age	25 to 44 years of age	> 45 years of age
1	Pedal cycling 332 (13.9)	Basketball 440 (20.9)	Basketball 256 (14.7)	Exercising/track 133 (24.1)
2	Basketball 261 (11.0)	Football 28 (13.7)	Pedal cycling 204 (11.7)	Recreation sport 112 (20.3)
3	Football 243 (10.2)	Exercising/track 172 (8.2)	Exercising/track 198 (11.4)	Water sport 44 (7.9)*
4	Playground equipment 219 (9.2)	Soccer 145 (6.9)	Baseball/softball 182 (10.4)	Skating/skateboarding 29 (5.2)*
5	Baseball/softball 185 (7.8)	Recreational sport 102 (4.9)	Recreational sport 146 (8.4)	Pedal cycling 27 (4.9)*
Remainder	1,114 (48.0)	958 (45.5)	754 (43.3)	208 (37.6)
Total	2,384 (100.0)	2,104 (100.0)	1,740 (100.0)	553 (100.0)

*Estimates may be unstable because they are based on fewer than 20 injuries or coefficient of variation > 30%.

(Adapted with permission from Conn JM, Annest JL, Gilchrist J: Sports- and recreation-related injury episodes in the US population. Inj Prev 2003;9:117-123.)

ness pertain to risk for sudden cardiac death among habitually sedentary versus habitually active men. An increased relative risk of sudden cardiac death occurs during exercise. Habitually active individuals experience only a small increase in risk, which is more than offset by the overall reduction in heart attacks associated with habitual exercise. One study reported that men who engaged in regular, moderate-intensity leisure time activity had one third the risk of primary cardiac arrest than those who did not engage in leisure time activity. The authors of this study previously reported that habitually sedentary men who sporadically engage in vigorous activity have up to a 100-fold increased risk of sudden cardiac death during exercise.

In clinical practice, familiarity with the specific sport and injury circumstances can provide important clues for a correct diagnosis. The concept of the body as a kinetic chain provides a working model for understanding, correcting, and preventing sport-specific patterns of overuse dysfunction. By relating the production and transfer of forces between the ground, body core, and extremities, this model explains why tennis players with lateral epicondylitis often will not recover without correction of underlying rotator cuff weakness, why baseball pitchers with elbow pain must be examined for weak quadriceps on their landing leg, and why runners must recover calf flexibility and eccentric calf strength to substantially improve plantar fasciitis symptoms. Specific sports have overuse and traumatic vulnerabilities. For example, young throwers with medial elbow pain can have a traction apophysitis, offensive linemen who

get rolled up in a pile can experience deltoid ligament injuries, and wrestlers more commonly experience lateral collateral ligament injuries. Although typically used for diagnosis and rehabilitation, knowledge of sport-specific injury mechanisms and sport-specific patterns for kinetic chain breakdown can also be implemented in injury prevention strategies.

The clinical evaluation of injuries involves the assessment of a patient's medical history, body type, level of competition, and previous injury status as well as the mechanism of injury. Academic discussions of injury epidemiology, however, typically divide risk factors into two broad categories: extrinsic and intrinsic risk factors. Extrinsic risk factors describe the influences of the environment on the athlete and typically include equipment, environment, errors in training, and rules governing play. Malalignment, inflexibility, fitness level, and movement (motor control) patterns represent intrinsic risk factors or factors that pertain to the individual athlete. The modification of extrinsic and intrinsic risk factors can prevent injury.

Extrinsic Risk Factors: The Effect of Environment on Injury Risk

Public policy efforts regarding injury prevention typically involve modification or elimination of extrinsic risk factors. Because alterations in a single extrinsic risk factor affect large populations of participants, these changes can result in significant financial and societal savings. But by the same token, poorly-informed prevention agendas—no matter how well intended—may result in significant costs without injury prevention benefits or may actually result in increased risk to the athletes they are designed to protect. Hence, policy changes must be based on solid scientific evidence and valid population statistics. Changing sport rules, mandating the use of protective equipment, taping and bracing of joints at risk, and altering the physical qualities of athletic equipment have all received considerable attention in sports medicine and public policy; however, there is a need for ongoing evaluation of these interventions to ensure that they continue to achieve the desired effects.

Rule Changes

The most famous and illustrative example of rule changes resulting in injury prevention occurred in the 1970s. During the late 1960s and early 1970s, on average 36 North American football players experienced catastrophic injuries (paralysis or death) each year. Using videotapes and a catastrophic injury registry, independent researchers and a National Collegiate Athletic Association commission determined that most of these injuries occurred when tacklers used the tops of their helmets to initiate contact (spear tackling). Led by Dr. Joseph Torg, these researchers performed biomechanical analyses demonstrating that spear tackling requires complete straightening of the cervical spine. By removing the usual protective, cushioning lordosis of the cervical spine and arranging the vertebrae into a straight column, spear tackling places potentially catastrophic compressive loads on the cervical vertebral bodies of the tackler. These findings led to rigid enforcement of previously existing but largely ignored rules. Beginning in the mid 1970s, spear tackling was severely penalized. Concurrently, player and coaching education programs encouraged "face-up" tackling techniques in which the initial contact is made with the chest and shoulder pads, rather than with the helmet. One study suggests that these two interventions have reduced the incidence of catastrophic injury in North America to essentially zero.

The effectiveness of rule changes in football spear tackling provides an excellent example of how epidemiologic data gathering, biomechanical analysis, and proper preventive interventions can lead to significant and proven injury prevention. Epidemiologic data gathering alone is insufficient. The problem of catastrophic neck injury in football was known before the publication of Dr. Torg's work. Previous solutions, however, including neck muscle strengthening programs, were not based on correct biomechanics and were therefore ineffective. Additionally, even good and effective preventive interventions can prove problematic. For example, football and hockey helmets and face masks were mandated and are effective in reducing injuries to the head and face; however, this preventive intervention altered the

way the game was played and led to the rise of a new injury in the kinetic chain. Virtually unheard of before the helmet mandate, catastrophic neck injuries claimed many lives as players began to use their helmets as weapons.

Hockey, soccer, and other sports have also adopted changes in rules governing player contact. Many of these efforts primarily attempt to reduce the number of concussions or mild traumatic brain injuries experienced by players. Although these rule changes appear to decrease the overall incidence of injuries that arise from the dangerous contact they proscribe, their effect on concussion prevention is more ambiguous. The uncertainty stems from the lack of consensus regarding the definition and evaluation of concussion. Attempts to measure concussion reduction are problematic at best. The recent use of brief standardized tools for balance testing, neurocognitive performance, and computerized neuropsychologic testing holds great promise for improved diagnosis and management of concussion. Repeated concussions may create detectable increases in the risk of subsequent concussion, suggesting that careful management of the initial injury is critical.

Protective Equipment

Helmets have been shown to decrease injury in the team sports of football, hockey, and baseball. In football and hockey, no conclusive evidence distinguishes one modern style or make of helmet as more protective than another. Proper fit, secure chin-strap wear, and adequate air-cell inflation are believed to maximize the protective benefit of helmets; however, there is little scientific evidence to support or refute this belief. Studies do show that helmets may prevent up to 85% of head and brain injury in motocross, skateboarding, and cycling.

Mouthguards have been proven to reduce many types of injury. Mouthguards stabilize dental structures during impact and distribute impact forces over the area of the appliance. This reduces the potential for dental injury and also the potential for penetrating injury to the soft orofacial tissues of the lips, mouth, tongue, and cheeks. Several analyses have demonstrated the efficacy of mouthguards in preventing maxillofacial injury. Mouthguards have also been postulated to protect against concussion by repositioning the condyles so that less force is transmitted to the base of the skull after a mandibular impact. Studies of mouthguard use for concussion reduction have contradictory findings, however. The major barrier to mouthguard use is compliance. Although a few organizations mandate the use of mouthguards during participation, larger population studies are needed to determine the cost consequences of mandating mouthguard use in specific youth sports.

Taping and Bracing

Most studies confirm the effectiveness of external ankle stabilization in reducing injury in high-risk sports. External ankle stabilization appears to have some efficacy in preventing the primary injury or first ankle sprain, especially for sports in which ankle injury is common. But studies more clearly document the success of external ankle support for preventing reinjury. Although taping has been the method of choice for ankle stabilization, rigid, semirigid, and neoprene ankle braces are now widely available. Limited studies with small populations have compared the efficacy of traditional ankle taping with external braces. The results of these studies are inconsistent, confounded by different taping methods and evaluation. The reported differences in injury rate are small. Presumed to be proprioceptive, the exact mechanism by which taping acts to reduce the risk of injury remains unclear. Biomechanical studies clearly demonstrate that the ability of the ankle tape to restrict range of motion is either significantly diminished or lost altogether after 20 minutes of moderate to vigorous exercise. Rigid support from an ankle brace should provide more ankle stability than athletic tape. The relative contributions of mechanical support versus proprioceptive aid provided by external ankle bracing have not been determined.

Despite the lack of clear efficacy data, many schools and organizations currently encourage the use of semirigid ankle braces. These ankle braces may be used repetitively throughout the season and do not require time from trainers or coaches for application, both of which result in significant cost savings. Some clinicians and trainers advocate the use of athletic taping plus an overlying external brace for injured athletes. Although no conclusive data indicate this to be a beneficial practice, external ankle supports are not associated with any increased rate of other injuries. Hence, the only apparent downside to the use of external ankle supports is their cost.

Several studies have examined the prophylactic use of knee braces in high-risk sports (including North American football). A promising application was reported in a study in which interior linemen used braces to reduce valgus strain injuries to the knee. The data in this study, however, demonstrate a definitive effect only for reserve players or those who play infrequently. Furthermore, other studies reported that bracing has no effect or a negative effect on knee injury. Biomechanical studies reveal some inherent limitations of knee braces both for primary injury prevention and reinjury protection. Braces made from soft materials provide no protection. Rigid or metallic-hinged braces offer the potential for collateral ligament protection, but they depend on stable, secure fixation to the knee, which is difficult to achieve. Considerable debate exists whether any external brace can adequately protect against the few millimeters of knee translation and rotation that precipitate most ligamentous injuries. Finally, rigid external knee braces alter muscle recruitment patterns, as well as result in increased rotational and angular forces at the knee joint. A consensus statement from the American Academy of Orthopaedic Surgeons confirms that there is no conclusive evidence that prophylactic knee braces can prevent knee ligament injuries.

Athletic Equipment Changes

Prevention of baseball and softball injuries is of special significance in injury epidemiology. Many injury prevention strategies such as safety (breakaway) bases, softer balls, and protective faceguards have all been shown to be very effective to possibly effective in recent confirmatory studies. Other proposed strategies do not have demonstrated efficacy, including the use of chest protectors to reduce the incidence of sudden cardiac death after being struck by a ball.

One classic study on decreasing sliding injury through the use of breakaway bases provides an example of good injury prevention research. In this study, the author demonstrated a substantial decrease in sliding injuries by using breakaway bases in softball. The use of breakaway bases resulted in dramatic injury reduction and substantial cost savings without affecting the sport.

Another study showed that both faceguards and safety balls were effective, although not perfect, in preventing youth baseball injuries. Of these two interventions, safety balls have the potential to prevent a larger number of injuries because defensive players experience 70% of all ball-related injuries. This study also demonstrates the minimal effect safety balls would have on "the feel of the game." When pitching, throwing, and batting under blinded conditions (with no identifying notation on the ball), adults cannot distinguish between a traditional ball and a modified ball that has as little as 20% of the traditional ball's hardness, and children (age 11 to 14 years) cannot distinguish between a traditional ball and a modified ball with as little as 15% of the traditional ball's hardness.

The use of chest protectors to protect against sudden cardiac death from being struck by a ball represents a well-intentioned but questionable injury prevention effect. Recent evidence suggests that sudden cardiac death is determined by the timing of impact in the cardiac cycle as well as by the force of the impact. Most critically, no available chest protector has been shown to be effective in reducing the force of impact, and there is no evidence that current chest protectors would offer any protection from sudden death resulting from commotio cordis.

Intrinsic Risk Factors: The Effect of Training and Individual Factors on Injury Prevention

Intrinsic risk factors typically pertain more to individual athletes than to entire populations of participants. Hence, intrinsic risk factors typically offer less opportunity for population cost savings, but modification of these risk factors can result in dramatically reducing injury risk in an individual or in a group of individuals with shared physical characteristics. Inherent difficulties complicate the measurement of intrinsic characteristics because human beings are less well suited for precise laboratory measurement than bats, balls, and other readily dissectible playthings. The athlete's injury history, level of fitness, joint alignment, and patterns of neuromuscular control represent a few intrinsic risk factors for injury.

History of Injury

Classic clinical teaching suggests that the previous injury history of an athlete is the most important predictor of future injury. Again, the model of the body as a kinetic chain is useful. Kinetic chains always break at their weakest link. A weak link may be caused by abnormal external forces that weaken an otherwise normal link. The demands of athletic activity place tremendous but predictable loads on the links of the kinetic chain. A broken link (or injury) may ensue because the particular link is biomechanically unable to withstand the normal demands of that sport; for instance, long-distance runners with varus knees have a higher incidence of osteoarthritis than long-distance runners with neutral alignment. Or, as is more commonly the case, the dysfunction of an upstream kinetic link results in an abnormal force that causes injury to a susceptible link downstream. As an example, inflexibility and loss of eccentric strength in the gastrocnemius-soleus complex causes abnormal forces to be transmitted to the ankle and foot. These abnormal forces can be associated with Achilles tendinopathy, plantar fasciitis, or bony stress fractures. Whether an athlete with an inflexible, weak soleus unit of the gastrocnemius-soleus complex will experience Achilles tendon pain, plantar injury, or stress fracture depends on the specific interaction of that athlete's kinetic chain with the environment and will be best predicted by that athlete's past pattern of injury.

Outside the area of sports injuries, studies document that previous back injury is a strong risk factor for predicting recurrent back injury. In military personnel, it has been shown that prior knee injury (measured by the need to obtain a medical waiver at time of recruitment) is strongly associated with a subsequent hospitalization for knee injury (relative risk, 8.0; 95% confidence interval, 2.1 to 29.9) and with risk of premature discharge for a knee condition (relative risk, 14.0; 95% confidence interval, 4.6 to 39.6). Although studied less often, similar effects of previous history predicting future injury have been observed in youth sports.

Fitness Level, Conditioning, and Stretching Programs

Although it is generally accepted that improved fitness and conditioning have considerable potential to reduce injury, conclusive evidence is lacking. One difficulty is the definition of fitness. Only a few studies prospectively examine the effect of fitness on injury incidence. One recent study collected data from New Zealand rugby players before the season and then tracked both the injury incidence and time lost from play over the course of the season. The measurements of preseason fitness yielded inconsistent injury prevention results. However, the authors of this study did find that players who started the season still recovering from injury were much more likely to be injured during that season than those without immediate injury history. Large-scale, controlled trials done in prospective fashion are needed. The same paucity of evidence exists for the role of stretching and warm-up programs in injury prevention.

Joint Alignment

Many large, population-based studies conclusively demonstrate that extremes in joint alignment predispose individuals to early or severe degenerative changes. The effect of valgus knees, anteverted hips, or flat feet on acute traumatic injuries is less studied and still poorly understood. For instance, one study demonstrated that US military recruits with pes planus have a twofold higher risk of lower extremity injury during 6 weeks of basic training compared with those with normal arches. Trainees with pes cavus experience a tenfold risk during that same time. No study, however, has determined whether interventions with corrective orthotics can decrease the risk of injury.

Motor (Neuromuscular) Control

The study of motor control or neuromuscular control seeks to explain how the central nervous system orchestrates complex, coordinated musculoskeletal movements. Knowledge of motor control and its relationship to injury is still rudimentary. Understanding how the brain controls the body offers an opportunity to train the brain to respond in a biomechanically safe manner when confronted by potentially dangerous situations. A better understanding of the central nervous system may represent the next great advance in modern medicine.

Movement patterns vary greatly between genders and among individuals. Certain movement patterns predispose individuals to specific injuries. Two studies have independently demonstrated evidence of gender differences in motor control patterns, suggesting that neuromuscular risk factors may be primarily responsible for the fact that women are at greater risk of anterior cruci-

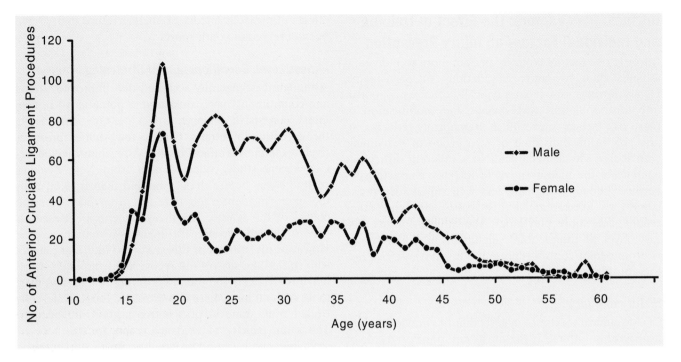

Figure 1 Graph illustrating the number of anterior cruciate ligament procedures done by candidates for certification by the American Board of Orthopaedic Surgeons in 2000. *(Adapted from Yu B, Kirkendall DT, Taft TN, Garret WE Jr: Lower extremity motor control-related and other risk factors for noncontact anterior cruciate ligament injuries. Instr Course Lect 2002;51:315-324.)*

ate ligament injury. Recent evidence, however, suggests that research in motor control and anterior cruciate ligament injury may need to focus on teenage subjects because the largest incidence of anterior cruciate ligament injury occurs between the ages of 15 and 18 years in both males and females (Figure 1). Unlike many other intrinsic risk factors for injury that would be difficult to modify (such as genu valgum, tibial torsion, and hormonal fluctuation), neuromuscular risk factors may be amenable to alteration via motor control retraining programs.

The Risks Versus Benefits of Exercise and Sports Participation

The overwhelming benefits of exercise in preventing obesity and complications from inactivity-related disease far outweigh the risks of exercise. But exercise does have risks, most notably sudden cardiac death and musculoskeletal injury. These risks can be greatly diminished by avoiding certain high-risk situations. As previously mentioned, habitually sedentary individuals have a 100-fold increased risk of sudden cardiac death when they exercise vigorously. However, moderate exercise offers all of the health benefits and a greatly reduced risk of sudden cardiac death to this same population. Similarly, the risk of musculoskeletal injury can be minimized by avoiding high-risk sports and common training errors (such as rapid increases in exercise frequency, intensity, and duration).

Physical inactivity and obesity are a growing problem. According to one study, nearly 75% of US adults report they are not regularly active or are inactive during leisure time. The Centers for Disease Control and Prevention recommends that adults accumulate at least 30 minutes of moderate physical activity most days of the week. Recent surveys indicate that less than 25% of US adults achieve this level of activity. American inactivity, along with other factors, has led to unprecedented levels of obesity and obesity-related disease. More than 33% of US adults are overweight, with more than 27% classified as obese. One study recently reported even more alarming data: childhood obesity increased by more than 10 percentage points between 1988 to 1994 and 1996 to 2000 for many groups of American children. These data indicate that the obesity epidemic is accelerating. The medical costs of treating obesity and obesity-related disease are similarly staggering. Direct costs from obesity are estimated to be as high as $24 billion (or 2.4% of all health care expenditures) annually. In measuring direct and indirect costs of obesity, one study estimated that $76.6 billion could be saved each year if all Americans over 15 years of age had a regular exercise program. Clearly, public health efforts to encourage physical activity should be supported by all physicians.

If the level of physical activity increases in the population, however, then a resulting upswing in the incidence of sports injuries may occur. The increase in injury incidence will need to be met with additional resources, including scientific investigation of potential prevention mechanisms and evaluation of prevention programs. Exercise prescription guidelines should be developed that minimize the risk of injury in sports and recreational activities, while maximizing the public health gain from the prevention of inactivity-related disease. These guidelines should be age and skill-level appropriate.

Future Directions in Injury Prevention

First, injury prevention strategies that work must be championed. For instance, helmets, mouthguards, and breakaway bases clearly prevent a significant number of serious injuries in a cost-effective manner without fundamental alterations to sport. Safety balls and face protectors may also prove effective. Yet despite overwhelming evidence of efficacy, these simple strategies are not implemented as often as they could be. Proven interventions should be championed and implemented as widely as possible within studied populations.

Second, prevention devices that have been proven ineffective must be clearly and decisively refuted. By clearly communicating this message to athletes, parents, coaches, and administrators, focus can be redirected to proven prevention strategies and efficacious ways to prevent these tragic incidents can be developed.

Areas with contradictory evidence present a unique challenge. Clearly, these areas should be addressed by carefully examining existing research and then designing solid research protocols and innovative collaborative trials. Consumer demand, however, can override these hostile factors. If consumers demand, and physicians educate patients to demand, solid evidence, then many of the increasing obstacles to good research can be overcome. If even a small portion of the resources presently spent on unproven modalities were redirected to research, a much clearer view of many now murky issues in sports injury prevention would result.

Finally, a fundamental understanding of neurologic and neuromuscular function is needed. Considerable and rational concern exists over the effects of mild brain injury from sport participation. Excellent strides have been made in some areas, such as quantifying the risk for repetitive heading of the ball in youth soccer. For concussion management, however, the progress is less encouraging. There is very little evidence that the many classification schemes truly improve management of the injury. If imperfect methods suggest a brain injury, the treatment armamentarium consists of little more than abstinence from future contact sports.

A similar paucity of knowledge exists in the understanding of motor control. Neuromuscular physiology dictates that instructions sent from the brain require approximately one half of a second before task completion to allow time for neuronal conduction and muscular contraction. There is currently no understanding of how these responses are anticipated, how these instructions are sent, and what happens when unexpected environmental changes interrupt a motor program already in transit or in progress. Imagine the rehabilitative potential if the central motor programs could be changed to incorporate more proprioceptive feedback from a previously injured limb, as well as the injury prevention benefit of a motor control program that placed the athlete in a more biomechanically safe position during landing, jumping, or cutting.

Summary

Sports medicine physicians play a critical role in sports injury prevention. Fundamental building blocks of injury prevention include understanding of the extrinsic and intrinsic risk factors for injury that affect individual or groups of athletes; awareness of proven, disproved, and controversial strategies in injury prevention; and resolve that future research meet appropriate evidence standards and answer questions that will increase knowledge of and the ability to design and implement sports injury prevention programs.

Annotated Bibliography

The Significance of Sports Injuries

Conn JM, Annest JL, Gilchrist J: Sports- and recreation-related injury episodes in the US population. *Inj Prev* 2003;9:117-123.

A summary of sports injury data collected by National Health Interview Survey (a face-to-face household survey), this report details the morbidity of sports injuries in the United States.

Sport-Specific Injury Patterns

Kibler WB, McMullen J: Scapular dyskinesis and its relation to shoulder pain. *J Am Acad Orthop Surg* 2003; 11:142-151.

The kinetic chain is well described here. Although originally applied to diagnosis, the kinetic chain also can be used to conceptualize and predict sport-specific injury patterns.

Extrinsic Risk Factors: The Effect of Environment on Injury Risk

Position Statement: The Use of Knee Braces. Rosemont, IL, American Academy of Orthopaedic Surgeons, 2004. Available at: http://www.aaos.org/wordhtml/papers/position/1124. Accessed May 17, 2004.

The American Academy of Orthopaedic Surgeons provides an informed assessment of the effectiveness of knee braces in the prevention and treatment of knee injuries and concludes that prophylactic knee braces have not been shown conclusively to prevent or reduce severity of injury.

Biasca N, Wirth S, Tegner Y: The avoidability of head and neck injuries in ice hockey: An historical review. *Br J Sports Med* 2002;36:410-427.

This thoughtful review details the history of attempts to reduce head injuries in hockey and examines the difficulties of preventing concussion, an injury about which relatively little is known.

Hume PA, Gerrard DF: Effectiveness of external ankle support: Bracing and taping in rugby union. *Sports Med* 1998;25:285-312.

This extensive review of the literature and specific trials involving rugby union players demonstrates that rigid lateral ankle support decreases reinjury rate.

Link MS, Maron BJ, Wang PJ, Pandian NG, VanderBrink BA, Estes NAM III: Reduced risk of sudden death from chest wall blows (commotio cordis) with safety baseballs. *Pediatrics* 2002;109:873-877.

This animal experiment with safety baseballs of different hardness demonstrates that softer baseballs reduce but do not eliminate the risk of commotio cordis from an ill-timed blow.

Marshall SW, Mueller FO, Kirby DT, Yang J: Evaluation of safety balls and face guards to prevent injury in youth baseball. *JAMA* 2003;289:568-574.

This cohort analysis showed that safety balls and face-guards are both effective in preventing ball-related and facial injury, respectively, in youth baseball.

Intrinsic Risk Factors: The Effect of Training and Individual Factors on Injury Prevention

Chappell JD, Kirkendall DJ, Yu B, Garrett WE: A comparison of knee kinetics between male and female recreational athletes in stop-jump tasks. *Am J Sports Med* 2002;30:261-267.

This study of knee kinematics in 20 recreational athletes shows clear differences in motor patterns between men and women during jump-stop maneuvers. Women landed with less knee flexion, more valgus force, and more anterior tibial sheer force than men.

Cox KA, Clark KL, Yuanzhang L, Powers TE, Krauss MR: Prior knee injury and risk of future hospitalization and discharge from military service. *Am J Prev Med* 2000;18(3 suppl):112-117.

This retrospective case-control study of 281 military recruits with a history of knee injury prior to active duty enlistment shows a greater than twofold increase in the likelihood of premature discharge for any reason and a 14-fold increase in premature discharge for a knee-related diagnosis in those with knee pain.

Huston L, Wojtys E: Neuromuscular differences between male and female athletes contributing to anterior cruciate ligament injuries, in Garrett WE Jr, Lester GE,

McGowan J, Kirkendall DT: (eds): *Women's Health in Sports and Exercise.* Rosemont, IL, American Academy of Orthopaedic Surgeons, 2000, pp 347-356.

This is a summary of multiple studies demonstrating differences in motor control patterns about the knee in male and female athletes.

Quarrie KL, Alsop JC, Waller AE, Bird YN, Marshall SW, Chalmers DJ: A prospective cohort study of risk factors for injury in Rugby Union football. *Br J Sports Med* 2001;35:157-166.

This is one of the only prospective, multiple regression studies of a cohort of rugby players. Risk factors studied included previous injury, hours of activity per week, smoking status, body mass index, and years of rugby participation. Previous injury was found to be predictive of future injury.

The Risks Versus Benefits of Exercise and Sports Participation

Lemaitre RN, Siscovick DS, Raghunathan TE, Weinmann S, Arbogast P, Lin DY: Leisure-time physical activity and the risk of primary cardiac arrest. *Arch Intern Med* 1999;159:686-690.

This case-control study assessed the risks of primary cardiac arrest in three groups: those who participate in moderate intensity leisure activities, those who participate in vigorous intensity leisure activities, and those who participate in no activity during leisure time. Both moderate and vigorous groups had an odds ratio of 0.36 for primary cardiac arrest when compared with the no activity group.

Ogden CL, Flegal KM, Carroll MD, Johnson CL: Prevalence and trends among overweight among US children and adolescents, 1999-2000. *JAMA* 2002;288:1728-1732.

This article provides new data on overweight children in America suggesting that childhood obesity is growing at an alarming rate among all groups of children and most rapidly in Mexican-American and non-Hispanic black adolescents.

Pratt M, Macera CA, Blanton C: Levels of physical activity and inactivity in children and adults in the United States: Current evidence and research issues. *Med Sci Sports Exerc* 1999;31(11 suppl):S526-S533.

This article provides the results of several combined surveys and shows worse than expected levels of activity in US children and adults.

Classic Bibliography

Albright JP, Powell JW, Smith W, et al: Medial collateral ligament knee sprains in college football: Effectiveness of preventive braces. *Am J Sports Med* 1994;22:12-18.

Garrick JG: Prevention of sports injuries. *Postgrad Med* 1972;51:125-129.

Garrick JG, Requa RK: Role of external support in the prevention of ankle sprains. *Med Sci Sports* 1973;5:200-203.

Hewett T, Stroupe A, Nance T, Noyes F: Plyometric training in female athletes: Decreased impact forces and increased hamstring torques. *Am J Sports Med* 1996;24:765-773.

Janda DH, Wojtys EM, Hankin FM, Benedict ME: Softball sliding injuries: A prospective study comparing standard and modified bases. *JAMA* 1988;259:1848-1850.

Jones BH, Bovee MW, Knapik JJ: Associations among body composition, physical fitness, and injury in men and women army trainees, in Marriott BM (ed): *Body Composition and Physical Performance*. Washington, DC, National Academy Press, 1992, pp 141-173.

Mueller FO, Cantu RC, Van Camp SP: *Catastrophic Injuries in High School and College Sports*. Champaign, IL, Human Kinetics, 1996, pp 42-47.

O'Connor FG, Howard TM, Fieseler CM, Nirschl RP: Managing overuse injuries: A systemic approach. *Phys Sportsmed* 1997;25:128-142.

Sitler M, Ryan J, Wheeler B, et al: The efficacy of a semi-rigid ankle stabilizer to reduce ankle injuries in basketball: A randomized clinical study at West Point. *Am J Sports Med* 1994;22:454-461.

Thompson DC, Rivara FP, Thompson RS: Effectiveness of bicycle safety helmets in preventing head injuries: A case-control study. *JAMA* 1996;276:1968-1973.

Torg JS, Sennett B, Pavlov H, Leventhal MR, Glasgow SG: Spear tackler's spine: An entity precluding participation in tackle football and collision activities that expose the cervical spine to axial energy inputs. *Am J Sports Med* 1993;21:640-649.

Chapter 32

Exercise in Pregnancy and Beyond: Benefits for Long-Term Health

Susanne L. Bathgate, MD

E. Britton Chahine, MD

John W. Larsen, MD

Charles J. Macri, MD

Introduction

New information has been identified that demonstrates the value of exercise for promoting women's health and well-being, both in pregnancy and in the long term. Because obesity has been identified as a major cause of poor health and is inversely related to the ability to exercise effectively, it is important for practicing physicians to encourage women to maintain healthy behaviors such as exercise programs and weight control to promote health. Preconception exercise may be encouraged to allow women to be in good physical condition before pregnancy and to allow them to reach their ideal body weight. Conditioned women should be encouraged to continue exercising during pregnancy, and all women should be encouraged to exercise regularly because of the benefits on the cardiovascular system and bone mass.

When making exercise recommendations, physicians should be aware of the health risks of obesity, including the recent demographic trends in the United States, prevalence of obesity, and management strategies, as well as the health benefits associated with exercise and physical fitness. When making exercise recommendations for pregnant women, physicians should understand the physiology of pregnancy and how aerobic exercise and weight training may enhance the physiologic changes of pregnancy. It is also important to understand the beneficial effects of exercise on fetal and placental development and the effects of exercise on maternal cardiorespiratory function and thermoregulation.

Some of the limitations and physical problems that the pregnant patient may encounter when exercising include increased joint laxity and instability, difficulty with balance, and cardiorespiratory changes. Physicians should know how to treat these problems and be up to date regarding the current pertinent recommendations for exercise from the National Institutes of Health (NIH), the Centers for Disease Control and Prevention (CDC), and the American College of Obstetricians and Gynecologists (ACOG).

What Is Exercise?

Exercise may be defined as a regular series of specific movements designed to strengthen or develop some part of the body or some faculty or an activity for training or developing the body or mind. Such systematic practice may include finger exercises for the pianist or bodily exertion for the sake of health.

Why It Is Important to Discuss Exercise With Patients

Obesity is a major cause of increasing morbidity and mortality in the United States. Although the percentage of overweight adults in the United States has been stable at about 33%, the percentage of obese adults has risen from approximately 16% in 1980 to more than 27% today. The prevalence of obesity among US adults increased by 1% each year during the 1990s. Women of racial and ethnic minorities are affected disproportionately by obesity, as are women of lower socioeconomic standing. For example, 69% of African-American women are overweight or obese compared with "only" 47% of non-Hispanic white women. The CDC estimates that obesity and related lifestyle issues cause 300,000 deaths per year and cost $117 billion in the year 2000. Exercise can be a part of lifestyle modification to decrease obesity and improve cardiovascular health.

Defining Obesity and the Risk for Obesity-Related Diseases

According to the NIH guidelines, the body mass index (BMI, calculated as the weight in kilograms divided by the square of height in meters) is the recommended method for measuring obesity in the clinical setting. It is believed that the BMI is an estimate of the amount of fat stored in the body. Patients who have a BMI of 25 to 29.9 are considered overweight, and those who have a BMI of 30 or more are considered obese. Large waist circumference (> 102 cm for men and > 88 cm for women) provides a practical means to identify increased fat and a strong cardiovascular risk factor. Based on these definitions, more than 60% of American adults are overweight or obese.

TABLE 1 | Cardiovascular Disease Risk Factors

Very high risk for cardiovascular disease occurs with:

Established heart disease or other atherosclerotic disease

Type 2 diabetes mellitus

Sleep apnea

Other risk factors for cardiovascular disease:

Cigarette smoking

Hypertension

High levels of low-density lipoprotein cholesterol

Low levels of high-density lipoprotein cholesterol

Impaired fasting glucose

Family history of premature coronary heart disease

Physical inactivity

High triglycerides

Age 45 years or older in men

Age 55 years or older in women

Presence of other diseases that may be associated with obesity (eg, osteoarthritis, gallstones, stress incontinence, and polycystic ovary syndrome)

(Adapted with permission from Serdula MK, Khan LK, Dietz WH: Weight loss counseling revisited. JAMA 2003;289:1747-1750.)

Although exercise can potentially benefit every individual, there may be modification of exercise intensity required because of a patient's risk for cardiovascular disease. Patients at risk may require a more thorough medical evaluation before initiation of a vigorous exercise program. Therefore, in addition to the anthropometric values noted above, obesity-associated diseases and cardiovascular disease risk factors should be sought and recorded for all patients before prescribing an exercise program (Table 1).

The Impact of Obesity on Health

The American Heart Association has cited obesity as a major modifiable risk factor for coronary heart disease, and it has been reported that the risk of developing coronary heart disease for a woman is increased threefold with a BMI greater than 29 compared with BMI less than 21.

The distribution of body fat has been identified as a significant independent risk factor for poor health. Waist circumference of greater than 102 cm or 40 inches in men and greater than 88 cm or 35 inches in women is associated with the presence of more visceral fat, a more atherogenic type of fat, and with reduced insulin sensitivity. In Gothenburg, Sweden, a longitudinal study showed that increased waist size positively correlated with an increased incidence of myocardial infarction, angina, and stroke independent of age or BMI.

Obesity predisposes individuals to a wide variety of diseases. Of special concern in women is the association of obesity with breast and endometrial cancers and disorders of reproduction. The link with uterine and breast cancer is believed to be the result of the increased amount of estrogen produced by adipose tissue, and in postmenopausal women this may be related to the amount of visceral fat.

Public Health Aspects of Obesity

It is generally accepted that a decrease in daily physical activity has been associated with the increased prevalence of obesity worldwide. Physical activity has decreased because of increasing mechanization on the job, laborsaving devices at home, and changing personal practices. Some authors recommend prescribing physical activity as a way to improve health. Numerous investigators have reported that changes in physical activity or cardiorespiratory fitness are predictors of weight change. Regular physical activity may be especially important for weight control for those with genetic predisposition for weight gain or those eating a high-fat diet. Following current guidelines, implementing a plant-based diet with no more than 30% of calories (energy) from fat may provide important health benefits and may reduce the risk of unhealthy weight gain. A minimum of 30 minutes of moderate-intensity physical activity over the course of most (preferably all) days of the week will lead to improved health and function and should aid in weight maintenance. The precise amount of activity necessary to prevent unhealthy weight gain is still unknown.

Benefits of Physical Activity

Daily physical activity is basic to good health. The benefits of regular exercise are well documented and include positive effects on mind, bone, lipid profile, endothelial function, risk for cancer, glucose tolerance, insulin sensitivity, and quality of life. The Nurses' Health Study documented a lower incidence of cardiovascular disease, including both coronary heart disease and stroke, with increasing physical activity in a dose-dependent manner. Even a moderate-intensity exercise such as walking was associated with a lower risk of disease. Lipid profiles are favorably affected by physical activity. Moderate- to high-level aerobic exercise has the most pronounced improvement on high-density lipoprotein cholesterol, with reductions in total cholesterol, low-density lipoprotein cholesterol, and triglycerides less frequently observed. Diet plus exercise led to significant reductions in low-density lipoprotein cholesterol in both men and women. It was noted that although the National Cholesterol Education Program step 2 diet alone was ineffective in reducing low-density lipoprotein cholesterol, exercise provided a powerful catalyst to improve lipid profiles. Because of the many benefits of exercise, the recommendation for aerobic activity has been raised from 20 minutes three times per week to 30 minutes on most, if not all, days of the week. This is the minimum recommendation; those wishing to lose weight should exceed this guideline. Yet, obese individuals who are not physically fit should be advised to build up to this recommendation incrementally because setting an exercise goal too high can result in rapid failure and discouragement.

Preconception and Pregnancy and Implementation of Healthy Lifestyle Changes

Women who are planning pregnancy actively seek information about healthy lifestyles and are more likely to interrupt unhealthy behaviors such as drinking alcohol and smoking cigarettes. They adopt favorable changes such as diet modification and increasing exercise in an attempt to improve pregnancy outcome. Weight loss before pregnancy associated with institution of a preconception exercise program may improve the pregnancy outcome and long-term health of women. When pregnant, many women extensively question and research food and activity options, trying to choose those that will be most conducive to giving birth to a healthy baby. Because of the substantial health benefits of exercise in general and also in pregnancy, continuation or initiation of exercise should be encouraged in pregnancy unless otherwise contraindicated.

Effects of Exercise on Pregnancy

Maternal Responses

Moderate exercise has no adverse effect on embryonic development, fetoplacental growth, prematurity, indices of fetal compromise, and condition during labor and at birth. Well-conditioned women who continue a regular running or aerobics regimen in the periconceptual period and throughout pregnancy do not experience an increase in the incidence of failure to conceive, abortion, congenital abnormalities, abnormal placentation, premature rupture of the membranes, or preterm labor. In fact, women who exercise regularly during pregnancy may experience shorter labors with less need for surgical delivery and less indications of fetal compromise during labor.

Cardiovascular Response

In normal pregnancy, women increase their circulating blood volume by about 40% by the third trimester, their resting heart rate by about 10 beats per minute, and their cardiac output by about 40%. Under the influence of increased circulating progesterone levels, they increase their minute ventilatory volume primarily by increasing tidal volume and not respiratory rate. Pregnant women may experience this as a sensation of shortness of breath. However, they should be reassured because resting oxygen uptake is increased with advancing pregnancy.

Light-headedness and frank syncope are common in normal pregnancy and are most often related to position and compression of the inferior vena cava by the gravid uterus, with decreased blood return to the heart and subsequent hypotension. Other causes of light-headedness include sudden position changes or prolonged standing in pregnancy. These symptoms may be more pronounced in pregnancy because of decreased systemic vascular resistance. Prolonged standing or sitting in the nonpregnant person can achieve the same effect.

Conditioned women may experience less significant physiologic changes than nonconditioned women. For example, as pregnancy progresses, similar amounts of activity produce increasing amounts of oxygen consumption, but this is less so with conditioned women. Subjective workload and maximum exercise performance are decreased, which is, again, less so with highly trained women. Of special importance is exercise-induced hemoconcentration. Pregnant women should be encouraged to drink fluids to maintain appropriate intravascular volume, especially when exercising in hot, humid climates.

Thermoregulation

Because of a hypothetical association of fetal teratogenic effects with high temperatures, thermoregulation has been closely monitored and studied during exercise in pregnancy. Despite the theoretic risks, no known study has demonstrated that birth defects are caused by exercise. Therefore, pregnant women may be encouraged to exercise.

Although basal metabolic rate and heat production increase during pregnancy, increases in core temperature are blunted. Pregnancy may confer thermal protection because of increased thermal inertia created by the increase in body weight. Pregnancy is also associated with an increase in plasma volume and skin blood flow, which helps to dissipate heat by convection and radiant heat loss through the skin. Furthermore, the sweat threshold progressively decreases throughout gestation, aiding evaporative heat loss. Because minute ventilation is increased during pregnancy, it is also possible that heat loss through the respiratory tract contributes to the thermal protection. Consequently, the physiologic changes that occur as a result of pregnancy appear to enhance heat dissipation during exercise and provide both maternal and fetal thermal protection.

Weight Gain

The ACOG generally suggests that a 25- to 35-lb weight gain is healthy for pregnant women beginning pregnancy at an average weight. Women should be counseled that fetal well-being depends on adequate maternal nutrition and fat stores, especially in early pregnancy. For women who exercise before pregnancy, however, continuing a regular exercise program throughout pregnancy does not appear to detrimentally limit the rate of early pregnancy weight gain or subcutaneous fat deposition. In studies of these exercising women, results show that weight gain and fat deposition slow in late pregnancy for those who continue to exercise, but the total weight gain is within the normal range. Because adequate fat stores are important as a source of fetal fuel for normal fetal growth and are required for successful lactation, exercising women should take into account the energy expended in exercise and consume adequate calories in addition to the additional 300 kcal/day required for those with a normal pregnancy in the second and third trimester.

Glucose Regulation

Glucose serves as a primary metabolic fuel for the fetus. Pregnancy is a state of relative insulin resistance, making glucose readily available as a source of energy substrate for the developing fetus. There are maternal counterregulatory mechanisms that limit maternal blood glucose elevations. Failure of these counterregulatory mechanisms leads to gestational diabetes and hyperglycemia in the fetus. Exercise may play a role in the primary prevention of gestational diabetes, especially in morbidly obese women. The American Diabetes Association has recognized exercise as a helpful adjunct therapy when diet alone is not sufficient to control blood glucose levels, especially in the gestational diabetic.

In the nonpregnant state, aerobic exercise produces an intensity-dependent rise in blood glucose. Pregnancy modifies this response such that by the middle of the first trimester a rise in glucose levels is seen only when exercise exceeds 80% of the maximum predicted heart rate based on age. Because weight training increases muscle mass, and muscle burns calories more efficiently than fat tissue, weight training may have an additive beneficial effect.

Fetal Response to Maternal Exercise

Fetal Heart Rate

The fetal heart rate has been used as an indicator of fetal well-being. Prolonged and recurrent episodes of fetal bradycardia or fetal tachycardia may be associated with fetal compromise. However, although studies observing fetal heart rate during maternal exercises have identified that transient fetal tachycardia occurs commonly and bradycardia occurs sporadically, neither of these conditions has been associated with poor pregnancy outcome. In a recent review of studies of the fetal heart rate during exercise, it was concluded that the fetal heart rate typically increases 10 to 30 beats per minute during exercise, regardless of gestational age or exercise intensity. Increased fetal heart rate may allow for increased fetal cardiac output and oxygen availability, thus serving as a reflex response to maternal exercise. One study reported that most of the subjects experienced fetal tachycardia during exercise, and suggested that this is a normal response not linked to fetal distress. Sporadic fetal bradycardia has also been described in healthy, exercising women but with no untoward outcome.

Doppler Studies and Fetal Activity

Two other measures of fetal well-being that have been studied in exercising pregnant women are the indirect measure of blood flow through the umbilical cord as measured by Doppler velocimetry and fetal activity. Fetal umbilical artery Doppler flow velocimetry studies have not shown significant changes in circulation in response to controlled episodes of exercise, but transiently elevated flow corresponding to fetal bradycardia has been reported. Similarly, several studies have reported a significant decrease in fetal breathing after maternal exercise by conditioned subjects, but these studies report no significant change in shoulder movements or kick response, confirming fetal well-being.

Newborn Outcomes

Size at Birth

Data regarding the effects of maternal exercise and fetal growth are inconsistent. The timing of the exercise may impact the effect of exercise on fetal growth in pregnancy. Beginning a moderate regimen of weight-bearing exercise in early pregnancy has been shown to enhance fetoplacental growth. Conversely, a high volume of moderate-intensity, weight-bearing exercise begun in middle or late pregnancy symmetrically reduces fetoplacental growth. Fetal growth seems to be influenced by the level of maternal activity as well. Some studies have reported that significantly bigger babies were born to moderately trained women than nontrained or heavily trained women. In the latter group, the reduction in the size of the babies born could be explained by a reduced neonatal fat mass.

Neurobehavioral Profile

Although data are limited, current studies show that the benefits of exercise during pregnancy may extend to the child even after birth. The newborn behavioral profile shows that infants of mothers who exercised regularly during pregnancy are better able to orient to environmental stimuli, regulate their state, and quiet themselves after sound and light stimuli than infants of mothers who did not exercise regularly. In one study, testing at 5 years of age showed children whose mothers exercised during pregnancy performed better on tests of oral language skills and intelligence. It is important to note, however, that these results may not be generalized to the overall population.

Effects of Pregnancy on the Exercising Woman

Although exercise is beneficial to a pregnant woman's physical and psychologic well-being and is safe for the fetus (Table 2), pregnant women experience physical and psychologic changes during pregnancy that may limit their ability to exercise.

Exercising pregnant women seem to have less musculoskeletal complaints in general. Although objective data are not conclusive, this may be a result of the stronger muscular core of the exercising pregnant woman. Improved muscle tone results in a more stable pelvis as well as decreased lordosis because of stronger abdominal and back muscles. In some women, however, the many physiologic changes that occur during pregnancy may lead to low back pain and hip pain.

Low Back Pain

One of the most important physiologic changes is the widening and increased mobility of the sacroiliac synchondroses and the symphysis pubis. This begins during the 10th to 12th week of pregnancy and is associated with increased relaxin, secreted by the corpus luteum. Widening of the symphysis pubis continues until full term, but it should always be less than 1 cm and may cause sliding and instability of the pelvic joints. In addition, there is considerable lordosis because of the increasing size of the uterus, which also contributes to the mobility of the sacroiliac joints.

The patient may experience discomfort ranging from point tenderness at the joint site or lumbar back pain to radiating pain that progresses down the back of the thighs or lower abdomen. In the evaluation of low back pain in pregnancy, it is important to remember that herniation of the lumbosacral disk is not uncommon in women of childbearing age.

Evaluation may include a three-view spine series after the first trimester or MRI at any gestational age. MRI has not been shown to have any detrimental effects on the fetus. It is recommended, however, that fetal exposure to ionizing radiation be kept as low as possible, and some specialists recommend delaying radiologic evaluation until after pregnancy.

Treatment of low back pain in pregnancy may include administration of acetaminophen, rest, and the application of local heat. In general, aspirin and nonsteroidal anti-inflammatory agents are not recommended for routine use in pregnancy. Once the acute pain is resolved, abdominal and back strengthening exercises may be recommended. Pregnant women should avoid exercising in the supine position after the first trimester because compression of the vena cava can cause hypotension. For some patients, the use of a support belt (trochanteric belt) may provide symptomatic relief of back pain.

TABLE 2	Guidelines for Exercise During Pregnancy

For all women of childbearing age, an accumulation of 30 minutes or more of moderate exercise a day should occur on most, if not all, days of the week. In the absence of either medical or obstetric complications, pregnant women should do so as well.

No exercise should be done in the supine position after the first trimester. Pregnant women should avoid prolonged periods of motionless standing.

Be aware of the changes and needs of pregnancy. Stop with fatigue; do not exercise to exhaustion. Modifications in exercise routine from weight bearing (eg, jogging) to non-weight-bearing (eg, stationary cycling and swimming) activities in later pregnancy may help with continuing exercise on a regular basis.

When good balance is necessary or abdominal trauma is a possibility, exercise should be avoided.

Pregnancy requires intake of an extra 300 kcal/day. Additional caloric requirements will be based on exercise duration and intensity.

Exercise in pregnancy requires appropriate hydration, clothing, and environment to dissipate heat.

Resuming exercise in the postpartum period is determined on a case-by-case basis and by physical limitation.

(Adapted with permission from ACOG Committee Opinion: No. 267. Exercise during pregnancy and the postpartum period. Obstet Gynecol 2002;99:171-173.)

Surgical treatment is generally reserved for patients with neurologic compromise from disk herniation accompanied by bowel or bladder incontinence. An orthopaedic surgeon, neurologist, or neurosurgeon with particular expertise in these disorders should evaluate patients with such neurologic involvement.

Hip Pain

Hip pain associated with pelvic instability is typically treated conservatively, but it must be differentiated from two uncommon disorders: osteonecrosis of the femoral head and osteoporosis of the hip. The etiology of osteonecrosis of the femoral head is not known, but it may be associated with the increased cortisol levels in pregnancy combined with increased interosseous pressure resulting from increased weight. The symptoms usually occur in the third trimester and may present as deep groin pain that radiates to the knee, thigh, or back. Plain radiography or MRI may be helpful for diagnosis. Treatment is identical to that for nonpregnant patients.

Osteoporosis of the hip may also occur in pregnancy, and patients with this disease often present with pain and limited hip mobility. An anteroposterior radiograph of the pelvis may demonstrate osteoporosis of the hip with preservation of the joint space. The pain may be sudden or gradual, occurring during weight bearing and progressing until the patient is bedridden. This is treated conservatively with crutches and reduced weight bear-

TABLE 3	Absolute Contraindications to Aerobic Exercise During Pregnancy

Hemodynamically significant heart disease

Restrictive lung disease

Incompetent cervix/cerclage

Multiple gestation at risk for premature labor

Persistent second or third trimester bleeding

Placenta previa after 26 weeks of gestation

Premature labor during the current pregnancy

Ruptured membranes

Preeclampsia/pregnancy-induced hypertension

(Adapted with permission from ACOG Committee Opinion: No. 267. Exercise during pregnancy and the postpartum period. Obstet Gynecol 2002;99:171-173.)

TABLE 4	Relative Contraindications to Aerobic Exercise During Pregnancy

Severe anemia

Unevaluated maternal cardiac arrhythmia

Chronic bronchitis

Poorly controlled type 1 diabetes mellitus

Extreme morbid obesity

Extreme underweight (BMI < 12)

History of extremely sedentary lifestyle

Intrauterine growth restriction in current pregnancy

Poorly controlled hypertension

Orthopaedic limitations

Poorly controlled seizure disorder

Poorly controlled hyperthyroidism

Heavy smoker

(Adapted with permission from ACOG Committee Opinion: No. 267. Exercise during pregnancy and the postpartum period. Obstet Gynecol 2002;99:171-173.)

TABLE 5	Warning Signs to Terminate Exercise During Pregnancy

Vaginal bleeding

Dyspnea before exertion

Dizziness

Headache

Chest pain

Muscle weakness

Calf pain or swelling (need to rule out thrombophlebitis)

Preterm labor

Decreased fetal movement

Amniotic fluid leakage

(Adapted with permission from ACOG Committee Opinion: No. 267. Exercise during pregnancy and the postpartum period. Obstet Gynecol 2002;99:171-173.)

ing to decrease the possibility of fracture of the femoral neck. If fracture does occur, surgical treatment is indicated.

Special Circumstances and Contraindications to Exercise

Under some circumstances, either the mother or fetus may poorly tolerate aerobic exercise, or some conditions may worsen with exercise, which the ACOG has divided into absolute and relative contraindications to exercise during pregnancy (Tables 3 and 4). In general, women may participate in a variety of physical activities during pregnancy, but each woman's overall health and each physical activity should be evaluated for potential risk. In women at risk for poor uteroplacental perfusion, such as those with hemodynamically significant heart disease, preeclampsia, pregnancy-induced hypertension, or intrauterine growth restriction, vigorous activities that can shunt blood flow away from the uterus should

be avoided. Women with existing obstetric complications who are at high risk for preterm delivery or premature placental separation, such as those with second or third trimester bleeding or incompetent cervix, should also avoid vigorous physical activity.

Individual activities should be evaluated for the risk of abdominal trauma or falls, and participation in sports with significant risk of abdominal trauma or falls should be discouraged. For example, contact sports such as ice hockey, soccer, and basketball could result in contact with the pregnant abdomen and result in subsequent premature placental separation and should therefore be avoided during pregnancy. Activities that pose a risk for falling, such as skiing and horseback riding, are also best avoided during pregnancy. Activities that are usually safe include low-impact aerobics, yoga, treadmill or stair machine use, walking, and swimming.

With advancing gestation, the enlarging uterus impedes blood return to the heart when pregnant women are in the supine position. This causes a decrease in cardiac output, which may result in lightheadedness for the pregnant woman and decreased uteroplacental blood flow. Activities involving motionless standing may also decrease cardiac output.

Pregnant women should be counseled against scuba diving because the fetus cannot filter bubbles formed in the bloodstream and is at risk for decompression sickness. Brief episodes of moderate exercise at altitudes up to 6,000 feet appear not to pose a significant risk to pregnant women or their fetuses.

The ACOG suggests that exercise be stopped under conditions suggestive of maternal, obstetrical, or fetal complications (Table 5). Maternal symptoms suggestive of preeclampsia or pulmonary embolism include headache, dizziness, and/or dyspnea before exertion and should be evaluated before continuing exercise. Amniotic fluid leakage, persistent preterm contractions, and decreased fetal movement may be obstetric or fetal complications and should also be investigated before continuing exercise.

Most studies of the effects of exercise on the pregnant woman and her fetus have been conducted at moderate ambient temperatures and with adequate hydration of the woman, typically for 30 minutes; therefore, these recommendations should not be extrapolated to extremes of temperature, exertion, or duration.

Summary

Obesity and a sedentary lifestyle are major risk factors for long-term health problems such as cardiovascular disease and cancer. Exercise has been shown to beneficially modify these risk factors. Women who are planning pregnancy actively seek information about healthy lifestyles and are more likely to interrupt unhealthy behaviors, such as drinking alcohol and smoking cigarettes. Furthermore, they typically adopt favorable changes, such as diet modification and increasing exercise, in an attempt to improve pregnancy outcome. Exercise should be encouraged before pregnancy, during pregnancy, and postpartum, unless otherwise individually thought detrimental.

Annotated Bibliography

General

Chakravarthy MV, Joyner MJ, Booth FW: An obligation for primary care physicians to prescribe physical activity to sedentary patients to reduce the risk of chronic health conditions. *Mayo Clin Proc* 2002;77:165-173.

The authors of this study present exercise recommendations for general health.

Fuscaldo JM: Prescribing physical activity in primary care. *W V Med J* 2002;98:250-253.

Health benefits of exercise for all people are discussed in this article.

Mayer-Davis EJ, Costacou T: Obesity and sedentary lifestyle: Modifiable risk factors for prevention of type 2 diabetes. *Curr Diab Rep* 2001;1:170-176.

The authors of this article discuss ways of preventing type 2 diabetes mellitus through exercise.

What Is Exercise?

Blair SN, Wei M: Sedentary habits, health, and function in older women and men. *Am J Health Promot* 2000;15:1-8.

The authors of this study discuss the health risks of a sedentary lifestyle.

Clinical guidelines on the identification, evaluation, and treatment of overweight and obesity in adults: The evidence report. National Institutes of Health. *Obes Res* 1998;6(suppl 2):51S-209S.

This report outlines the guidelines for the evaluation and treatment of obesity.

DiPietro L, Kohl HW III, Barlow CE, Blair SN: Improvements in cardiorespiratory fitness attenuate age-related weight gain in healthy men and women: The Aerobics Center Longitudinal Study. *Int J Obes Relat Metab Disord* 1998;22:55-62.

The authors of this study discuss ways to prevent weight gain through exercise.

Guo SS, Zeller C, Chumlea WC, Siervogel RM: Aging, body composition, and lifestyle: The Fels Longitudinal Study. *Am J Clin Nutr* 1999;70:405-411.

The authors of this study examined patterns of change in body composition and determined the effects of long-term patterns of change in physical activity in older men and women and in menopausal status and estrogen use in women. They report that increased physical activity can improve low fat-free mass, the effects of an intervention program on body composition can be masked if only body weight or BMI is measured, the effects of physical activity can be more profound in postmenopausal than in premenopausal women, and estrogen use can have beneficial effects on body composition.

Heim DL, Holcomb CA, Loughin TM: Exercise mitigates the association of abdominal obesity with high-density lipoprotein cholesterol in premenopausal women: Results from the third National Health and Nutrition Examination Survey. *J Am Diet Assoc* 2000;100:1347-1353.

The authors of this study report that exercise can effectively decrease abdominal obesity.

Hu FB, Stampfer MJ, Colditz GA, et al: Physical activity and risk of stroke in women. *JAMA* 2000;283:2961-2967.

This study was conducted to examine the association between physical activity and risk of total stroke and stroke subtypes in women. The authors report that exercise decreases the risk of stroke in women.

Klauer J, Aronne LJ: Managing overweight and obesity in women. *Clin Obstet Gynecol* 2002;45:1080-1088.

The authors of this article report that the risk of developing coronary heart disease is increased by three-fold when the BMI is 29 compared with a BMI of 21.

Krauss RM, Eckel RH, Howard B, et al: AHA Dietary Guidelines: Revision 2000. A statement for healthcare professionals from the Nutrition Committee of the American Heart Association. *Stroke* 2000;31:2751-2766.

The authors of this article discuss the health benefits of caloric restriction.

Nestle M, Jacobson MF: Halting the obesity epidemic: A public health policy approach. *Public Health Rep* 2000; 115:12-24.

The authors of this article discuss the use of exercise as a way of decreasing obesity.

Serdula MK, Khan LK, Dietz WH: Weight loss counseling revisited. *JAMA* 2003;289:1747-1750.

The authors of this article discuss how weight loss counseling can affect weight loss.

Stefanick ML, Mackey S, Sheehan M, Ellsworth N, Haskell WL, Wood PD: Effects of diet and exercise in men and postmenopausal women with low levels of HDL cholesterol and high levels of LDL cholesterol. *N Engl J Med* 1998;339:12-20.

The authors of this study report that exercise can improve cardiovascular profile.

Effects of Exercise on Pregnancy

Clapp JF III: Exercise during pregnancy: A clinical update. *Clin Sports Med* 2000;19:273-286.

The author of this article reports that exercise is safe and beneficial during pregnancy.

Clapp JF III, Kim H, Burciu B, Schmidt S, Petry K, Lopez B: Continuing regular exercise during pregnancy: Effect of exercise volume on fetoplacental growth. *Am J Obstet Gynecol* 2002;186:142-147.

This study was conducted to determine whether the volume of exercise at different times during pregnancy has any effect on fetoplacental growth. The authors conclude that a high volume of moderate-intensity, weight-bearing exercise in mid and late pregnancy symmetrically reduces fetoplacental growth, whereas a reduction in exercise volume enhances fetoplacental growth with a proportionally greater increase in fat mass than in lean body mass.

Classic Bibliography

Bild DE, Sholinsky P, Smith DE, Lewis CE, Hardin JM, Burke GL: Correlates and predictors of weight loss in young adults: The CARDIA study. *Int J Obes Relat Metab Disord* 1996;20:47-55.

Bung P, Artal R, Khodiguian N: Regular exercise therapy in disorders of carbohydrate metabolism in pregnancy: Results of a prospective, randomized longitudinal study. [German]. *Geburtshilfe Frauenheilkd* 1993;53:188-193.

Bung P, Bung C, Artal R, Khodiguian N, Fallenstein F, Spatling L: Therapeutic exercise for insulin-requiring gestational diabetics: Effects on the fetus. Results of a randomized prospective longitudinal study. *J Perinat Med* 1993;21:125-137.

Carpenter MW, Sady SP, Hoegsberg B, et al: Fetal heart rate response to maternal exertion. *JAMA* 1988;259: 3006-3009.

Clapp JF III: Morphometric and neurodevelopmental outcome at age five years of the offspring of women who continued to exercise regularly throughout pregnancy. *J Pediatr* 1996;129:856-863.

Clapp JF III: The changing thermal response to endurance exercise during pregnancy. *Am J Obstet Gynecol* 1991;165:1684-1689.

Clapp JF III, Capeless EL: The changing glycemic response to exercise during pregnancy. *Am J Obstet Gynecol* 1991;165:1678-1683.

Clapp JF III, Little KD: Effect of recreational exercise on pregnancy weight gain and subcutaneous fat deposition. *Med Sci Sports Exerc* 1995;27:170-177.

Clapp JF III, Little KD, Capeless EL: Fetal heart rate response to sustained recreational exercise. *Am J Obstet Gynecol* 1993;168:198-206.

Despres JP, Kraus R: Obesity and lipoprotein metabolism, in Bray GA, Bouchard C, James WP (eds): *Handbook of Obesity*. New York, NY, Marcel Dekker, 1997, pp 651-675.

Fletcher GF, Balady G, Blair SN, et al: Statement on exercise: Benefits and recommendations for physical activity programs for all Americans. A statement for health professionals by the Committee on Exercise and Cardiac Rehabilitation of the Council on Clinical Cardiology, American Heart Association. *Circulation* 1996;94: 857-862.

Haapanen N, Miilunpalo S, Pasanen M, Oja P, Vuori I: Association between leisure time physical activity and 10-year body mass change among working-aged men and women. *Int J Obes Relat Metab Disord* 1997;21:288-296.

Haskell WL: Physical activity, sport, and health: Toward the next century. *Res Q Exerc Sport* 1996;67(3 suppl): S37-S47.

Hatoum N, Clapp JF III, Newman MR, Dajani N, Amini SB: Effects of maternal exercise on fetal activity in late gestation. *J Matern Fetal Med* 1997;6:134-139.

Heitmann BL, Kaprio J, Harris JR, Rissanen A, Korkeila M, Koskenvuo M: Are genetic determinants of weight gain modified by leisure-time physical activity? A prospective study of Finnish twins. *Am J Clin Nutr* 1997;66:672-678.

Jovanovic L, Kessler A, Peterson CM: Human maternal and fetal response to graded exercise. *J Appl Physiol* 1985;58:1719-1722.

Katz VL: Physiologic changes during normal pregnancy. *Curr Opin Obstet Gynecol* 1991;3:750-758.

Katz VL, McMurray R, Goodwin WE, Cefalo RC: Non-weightbearing exercise during pregnancy on land and during immersion: A comparative study. *Am J Perinatol* 1990;7:281-284.

Lapidus L, Bengtsson C, Larsson B, Pennert K, Rybo E, Sjostrom L: Distribution of adipose tissue and risk of cardiovascular disease and death: A 12 year follow up of participants in the population study of women in Gothenburg, Sweden. *Br Med J (Clin Res Ed)* 1984;289:1257-1261.

Lissner L, Heitmann BL, Bengtsson C: Low-fat diets may prevent weight gain in sedentary women: Prospective observations from the population study of women in Gothenburg, Sweden. *Obes Res* 1997;5:43-48.

Lotgering FK, Gilbert RD, Longo LD: Maternal and fetal responses to exercise during pregnancy. *Physiol Rev* 1985;65:1-36.

McMurray RG, Mottola MF, Wolfe LA, Artal R, Millar L, Pivarnik JM: Recent advances in understanding maternal and fetal responses to exercise. *Med Sci Sports Exerc* 1993;25:1305-1321.

O'Neill ME: Maternal rectal temperature and fetal heart rate responses to upright cycling in late pregnancy. *Br J Sports Med* 1996;30:32-35.

Pate RR, Pratt M, Blair SN, et al: Physical activity and public health: A recommendation from the Centers for Disease Control and Prevention and the American College of Sports Medicine. *JAMA* 1995;273:402-407.

Sady SP, Carpenter MW, Sady MA, et al: Prediction of VO_2max during cycle exercise in pregnant women. *J Appl Physiol* 1988;65:657-666.

Schapira DV, Clark RA, Wolff PA, Jarrett AR, Kumar NB, Aziz NM: Visceral obesity and breast cancer risk. *Cancer* 1994;74:632-639.

Spinnewijn WE, Lotgering FK, Struijk PC, Wallenburg HC: Fetal heart rate and uterine contractility during maternal exercise at term. *Am J Obstet Gynecol* 1996;174:43-48.

Webb KA, Wolfe LA, McGrath MJ: Effects of acute and chronic maternal exercise on fetal heart rate. *J Appl Physiol* 1994;77:2207-2213.

Chapter 33

Drug Testing

Edward R. McDevitt, MD

Introduction

The concept of aiding athletic performance by taking drugs is not new. Physicians caring for athletes must be aware that some athletes will take substances, including poisons, to achieve success. Drugs ingested to increase an athlete's performance are called ergogenic drugs. The use of illegal ergogenic drugs is called doping.

The term doping comes from the South African word "dop," which referred to an herbal drink imbibed by tribal members in 19th Century South African ceremonies. The definition of the word doping has been extended not only to the practice of misusing drugs for athletic advantage, but also to include any method of illegally improving performance. Most sports have based their definition of doping on the definition developed by the International Olympic Committee (IOC). The IOC Charter states that doping is forbidden and that the IOC Medical Commission shall prepare a list of prohibited classes of drugs and banned procedures. The most recent definition of doping, which is included in the 1999 *Olympic Movement Anti-Doping Code*, states that doping is the use of an expedient (substance or method) that is potentially harmful to the athletes' health and/or capable of enhancing their performance or the presence in an athlete's body of a prohibited substance or evidence of the use thereof or evidence of the use of a prohibited method.

Defining doping in terms of the use of prohibited substances emphasizes the importance of drug testing for these substances. It is critical for athletes to be aware of the list of banned drugs and to avoid taking any drug that includes a banned substance. The current IOC list of prohibited substances and methods is listed in Table 1.

The US Anti-Doping Agency provides a wallet-sized card that lists the substances that are prohibited as well as medications that are allowed on its Web site (Table 2). The list of prohibited substances is based on the IOC list of banned substances, but it contains additional information, including listing inhalers (used to treat asthma) and insulin (used to treat type 1 diabetes mellitus) among the prohibited drugs. Use of these medications is allowed, however, if medically necessary and documentation regarding medical necessity is provided to the testing authority. It is the responsibility of an athlete's team physician to be aware of which drugs are allowed or prohibited and to prevent an athlete from having to deal with the consequences of an inadvertent and preventable positive drug result.

Surveys have been conducted for the past 20 years asking Olympic athletes a simple question: Would they take a pill that would guarantee the athlete an Olympic gold medal but would also guarantee the athlete's death from adverse effects within 5 years? For each Olympic event, the results of the survey have been consistent. More than 50% of the athletes answered that they would take such a pill. If the athlete is willing to die to win an Olympic gold medal, what is the team physician to do to help the athlete? The team physician must first become aware that an athlete taking ergogenic drugs is cheating and that the drugs the athlete ingests potentially threaten the athlete's health and well-being. The use of illegal drugs also threatens the integrity of sports. It is important, therefore, for the team physician to understand the vast choices of legal and illegal drugs that are available to athletes and help athletes know the dangers of drug use as well as the mechanics and limitations of drug testing.

It is clear from various sources that ergogenic drugs are widely used by both amateur and professional athletes. It was recently discovered that East Germany had a government-sponsored program that gave male and female athletes ergogenic drugs without the athletes' knowledge. East German athletes were given a daily "vitamin." It was later discovered that this "vitamin" was an anabolic steroid. Other governments, including the United States, although not sanctioning the use of ergogenic drugs, often looked the other way while cognizant of their own country's athletes' ubiquitous use of ergogenic drugs. International sporting groups often claim that widespread testing of athletes is too costly because each urine test costs approximately $100 to process.

TABLE 1 | Current International Olympic Committee List of Prohibited Substances and Methods

Prohibited Classes of Substances

Stimulants

Narcotics

Anabolic agents

Diuretics

Peptide hormones, mimetics and analogs

Agents with an antiestrogenic activity

Masking agents

Prohibited methods

Blood doping

Administering artificial oxygen carriers or plasma expanders

Pharmacologic, chemical, and physical manipulation

Gene doping

Classes of Prohibited Substances in Certain Circumstances

Alcohol

Cannabinoids

Local anesthetics

Glucocorticoids

Beta-blockers

TABLE 2 | Internet Resources on Banned Substances and Drug Testing in Athletics

http://www.usantidoping.org/	This Web site of the US Anti-Doping Agency has downloadable wallet cards that list the banned substances.
http://www.wada-ama.org/en/t1.asp	This Web site of WADA is a valuable resource on what is new in drug testing.
http://www.ncaa.org/	This Web site of the NCAA is particularly invaluable for team physicians at the college level who must deal with the intricacies of drug testing.

The IOC has attempted to bring about a concensus among the various athletic organizations on a definition of doping and to agree to a list of substances that are to be banned because of their ability to enhance athletic performance. The seminal event in sports competition that stimulated a general consensus regarding drug testing was the 1998 Tour de France cycling competition. In this competition, drug testing was extensively used and the French police decided to act on the results obtained. Cameras captured athletes being taken off their bicycles to jail for testing positive for ergogenic drugs. As a result, The World Anti-Doping Agency (WADA) was commissioned to develop consensus among the various sporting organizations. In March 2003, all major sports federations and nearly 80 governments gave their approval to the first World Anti-Doping Code by backing a resolution that accepts the World Anti-Doping Code

as the basis for the condemnation of doping in athletics. The IOC adopted the code formally in July 2003.

History of Drug Testing

During World War II amphetamines were used widely to enhance the performance and prevent fatigue of combat troops. Athletes soon began using amphetamines in an attempt to stimulate athletic performance. A cyclist died in the 1960 Olympics after ingesting amphetamines. In 1964, the IOC voted unanimously to ban performance-enhancing drugs. It was not until 1967 that the IOC established a medical committee to initiate drug testing of Olympic athletes. Full-scale drug testing was established in 1972 for both the summer and winter Olympics and has continued with improved methods of detection of the ever-growing number of banned substances. The National Collegiate Athletic Association (NCAA) began a testing program in 1986 that was first limited to testing at championship games or major football bowl games but has since expanded to include off-season testing. The National Football League started testing its players for drugs in training camps in 1982 and started anabolic steroid testing in 1987. As sporting organizations developed their own testing programs, they also identified different definitions of what was considered illegal. There was little consensus.

Laboratory Testing Methods

It was not until the development of complex radioimmunoassay (RIA) screening techniques that testing for anabolic steroids was first done at the 1976 Olympics. RIA is an assay in which a radioactive tracer is used to detect antibodies to specific steroid receptors. RIA techniques, however, have very poor specificity and produce many false-positive results. In the 1976 Olympics, RIA was used, but only 15% of the samples could be tested, and only 8 positive results were reported. A more specific test needed to be developed.

Gas chromatography-mass spectrometry (GC-MS) was adopted as both the screening and confirmatory method of detecting the presence of anabolic steroids in athletes participating in the 1984 Olympics because of its increased specificity . Although most anti-doping laboratories use GC-MS techniques, which, as with RIA techniques, also test an athlete's urine, the cost (approximately $100 per test) was still considered prohibitive. Therefore, newer techniques such as liquid chromatography-mass spectrometry (LC-MS) were developed for detecting doping. LC-MS is similar to GC-MS, but the urine sample is passed through the separation column in liquid rather than the gas phase. LC-MS has many advantages over GC-MC. Because the sample does not have to be heated, unstable, polar, and natural hormones with a larger molecular weight such as human growth hormone (hGH) and a blood cell simulating hormone called erythropoietin (EPO) can be detected. Another testing method being proposed is isotope ratio mass spectrometry. This technique uses carbon isotope ratio methods to determine whether urinary steroids are endogenous or exogenous. The testing is based on the fact that carbon 13, a naturally occurring, nonradioactive isotope of carbon, is found in approximately 1% of the endogenous testosterone made in the body from dietary carbon plant and animal sources. Because the percentage of carbon 13 in synthetic anabolic steroids is significantly greater than that which occurs naturally in the body, the illegal use of anabolic steroids can be determined using this method. The isotope ratio mass spectrometry machine, however, currently costs $100,000, limiting its widespread use.

Blood tests are much more specific and have much greater ability to detect abnormalities in the athlete's system, but they have not been widely done for several reasons. Blood testing was believed to be a much more invasive procedure that was not only dreaded by many athletes but also considered expensive and complex. More medically skilled personnel are required to obtain blood samples and to treat athletes who have vagal reactions when giving blood. Although most athletes do not particularly relish giving urine samples, many athletes refuse, often on religious grounds, to allow blood samples to be taken. Athletes have even threatened to sue the IOC if injured when giving blood.

Much more specific testing can be done on blood samples than urine; therefore, blood tests to screen for certain banned substances such as hGH and EPO are being developed. There are currently no urine tests that can determine whether an athlete has used either of these two substances. Because the costs for developing a blood test to screen for hGH and EPO use are substantial, the IOC committed $2 million and the Growth Hormone 2000 Group committed $5 million to develop a reliable test to screen for hGH use. WADA has made the development of an hGH blood test a high priority. Comparable funding has been secured to develop a blood test to screen for EPO use.

Hair analysis has been proposed as a relatively painless technique for detecting the presence of doping agents in athletes. Because hair analysis had been used successfully for toxicologic analysis, it was hoped that it could provide a specific, simple, atraumatic method of screening for the presence of illegal substances. Drugs remain in the keratin matrix for a long period, allowing a much wider window of opportunity for discovering illicit ergogenic drug use than what is available with urine or blood testing.

Hair consists primarily of keratin, and it grows on average 1 cm per month. The lifespan of a hair varies from 4 months to 4 years; therefore, sectional analysis of hair can provide reasonable analysis of the duration and timing of drug ingestion. Only a small amount of hair needs to be collected for drug screening. Hair can be stored at room temperature in paper, plastic, or in glass or paper tubes. After extraction and processing, gas chromatography techniques are used to detect doping substances.

Unfortunately, several problems currently exist when using hair analysis to detect the presence of doping substances. First, although qualitative and quantitative analytic standards are available for many drugs, not all ergogenic drugs can be detected using hair analysis. Second, the relationship between urine, blood, and hair quantitative results is not clearly established and additional research is needed to establish the accuracy of hair analysis. Third, athletes have discovered that dying, tinting, and cutting the hair closely can affect the results of hair analysis. Fourth, hair pigmentation and gender differences also influence the concentration of drug measured in hair. African-American female hair binds to cocaine 157 times greater than it does in Caucasian blonde hair. Stanazole, one of the most frequently abused anabolic steroids, is incorporated in highly pigmented hair in much greater concentrations than in nonpigmented hair.

Athletic Education and Drug Testing Procedures

One important aspect of athletic education is the understanding of drug testing procedures. Worldwide, over 100,000 drug tests designed to detect the presence of ergogenic drugs in athletes are conducted annually at a cost of more than $35 million. The penalties for a positive drug test result can be severe, and athletes must understand the mechanics of the drug testing process. NCAA and Olympic athletes are required to sign a consent form, which indicates their understanding and compliance with the rules. Failure to sign the consent form leads to loss of eligibility to compete. The team physician should review the rules of drug testing with team members, explain how athletes are tested, and emphasize the consequences of a positive drug test result. Details concerning the chain of custody must be stressed. Athletes must understand that they have rights that help prevent the commitment of an inadvertent wrong.

Athletes must understand that drug testing may be done at any time. Year-round, short-notice, and no-notice testing have been found to be the most effective means to detect the use of ergogenic drugs. In the United States, the National Football League and the NCAA have short-notice (1 to 2 days) programs, and the IOC has implemented a no-notice program. If an athlete is selected to be tested, the athlete is obligated to report to the testing site. Once an athlete arrives at the testing site, the athlete must be under the direct supervision and observation of a member of the drug testing committee until the sample is collected and sealed.

The majority of drug testing programs use urine samples. The athlete must list on the testing form any medications or supplements used within the past 7 days. To ensure that the urine sample actually comes from the athlete, the testing officer must be able to see the urine flow from the athlete and into the bottle. This is true for both male and female athletes.

After the 70 mL sample is obtained, the athlete, under direct supervision, divides the urine into two containers. The samples are labeled, sealed, and placed into two separate boxes. Once sealed, the boxes are not opened until they are ready for testing at the laboratory. Each sealed urine box receives a unique serial number with no mention of the athlete's name. A matching list should be kept locked in a safe. These precautions in the chain of custody are necessary to eliminate any manipulation of the samples or mislabeling of an athlete's urine. The second sample is kept in reserve for additional testing if the first is found to be positive for the presence of illegal drugs or if questions regarding the handling of the sample in the laboratory are raised by the athlete or the athlete's representatives. If the first urine sample tests positive, the laboratory contacts the governing body, which will then notify the athlete. The athlete has the right to have the second sample analyzed, and the athlete or the athlete's representative may observe the analysis. A different laboratory team from the same accredited laboratory will analyze the second sample. The athlete is usually suspended from competition pending the outcome of the analysis of the second urine sample.

Testing for Specific Ergogenic Drugs

Testosterone and Anabolic Steroids

Anabolic steroids are considered to be the most commonly abused ergogenic drugs. Anabolic steroids are synthetic derivatives of testosterone and are used to increase muscle mass, increase muscle strength, and reduce the recovery time after exercise.

The problem with anabolic steroids is that these drugs are not purely anabolic nor purely androgenic. Anabolic steroids have anabolic effects or androgenic effects that are dependent on the target organ. Although methandrostenolone (Dianabol), was developed in the 1960s as a significant improvement over testosterone, the adverse androgenic effects were not eliminated. Once use of anabolic steroids became ubiquitous in the sporting world, drug companies worked to alter the testosterone molecule to find a stronger, safer, and, after the advent of drug testing, a less detectable drug. It was not until later in the 1960s that the use of anabolic steroids was banned, and it was not until 1972 that full-scale drug testing was implemented by the IOC.

Anabolic Steroid Synthesis and Development of Exogenous Analogs

In the body, testosterone is synthesized through the conversion of cholesterol via five enzymatic steps. The rate-limiting step in testosterone synthesis is the first step in cholesterol metabolism. Cholesterol is cleaved in size from a 27-carbon molecule to a 19-carbon molecule as it is converted to pregnenolone and then to progesterone. Further enzymatic processes result in the conversion to 17-OH-progesterone, androstenedione, and subsequently testosterone, a 17-carbon molecule. Athletes have taken many of the precursors of testosterone. The precursors are not specifically destined to synthesize testosterone, however, and may go down a parallel path to estrogen synthesis. Scientists have altered the testosterone molecule in an attempt to synthesize more potent and safer compounds. One problem in testosterone administration is that oral preparations of testosterone are quickly metabolized in the liver. Parenteral injections provide higher systemic levels. Gels or dermal patches may allow slower absorption, but molecular modification has provided a more potent means of anabolic steroid delivery.

The three most common means of testosterone modification are esterization of the 17β-hydroxy groups, alkylation at the 17α-groups, or modification of the molecular rings. Esterization of the 17β-hydroxy groups makes the molecule less polar, more soluble in the fat vehicles used for injection, and prolongs the effect of the drug. The more carboxylic groups that are added to the molecule for esterization, the longer the compound lasts in the body. All esters need to be injected, and all are detectable in plasma. Alkylation of the 17α-hydroxy groups was done in an attempt to increase the anabolic properties while simultaneously decreasing the metabolic degradation of the compound in the liver. Test results showed that 17α-alkyl-substituted anabolic steroids had higher anabolic properties and decreased androgenic properties, but also higher toxicities than unsubstituted anabolic steroids. Further changes in the testosterone molecule have led to compounds called designer steroids, which are compounds with high anabolic properties that were designed to not be detectable by standard drug testing procedures.

An interesting discovery occurred in 2003. An American female athlete who was tested for anabolic steroids had a urine sample in which the level of natural hormones was almost zero. Because exogenous steroids administered to athletes will suppress endogenous production, it was suspected that this athlete was using a steroid that was not being screened for with standard testing techniques. This new steroid, it was thought, would suppress the production of endogenous hormones normally found in the urine of both male and female athletes. The testers suspected that they were looking for a new designer drug. What they discovered was that the athlete was taking a drug, norbolethone, an anabolic steroid of high anabolic potency developed in the early 1960s but never manufactured in any quantity because it was thought that it was not marketable. Because it was never commercially manufactured, athletes were not being screened for norbolethone use in standard laboratories; therefore, it became an ideal designer drug for an athlete to take to beat the testing system. It now appears that norbolethone was manufactured in China and has been used by athletes for years. Testers had hoped that they could retest the urine samples of athletes who competed in the 2000 Sydney Summer Olympics for norbolethone, but the urine samples had been discarded. As some athletes continue to look for ways to beat the testing systems, laboratories continue to improve their testing methods to look for newly designed or newly discovered anabolic steroids.

In the summer of 2003, an anonymous tipster, identifying himself as a high-profile but disgruntled coach, sent a vial of a substance to the University of California Los Angeles laboratory testing facility. The coach claimed the substance was a designer steroid being sold to athletes as an anabolic steroid compound that had been structurally altered to make it undetectable to laboratory testing. After a month of analysis, the laboratory determined that the compound substance was a previously unknown anabolic steroid, a true designer steroid, with anabolic properties and no means of detection. The University of California Los Angeles laboratory analyzed the drug, discovered its structure, and proceeded to manufacture the drug. They named the newly discovered steroid tetrahydogestrinone (THG). THG is a 19 nor-steroid structurally related to gestrinone, a drug that had been used for the treatment of endometriosis. Because it was a new compound, previous laboratory tests would not have discovered its use by athletes. Once the structure was identified, testing was possible, and many athletes were soon testing positive for THG.

Many of the athletes caught using THG admitted obtaining the drug from the Bay Area Laboratory Cooperative (BALCO). These athletes claimed that the owner of BALCO promised them that the drug would deliver impressive performance-enhancing effects with the bonus of being totally undetectable. High-profile athletes in professional baseball, football, boxing, and Olympic track and swimming athletes were detected using THG. THG was soon banned by the IOC, but many ethical dilemmas remain. Because urine samples have been saved from many past Olympic games, it is now being debated whether the saved urine samples should be retested for the presence of THG. It is possible that THG is just one of many designer steroids being used by athletes. How many drugs are available to athletes that have been designed specifically to beat the present drug testing system has yet to be determined.

Androgens for pharmaceutical use are made via the semisynthesis of starting compounds derived from plants. These compounds have fewer 13-carbon molecules than their endogenous homologs. Urinary steroids with a low 13-carbon molecule/12-carbon molecule ratio are likely to have originated from plant sources. Testing consists of measuring both testosterone and epitestosterone (the epimeric form of testosterone) in the same sample. Testosterone and epitestosterone are normally present in the urine in an approximate 1:1 ratio (T:E ratio) for both males and females. Exogenously administered testosterone, however, forms little or no epitestosterone and thus significantly raises the T:E ratio. Initially, a T:E ratio of greater than 6:1 was considered a positive test result for the presence of exogenous testosterone, but exceptions to this threshold have appeared and now a T:E ratio of greater than 6:1 is considered suspicious and a T:E ratio greater than 10:1 is considered a positive test result.

In an attempt to achieve negative test results, some athletes using anabolic steroids attempt to diminish their T:E ratio by adding epitestosterone to the urine or blood. The East German athletes were the first to do this on a regular basis. They added enough epitestosterone to keep the T:E ratio within allowable limits. Because epitestosterone has minimal androgenic activity, testing laboratories caught on to this manipulation when they started to measure the epitestosterone levels in the urine. It was determined that urinary levels exceeding 200 ng/mL were abnormal and provided evidence of illegal tampering. Epitestosterone is not available in the United States because it is not an approved pharmaceutical substance. Because of its potential to be used as a urine-manipulating substance, epitestosterone was banned by the IOC.

To understand the variety of anabolic steroids that are consumed by athletes, it is important to understand the synthesis in the body of testosterone from cholesterol from the most common pathway. Cholesterol is converted to pregnanediol, which is converted to 17-OH-pregnanediol, which is converted to dehydroepiandrosterone, which is converted to androstenedione, which is converted to testosterone. Athletes have attempted to boost testosterone "legally" by using the precursors, which are in many cases "legal." But the path from cholesterol to androgens also has precursors with the pathway from cholesterol to estrogens, and some athletes may inadvertently increase their female hormones when attempting to stimulate their male hormones. And even if "legally" obtained and used, any compound that leads to increased testosterone production will lead to a positive drug test result when the precursor is taken in sufficient quantity.

Human Growth Hormone
Despite its high costs and potential adverse effects, hGH has been widely used by elite athletes for ergo-

genic purposes; moreover, it cannot be detected via current laboratory testing procedures. The use hGH may be tempting because it is a potent anabolic as well as lipolytic agent. Although hGH secretion peaks at puberty for both men and women, hGH is secreted throughout a person's lifetime. hGH secretion varies throughout the day, with the highest levels occurring during sleep. Because the levels of hGH vary widely throughout the day for each individual, attempting to find a "normal" level of hGH in an athlete's body is complicated by the daily wide fluctuations. And unlike anabolic steroids, which can be detected for months after they are used, hGH is rapidly metabolized, so it is difficult to determine whether extra hGH has been taken. hGH is also metabolized to insulin-like growth factor-I (IGF-I). IGF-I is another drug that is used by athletes because it is anabolic, lipolytic, and, as with hGH, not detectable via current laboratory testing procedures. Although not studied extensively in athletes, hGH is associated with many adverse effects; the biggest deterrent to its use by athletes, however, is its cost (more than $1,000 per month) and the need to inject the compound because the oral forms are quickly deactivated in the stomach. Nevertheless, athletes use both hGH and IGF-I and often inject them in tandem. Because they are closely related, hGH and IGF-I levels vary in individual athletes from day to day and from hour to hour, making laboratory analysis of abnormally high levels difficult. Extensive research is currently underway to find a laboratory test that is sensitive and specific to the illegal use of hGH and IGF-I.

Erythropoietin

Because blood oxygenation is a fundamental factor in optimizing muscular activity, the enhancement of oxygen delivery to tissues is associated with substantial improvement in athletic performance, particularly in endurance sports. To accomplish this, some athletes get blood transfusions, take blood substitutes, and stimulate the endogenous production of red blood cells with altitude, EPOs, EPO gene therapy, or EPO mimetics. Progress in medical research has led to the identification of new chemicals for the treatment of severe anemia. These chemicals have, in turn, been used for doping athletes.

As with the other ergogenic drugs mentioned, some athletes will try such techniques and take new chemicals such as EPOs before safety tests have been completed. As a result, these athletes are taking great health risks. New chemicals such as EPOs have also created the need for the development of new instrumental strategies in doping control laboratories, but not all of these chemicals are detectable. EPO has been one of the most widely abused drugs among athletes. It is effective in stimulating red blood cell production, and until recently, it was undetectable using standard laboratory testing

procedures. The main disadvantages of EPOs are the adverse effects resulting from increased viscosity, which can lead to myocardial injury and cerebrovascular accident.

Two more methods of increasing red blood cell concentration for use in medicine have been developed, and evidence suggests that some athletes are already adapting these new methods for their benefit. Hemoglobin oxygen carriers and perfluorocarbons, each having a different structure, allow oxygen to be delivered to the tissues. Hemoglobin oxygen carriers physically alter the hemoglobin molecule by several methods so that complications such as renal toxicity are obviated. Perfluorocarbons belong to a group of synthetic compounds containing hydrocarbons to which fluorine is added.

When it was realized in the late 1990s that some athletes, especially cyclists, were using EPOs, international sporting federations began random blood testing to screen for abnormally high hematocrit levels in these athletes, which is indirect evidence of blood boosting by transfusions or by using EPOs. This testing methodology was widely criticized because hematocrit levels are affected by shifts in body hydration as well as the training status of the athlete. Hematocrit levels have been reported to be lower in athletes during intense training periods and, therefore, subject to variations other than those directly related to illegal activity. Screening for EPOs using urine or blood testing has also been limited by the short half-life of injected EPO (between 8 and 20 hours).

It has been estimated that DNA-recombinant human EPO (rhEPO) has been used as a pharmacologic ergogenic aid for the enhancement of aerobic performance by at least 7% of elite athletes. rhEPO is nearly identical immunologically and biochemically to endogenous EPO. The results of a limited number of human studies have suggested that rhEPO provides a significant erythropoietic and ergogenic benefit in trained athletes because it can increase hemoglobin and hematocrit levels, maximal oxygen uptake, and exercise endurance time. These findings led to a surge in the illicit use of rhEPO in athletes. As a result, the IOC banned rhEPO in 1990. Since that time, several methods have been proposed to detect the illegal use of rhEPO, most of which use indirect markers such as macrocytic hypochromatic erythrocytes and serum soluble transferrin receptor concentration to detect rhEPO in blood samples. Another indirect technique uses five markers of enhanced erythropoiesis to detect rhEPO. The electrophoretic mobility technique directly measures urine and serum levels of rhEPO. Isoelectric patterning/focusing has recently been developed to directly analyze rhEPO in urine. Of these various techniques, the indirect method that uses multiple markers of enhanced erythropoiesis seems to be the most reliable and valid technique for the detection of rhEPO in athletes. In August 2000, this protocol was approved by the IOC Medical Commission, and it was subsequently used along with isoelectric patterning to identify the presence of rhEPO in athletes competing in the 2000 Sydney Summer Olympics. Although performing combined blood and urine tests for the 2000 Sydney Summer Olympics was challenging and several athletes dropped out when they learned they would be tested for rhEPO, there were no positive drug test results. During the 2002 Salt Lake City Winter Olympics, there was one positive drug test result. Nevertheless, the decision by the IOC to perform blood testing, however limited, provided additional opportunities to identify banned substance users.

Summary

The Olympic motto is "swifter, higher, stronger"; unfortunately, many athletes look to any method, no matter how dangerous or illegal, to improve athletic performance. The establishment of WADA to establish a fair and effective testing program for athletes is a tremendous step toward creating a safe and equitable playing field for all athletes. It must be realized, however, that many athletes are willing to cheat and perhaps die to achieve their athletic goals. Testing for ergogenic drugs must also continue to develop and to adapt to new techniques of avoiding ergogenic drug use detection. Moreover, punishments for the illegal use of ergogenic drugs must be severe and reflect the worldwide effort to ensure drug-free competition, and physicians must educate athletes, parents, and coaches at the entry level of sport regarding the dangers and ethics of using ergogenic drugs.

Annotated Bibliography

History of Drug Testing

McDevitt E: Ergogenic drugs and growth hormones, in DeLee JC, Drez D Jr, Miller MD (eds): *DeLee and Drez's Orthopaedic Sports Medicine: Principles and Practice*, ed 2. New York, NY, WB Saunders, 2003, pp 475-483.
This chapter provides a history of athletic drug use and discusses the various drugs used by athletes to improve performance.

Prendergast H: The toxic torch of the modern Olympic Games. *Vet Hum Toxicol* 2003;45:97-102.
This article reviews drugs in sports and suggests that the Olympic games are becomingly increasingly poisoned by drugs as the pressures of winning at all costs are combined with tremendous financial gains for winning athletes.

Tuffs A: Doped East German athletes to receive compensation. *BMJ* 2002;324:1544.
This article provides a review of the East German government's 20-year program of systematic doping of their athletes,

the full story of which may be found in Steven Ungerleider's book, *Faust's Gold* (New York, NY, St. Martin's Press, 2001).

Laboratory Testing Methods

Delbeke F: Prohormones and sport. *J Steroid Biochem Mol Biol* 2002;83:245-251.
This article concludes that athletes taking legally obtained precursors of testosterone may have positive results when tested for illegal anabolic steroids.

Ehrnborg C: The growth hormone/insulin-like growth factor-I axis hormones and bone markers in elite athletes in response to a maximum exercise test. *J Clin Endocrinol Metab* 2003;88:394-401.
This article discusses the hGH-IGF-I axis and the implications of testing for bone markers.

Midio AF: The possibilities of hair analysis in the determination of involuntary doping in sports. *Sports Med* 2001;31:321-324.
The author of this article discusses the use of hair analysis to detect the presence of many ergogenic drugs.

Athletic Education and Drug Testing Procedures

Bidlingmaier M: Doping with growth hormone. *J Pediatr Endocrinol Metab* 2001;14:1077-1083.
This article addresses the question that if there is not one scientific study proving hGH aids athletic performance, why do athletes abuse it?

Koch J: Performance-enhancing substances and their use among adolescent athletes. *Pediatr Rev* 2002;23:310-317.
The author of this article argues that, as with Olympic athletes, adolescent athletes are drawn to the lure of using ergogenic drugs to boost athletic performance.

Yesalis CE, Bahrke MS: Anabolic-androgenic steroids and related substances. *Curr Sports Med Rep* 2002;1:246-252.
The authors of this article report that the long-term effects of androstenedione supplementation are unknown and that DHEA supplementation does not increase serum testosterone levels or strength in men and may have a virilizing effect on women.

Testing for Specific Ergogenic Drugs

Dean H: Does exogenous growth hormone improve athletic performance? *Clin J Sport Med* 2002;12:250-253.
The author of this article not only argues that hGH is dangerous and illegal, but also questions whether it actually aids athletic performance.

Gaudard A: Drugs for increasing oxygen and their potential use in doping: A review. *Sports Med* 2003;33:187-212.

The author of this article reviews many of the ways athletes attempt to increase their aerobic capacity, many of which are illegal.

Kniess A: Potential parameters for the detection of hGH doping. *Anal Bioanal Chem* 2003;376:696-700.

This article provides new information regarding drug testing for the elusive hGH.

Saugy M: Test methods: Anabolics. *Baillieres Best Pract Res Clin Endocrinol Metab* 2000;14:111-133.

The author of this article discusses testing techniques for the presence of anabolic steroids.

Thieme D: Analytical strategy for detecting doping agents in hair. *Forensic Sci Int* 2000;107:335-345.

This is another well-written article on the analysis of hair to detect the presence of doping agents.

Wilber RL: Detection of DNA-recombinant human epoetin-alfa as a pharmacological ergogenic aid. *Sports Med* 2002;32:125-142.

The author of this article discusses the new methods of testing for the presence of EPO.

Classic Bibliography

Bergman R, Leach RE: The use and abuse of anabolic steroids in Olympic-caliber athletes. *Clin Orthop* 1985; 198:169-172.

Cowart VS: Athlete drug testing receiving more attention than ever before in history of competition. *JAMA* 1989;261:3510-3511, 3516.

Gunby P: Olympics drug testing: Basis for future study. *JAMA* 1984;252:454-455, 459-460.

Puffer JC: The use of drugs in swimming. *Clin Sports Med* 1986;5:77-89.

Chapter 34

Legal Aspects of Sports Medicine

John S. Baxter, MD, JD

Introduction

Sports medicine is becoming a rapidly expanding specialty as athletics become a greater part of life. Sports teams now thrive at every educational and performance level. Therefore, the team physician plays an ever more important role. From the preparticipation physical examination to the all-important decision whether to permit an athlete with an injury to compete, the legal issues faced by the team physician are becoming more complex.

Sports Injuries in a Litigious Society

The level of play has steadily advanced over the years. Concomitantly, the number of sports-related injuries in children is rising. According to the Centers for Disease Control and Prevention (CDC), sports-related injuries are the leading reason for emergency department visits among US teenagers 14 to 17 years of age. Contact sports, including football, basketball, baseball, and soccer, account for almost 80% of all sports injuries requiring emergency department visits in children 5 to 14 years old. The CDC also estimates that up to half of sports-related injuries could be prevented. Ominously, the incidence of sudden cardiac death has risen 10% over the past decade in people 15 to 34 years old. Heat-related deaths in football have steadily increased, replacing traumatic injuries as that sport's biggest danger. Consequently, increasingly comprehensive preparticipation physical examinations are recommended by the American Academy of Pediatrics (AAP), the American College of Sports Medicine, the American Orthopaedic Society for Sports Medicine, and other organizations. There has been a steady increase in the number of legal cases involving not only sports medicine physicians but also coaches, trainers, supervisors, and even the sellers, lessors, and maintainers of equipment used in sporting events.

The Psychologic Aspects of Athletics

Athletes are competitive by nature. Often, they will not be receptive to advice that they sit out or that they not play because of an injury. Similarly, they may shun the use of readily available protective equipment despite serious danger. The Italian cyclist Fabio Casartelli died when he crashed in the Tour de France in 1995. He was not wearing a helmet. Even today, many riders in the Tour de France refuse to wear helmets despite the undeniable protection they provide. To build rapport with and earn compliance by patients, sports physicians must fully understand this psychologic aspect of the athlete and their desire to sometimes "play through the pain." The win-at-all-costs attitude held by some athletes places a special burden on the sports medicine physician: to protect athletes from themselves. This is not only the right thing to do from an ethical standpoint, but it is essential in avoiding legal liability and allegations of negligence.

Negligence

When injuries occur, the legal issues faced by sports medicine physicians primarily involve negligence and are likely to involve whether the physician exercised a reasonable level of care in the screening, treatment, and decision-making regarding the athlete's participation.

Torts are actionable civil wrongs that do not include breach of contract. They are divided into two broad categories: intentional torts and negligence. Intentional torts include assault and battery and conversion (theft). The majority of torts, however, are those of the nonintentional type, commonly referred to as negligence. In medicine, negligence is often referred to as medical malpractice. Sports medicine physicians must become familiar with negligence to minimize any factors that might be construed as negligence.

Elements of Negligence

To establish the civil wrong of negligence four elements are necessary. First, there must be a duty of care. This means simply that one must exercise due care not to harm (physically or otherwise) those who might foreseeably be injured. Second, there must be a breach of the standard of care. The standard of care is the reasonable exercise of due diligence under the circumstances, often defined by reasonable practices in the community.

Third, the breach must cause the injury to the aggrieved party. Fourth, there must be damages or harm (physical or otherwise) to the injured party. This is a simplified overview of the subject. Each element has many nuances and exceptions.

Duty of Care

The first element required to establish negligence is that a duty of care exists. If a physician does not owe a duty of care to the injured party, then a tort in negligence cannot be established against the physician. In most cases involving a physician and patient, there clearly exists a duty of care simply because a physician-patient relationship exists. When a patient seeks advice or treatment from a physician, the physician quite logically owes the patient a duty to exercise reasonable care in providing medical advice and treatment. However, consider the case of a physician attending a sports event who is a spectator only. If that physician fails to come to the aid of a player down on the field, the traditional and common law view holds that the physician did not owe a duty of care to that player. This may be surprising to some, but the US legal system does not recognize either a federal constitutional or a legal right to rescue, not even an emergency rescue by the government itself in instances in which public officials are aware of life-threatening situations. The physician in the scenario presented above is not the team physician and does not have any other preexisting physician-patient relationship with the player. Furthermore, under the common law, if a spectator does undertake to help an injured party, then a duty of care would be established; if an adverse outcome results, liability might be established. This obviously discourages some from coming to the aid of injured parties.

This common law rule thus gave rise to what are known as Good Samaritan statutes. In general, these statutes relieve from liability those who come to the aid of injured people in need of assistance. They generally protect against simple negligence but do not relieve a rescuer from liability if the rescuer has been grossly negligent or has engaged in willful or wanton misconduct. In addition, all physicians should be aware that statutes and case law are trending toward establishment of duties to provide care in other areas in which none existed under common law. In particular, the Emergency Medical Treatment and Active Labor Act of 1986, Title VI of the 1964 Civil Rights Act, and the Americans with Disabilities Act have all been held to establish widespread duties to provide care in a variety of situations in which none previously existed under common law.

Breach of Duty

The second element necessary to establish negligence is breach of duty. There must be a breach of the standard

of care; in other words, there is a failure to exercise that level of care and due diligence required by the situation and expected of those with similar training under the circumstances. This is the area in which most active litigation cases involving sports medicine take place, just as with most other negligence cases. The controversy almost always involves whether the standard of care was met. Typical questions in sports medicine include the following: Did the physician perform an adequate preparticipation physical examination? Did the physician correctly advise the patient of the nature and severity of the injury and of the consequences that might result from competing with that injury? Should the physician have disallowed further participation after an injury?

Standard of Care

The standard of care is usually held to be the level of care that a similarly qualified person under similar circumstances would exercise. The standard may be different for an internist who volunteers as a high school team physician in a rural area than it would be for an orthopaedist trained in sports medicine who serves as the team physician for a professional sports team. The applicable standard of care is closely intertwined with the determination whether a breach of the standard occurred. In medical cases, the courts often look to the practices in the local community in establishing the appropriate standard of care.

Causation

The third element is causation. To establish liability in tort, the wrongful (negligent) act or omission must be both the actual and the legal or proximate cause of the injury. If a physician negligently advises a patient, and the patient acts on the advice and subsequently suffers an injury, it is usually fairly easy to establish that the negligent act or omission by the physician was the cause-in-fact of the injury. The negligent act or omission, however, must also be what is known as the proximate cause of the injury. There is no exact test for establishing proximate cause. Essentially, the injury that occurred must have been a reasonably foreseeable result of the negligent act or omission. Sports medicine physicians should therefore focus efforts on ensuring that due care is used in the advice and treatment they render to the players under their care, and they are well advised to err on the side of caution when making decisions to protect an athlete's health.

Damages

The final element needed to establish liability in a negligence case is that of injury to the aggrieved party (the plaintiff). This element is known as damages. In cases involving athletes, this usually includes elements such as pain and suffering (to which a monetary value will be computed) and loss of earning capacity. In instances in which professional athletes and athletes with professional prospects are involved, damages may be quite substantial. Even where the direct earnings of professional athletics are not involved, however, plaintiffs will commonly sue for loss of earning capacity on other grounds. They may allege that the injury prevented them from gaining admission to certain universities or that a permanent injury impaired their lifetime earning capacity. Children may suffer growth plate or other injuries that impair development. Damages in such cases can be understandably high. There are cases, sometimes referred to as negligence in the air, in which a negligent act or omission occurred but no injury resulted. Lawsuits for such acts or omissions are not sustainable because there are no damages. Such incidents may, nevertheless, affect physicians' credentials and have other undesirable effects on their professional lives.

Defenses

There are common defenses to allegations of negligence. Perhaps most important in athletic cases is that of assumption of risk. This defense is based on the doctrine of implied consent and has been recognized by the courts for many years. The basis of the defense is that participation in sports can be inherently dangerous and that one who chooses to participate must assume the risk of injury. Some injuries are accepted as commonplace, such as bruises in football. Some injuries are not accepted as commonplace, however, such as those experienced when playing without proper protection and against a grossly mismatched opponent and contracting human immunodeficiency virus (HIV) from an infected opponent. Similarly, quadriplegia and death are not risks ordinarily assumed by participants in athletic activities.

A few states, including Virginia, Georgia, and California, have enacted statutes that give immunity to physicians volunteering services to nonprofessional teams. These statutes offer a defense to charges of simple negligence in those jurisdictions. Like the Good Samaritan statutes, these statutes generally do not provide protection in cases of gross negligence or willful or wanton misconduct.

Waivers and Assumption of Risk

Participation in sports can be inherently dangerous. Injuries can be traumatic, environmental (caused by heat stroke or frostbite, for example), or result from preexisting medical conditions (such as in athletes with a single kidney or testicle). In all of these instances, the better practice is to require the athlete to assign a simply worded waiver and release of liability as a condition to allowing the athlete to participate in athletic activities.

Although this does not guarantee that courts will deny liability in the case of a lawsuit arising from an injury, it is advisable for several reasons. First, it demonstrates recognition of the risk and that the athlete was clearly on notice of the risk. Second, the fact that the waiver and release were obtained may serve to deter the athlete from initiating a lawsuit. Third, if a lawsuit is initiated, the waiver may serve to limit damages by showing that at least the athlete should assume some of the responsibility. Fourth, the waiver and release may be upheld, thus relieving the defendant from any liability.

The physician and coaching staff can improve the chances that the waiver will be upheld by wording the waiver specifically and in plain, understandable language. In other words, long, preprinted forms with excessive legal jargon should be avoided. The reason for the waiver should be specifically stated. For example, if an athlete has a single testicle, this should be clearly specified in the waiver. Additionally, the waiver should detail the fact that damage could occur to the testicle if the athlete chooses to participate in athletic activity and that such damage could likely result in the loss of the ability to father children (it is preferable to use this simple language rather that the phrase "loss of reproductive capacity"). It should be noted that this example couches the waiver in terms of the athlete's "choosing to play," highlighting that the athlete had the freedom of choice in the matter. Other techniques used to demonstrate understanding on the part of the athlete include requiring the athlete to initial each paragraph that contains a specific risk, providing a paragraph that asks the athlete to write in his or her own words the risk or condition that they understand they are waiving, and making sure the waiver contains a place for the athlete to indicate whether they understand the document and whether they have any questions. These features should not merely permit the athlete to check "yes" or "no," but blanks should be provided for the athlete to actually write "yes" or "no." Plaintiffs are unlikely to make the assertion that they did not know what they were signing when they have actually answered questions in their own handwriting. Finally, the waiver should be witnessed. In addition to the actual mechanics of the waiver document, the institution should act in good faith to protect the health of the athlete. If an injury occurs in the presence of significant negligence on the part of the institution, courts are more likely to consider the waiver invalid for the reason that shielding negligent parties who injure others is against public policy.

Privacy

Patients have a right to privacy with regard to their medical conditions and medical records. Although this has always been true, the issue of confidentiality has received increased attention over time. All sports to some

TABLE 1 | HIPAA and FERPA Resources

Department of Health and Human Services Office of Civil Rights guidance and technical assistance	http://www.hhs.gov/ocr/hipaa
HIPAA news and other links	http://www.hipaadvisory.com and http://www.hipaacomply.com
EDUCAUSE	http://www.educause.edu/issues/hipaa.html
Department of Education Family Policy Compliance Online	http://www.ed.gov/offices/OM/fpco/ferpa

(Reproduced with permission from Magee JT, Almekinders LC, Taft TN: HIPAA and the team physician. Sports Medicine Update *March-April 2003, p 7.)*

degree have a public aspect. Thus, consent forms are sometimes signed to allow some limited release of medical information. Without signed consent, commentators and others would be constrained from describing the results of on-field and other medical evaluations. After all, for better or worse, the status of a player's knee ligaments is often the subject of living room discussions across America. It should also be noted that the Health Insurance Portability and Accountability Act (HIPAA) became effective as of April 14, 2003. HIPAA mandates sweeping new protections for patient medical information. It includes both civil and criminal penalties for noncompliance. Sports medicine physicians, as with colleagues in other fields, must ensure practices are in compliance with HIPAA. HIPAA states that any health plan or provider who maintains or transmits health information shall maintain reasonable and appropriate administrative, technical, and physical safeguards to ensure the integrity and confidentiality of the information to protect against any reasonably anticipated threats or hazards to the security or integrity of the information and unauthorized uses or disclosures of the information and otherwise to ensure the compliance with this part by the officers and employees of such person.

Under HIPAA, written authorization generally must be obtained for any uses of "individually identifiable health information" other than treatment, payment, and health care operation activities. This raises obvious issues for athletes who usually have many people involved in their athletic endeavors. Coaches, trainers, athletic directors, public affairs officers, other health care providers, parents and guardians, hospitals and/or medical clinics and laboratories, academic counselors, university administrators, and others require some knowledge of the athlete's individual health information in order to perform their duties and to protect the athlete. The best solution, and the one most widely used since HIPAA was implemented, is to request that the athlete execute a consent form to cover the common releases of medical information that are likely to be needed. It should be noted that athletes who are students are usually governed by the Family Educational Rights and Privacy Act (FERPA). FERPA, which applies to all institutions that receive federal funds, requires that student athletes must sign a consent before their personal medical information can be released. Additional resources for information about HIPAA and FERPA are listed in Table 1.

Other Issues

As discussed previously, athletes assume the foreseeable risks attendant to vigorous athletics. In the past decade, the question has arisen regarding the status of athletes infected with HIV. Infection resulting from contact with a player with HIV or another blood-borne viral pathogen such as hepatitis B is not a risk that was foreseeable in the past. Although there are no right or wrong answers in such a controversial topic, the AAP issued a policy statement in 1999. Essentially, the AAP recommends allowing infected athletes to play and recommends against disclosure of the athlete's infection to other athletes or to coaching and other staff. Physicians are encouraged to counsel infected athletes that they do run a small risk of infecting other athletes. Infected athletes are encouraged to consider participating in sports in which the risk of transmission is relatively low. Finally, all athletes are to be advised that the sport is being conducted under the above rules.

Recommendations for Sports Medicine Physicians

Physicians treating athletes must strike a reasoned balance between protecting athletes from injury and allowing them to participate in a vigorous and competitive manner. The following are some general recommendations (Table 2). (1) An age- and risk-appropriate preparticipation physical examination should be performed before participation in training or competition. Some common sense should be used. For example, the preparticipation physical examination for a college basketball player might be somewhat more comprehensive than for a high school golfer. Additionally, specific care should be exercised with regard to history of cardiac problems, syncope, and family history of sudden cardiac death. Any history of such, with or without physical findings, warrants further investigation either by or in conjunction with a cardiologist. The AAP issued specific recommendations on this topic in 1995. (2) A waiver should be discussed with the athlete (and with the athlete's parents if the athlete is a minor), and the waiver should be executed after the athlete (and the athlete's parents, if applicable) fully understands the risks of participation. (3) The athlete should wear properly designed and functioning protective equipment. In baseball alone, the US Consumer Product Safety

TABLE 2 | General Recommendations for Sports Medicine Physicians and Athletes

An age- and risk-appropriate preparticipation physical examination should be performed before participation in athletic training or competition.

A waiver should be discussed with the athlete (and with the athlete's parents if the athlete is a minor), and the waiver should be executed after the athlete (and the athlete's parents, if applicable) fully understands the risks of participation.

The athlete should wear properly designed and functioning protective equipment.

The athlete should practice and compete only under qualified supervision.

The athletic field and equipment used should be properly maintained and safe.

No performance-enhancing substances should be used by the athlete.

The athlete should be properly trained and conditioned before participation in competition.

A professional who is trained in injury recognition should evaluate injuries; injuries with potentially serious consequences should be thoroughly and adequately evaluated before a decision is made to allow the athlete to return to play.

The athlete's privacy should be meticulously protected unless the athlete has specifically consented in writing to disclosure of medical information.

Decision making by sports physicians should be documented, particularly when serious medical conditions are involved.

Commission found that protective equipment currently on the market could reduce or prevent up to 36% of the 162,100 baseball injuries that occur in children treated in emergency departments each year. (4) The athlete should practice and compete only under qualified supervision. (5) The athletic field and equipment used should be properly maintained and safe. (6) No performance-enhancing substances should be used. (7) Athletes should be properly trained and conditioned before participation in competition. (8) Injuries should be evaluated by a professional trained in injury recognition. Injuries with potentially serious consequences should be thoroughly and adequately evaluated before a decision is made to allow the athlete to return to play. In all cases, the athlete's long-term health must be the primary consideration. Moreover, the physician must always be aware that motivated athletes often will not be receptive to decisions not to allow further athletic participation. Having built good rapport with patients before the injury can be most helpful when the occasion arises in which the physician must advise against further athletic participation. Athletes who do not accept prohibitions from athletic participation sometimes resort to litigation. Courts have held that barring athletes from play in certain circumstances can be a violation of their civil rights. Motivated players may also seek the opinions of

other physicians who may support their desire to continue participation in athletic competition. Conflicting medical opinions will, of course, further complicate the issue. (9) The athlete's privacy should be meticulously protected unless the athlete has specifically consented in writing to disclosure of medical information. Compliance with HIPAA is federally mandated and must be maintained. (10) Decision making by sports physicians should be documented, particularly when serious medical conditions are involved.

Summary

With the rising incidence of sports-related injuries and sudden cardiac death, sports medicine physicians must err on the side of caution to ensure that proper evaluation and treatment are accomplished before athletes are allowed to participate in athletic activities. If one rule could always be followed, it should be to always act in the best interest of the athlete, no matter how great the pressure from that athlete or other interested parties. Adherence to this one rule is perhaps the best protection against legal problems. In addition, to avoid allegations of negligence, sports medicine physicians must be astute in medical diagnosis and treatment and should also be very attentive to patient privacy and documentation. In a worst-case scenario where an injured athlete sues, the well-prepared sports medicine physician will have good documentation of care and a well-drafted waiver. These documents, if prepared correctly, will demonstrate that appropriate care and advice were given, and they will aid greatly in demonstrating that the injured plaintiff understood the risks of the sport and chose to assume those risks.

Annotated Bibliography

Sports Injuries in a Litigious Society

American Academy of Pediatrics: Sports injuries: A growing problem in kids. *USA Today* October 18-20, 2002, Kids Health Supplement. Available at: http://www.aap.org/advocacy/releases/sportsinjury.htm. Accessed April 28, 2004.

This article specifically discusses the growing problem of athletic overuse injuries in children and adolescents and provides tips on how these injuries can be prevented.

Sports and recreation related injuries. Centers for Disease Control and Prevention Web site. Available at: http://www.cdc.gov/communication/tips/sports.htm. Accessed March 15, 2004.

This article discusses the risks associated with sports and recreational activities as well as steps that can be taken to prevent sports-related injuries.

Cardiac deaths increase among the young: CDC report shows greatest increase in deaths among young women.

Available at: http://usgovinfo.about.com/library/weekly/ aa030301a.htm. Accessed March 15, 2004.

In response to a CDC report showing a 10% increase in sudden cardiac deaths in persons between ages 15 and 34 years over the last decade (from 2,719 in 1989 to 3,000 in 1996), this article discusses the causes of sudden cardiac death as well as methods of prevention.

Lillard M: Study tallies 23 football deaths in 2001. *Savannah Now* [serial online], July 25, 2002. Available at: http://www.savannahnow.com/stories/072502/ SPTheatstudy.shtml. Accessed March 15, 2004.

This article points out that heat-related football deaths at all levels have steadily increased and have replaced direct fatal injuries as football's greatest on-field safety risk.

Pre-participation physical examinations: American College of Sports Medicine Web site. Available at: http:// www.acsm.org/pdf/prepart022702.pdf. Accessed March 15, 2004.

This document provides specific guidelines for performing preparticipation physical examinations for athletes.

American College of Legal Medicine: *Legal Medicine*, ed 5. St. Louis, MO, Mosby, 2001, pp 448-450.

This book explores and illustrates the legal implications of medical practice and the special legal issues arising from managed care.

Negligence

Rosenbaum S: The impact of United States law on medicine as a profession. *JAMA* 2003;289:1546-1556.

This article discusses the evolution of the no duty to treat principle and the role of modern health care financing and civil rights law in altering this rule. Also discussed are the manner in which advances in medicine led courts and legislatures to change the standards against which professional medical liability is measured and the basic loss of highly preferential treatment under US laws aimed at preventing anticompetitive conduct by businesses.

Privacy

Magee JT, Almekinders LC, Taft TN: HIPAA and the team physician. *Sports Medicine Update* March-April

2003, pp 4-7. Available at: www.aossm.org/downloads/ pdf/SMU2003MarApr.pdf. Accessed April 29, 2004.

This article outlines the new HIPAA privacy regulations that place provisions and limits on the disclosure of health information.

Other Issues

Human immunodeficiency virus and other blood-borne viral pathogens in the athletic setting: Committee on Sports Medicine and Fitness. American Academy of Pediatrics. *Pediatrics* 1999;104:1400-1403.

This statement updates a previous position statement of the AAP and discusses sports participation for athletes infected with HIV and other blood-borne pathogens and the precautions needed to reduce the risk of infection to others in the athletic setting.

Classic Bibliography

Cardiac dysrhythmias and sports: Committee on Sports Medicine and Fitness. American Academy of Pediatrics. *Pediatrics* 1995;95:786-788.

Family Educational Rights and Privacy Act (FERPA), 20 USC, Chapter 31 §1232(g).

Health Insurance Portability and Accountability Act, PL §104-191 (1996).

Tolman L: Use your head: Wear a helmet. *Worcester Telegram & Gazette.* August 13, 1995.

US Consumer Product Safety Commission: Office of Information and Public Affairs: CPSC releases study of protective equipment for baseball. [US Consumer Product Safety Commission Web site]. June 4, 1996, Release #96-140. Available at: http://www.cpsc.gov/CPSCPUB/ PREREL/PRHTML96/96140.html. Accessed March 15, 2004.

US Department of Health and Human Services: The Health Insurance Portability and Accountability Act of 1996 (HIPAA), Public Law 104-191. Available at: http:// www.hhs.gov/ocr/hipaa. Accessed March 15, 2004.

Chapter 35

Anterior Cruciate Ligament Injuries in Female Athletes

Marlene DeMaio, MD, CAPT, MC, USN

Kathleen McHale, MD, FACS, COL, MC, USA

Introduction

The recent focus on women's health issues has brought the relationship between gender and disease to the attention of orthopaedic surgeons. Although injury patterns among men and women are generally similar, and researchers have determined that injury patterns are generally sport-specific, exceptions have been noted. For example, studies and data on anterior cruciate ligament (ACL) injuries indicate that these injuries are particularly problematic for women and that there is, as yet, no conclusive evidence to explain the gender difference prevalence. The medical literature is replete with studies on conditions such as osteoporosis, stress fractures, patellofemoral syndromes, and bunions that reflect a female predominance. Although some injuries are more difficult to explain by gender division, ACL injuries provide a striking example in which the injuries of men and women are truly different.

Epidemiology

Both retrospective and prospective studies show that higher rates of ACL tears occur in women than men. Although rates of ACL injuries vary among sports, they may be as high as two to eight times higher in women who participate in jumping and cutting activities than men. A survey of National Collegiate Athletic Association Division 1 teams from 1989 to 1993 showed that the risk of ACL injury in women who play basketball and soccer was two and four times higher, respectively, in women than in men. Another study reported a comparable increase in the rate of ACL injuries in women playing volleyball.

The most common mechanism of ACL injury in women appears to be of a noncontact nature both in the sports setting and in military training. At the amateur athletic level, however, contact injuries appear to be more prevalent. A review of female soccer players in Sweden showed that the majority of ACL injuries in senior level competition occurred in a contact situation in players younger than 16 years. This study suggests that contact may be the mechanism of injury in the physically immature individual who participates at a higher level of play.

Risk Factors

The susceptibility of female athletes to experience ACL injuries appears to be multifactorial. Intrinsic factors involve the biomechanics, biochemistry, and anatomic structure of the ligament and knee joint itself. Extrinsic factors include neuromuscular composition, body movement with shoe surface interface, and skill level.

Intrinsic Factors

The biomechanics of the female ACL ligament (for example, the relationship of knee laxity to ligament injury) are not well understood. Knee stiffness, measured as force over the amount of displacement of the proximal tibia, may be a factor in preventing injury. In a study comparing male and female athletes to control subjects, the authors reported that the knees of athletes were tighter than those of the control subjects and that the knees of women were looser than those of men. Volitional contraction of the knee musculature is known to increase the resistance of the knee to shear deformation. This contraction, however, increases shear stiffness to a greater extent in men, even when body weight is considered. Therefore, the "protection" of the ACL from the thigh musculature may be less in women.

The biochemistry of ACL function focuses on hormonal effects on the ligament and the fact that there are estrogen and progesterone receptors on the human ACL. Estrogen effects seem most important in influencing the laxity and injury rates that vary with the menstrual cycle. High- and low-risk intervals are associated with the follicular and luteal phases. In a multicenter study of female athletes who experienced acute ACL injuries, the results from hormone assays indicated that there was a greater than expected percentage of ACL injuries when estrogen levels were at their highest during ovulation. Conversely, during the ebb of estrogen levels in the luteal phase, there was less than the expected number of ACL injuries. Oral contraceptive use

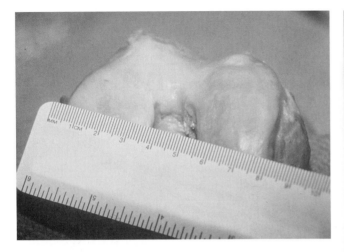

Figure 1 Anatomic measurement of the notch width on a cadaveric knee at the level of the popliteal hiatus.

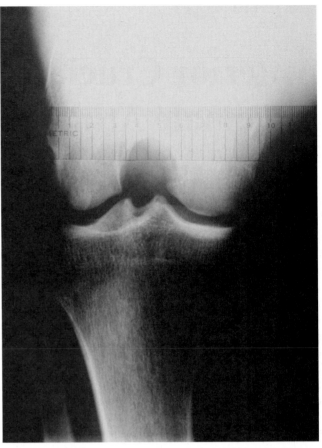

Figure 2 Radiographic measurement of the notch width at the level of the popliteal hiatus.

that prevents ovulation also diminished the significant association between ACL tear distribution and ovulation. In another study, the use of oral contraceptives appeared to shift the risk to the beginning of the cycle (ie, the follicular phase).

It has been hypothesized that estrogen increases ligamentous laxity. There is evidence that anterior translation of the knee when stressed (laxity) is highest when circulating estrogen is at its peak level. In one study of young women with normal menstrual cycles, the anterior displacement using a KT-2000 arthrometer (MEDmetric, San Diego, CA) was shown to vary between the follicular and ovulatory phases and between the follicular and luteal phases. Another study measuring anterior translation with the KT-1000 arthrometer (MEDmetric) showed a statistically significant increase in laxity in the third trimester of pregnancy when estrogen (estradiol) levels are extremely high compared with postpartum. Differences in results have been reported, however, in animal studies when anterior translation stress is taken to failure. In a study comparing two groups of ovariectomized New Zealand white rabbits that were treated with estradiol or untreated, the authors showed that the estradiol-treated group, which had a 50% higher estrogen level than the untreated group, required smaller loads to result in failure. Conversely, another study showed no differences in energy to failure, maximum force, stiffness, or failure site when comparing ovariectomized female sheep that were treated with estradiol or untreated. In the same study, however, the ultimate energy to failure was significantly higher in male sheep than in female sheep. It has also been suggested that relaxin, the receptors of which have been discovered in the ACL, poses another possible hormonal risk factor for female ACL injury. Thus far, however, there has

been no demonstrable evidence of increase in anterior translation related to levels of relaxin in nongravid subjects.

The anatomic structure of the female knee joint has been analyzed as a significant factor in predisposition to ACL injuries, and a small femoral notch width repeatedly has been shown to be associated with such injuries (Figures 1 and 2). A notch width of less than 15 mm is considered a risk factor for ACL tears. Women have smaller notch widths, even after adjusting for height and weight. A study of fresh-frozen cadaveric knee specimens revealed both smaller ACL widths and smaller femoral intercondylar notch widths in specimens obtained from females. Although this suggests that the comparatively smaller size of the female ACL may predispose it to injury, it has been argued that the ratio of the width of the ACL to the femoral intercondylar notch width, which was smaller in females in this study, may be the predisposing factor. The width of the femoral intercondylar notch as it relates to the size of the distal femur does not appear to correlate with the incidence of ACL injuries. The notch width index is the ratio of the femoral intercondylar notch width to the width of the femur at the level of the popliteus in a

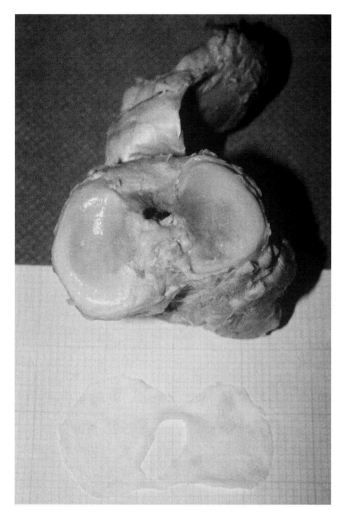

Figure 3 Photograph of a cadaveric knee showing the surface area of the insertion of the ACL on the tibia and the surface area of the tibial plateau.

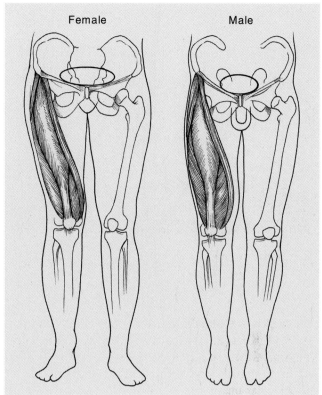

Figure 4 In general, when compared with men of equal ages, women have wider pelvises as well as greater hip varus, knee valgus, and foot pronation. *(Reproduced from Griffin LY, Agel J, Albohm MJ, et al: Noncontact anterior cruciate ligament injuries: Risk factors and prevention strategies. J Am Acad Orthop Surg 2000;8:141-150.)*

non–weight-bearing tunnel view. In a study of 20 men and 20 women with noncontact ACL tears and matched controls, there was no difference in the notch width index between groups with tears or with intact ACLs regardless of gender. The caudal slope of the plateau, tibial eminence width, and ratio of the tibial spines to the plateau width have also been examined for their relationship to female ACL injuries, but these anatomic features of the knee have not been shown to correlate positively with ACL injury (Figure 3).

Limb alignment in females may contribute to ACL injury susceptibility. Females have a wider pelvis, lower center of gravity, and greater knee valgus—all of which may contribute to the difference in knee ligament mechanics (Figure 4). Rotational alignment differences in females may contribute to ACL injury risk, but ACL injury risk has not been shown to be associated with femoral anteversion and quadriceps angle (Figures 5 and 6). Nevertheless, there does appear to be a tendency for having a higher thigh-foot angle in females with ACL tears, suggesting increased external rotation when plant-

ing the foot. Angular differences in the coronal and sagittal planes also have been examined as contributing factors to ACL injury risk. In a study of the static posture of 20 females with ACL tears and 20 control subjects, seven variables were assessed: standing pelvic position, hip position, standing sag knee position, standing frontal knee position, hamstring length, prone subtalar joint position, and navicular drop test. With regression analysis, knee recurvatum, navicular drop, and prone subtalar joint pronation were found to be associated with ACL injury.

Extrinsic Factors

Neuromuscular and muscle function factors that impact control, muscle strength, and muscle endurance have a significant effect on ACL injury rates. Women have less potential for muscular protection of passive structures of the knee in anterior tibial translation than men for three reasons. First, the knee control contributed by the thigh muscles may be relatively less in women than men because there is some evidence that skeletal muscle fiber types are different in men and women, and muscle elasticity appears to be relatively higher in women. One study showed that female muscles were looser than male muscles on dynamic stress testing, and another

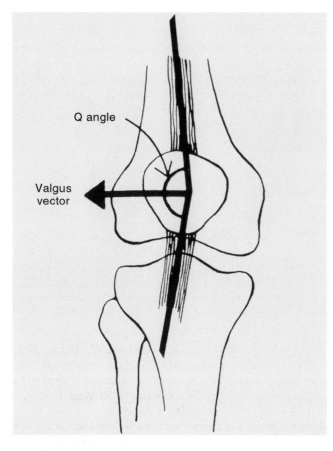

Figure 5 Illustration of the measurement of the Q angle.

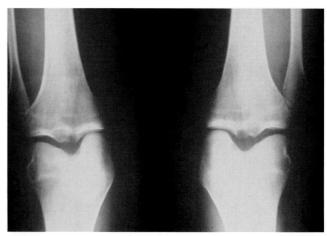

Figure 6 Radiographic estimation of the Q angle on weight-bearing PA (Rosenberg) view.

study demonstrated that female muscles had a longer electromechanical delay than male muscles. Second, relative muscle strength may be less in women than men. Women need more time than men to produce the same absolute muscle force, even when results are adjusted for body weight. Electromechanical delay of the hamstrings may be the reason why female athletes protect against anterior tibial translation. The order of muscle recruitment is the same in men and women; however, a shorter latency in quadriceps activation occurs in women. Increased quadriceps coactivation in women may increase anterior tibial loads under dynamic conditions, thus placing the female ACLs at higher risk. Third, endurance of women may be less than that of men. Early gastrocnemius-soleus complex activation has been shown to occur after fatigue of the quadriceps with eccentric contraction in female track athletes. There does not appear to be a difference in aerobic capacity, anaerobic capacity, aerobic endurance, or muscle strength in any specific menstrual cycle phase.

Body movements or kinematics of the knee and the entire lower extremity appear to be different in women and men. Studies have focused on common body positions that occur in athletics. One such position is landing from a jump. In one study, female athletes demonstrated

a more erect landing posture, greater hip and ankle joint range of motion, maximum joint angular velocities, and greater energy absorption from knee extensors and ankle dorsiflexors than male athletes in a drop landing. Female athletes may be at risk for ACL injuries because of their energy absorption strategy. During stop-jump tasks, female athletes exhibit greater proximal shear force with greater knee extension and valgus moments than male athletes during the landing phase. Female athletes display muscle synchrony that is less protective of the ACL than male athletes, possibly increasing the susceptibility in noncontact injuries. Another position frequently assumed in athletic activity is the single-legged squat. In this position, female athletes demonstrate significantly more ankle dorsiflexion and pronation; more hip adduction, flexion, and external rotation; and less trunk flexion than male athletes; therefore, female athletes have less ability to maintain the knee in a varus position. It appears that under physiologic load in this position female athletes tend to position the lower extremity and activate muscles in a way that can increase strain on the ACL. With other common athletic activities such as running, side-cutting, and cross-cutting, female athletes appear to have smaller knee flexion angles, larger knee valgus angles, greater quadriceps activation, and lower hamstring activation when compared with male athletes. Loading of a valgus knee, particularly with the female pattern of muscle synchrony, will increase strain on the ACL.

In a study of collegiate basketball players, female athletes were shown to land with greater knee flexion angles and greater knee flexion accelerations than male athletes. The authors suggest that this knee flexion is protective and does not significantly predispose female athletes to ACL injuries. Hamstring muscle activation, however, was similar in both male and female athletes, which raises the issue that protection may be provided by specific training.

The relationship of athletic skill level to ACL injury risk is unclear. Although ACL tear rates do not appear to correlate with athletic skill levels, neuromuscular training has been shown to decrease the rate of ACL tears. Several studies have reported that sport-specific training can significantly decrease injury rates.

Treatment

Male and female athletes with ACL injuries do not require different types of rehabilitation or reconstruction. Studies have shown that autogenous bone-patella tendon-bone ACL reconstruction appears to be equally successful in well-matched populations of males and females. In a study of ACL reconstructions using different autografts, hamstring grafts had more failures, more clinical laxity, and more frequent KT-1000 arthrometer differences than patellar tendon grafts. Although these results were not statistically significant, they show a trend toward graft or knee laxity with hamstring grafts. Other intra-articular pathology such as meniscal tears and medial femoral condyle injuries are less frequent in female athletes with ACL tears. If intra-articular injuries are a risk factor for poor long-term outcome, women may actually have a better prognosis after reconstruction.

Summary

Female athletes are more susceptible to ACL injuries than male athletes for several reasons. The ACL and knee are more lax in females than in males. Additionally, the ACL has estrogen receptors, resulting in an increased ACL vulnerability during the ovulation phase of the menstrual cycle when estrogen is at its highest. The hamstring muscles in female athletes are slower to respond than those in male athletes; thus, the knees of female athletes are less able to increase stiffness. Valgus orientation of the knees of female athletes is more prone to preload of the ACL. The thigh muscles of female athletes are less capable of absorbing load, which increases the risk of overloading the ACL. Specific training has been shown to decrease the incidence of ACL injuries in both men and women. Reconstruction of the knee after ACL injury has also been shown to be as satisfactory in women as it is in men.

Annotated Bibliography

General

Statement of Michael Ehrlich, MD, Chairman, Committee on Research, American Academy of Orthopaedic Surgeons, on the Fiscal Year 1999 appropriation for the National Institute of Arthritis and Musculoskeletal and Skin Diseases to the House Labor/Health and Human Services/Education Subcommittee on Appropriations on February 4, 1998. American Academy of Orthopaedic Surgeons Web site. Available at: http://www.aaos.org/wordhtml/ehrlic98.htm. Accessed March 17, 2004.

The author emphasizes that several prevalent diseases of the musculoskeletal system are disorders that occur predominantly in women, including arthritis, osteoporosis, and sports injuries.

Epidemiology

Soderman K, Pietila T, Alfredson H, Werner S: Anterior cruciate ligament injuries in young females playing soccer at senior levels. *Scand J Med Sci Sports* 2002;12:65-68.

Three hundred ninety-eight Swedish female soccer players who had an ACL injury before age 19 years were investigated. Of these, 38% were injured before age 16 years. The authors conclude that female soccer players younger than 16 years should be allowed to participate only in practice but not games at the senior level.

Uhorchak JM, Scoville CR, Williams GN, Arciero RA, St. Pierre P, Taylor DC: Risk factors associated with noncontact injury of the anterior cruciate ligament: A prospective four-year evaluation of 859 West Point cadets. *Am J Sports Med* 2003;31:831-842.

The results of this prospective study of knee injuries in West Point cadets showed that female cadets who had some combination of risk factors (small femoral notch width, joint laxity, higher than normal body mass index, and low or high KT-2000 arthrometer values) sustained more noncontact ACL injuries than their male counterparts, suggesting that some combination of factors render the knees of female cadets more susceptible to injury.

Risk Factors

Arendt EA, Bershadsky B, Agel J: Periodicity of noncontact anterior cruciate ligament injuries during the menstrual cycle. *J Gend Specif Med* 2002;5:19-26.

Eighty-three female collegiate athletes participated in this study that analyzed the 28-day periodicity of ACL injuries. Twenty-five athletes were taking oral contraceptives and 58 were not. The authors concluded that there appears to be a significant relationship between ACL injury occurrence and the menstrual cycle regardless of oral contraceptive usage.

Arnold C, Van Bell C, Rogers V, Cooney T: The relationship between serum relaxin and knee joint laxity in female athletes. *Orthopedics* 2002;25:669-673.

This study examined the relationship between serum relaxin levels and joint laxity. Serum relaxin levels and knee arthrometry were done on a group of 57 college women; among them were athletes, ACL-injured athletes, and nonathletes. A group of five men served as a control. The authors reported a significant change in weekly serum relaxin levels but not in anterior translation in women and concluded that relaxin does not affect knee laxity.

Chappell JD, Yu B, Kirkendall DT, Garrett WE: A comparison of knee kinetics between male and female recreational athletes in stop-jump tasks. *Am J Sports Med* 2002;30:261-267.

Three-dimensional videography was done and force-plate data recorded for three different stop-jump tasks in recreational athletes. The landing phase produced more stress on the ACL than the take-off phase in both men and women; however, women showed greater proximal anterior shear force and greater knee extension and valgus moments during landing phase than men. These results suggest that female recreational athletes use motor strategies that produce knee positions that make the ACL susceptible to injury.

Charlton WP, Coslett-Charlton LM, Ciccotti MG: Correlation of estradiol in pregnancy and anterior cruciate ligament laxity. *Clin Orthop* 2001;387:165-170.

Estradiol levels and anterior tibial translation were measured in 40 human subjects during the third trimester of pregnancy and then again postpartum. The authors report a statistically significant decrease in anterior tibial translation that corresponds to the return of serum estradiol to nonpregnant levels after delivery.

Cowling EJ, Steele JR: Is lower limb muscle synchrony during landing affected by gender? Implications for variations in ACL injury rates. *J Electomyogr Kinesiol* 2001;11:263-268.

Ground reaction force, electromyographic, sagittal plane motion, knee joint reaction force, and sagittal planar net moments of force data were collected for 7 male and 11 female athletes in single-limb stance after receiving a chest-height netball pass and decelerating abruptly. The authors report that semimembranous muscle in male athletes had a delayed onset at ground contact and a delayed time to peak force compared with that of female athletes.

Decker MJ, Torry MR, Wyland DJ, Sterett WI, Richard Steadman J: Gender differences in lower extremity kinematics, kinetics, and energy absorption during landing. *Clin Biomech (Bristol, Avon)* 2003;18:662-669.

In this study of landing strategies, women demonstrated a more erect landing posture with greater hip and ankle joint range of motion and maximum joint angular velocities than men. Women had greater energy absorption from knee extension and plantar flexors than men. The authors conclude that women may land in a more erect posture to maximize the energy absorption from the joints nearest the ground contact and that this energy absorption strategy may put the female ACL at greater risk for injury.

Deie M, Sakamaki Y, Sumen Y, Urabe Y, Ikuta Y: Anterior knee laxity in young women varies with their menstrual cycle. *Int Orthop* 2002;26:154-156.

Sixteen women underwent measurement of basal body temperature and serum estradiol and progesterone levels to determine the follicular, ovulatory, and luteal phases of the menstrual cycle. A group of men served as controls. KT-2000 arthrometry was used to measure anterior displacement of the knee several times over a 4-week period. The authors report that in women there were statistically significant differences in anterior translation for menstrual phases at both low and high forces. They concluded that ACL laxity in women may depend on hormonal concentration.

Dragoo JL, Lee RS, Benhaim P, Finerman GA, Hame SL: Relaxin receptors in the human female anterior cruciate ligament. *Am J Sports Med* 2003;31:577-584.

Specimens of ACLs from five men and five women were obtained during ligament reconstruction. The ACL specimens from the women revealed the specific binding of relaxin to relaxin receptors, but those of the men did not.

Fagenbaum R, Darling WG: Jump landing strategies in male and female college athletes and the implications of such strategies for anterior cruciate ligament injury. *Am J Sports Med* 2003;31:233-240.

Male and female collegiate varsity basketball players underwent knee joint angle measurement and surface electrode electromyography of the quadriceps, hamstrings, and gastrocnemius muscles during jump landings from a platform. The women landed with greater knee flexion angles and knee flexion accelerations than the men; however, knee muscle activation patterns in this study were similar in men and women.

Lebrun CM, Rumball JS: Relationship between athletic performance and menstrual cycle. *Curr Womens Health Rep* 2001;1:232-240.

The authors of this article reviewed the effects of female sex steroid hormones on various body systems and structures, including the ACL. The authors suggest that current science has not consistently shown that there are significant differences in aerobic capacity, anaerobic capacity, aerobic endurance, muscle strength, or susceptibility to ACL injuries in the specific phases of the menstrual cycle.

Malinzak RA, Colby SM, Kirkendall DT, Yu B, Garrett WE: A comparison of knee joint motion patterns between men and women in selected athletic tasks. *Clin Biomech (Bristol, Avon)* 2001;16:438-445.

The authors of this study examined the patterns of knee kinematics and electromyographic data in men and women during running, side-cutting, and cross-cutting. They report that women had smaller knee flexion angles, greater knee valgus, greater quadriceps activation, and less hamstring activation than men in each activity. They concluded, therefore, that women may have altered knee motion patterns that predispose to ACL injuries.

Rizzo M, Holler SB, Bassett FH III: Comparison of males' and females' ratios of anterior-cruciate-ligament width to femoral-intercondylar notch width: A cadaveric study. *Am J Orthop* 2001;30:660-664.

The authors of this study examined fresh-frozen cadaver knees and found that the ACL width and the ratio of ACL width to femoral intercondylar notch width are significantly smaller in females than males. The authors concluded that this size difference may be the factor that predisposes the female knee to ACL injury.

Shelbourne KD, Davis TJ, Klootwyk T: The relationship between intercondylar notch width of the femur and the incidence of anterior cruciate ligament tears. *Am J Sports Med* 1998;26:402-408.

In this prospective study, the authors assessed postoperative tears of ACL grafts or contralateral ACL tears and found that intercondylar notch widths smaller than 15 mm were associated with significantly more injuries. With height and weight taken into account, women still had smaller intercondylar notch widths than men.

Shultz SJ, Perrin DH, Adams MJ, Arnold BL, Gansneder BM, Granata KP: Neuromuscular response characteristics in men and women after knee perturbation in a single-leg, weight-bearing stance. *J Athl Train* 2001;36:37-43.

In this study, 32 female (19 lacrosse and 13 soccer players) and 32 male (all lacrosse players) intercollegiate athletes used a lower extremity perturbation device to produce sudden, forward, and rotational moment of the trunk and femur relative to the weight-bearing tibia. Surface electromyography was used to record long latency reflex times of the thigh muscles and the gastrocnemius-soleus complex. The order of muscle recruitment was the same in men and women; however, women responded faster than men because of a shorter latency in quadriceps activation.

Slauterbeck JR, Hardy DM: Sex hormones and knee ligament injuries in female athletes. *Am J Med Sci* 2001; 322:196-199.

The authors of this study report that gender differences in matrix metalloproteinases and their inhibitors may be contributing factors in the susceptibility of female athletes ACL to injury.

Strickland SM, Belknap TW, Turner SA, Wright TM, Hannafin JA: Lack of hormonal influences on mechanical properties of sheep. *Am J Sports Med* 2003;31:210-215.

Mature female sheep were divided into the following five groups: those that underwent sham operations, ovariectomy, or ovariectomy and estradiol implant and those that received low-dose raloxifene or high-dose raloxifene. After 6 months the animals were killed and no differences were found in treatment groups for maximum force, stiffness, energy to failure, or failure site. Male sheep had greater stress to failure than female sheep. The authors concluded that estrogen and estrogen receptor agonists at physiologic levels do not lead to decreased knee ligament strength.

White KK, Lee SS, Cutuk A, Hargens AR, Pedowitz RA: EMG power spectra of intercollegiate athletes and anterior cruciate ligament injury risk in females. *Med Sci Sports Exerc* 2003;35:371-376.

This study evaluates electromyographic power spectra of the quadriceps and hamstring muscles during dynamic, fatiguing exercise to examine differences between male (26) and female (25) intercollegiate athletes. Maximum voluntary contraction was determined for knee flexion and extension. The authors report that maximum voluntary contraction normalized to body weight was significantly greater in male than in female athletes for the quadriceps ($P < 0.01$) and that quadriceps coactivation ratios were significantly higher in female athletes than in male athletes during knee flexion exercises ($P < 0.01$).

Wojtys EM, Ashton-Miller JA, Huston LJ: A gender-related difference in the contribution of the knee musculature to sagittal-plane shear stiffness in subjects with similar knee laxity. *J Bone Joint Surg Am* 2002;84:10-16.

Ten male and 13 female volunteers showed that maximum cocontraction of the knee musculature significantly decreased mean anterior tibial translation in both men and women. The corresponding percentage increase in shear stiffness of the knee, however, was greater in men than in women ($P = 0.003$), even with load adjusted for body weight.

Wojtys EM, Huston LJ, Boynton MD, Spindler KP, Lindenfeld TN: The effect of the menstrual cycle on anterior cruciate ligament injuries in women as determined by hormone levels. *Am J Sports Med* 2002;30:182-188.

In this study, 69 female athletes had hormonal assays done to confirm menstrual phase. The authors report a significantly greater than expected percentage of ACL injuries during midcycle (ovulatory phase) and a lower than expected percentage of ACL injuries during the luteal phase. Oral contraceptive use appeared to decrease the association of ACL injuries and the ovulatory phase.

Zeller BL, McCrory JL, Kibler WB, Uhl TL: Differences in kinematics and electromyographic activity between men and women during the single-legged squat. *Am J Sports Med* 2003;31:449-456.

The authors of this study assessed the kinematics and electromyographic data of men and women performing a single-legged squat activity. The authors report that women showed more ankle dorsiflexion, ankle pronation, hip adduction, hip flexion, and hip external rotation and less lateral flexion of the trunk than men. Thus, women were less able to maintain a varus knee position. Women also had greater muscle activation than men. The authors concluded that the positioning of the female lower extremity and muscle activation under load may increase strain on the ACL.

Treatment

Barrett GR, Noojin FK, Hartzog CW, Nash CR: Reconstruction of the anterior cruciate ligament in females: A comparison of hamstring versus patellar tendon autograft. *Arthroscopy* 2002;18:46-54.

This study compared ACL reconstruction in females using quadruple-looped hamstring autograft versus patellar tendon autograft. The authors reported that at greater than 2-year follow-up, outcome differences were not statistically significant; however, the hamstring group had more failures, more laxity on clinical examination, and more patients with larger KT-1000 differences.

Hewett TE, Lindenfeld TN, Riccobene JV, Noyes FR: The effect of neuromuscular training on the incidence of knee injury in female athletes: A prospective study. *Am J Sports Med* 1999;27:699-706.

This study prospectively evaluated the effects of specific training on ACL injuries in female high school soccer, basketball, and volleyball players as compared with male control subjects. Female athletes were divided into two groups: one group was trained, and the other group was untrained. All of the male control subjects were untrained. There were 1,263 participants and 14 ACL injuries. In the untrained female group, the rate of injury was 0.43 incidents per 1,000 athlete exposures, which was 3.6 times higher ($P = 0.05$) than the 0.12 rate of injury in the trained female group. The male control subjects had a 0.09 rate of injury.

Myklebus G, Engebretsen L, Braekken IH, Skjolberg A, Olsen OE, Bahr R: Prevention of anterior cruciate ligament injuries in female team handball players: A prospective intervention study over three seasons. *Clin J Sport Med* 2003;13:71-78.

In this study, female handball players from the three top divisions underwent a five-phase program (duration, 15 minutes) with three balance exercises focusing on neuromuscular control and planting and landing skills over three seasons (more than 850 players each season). The incidence of injury decreased over the first and second interventional years. This decrease was statistically significant in the elite group who completed the ACL injury prevention program compared with those who did not.

Ott SM, Ireland ML, Ballantyne BT, Willson JD, McClay Davis IS: Comparison of outcomes between males and females after anterior cruciate ligament reconstruction. *Knee Surg Sports Traumatol Arthrosc* 2003;11:75-80.

The authors of this study conducted a statistical analysis of autogenous bone-patella tendon-bone ACL reconstruction and found no difference in ACL quality of life scale scores when comparing women and men. On the Tegner scale, women reported that they had a higher activity level before surgery; no other differences were noted. On the Cincinnati scale, women had lower scores than men, with a trend toward lower scores in female patients age 12 to 18 years and those older than 24 years. The authors concluded that this technique

of ACL reconstruction is equally successful in matched populations of men and women.

Piasecki DP, Spindler KP, Warren TA, Andrish JT, Parker RD: Intraarticular injuries associated with anterior cruciate ligament tear: Findings at ligament reconstruction in high school and recreational athletes. An analysis of sex-based differences. *Am J Sports Med* 2003; 31:601-605.

The authors of this study assessed 221 high school athletes who underwent ACL reconstruction. The mechanism of injury was similar for male and female athletes. Fewer additional intra-articular injuries occurred in female athletes. Female basketball players had fewer lateral meniscus tears and medial femoral condylar injuries than their male counterparts, and female soccer players had fewer medial meniscus tears than their male counterparts.

Classic Bibliography

Arendt E, Dick R: Knee injury patterns among men and women in collegiate basketball and soccer: NCAA data and review of literature. *Am J Sports Med* 1995;23:694-701.

Ferreti A, Papandrea P, Conteduca F, Mariani PP: Knee ligament injuries in volleyball players. *Am J Sports Med* 1992;20:203-207.

Hakkinen K: Force production characteristics of leg extensor, trunk flexor, and extensor muscles in male and female basketball players. *J Sports Med Phys Fitness* 1991;31:325-331.

Huston LJ, Wojtys EM: Neuromuscular performance characteristics of elite female athletes. *Am J Sports Med* 1996;24:427-435.

Loudon JK, Jenkins W, Loudon KL: The relationship between static posture and ACL injury in female athletes. *J Orthop Sports Phys Ther* 1996;24:91-97.

Shelbourne KD, Facibene WA, Hunt JJ: Radiographic and intraoperative intercondylar notch width measurements in men and women with unilateral and bilateral anterior cruciate ligament tears. *Knee Surg Sports Traum Arthrosc* 1997;5:229-233.

Teitz CC, Lind BK, Sacks BM: Symmetry of the femoral notch width index. *Am J Sports Med* 1997;25:687-690.

Winter GJ, Murphy AJ, Pryor JF: Musculotendinous stiffness: Its relationship to eccentric, isometric, and concentric performance. *J Appl Physiol* 1994;76:2714-2719.

Appendix

AOSSM Education Curriculum

Explanation of the Orthopaedic Sports Medicine Curriculum for American Orthopaedic Society for Sports Medicine Members

Overview

This curriculum for learning in sports medicine contains organized and prioritized topics for continuing education. We have rated topic areas in two ways: knowledge and instruction.

Fundamentally, there are three types of knowledge: (1) knowing what (declarative knowledge), (2) knowing how (procedural knowledge), and (3) knowing when and why (conditional knowledge). A command of all three types of knowledge is required for surgical practice. Procedural knowledge (ie, knowing the steps one is to follow in doing a particular procedure as described in *Campbell's*) and being able to do the procedure are very distinct. Knowing the relevant declarative, procedural, and conditional knowledge is necessary but not sufficient for being able to practice orthopaedic sports medicine proficiently.

A "scoring key" was developed to break down the curriculum topics into functional (depth of knowledge) and instructional (instructional guide) rating categories. The curriculum is designed to separate topics that should be mastered by all sports medicine practitioners (rating of 1) and those topics in which mastery is expected only in subspecialists who have a particular interest in that area (rating of 2). The instructional rating describes the level to which our association should plan instruction. Instruction for topics with an "A" rating should not only deal with declarative, procedural, and conditional knowledge, but it should also provide psychomotor skills training. Instruction for topics with a "B" rating should deal with declarative, procedural, and conditional knowledge, but it does not require psychomotor skills training. Topics rated "C" are suitable for electronic or print media.

Particular care needs to be taken in advertising and introducing hands-on surgical continuing medical education (CME) courses to warn participants that what they learn in a particular course is intended to contribute to becoming proficient in using particular types of equipment and/or doing specific types of procedures. The course is not, however, intended to, nor should it be construed to, guarantee proficiency. For such proficiency to be attained, additional learning may be necessary, and engaging in that additional learning is each participant's responsibility. Professional societies, such as the American Orthopaedic Society for Sports Medicine (AOSSM), may or may not choose to provide some or all of the needed, additional learning experiences to fill that gap.

The Curriculum and Its Use

In their responses to the 1996 membership survey, AOSSM members put a relatively high priority on the educational offerings of the AOSSM. Many such offerings are made available each year. Most of them have been presented in traditional CME formats, such as slide talks in large sessions, panel presentations, and instructional courses (didactic with or without hands-on experiences). Some offerings have used less traditional formats, such as anomaly-based workshops, traveling fellowships, and one-on-one or small group, AOSSM-sponsored several day apprenticeships with experts.

Educational offerings of the AOSSM have tended to be based on what was assumed to have been needed, what has been well received, and/or what popular and, in some cases, what charismatic presenters have wanted to or were willing to present. The AOSSM leaders feel that significant improvement in the current system can be made by better prioritizing its educational programs by developing a curriculum that more systematically addresses the needs of its members. The goal of the Education Subcommittee has been to provide such a curriculum along with a recommended strategic plan to implement and periodically update it.

The term "curriculum" is potentially confusing. A CME curriculum is different from a schooling curriculum (kindergarten through university level including residency and fellowship training). A CME curriculum is a program or sequence of courses or other instructional activities covering several years (Good, 1959).

The development of the Orthopaedic Sports Medicine Curriculum for AOSSM members used concepts and formats from previously developed orthopaedic education curricula, including Noyes and Farmer, 1992; Green, Herndon, and Farmer, 1991; Gross and Farmer, 1990; and those published in 1991 by the Arthroscopy Association of North America and in 1989 by the Canadian Orthopaedic Association. All of those curricula pertained to resident or fellowship training. In contrast, the Orthopaedic Sports Medicine Curriculum for AOSSM members pertains to CME.

In order for a sound CME curriculum to be developed and updated, it is necessary that the nature and extent of potential content and alternative ways of delivering such content be made explicit along with a plan for prioritizing potential offerings and related strategic decisions. Deciding what educational content to offer and how without a sound curriculum is like doing research without making explicit the population from which the sample is selected.

Much of what is needed (Ruesch, 1975; Baskett and Marsick, 1992; Eraut, 1994, 1985) in orthopaedic practice generally and orthopaedic sports medicine specifically is "knowledge in action" and not merely knowledge or action. When developing, updating, and implementing sound CME curricula, it is essential to determine whether knowing about something (ie, sports and sports rules) is necessary and sufficient or whether knowing and being able to do something (ie, perform an arthroscopic ligament repair) proficiently and knowledgeably is necessary (Ruesch, 1975; Baskett and Marsick, 1992; Eraut, 1985, 1994) for particular types of orthopaedic sports medicine providers.

Being able to understand and deal with a particular type of injury or illness proficiently means using one or more acceptable (as defined by the profession) procedures or processes and avoiding unacceptable practices. Expertise may evolve from such proficiency as a result of extensive experience and, in some cases, specialized training. The basic goal of CME is establishing proficiency, as necessary, and maintaining it. Developing expertise is a specialized goal. This means that all AOSSM members should be helped to develop (as necessary) and retain proficiency as orthopaedic sport medicine providers and that those who choose to do so should be helped to attain expertise in specialized aspects of orthopaedic sports medicine.

Major topics covered in the curriculum include sports medicine education and inquiry, research, general sports medicine, and musculoskeletal topics. For the musculoskeletal section, a template was developed to cover each anatomic area (eg, ligament, cartilage, tendon, muscle, bone, nerve, and vessel) of each specific joint. For each anatomic area, consideration is given to the relevant basic science (anatomy, biomechanics, and biology) and clinical topics including classification of injury/disease, evaluation and management (nonsurgical and surgical). Ratings of specific topics take into consideration issues that are unique to orthopaedic sports medicine such as return to play and sport-specific outcomes research.

Reportedly, many general surgeons were taught how to make diagnoses and perform certain abdominal surgical procedures using endoscopic techniques (eg, cholecystectomy). The main way they were taught was through short, AOSSM-sponsored CME courses that included didactic presentations supplemented by hands-on experience. Unfortunately, this new technology leads to an alarming increase in the number of intraoperative and postoperative complications (Soper, Brunt, and Kerbel, 1994). When the matter was reviewed, it was concluded that these surgeons had become somewhat knowledgeable about the use of such equipment but not technically proficient as a result of what they learned mainly in the short CME courses.

A valid orthopaedic sports medicine curriculum intersects content in other curricula (ie, arthroscopic surgery, foot and ankle, pediatric medicine, and nonorthopaedic sports medicine). Nevertheless, the intersecting content takes on specialized meaning and is often used somewhat differently because of it being related to sports, on the one hand, and orthopaedics, on the other.

Christopher D. Harner, MD
Professor, Department of Orthopaedic Surgery
University of Pittsburgh School of Medicine
Chairman, Education Committee, 1998-2001

James A. Farmer Jr, EdD
Professor Emeritus of Continuing Education
University of Illinois at Champaign-Urbana
Educational Consultant to the AOSSM

References

Baskett, HK, Marsick VJ (eds): Professionals' ways of knowing: New findings on how to improve professional education, in *New Directions for Adult and Continuing Education*, 55, Fall. San Francisco, CA, Jossey-Bass, 1992.

Eraut M: Knowledge creation and knowledge use in professional contexts. *Studies in Higher Education* 1985; 10:117-133.

Good CV (ed): *Dictionary of Education*, ed 2. New York, NY, McGraw-Hill, 1959.

Green NE, Herndon JH, Farmer JA: *A Clinical Curriculum for Orthopaedic Surgery Residency Programs*. American Board of Orthopaedic Surgery and Academic Orthopaedic Society, 1992.

Gross RH, Farmer JA: *Core Curriculum for Pediatric Orthopaedic Residency Training.* Pediatric Orthopaedic Society of North America, 1990.

Noyes FR, Farmer JA: *Committee Report on Sports Medicine Fellowship Curriculum and Structure.* American Society of Orthopaedic Sports Medicine Fellowship Directors and the American Orthopaedic Society for Sports Medicine, 1992.

Ruesch J: *Knowledge in Action: Communication, Social Operations, and Management.* New York, NY, Jason Aronson, 1975.

Soper NJ, Brunt LM, Kerble K: Laparoscopic general surgery. *N Engl J Med* 1994;330:409-419.

Fellowship Core Curriculum. Arthroscopy Association of North America, 1991.

Postgraduate Orthopaedic Educational Objectives. Canadian Orthopaedic Association, 1989.

AOSSM
Educational Curriculum

Developed by the Education Committee and Approved by the Collective Leadership of the AOSSM; Funding provided by education and research funds of the AOSSM formerly, the Foundation for Sports Medicine Education and Research. Last Revision: April, 2000.

Scoring Key

Topic Scoring

Depth of Knowledge:

1 = All should have in-depth knowledge.

2 = All should be aware of this item, but only those who subspecialize in a particular aspect of orthopaedic sports medicine need in-depth knowledge.

Instructional Guidelines:

A = In-depth instruction provided, including psychomotor skill development.

B = In-depth instruction provided, without psychomotor skill development.

C = Instruction provided through the use of electronic or print media.

Musculoskeletal

Basic Science*:

Anatomy
  gross
  functional
Biomechancis
  mechancial properties
  kinematics
  In situ forces
Biology of Healing
  injury
  healing
  repair

Evaluation**:

History
Physical Exam
Imaging
Additional Studies

Management***:

Non-Operative^A
  medication/injection
  brace/splint/cast
  rehabilitation
  return to play
  outcomes
Operative^B
  indications
  techniques
  rehabilitation
  complications
  return to play
  special considerations
  outcomes

General Sports Medicine Topics

TOPIC	SCORE	
	Knowledge	**Instruction**
I. Medical Aspects of Sports Medicine		
A. Cardiac	2	C
B. Dermatology	2	C
C. Pulmonary	2	C
D. Infection	2	C
E. Nutrition		
1. Eating Disorders	2	C
2. Hydration	1	C
3. Anabolic Steroids	1	C
4. Nutritional Supplements	2	C
5. Ergogenic Aids	2	C
F. Drug Testing/Banned Substances	2	C
G. Environmental Exposure		
1. Hypothermia	2	C
2. Heat Injuries	1	B
3. Altitude Sickness	2	C
4. Decompression Sickness	2	C
II. Exercise Physiology		
A. Response to Exercise	2	C
B. Fitness Level	2	C
C. Training	2	C
D. Adaptation	2	C
E. Motor Skills	2	C
F. Performance Factors	2	C
III. Athletic Populations		
A. Female Athletes	1	B
B. Disabled Athletes	1	B
C. Aging Athletes	1	B
IV. Pediatric and Adolescent Issues in Sports	1	B
V. Preventative Sports Medicine		
A. Pre-participation Guidelines	1	C
B. Rules of Sports	2	C
C. Protective Equipment	1	C
VI. Sports Specific Trauma		
A. Eye, Ear, Mouth & Face	2	B
B. Head: Concussion, Closed Head Injury	1	B
C. Chest		
1. Rib	1	B
2. Cardiac Contusion	2	B
3. Pneumothorax	2	B
D. Abdomen		
1. Spleen	2	B
2. Liver	2	B
4. Other Organ Injury	2	B
E. Genito-Urinary		
1. Male	2	B
2. Female	2	B

TOPIC	SCORE	
	Knowledge	**Instruction**
VII. Protective Equipment Including Braces		
A. Head Gear - Football Helmet		
1. Design	1	B
2. Removal	1	B
3. Protective Effect	1	B
B. Head Gear - Other Sports (Hockey, Boxing, etc.)		
1. Design	1	C
2. Protective Effect	1	C
C. Neck - Soft Orthoses		
1. Use of Collars in Football	1	B
2. Use of Rolls in Football	1	B
D. Neck - Spine Boards		
1. Indications for Use	1	B
2. How to Apply	1	B
3. How to Transport	1	B
E. Lumbar Spine		
1. Corset	1	B
2. Brace for Spondylosis in Adolescent Adults	1	B
F. Ribs		
1. Flak Jacket	1	B
G. Shoulder		
1. Use of Harness to Prevent Glenohumeral Instability in Football, Hockey, etc.	1	B
H. Elbow		
1. Hyperextension Brace	1	B
I. Hand & Wrist		
1. Plastic and Silicone Materials for Navicular Fractures and Game Keepers Thumb in Football, Skiing, etc.	1	B
J. Knee		
1. Patella Brace		
a. How to Apply	1	B
b. Function	1	B
2. Sleeves	1	B
3. Ligament Brace		
a. Classification		
i. Prophylactic	1	B
ii. Rehabilitation	1	B
iii. Functional	1	B
b. Design	2	C
c. Objective Data		
i. Biomechanical	1	B
ii. Clinical	1	B
K. Ankle		
1. Taping		
a. Techniques	1	B
b. Effects	1	B
c. Results	1	B
2. Air Stirrup Brace	1	B
3. Lace-up Support	1	B

TOPIC	SCORE	
	Knowledge	Instruction
L. Foot		
1. Orthoses for Runners		
a. Different Materials	1	B
b. Indications	1	B
2. Heel Protectors	1	B
3. Foot Wear	1	B
4. Plantar Fascia Braces	1	B
VIII. Team Physician Issues		
A. Traveling Team Physician	1	C
B. Pre-participation Physical	1	C
C. Medical/Legal Issues	1	C
D. Ethics	1	C
E. Re-certification	1	C
F. Sports Environment and Facilities	2	C
G. Interaction with Ancillary Medical Personnel	2	C
H. Policies on Blood Borne Pathogens	2	C
I. Policies on Drug Abuse	2	C
J. Rules of Sports as it Pertains to Medical Coverage	1	C
K. Emergency Plans at Sporting Events	1	C
L. Medical Guidelines		
1. State High School	2	B
2. NCAA/Collegiate	2	B
3. Professional Sports	2	B
IX. Practice Management		
A. Office	1	B
B. Billing/coding	1	B
X. Information Technology	1	B

Sports Medicine Research

TOPIC	SCORE	
	Knowledge	**Instruction**
I. Critical Appraisal of Literature	1	B
II. Bias	1	B
III. Study Design	1	B
IV. Statistics	1	C
V. Computers	1	B

Sports Medicine Education and Inquiry

TOPIC	SCORE	
	Knowledge	Instruction

I. Educating the members about how to educate the following about orthopaedic sports medicine: 　　Knowledge 2　Instruction B
  A. Medical Students
  B. Residents
  C. Fellows
  D. AOSSM Members
  E. Other Physicians and Surgeons
  F. Other Allied Health Personnel (ATCs, PTs, EMTs, etc.)
  G. Patients
  H. Coaches
  I. The Public
  J. The Media

II. Helping members engage in inquiry* about important aspects of orthopaedic sports medicine about which:　2　B
  A. Little is known
  B. What is known is problematic

* In the past decade, AOSSM has sponsored such inquiry which was conducted in anomaly-based workshops on topics such as the female athlete, sports-induced soft-tissue inflammation, extra-articular support of the ACL, therapeutic modalities for sports injuries, intensive participation in children's sports, and strength training for pre-pubescent athletes.

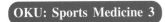
Musculoskeletal

See Template for the Musculoskeletal Section of the Educational Curriculum for an explanation of this section's format.

TOPIC	SCORE	
	Knowledge	**Instruction**
SHOULDER/glenohumeral		
I. Ligament (IGHL, MGHL, SGHL, Labrum)		
A. Basic Science*	1	B
B. Clinical - Instability		
1. Classification of Injury/Disease	1	B
a. Traumatic		
i. Instability		
aa. Direction	1	B
bb. Degree	1	B
cc. Timing	1	B
dd. Acute/chronic	1	B
ee. Associated pathology	1	B
ff. Frequency	1	B
b. Inflammatory		
i. Adhesive capsulitis		
ii. Post-trauma/surgery		
c. Other		
2. Evaluation**	1	A
3. Management***		
a. Non-Operative^A		
i. Unidirectional		
aa. Anterior	1	B
bb. Posterior	1	B
cc. Inferior	1	B
ii. Multidirectional	1	B
iii. Adhesive capsulitis	1	B
b. Operative^B (open/arthroscopic)		
i. Unidirectional		
aa. Anterior	1	A
bb. Posterior	2	A
cc. Inferior	2	A
ii. Multidirectional	2	A
iii. Adhesive capsulitis	2	A
II. Cartilage		
A. Articular (chondral, osteochondral)		
1. Basic Science*	1	B
2. Clinical		
a. Classification of Injury/Disease	1	B
i. Etiology		
aa. Traumatic	1	B
bb. Degenerative	1	B
cc. Inflammatory	1	B
dd. Other (tumor, infection, OCD, AVN)	1	B
ii. Location (size/depth)	1	B
b. Evaluation**	1	B

TOPIC	SCORE	
	Knowledge	Instruction
c. Management***		
i. Non-Operative^A		
aa. Traumatic	1	B
bb. Degenerative	1	B
cc. Inflammatory	2	B
dd. Other (OCD, etc.)	2	B
b. Operative^B		
aa. Traumatic	2	A
bb. Degenerative	2	A
cc. Inflammatory	2	A
dd. Other	2	C
B. Labral (superior, anterior, posterior)		
1. Basic Science*	1	B
2. Clinical		
a. Classification of Injury/Disease		
1. Traumatic (SLAP, Bankart)	1	A
2. Degenerative	1	A
b. Evaluation**	1	B
c. Management***		
i. Non-Operative^A	1	B
ii. Operative^B		
aa. Traumatic (SLAP, Bankart)	1	B
bb. Degenerative	2	B
III. Tendon (rotator cuff, biceps)		
A. Basic Science*	1	B
B. Clinical		
1. Classification of Injury/Disease		
a. Traumatic-tear	1	B
b. Inflammatory		
i. Mech. impingement	1	B
ii. Calcific tendonitis	1	B
iii. Assoc. pathology		
aa. GH arthritis (cuff arthopathy)	1	B
bb. AC joint arthritis	1	B
cc. Bicep tendon	1	B
dd. GH instability	1	B
c. Other - tumor	1	B
2. Evaluation**	1	B
3. Management***		
a. Non-Operative^A		
i. Impingement/tendonitis	1	B
ii. Rotator cuff tear (partial to full)	1	B
iii. Rotator cuff arthropathy	1	B
iv. Instability/tendonitis	1	B
v. Bicep tendonitis/rupture	1	B
b. Operative^B		
i. Impingement/tendonitis	1	A
ii. Rotator cuff tear (partial to full)	1	A
iii. Rotator cuff arthropathy	2	B
iv. Instability/tendonitis	1	A

TOPIC	SCORE	
	Knowledge	**Instruction**
v. Bicep tendonitis/rupture	1	A
IV. Muscle (extrinsic muscles [i.e. not rotator cuff] Pec major, deltoid, trapezius)		
A. Basic Science*	1	B
B. Clinical		
1. Classification of Injury/Disease (traumatic, inflammatory, tumor)	1	B
a. Traumatic		
b. Inflammatory		
c. Other - tumor		
2. Evaluation**	1	B
3. Management***		
a. Non-Operative^A		
i. Strains/ruptures (eg. pec major)	1	B
ii. Tumors	2	C
b. Operative^B		
i. Strains/ruptures	1	B
ii. Tumors	2	C
V. Bone (humerus)		
A. Basic Science*	1	B
B. Clinical		
1. Classification of Injury/Disease		
a. Traumatic (intra-articular, extra-articular)		
i. Stress fracture	1	B
ii. Macro fracture	1	B
b. Disease		
i. Metabolic	2	C
ii. Infectious	2	C
iii. Tumors	2	C
2. Evaluation**	1	B
3. Management***		
a. Non-Operative^A		
i. Traumatic		
aa. Intra-articular (glenohumeral)	1	B
bb. Extra-articular (humerus, tuberosities)	1	B
ii. Disease		
aa. Metabolic	2	C
bb. Infectious	2	C
cc. Tumors	2	C
b. Operative^B		
i. Traumatic		
aa. Intra-articular (glenohumeral)	2	B
bb. Extra-articular		
Humerus (stress function, macro function)	2	B
Tuberosities	2	B
IV. Nerve (Brachial plexus, peripheral, axillary, supra scapular nerve, long throacic nerve)		
A. Basic Science*	1	B
B. Clinical		
1. Classification of Injury/Disease		
a. Traumatic	2	C
b. Inflammatory	2	C
c. Other - tumor	2	C

TOPIC	SCORE	
	Knowledge	**Instruction**
2. Evaluation**	1	C
3. Management***		
a. Non-Operative^A		
i. Traumatic (neuropraxia to axonotmesis)		
aa. Brachial plexus	1	B
i. Stingers		
ii. Thoracic outlet	2	C
bb. Suprascapular nerve entrapment	2	B
cc. Long thoracic nerve	2	B
ii. Inflammatory		
aa. Brachial plexopathy	2	C
iii. Tumor	2	C
b. Operative^B		
i. Traumatic (neuropraxia to axonotmesis)		
aa. Brachial plexus	2	C
bb. Suprascapular nerve entrapment	2	C
cc. Long thoracic nerve	2	C
ii. Inflammatory	2	C
iii. Tumor	2	C
VII. Vessel (subclavian, axillary)		
A. Basic Science*	1	C
B. Clinical		
1. Classification of Injury/Disease		
a. Traumatic (rupture, external compression)	1	C
b. Inflammatory (included occlusion)	2	C
c. Tumor	2	C
2. Evaluation**	1	C
3. Management***		
a. Non-Operative^A		
i. Traumatic	1	C
ii. Inflammatory	2	C
iii. Tumor	2	C
b. Operative^B		
i. Traumatic	2	C
ii. Inflammatory	2	C
iii. Tumor	2	C
SHOULDER/acromioclavicular		
I. Ligament		
A. Basic Science*	1	B
B. Clinical		
1. Classification of Injury/Disease		
a. Traumatic (sprains/separations (I-IV))	1	B
b. Inflammatory	1	B
c. Tumor	1	B
2. Evaluation**	1	B
3. Management***		
a. Non-Operative^A		
i. Traumatic (sprains/strains)	1	B
ii. Inflammatory	1	B
iii. Tumor	2	C

TOPIC	SCORE	
	Knowledge	**Instruction**
b. Operative[B]		
i. Traumatic	1	B
ii. Inflammatory	1	B
iii. Tumor	2	C
II. Cartilage (articular, meniscal)		
A. Basic Science*	1	B
B. Clinical		
1. Classification of Injury/Disease		
a. Traumatic (post-traumatic, OA)	1	B
b. Inflammatory (DJD, osteolysis, etc.)	1	B
c. Tumor	2	C
2. Evaluation**		
3. Management***		
a. Non-Operative[A]		
i. Traumatic	1	B
ii. Inflammatory (DJD, osteolysis, etc.)	1	B
iii. Tumor	2	C
b. Operative[B]		
i. Traumatic	1	B
ii. Inflammatory	1	B
iii. Tumor	2	C
III. Tendon - Not applicable		
IV. Muscle - Not applicable		
V. Bone (includes acromion, clavicle and joint)		
A. Basic Science*	1	B
B. Clinical		
1. Classification of Injury/Disease		
a. Traumatic - fractures, non-unions		
i. Intra-articular	1	B
ii. Extra-articular	1	B
b. Inflammatory		
i. Osteolysis	1	B
ii. Os acromiale	1	B
c. Tumor	2	C
2. Evaluation**	1	B
3. Management***		
a. Non-Operative[A]		
i. Traumatic (fractures)		
aa. Intra-articular	1	B
bb. Extra-articular		
Clavicle	1	B
Acromion	1	B
ii. Inflammatory		
aa. Osteolysis	1	B
bb. Os acromiale	1	B
iii. Tumor	2	C
b. Operative[B]		
i. Traumatic (fracture)		
aa. Intra-articular	2	C

TOPIC	SCORE	
	Knowledge	Instruction
bb. Extra-articular		
Clavicule	1	B
Acromion	1	B
ii. Tumor	2	C

VI. Nerve

VII. Vessel

SHOULDER/scapulothoracic

I. Ligament - Not applicable

II. Cartilage - Not applicable

III. Tendon - Not applicable

IV. Muscle -

A. Basic Science*	2	C
B. Clinical		
1. Classification of Injury/Disease		
a. Traumatic	1	B
b. Inflammatory	1	B
c. Tumor	2	C
2. Evaluation**		
3. Management***		
a. Non-Operative[A]		
i. Traumatic	2	C
ii. Inflammatory	2	C
iii. Tumor	2	C
b. Operative[B]		
i. Traumatic	2	C
ii. Inflammatory	2	C
iii. Tumor	2	C

V. Bone

A. Basic Science*	2	C
B. Clinical		
1. Classification of Injury/Disease		
a. Traumatic fractures		
i. Scapula fractures	1	B
ii. Rib fractures	1	B
b. Inflammatory (bursitis)	1	B
c. Tumor	2	C
2. Evaluation**	1	B
3. Management***		
a. Non-Operative[A]		
i. Traumatic	2	C
aa. Scapula fracture	1	C
bb. Rib fracture	1	C
ii. Inflammatory (bursitis)	1	C
iii. Tumor	2	C
b. Operative[B]		
i. Traumatic	2	C
aa. Scapula fracture	2	C
bb. Rib fracture	2	C
ii. Inflammatory (bursitis)	2	C
iii. Tumor	2	C

TOPIC	SCORE	
	Knowledge	**Instruction**
VI. Nerve		
A. Basic Science*	1	B
B. Clinical		
1. Classification of Injury/Disease		
a. Traumatic (winging of the scapula)	1	B
b. Inflammatory	1	B
c. Tumor	2	C
2. Evaluation**	1	B
3. Management***		
a. Non-Operative[A]	1	B
b. Operative[B]	1	B
VII. Vessel - See Glenohumeral Joint		
SHOULDER/sternoclavicular		
I. Ligament		
A. Basic Science*	1	B
B. Clinical		
1. Classification of Injury/Disease		
a. Traumatic	1	B
b. Inflammatory	1	B
c. Other - tumor	2	C
2. Evaluation**	1	B
3. Management***		
a. Non-Operative[A]		
i. Traumatic		
aa. Strains/sprains	1	B
ii. Inflammatory	1	C
iii. Tumor	2	C
b. Operative[B]		
i. Traumatic		
aa. Strains/sprains	2	C
ii. Inflammatory	2	C
iii. Tumor	2	C
II. Cartilage		
A. Basic Science*	1	B
B. Clinical		
1. Classification of Injury/Disease		
a. Traumatic	1	B
b. Inflammatory	1	B
c. Other - tumor	2	C
2. Evaluation**	1	B
3. Management***		
a. Non-Operative[A]		
i. Traumatic	1	B
ii. Inflammatory (arthritis,infection)	1	B
iii. Tumor	2	C
b. Operative[B]		
i. Traumatic	2	C
ii. Inflammatory	2	C
iii. Tumor	2	C
III. Tendon - Not applicable		

TOPIC	SCORE	
	Knowledge	**Instruction**
IV. Muscle - Not applicable		
V. Bone		
A. Basic Science*	1	B
B. Clinical		
1. Classification of Injury/Disease		
a. Traumatic	1	B
b. Inflammatory	1	B
c. Other - tumor	2	C
2. Evaluation**	1	B
3. Management***		
a. Non-Operative[A]		
i. Traumatic (fractures)		
aa. Intra-articular	1	B
bb. Epiphyseal	1	B
ii. Inflammatory	1	B
iii. Tumor	2	C
b. Operative[B]		
i. Traumatic	2	C
ii. Inflammatory	2	C
iii. Tumor	2	C
VI. Nerve - See Glenohumeral Joint		
VII. Vessel - See Glenohumeral Joint		

TOPIC	SCORE	
	Knowledge	**Instruction**

ELBOW

I. Ligament

    A. Basic Science*   1   B

    B. Clinical

        1. Classification of Injury/Disease   1   B

        2. Evaluation**   1   A

        3. Management***

             a. Non-Operative[A]

                  i. Acute medial rupture   1   B

                  ii. Chronic medial instability   2   B

                  iii. Dislocations   1   C

             b. Operative[B]

                  i. Acute medial rupture   2   B

                  ii. Acute lateral rupture   2   B

                  iii. Chronic medial instability   2   B

                  iv. Dislocation   2   C

II. Cartilage

    A. Basic Science*   1   C

    B. Clinical

        1. Classification of Injury/Disease

             a. OCD (Loose bodies)   1   B

             b. DJD   2   C

        2. Evaluation**   1   B

        3. Management***

             a. Non-Operative[A]

                  i. OCD   1   B

                  ii. DJD   2   C

             b. Operative[B] (open/arthroscopic)

                  i. OCD   2   B

                  ii. DJD   2   C

III. Tendon

    A. Basic Science*   1   B

    B. Clinical

        1. Classification of Injury/Disease

             a. Epicondylitis   1   B

             b. Biceps/triceps - tendinitis   1   B

             c. Biceps/triceps - ruptures   1   B

        2. Evaluation**   1   B

        3. Management***

             a. Non-Operative[A]

                  i. Lateral epicondylitis   1   B

                  ii. Medial (Flexor/Pronator) tendinitis 1   B

                  iii. Biceps tendinitis/triceps   1   C

                  iv. Tendon rupture   1   C

TOPIC	SCORE	
	Knowledge	**Instruction**
b. Operative^B		
i. Lateral epicondylitis	2	B
ii. Medial tendinitis	2	B
iii. Biceps rupture	2	B
iv. Tendon rupture	2	B
IV. Muscle - Not applicable		
V. Bone		
A. Basic Science*	1	B
B. Clinical		
1. Classification of Injury/Disease		
a. Supracondylar fracture	1	C
b. Radial head fracture	1	C
c. Olecranon fracture	1	C
2. Evaluation**	1	B
3. Management***		
a. Non-Operative^A		
i. Supracondylar fracture	1	B
ii. Radial head fracture	1	B
iii. Olecranon fracture	1	B
iv. Coronoid fracture	1	B
v. Tumors (benign)	2	C
b. Operative^B		
i. Supracondylar fracture	2	C
ii. Radial head fracture	2	B
iii. Olecranon fracture	2	C
iv. Coronoid fracture	2	C
v. Tumors (benign)	2	C
vi. Tumors (malignant)	2	C
VI. Nerve		
A. Basic Science*	1	B
B. Clinical		
1. Classification of Injury/Disease	1	B
2. Evaluation**	1	B
3. Management***		
a. Non-Operative^A		
i. Ulnar nerve entrapment	2	B
ii. Posterior interosseous nerve entrapment	2	B
b. Operative^B		
i. Ulnar nerve entrapment	2	B
ii. Posterior interosseous nerve entrapment	2	C
VII. Vessel - Not applicable		

TOPIC	SCORE	
	Knowledge	Instruction

WRIST/HAND

I. Ligament

    A. Basic Science*   1   B

    B. Clinical

        1. Classification of Injury/Disease

            a. Carpal instability   2   B

            b. Thumb MCP instability   2   B

        2. Evaluation**   1   B

        3. Management***

            a. Non-Operative[A]

                i. Wrist sprain   1   B

                ii. DRUJ sprain   2   B

                iii. Thumb MCP sprain   1   B

                iv. Finger sprain   1   C

                v. Finger dislocation   1   C

            b. Operative[B]

                i. Wrist instability (acute/chronic)   2   C

                ii. DRUJ instability (acute/chronic)   2   C

                iii. Skier's thumb (Thumb UCL Sprain)   2   B

                iv. Thumb RCL sprain   2   C

                v. Finger dislocation   1   C

II. Cartilage

    A. Basic Science*   1   B

    B. Clinical

        1. Classification of Injury/Disease   2   C

        2. Evaluation**   1   B

        3. Management***

            a. Non-Operative[A]

                i. TFC tear   2   B

                ii. DJD - thumb - CMC   2   C

                iii. DJD - carpals   2   C

                iv. DJD - fingers   2   C

            b. Operative[B] (open/arthroscopic)

                i. TFC tears   2   B

                ii. DJD - thumb - CMC   2   C

                iii. DJD - fingers   2   C

III. Tendon

    A. Basic Science*   1   B

    B. Clinical

        1. Classification of Injury/Disease

            a. Hand lacerations   1   B

        2. Evaluation**   1   B

        3. Management***

            a. Non-Operative[A]

                i. DeQuervain's   2   C

                ii. Flexor strains   2   B

                iii. Extensor strains   2   B

                iv. Mallet finger   1   C

TOPIC	SCORE	
	Knowledge	**Instruction**
v. Lacerations	2	B
vi. Trigger finger	2	C
b. Operative[B]		
i. DeQuervain's	2	C
ii. Mallet finger	2	B
iii. Lacerations	2	C
iv. Trigger finger	2	C
IV. Muscle		
V. Bone		
A. Basic Science*	1	B
B. Clinical		
1. Classification of Injury/Disease		
a. Distal radial	1	B
b. Thumb MC	2	B
c. Finger	1	C
d. Scaphoid	1	C
2. Evaluation**	1	B
3. Management***		
a. Non-Operative[A]		
i. Distal radial fracture	1	B
ii. Scaphoid fracture	2	B
iii. Hamate fracture	2	B
iv. Thumb MC fracture	2	B
v. MC fracture	2	C
vi. Phalanx fracture	1	C
vii. Lunate AVN (Kienbock's)	2	C
viii. Tumors (benign)	2	C
b. Operative[B]		
i. Distal radial fracture	1	B
ii. Scaphoid fracture	2	C
iii. Hamate fracture	2	B
iv. Thumb MC fracture	1	C
v. Phalanx fracture	1	C
vi. Lunate AVN	2	C
vii. Tumors (benign)	2	C
viii. Tumors (malignant)	2	C
VI. Nerve		
A. Basic Science*	1	B
B. Clinical		
1. Classification of Injury/Disease	1	C
2. Evaluation**	1	B
3. Management***		
a. Non-Operative[A]		
i. Carpal tunnel	1	C
ii. Ulnar nerve compression	1	C
b. Operative[B]		
i. Carpal tunnel	2	B
ii. Ulnar nerve compression	2	C
iii. Digital nerve laceration	2	C
VII. Vessel		

TOPIC	SCORE	
	Knowledge	Instruction
A. Basic Science*	1	B
B. Clinical		
1. Evaluation**	1	B
2. Management***		
a. Non-Operative[A]		
i. Raynaud's Syndrome	2	C
ii. Thrombosis	2	C
iii. Laceration	1	C
b. Operative[B]		
i. Laceration	2	C

TOPIC	SCORE	
	Knowledge	Instruction

HIP

I. Ligament

    A. Basic Science*

    B. Clinical

        1. Classification of Injury/Disease

            a. SI sprain

            b. Hip subluxation/dislocation

            c. Osteitis pubis

        2. Evaluation**

        3. Management***

            a. Non-Operative[A]

                i. Ligamentous sprain

                ii. SI joint sprain

                iii. Osteitis pubis

            b. Operative[B]

                i. Osteitis pubis

Topic	Knowledge	Instruction
I. Ligament A. Basic Science*	1	B
a. SI sprain	1	B
b. Hip subluxation/dislocation	1	B
c. Osteitis pubis	1	B
2. Evaluation**	1	B
i. Ligamentous sprain	1	B
ii. SI joint sprain	1	B
iii. Osteitis pubis	1	B
i. Osteitis pubis (Operative)	2	C

II. Cartilage and Labral Injuries

    A. Basic Science*

    B. Clinical

        1. Classification of Injury/Disease

        2. Evaluation**

        3. Management***

            a. Non-Operative[A]

                i. Loose bodies

                ii. Chondral lesions

                iii. Degenerative arthritis

                iv. Labral tear

            b. Operative[B]

                i. Loose bodies

                ii. Chondral lesions

                iii. Degenerative arthritis

                iv. Labral tear

Topic	Knowledge	Instruction
II. Cartilage and Labral Injuries A. Basic Science*	1	B
2. Evaluation**	1	B
i. Loose bodies	1	B
ii. Chondral lesions	1	B
iii. Degenerative arthritis	1	B
iv. Labral tear	1	B
i. Loose bodies (Operative)	2	C
ii. Chondral lesions (Operative)	2	C
iii. Degenerative arthritis (Operative)	2	C
iv. Labral tear (Operative)	2	C

III. Tendon

    A. Basic Science*

    B. Clinical

        1. Classification of Injury/Disease

        2. Evaluation**

        3. Management***

            a. Non-Operative[A]

                i. Greater trochanteric bursitis

                ii. Snapping hip syndrome

            b. Operative[B]

                i. Greater trochanteric bursitis

                ii. Snapping hip syndrome

Topic	Knowledge	Instruction
III. Tendon A. Basic Science*	1	B
2. Evaluation**	1	B
i. Greater trochanteric bursitis	1	B
ii. Snapping hip syndrome	1	B
i. Greater trochanteric bursitis (Operative)	2	C
ii. Snapping hip syndrome (Operative)	2	C

TOPIC	SCORE	
	Knowledge	**Instruction**
IV. Muscle		
A. Basic Science*	1	B
B. Clinical		
1. Classification of Injury/Disease		
a. Strain	1	B
b. Contusion	1	B
2. Evaluation**	1	B
3. Management***		
a. Non-Operative[A]		
i. Strain	1	B
ii. Contusion	1	B
V. Bone		
A. Basic Science*		
B. Clinical		
1. Classification of Injury/Disease		
a. Pelvic ring fractures	1	B
b. Avulsion fractures	1	B
c. Hip fractures	1	B
d. Stress fractures	1	B
e. Hip dislocations	1	B
f. Avascular necrosis	1	B
g. Slipped capital femoral epiphysis	1	B
2. Evaluation**		
3. Management***		
a. Non-Operative[A]		
i. Pelvic ring fractures	1	B
ii. Avulsion fractures	1	B
iii. Acetabular fractures	1	B
iv. Femoral head fractures	1	B
v. Femoral neck fracture	1	B
vi. Trochaneric fractures	1	B
vii. Hip dislocation	1	B
viii. Avascular necrosis	1	B
ix. Slipped capital femoral epiphysis	1	B
b. Operative[B]		
i. Pelvic ring fractures	2	C
ii. Avulsion fractures	2	C
iii. Acetabular fractures	2	C
iv. Femoral head fractures	2	C
v. Femoral neck fracture	2	C
vi. Pertrochaneric fractures	2	C
vii. Hip dislocation	2	C
viii. Avascular necrosis	2	C
ix. Slipped capital femoral epiphysis	2	C
VI. Nerve		
A. Basic Science*	1	B
B. Clinical		
1. Classification of Injury/Disease		
2. Evaluation**	1	B
3. Management***		

TOPIC	SCORE	
	Knowledge	**Instruction**
a. Non-Operative[A]		
i. Femoral nerve	1	B
ii. Sciatic nerve	1	B
iii. Obturator nerve	1	B
b. Operative[B]		
i. Femoral nerve	2	C
ii. Sciatic nerve	2	C
iii. Obturator nerve	2	C
VII. Vascular Injuries		
A. Basic Science*	1	B
B. Clinical		
1. Classification of Injury/Disease		
2. Evaluation**	1	B
3. Management***		
a. Non-Operative[A]		
i. Femoral artery and vein	1	B
b. Operative[B]		
i. Femoral artery and vein	2	C

TOPIC	SCORE	
	Knowledge	Instruction
KNEE/tibiofemoral		
I. Ligament (ACL, PCL, MCL, LCL/posterolateral corner)		
A. Basic Science*	1	B
B. Clinical		
1. Classification of Injury/Disease (traumatic, inflammatory, tumor)	1	B
2. Evaluation**	1	B
3. Management***		
a. Non-Operative[A]		
i. Isolated		
aa. ACL	1	A
bb. PCL	1	A
cc. MCL	1	A
dd. LCL/Posterolateral	1	A
ii. Combined injuries	1	A
iii. Dislocated knee	2	A
iv. Arthritis/Instability	2	A
b. Operative[B]		
i. Isolated		
aa. ACL	1	A
bb. PCL	2	A
cc. MCL	2	A
dd. Posterolateral	2	A
ii. Combined injuries		
aa. ACL/medial	2	A
bb. ACL/lateral	2	A
cc. PCL/medial	2	A
dd. PCL/lateral	2	A
iii. Dislocated knee	2	A
iv. Arthritis/Instability	2	A
II. Cartilage/Articular (chondral, osteochondral)		
A. Basic Science*	1	B
B. Clinical		
1. Classification of Injury/Disease	1	B
a. Etiology		
i. Traumatic	1	C
ii. Degenerative	1	C
iii. Inflammatory	1	C
iv. Tumor	1	C
v. Other	1	C
b. Timing		
i. Acute versus chronic		
c. Location		
i. Depth/size		
2. Evaluation**	1	B
3. Management***		
a. Non-Operative[A]	1	B
b. Operative[B]		
i. Traumatic (acute/chronic)		
aa. Chondral	1	A

TOPIC	SCORE	
	Knowledge	**Instruction**
bb. Osteochondral	1	A
ii. Degenerative	1	A
iii. Inflammatory	1	A
III. Meniscal		
A. Basic Science*	1	B
B. Clinical		
1. Classification of Injury/Disease (see articular cartilage)	1	B
2. Evaluation**	1	B
3. Management***		
a. Non-Operative^A	1	B
b. Operative^B		
i. Meniscectomy	1	A
ii. Meniscal repair	1	A
iii. Meniscal replacement	2	A
IV. Tendon (quadriceps, patellar, hamstring, popliteus)		
A. Basic Science*	1	B
B. Clinical		
1. Classification of Injury/Disease (traumtic, inflammatory, other)	1	B
2. Evaluation**	1	B
3. Management***		
a. Non-Operative^A		
i. Traumatic		
aa. Partial tear	1	B
bb. Complete tear	1	B
ii. Inflammatory (tendinitis, bursitis)		
aa. Acute	1	B
bb. Chronic	1	B
iii. Other	2	C
b. Operative^B		
i. Traumatic		
aa. Partial tear	2	B
bb. Complete tear	2	B
ii. Inflammatory (tendinitis, bursitis)		
aa. Acute	2	B
bb. Chronic	2	B
iii. Other	2	C
V. Muscle (thigh, lower leg)		
A. Basic Science*	1	B
B. Clinical		
1. Classification of Injury/Disease		
a. Traumatic		
i. Strain	1	B
ii. Contusion	1	B
b. Inflammatory	1	B
c. Disease	1	B
2. Evaluation**	1	B
3. Management***		
a. Non-Operative^A		
i. Traumatic		
aa. Strain	1	B

TOPIC			SCORE	
			Knowledge	Instruction
		bb. Contusion	1	B
		cc. Compartment syndrome - chronic & acute	1	B
	ii. Inflammatory			
		aa. Post exercise	1	B
	iii. Disease			
		aa. Tumor	2	C
		bb. Infection	2	C
		cc. Neuropathic	2	C
b. Operative[B]				
	i. Traumatic			
		aa. Strain	2	B
		bb. Contusion	2	B
	ii. Inflammatory		2	C
	iii. Disease			
		aa. Tumor	2	C
		bb. Infection	2	C
		cc. Neuropathic	2	C
VI. Bone (femur, intra-articular, tibia, fibula)				
A. Basic Science*			2	B
B. Clinical				
1. Classification of Injury/Disease				
a. Traumatic (intra-articular, extra-articular)				
	i. Fracture		1	B
	ii. Stress fracture		1	B
b. Disease				
	i. Metabolic		1	B
	ii. Infectious		1	B
	iii. Tumors		2	C
2. Evaluation**			1	B
3. Management***				
a. Non-Operative[A]				
	i. Traumatic			
		aa. Fracture	1	B
		bb. Stress fracture	1	B
	ii. Disease			
		aa. Metabolic	2	C
		bb. Infectious	2	C
		cc. Tumors	2	C
b. Operative[B]				
	i. Traumatic			
		aa. Fracture	1	B
		bb. Stress fracture	1	B
	ii. Disease			
		aa. Metabolic	2	C
		bb. Infectious	2	C
		cc. Tumors	2	C
VII. Nerve (sciatic, femoral, tibial, peroneal)				
A. Basic Science*			1	C
B. Clinical				
1. Classification of Injury/Disease (traumatic, inflammatory)			1	C

TOPIC	SCORE	
	Knowledge	Instruction
2. Evaluation**	1	C
3. Management***		
a. Non-Operative^A		
i. Injury		
aa. Rupture	2	C
bb. Entrapment	2	C
ii. Disease		
aa. Inflammatory	2	C
bb. Tumor	2	C
iii. Other		
b. Operative^B		
i. Injury		
aa. Rupture	2	C
bb. Entrapment	2	C
ii. Disease		
aa. Inflammatory	2	C
bb. Tumor	2	C
VIII. Vessel (popliteal, geniculates, tibial)		
A. Basic Science*	2	C
B. Clinical		
1. Classification of Injury/Disease		
a. Traumatic	1	B
b. Inflammatory	1	B
c. Tumor	2	C
2. Evaluation**	1	B
3. Management***		
a. Non-Operative^A		
i. Traumatic		
aa. Partial rupture (intimal tear)	1	B
bb. Complete	1	B
ii. Inflammatory (incl. occlusion) (e.g. PUT, arterial orcle)	1	C
iii. Tumors	2	C
b. Operative^B		
i. Traumatic		
aa. Partial rupture (intimal tear)	2	C
bb. Complete	2	C
ii. Inflammatory (incl. occlusion)	2	C
iii. Tumors	2	C
KNEE/patellofemoral		
I. Ligament (ACL, PCL, MCL, LCL/posterolateral corner)		
A. Basic Science*	1	B
B. Clinical		
1. Classification of Injury/Disease(traumatic, inflammatory, tumor)	1	B
2. Evaluation**	1	B
3. Management***		
a. Non-Operative^A		
i. Isolated		
aa. ACL	1	A
bb. PCL	1	A
cc. MCL	1	A

TOPIC	SCORE Knowledge	Instruction
dd. LCL/Posterolateral	1	A
ii. Combined injuries	1	A
iii. Dislocated knee	2	A
iv. Arthritis/Instability	2	A
b. Operative[B]		
i. Isolated		
aa. ACL	1	A
bb. PCL	2	A
cc. MCL	2	A
dd. Posterolateral	2	A
ii. Combined injuries		
aa. ACL/medial	2	A
bb. ACL/lateral	2	A
cc. PCL/medial	2	A
dd. PCL/lateral	2	A
iii. Dislocated knee	2	A
iv. Arthritis/Instability	2	A
II. Cartilage/Articular (chondral, osteochondral)		
A. Basic Science*	1	B
B. Clinical		
1. Classification of Injury/Disease	1	B
a. Etiology		
i. Traumatic	1	C
ii. Degenerative	1	C
iii. Inflammatory	1	C
iv. Tumor	1	C
v. Other	1	C
b. Timing		
i. Acute vs. chronic	1	B
c. Location		
i. Depth/size	1	B
2. Evaluation**	1	B
3. Management***		
a. Non-Operative[A]	1	B
b. Operative[B]		
i. Traumatic (acute/chronic)		
aa. Chondral	1	A
bb. Osteochondral	1	A
ii. Degenerative	1	A
iii. Inflammatory	1	A
III. Meniscal		
A. Basic Science*	1	B
B. Clinical		
1. Classification of Injury/Disease (see articular cartilage)	1	B
2. Evaluation**	1	B
3. Management***		
a. Non-Operative[A]	1	B
b. Operative[B]		
i. Meniscectomy	1	A
ii. Meniscal repair	1	A

TOPIC	SCORE	
	Knowledge	**Instruction**
iii. Meniscal replacement	2	A
IV. Tendon (quadriceps, patellar, hamstring, popliteus)		
A. Basic Science*	1	B
B. Clinical		
1. Classification of Injury/Disease (traumatic, inflammatory, other)	1	B
2. Evaluation**	1	B
3. Management***		
a. Non-Operative^A		
i. Traumatic		
aa. Partial tear	1	B
bb. Complete tear	1	B
ii. Inflammatory (tendinitis, bursitis)		
aa. Acute	1	B
bb. Chronic	1	B
iii. Other	2	C
b. Operative^B		
i. Traumatic		
aa. Partial tear	2	B
bb. Complete tear	2	B
ii. Inflammatory (tendinitis, bursitis)		
aa. Acute	2	B
bb. Chronic	2	B
iii. Other	2	C
V. Muscle (thigh, lower leg)		
A. Basic Science*	1	B
B. Clinical		
1. Classification of Injury/Disease		
a. Traumatic		
i. Strain	1	B
ii. Contusion	1	B
b. Inflammatory	1	B
c. Disease	1	B
2. Evaluation**	1	B
3. Management***		
a. Non-Operative^A		
i. Traumatic		
aa. Strain	1	B
bb. Contusion	1	B
cc. Compartment syndrome - chronic & acute	1	B
ii. Inflammatory		
aa. Post exercise	1	B
iii. Disease		
aa. Tumor	2	C
bb. Infection	2	C
cc. Neuropathic	2	C
b. Operative^B		
i. Traumatic		
aa. Strain	2	B
bb. Contusion	2	B
ii. Inflammatory	2	C

TOPIC	SCORE	
	Knowledge	Instruction
iii. Disease		
aa. Tumor	2	C
bb. Infection	2	C
cc. Neuropathic	2	C
VI. Bone (femur, intra-articular, tibia, fibula)		
A. Basic Science*	2	B
B. Clinical		
1. Classification of Injury/Disease	1	B
a. Traumatic (intra-articular, extra-articular)		
i. Fracture		
ii. Stress fracture		
b. Disease		
i. Metabolic		
ii. Infectious		
iii. Tumors		
2. Evaluation**	1	B
3. Management***		
a. Non-Operative[A]		
i. Traumatic		
aa. Fracture	1	B
bb. Stress fracture	1	B
ii. Disease		
aa. Metabolic	2	C
bb. Infectious	2	C
cc. Tumors	2	C
b. Operative[B]		
i. Traumatic		
aa. Fracture	1	B
bb. Stress fracture	1	B
ii. Disease		
aa. Metabolic	2	C
bb. Infectious	2	C
cc. Tumors	2	C
VII. Nerve (sciatic, femoral, tibial, peroneal)		
A. Basic Science*	1	C
B. Clinical		
1. Classification of Injury/Disease (traumatic, inflammatory)	1	C
2. Evaluation**	1	C
3. Management***		
a. Non-Operative[A]		
i. Injury		
aa. Rupture	2	C
bb. Entrapment	2	C
ii. Disease		
aa. Inflammatory	2	C
bb. Tumor	2	C
iii. Other		
b. Operative[B]		
i. Injury		
aa. Rupture	2	C

TOPIC	SCORE	
	Knowledge	**Instruction**
bb. Entrapment	2	C
ii. Disease		
aa. Inflammatory	2	C
bb. Tumor	2	C
VIII. Vessel (popliteal, geniculates, tibial)		
A. Basic Science*	2	C
B. Clinical		
1. Classification of Injury/Disease		
a. Traumatic	1	B
b. Inflammatory	1	B
c. Tumor	2	C
2. Evaluation**	1	B
3. Management***		
a. Non-Operative[A]		
i. Traumatic		
aa. Partial rupture (intimal tear)	1	B
bb. Complete	1	B
ii. Inflammatory (incl. occlusion) (e.g. PUT, arterial orcle)	1	C
iii. Tumors	2	C
b. Operative[B]		
i. Traumatic		
aa. Partial rupture (intimal tear)	2	C
bb. Complete	2	C
ii. Inflammatory (incl. occlusion)	2	C
iii. Tumors	2	C

TOPIC	SCORE	
	Knowledge	Instruction

TIBIA/FIBULA (proximal)

I. Ligament - Not applicable

II. Cartilage - Not applicable

III. Tendon - Not applicable

IV. Muscle

	Knowledge	Instruction
A. Basic Science*	1	B
B. Clinical		
1. Classification of Injury/Disease		
2. Evaluation**	1	B
3. Management***		
a. Non-Operative[A]		
i. Posterior tibial tendonitis	1	B
ii. Peroneal tendonitis	1	B
iii. Compartment syndromes	1	B
iv. Gastrocsoleus muscle tendon injuries	1	B
b. Operative[B]		
i. Posterior tibial tendonitis	1	A
ii. Peroneal tendonitis	1	A
iii. Compartment syndromes	1	A
iv. Gastrocsoleus muscle tendon injuries	1	A

V. Bone

	Knowledge	Instruction
A. Basic Science*	1	B
B. Clinical		
1. Classification of Injury/Disease		
a. Fractures of the lower leg	1	B
2. Evaluation**	1	B
3. Management***		
a. Non-Operative[A]		
i. Stress reactions	1	B
ii. Stress fractures	1	B
iii. Fractures	1	B
b. Operative[B]		
i. Stress fractures	1	A
ii. Fractures	1	A

VI. Nerve - Not applicable

VII. Vessel - Not applicable

TOPIC	SCORE	
	Knowledge	Instruction

ANKLE

I. Ligament

    A. Basic Science* — 1 — B

    B. Clinical

        1. Classification of Injury/Disease

        2. Evaluation** — 1 — B

        3. Management***

            a. Non-Operative^A

                i. Ankle sprains — 1 — B

            b. Operative^B

                i. Ankle sprains

                    aa. Acute — 1 — A

                    bb. Chronic — 1 — A

II. Cartilage

    A. Basic Science* — 1 — B

    B. Clinical

        1. Classification of Injury/Disease

            a. Traumatic

                i. OCD — 1 — B

                ii. Osteochondral fractures — 1 — B

                iii. Chondral injury — 1 — B

            b. Degenerative

                i. DJD — 1 — B

                ii. Loose bodies — 1 — B

        2. Evaluation** — 1 — B

        3. Management***

            a. Non-Operative^A — 1 — B

            b. Operative^B

                i. Open/arthroscopic — 1 — A

III. Tendon

    A. Basic Science* — 1 — B

    B. Clinical

        1. Classification of Injury/Disease

        2. Evaluation** — 1 — B

        3. Management***

            a. Non-Operative^A

                i. Tendonitis

                    aa. Achilles — 1 — B

                    bb. Posterior tibial — 1 — B

                    cc. Peroneal — 1 — B

                    dd. Bursitis — 1 — B

                    ee. Retrocalcaneal bursitis — 1 — B

            b. Operative^B

                i. Achilles tendon rupture/tendinitis — 1 — A

                ii. Posterior tibial tendinitis/rupture — 1 — A

                iii. Peroneal tendinitis/rupture — 1 — A

                iv. Retrocalcaneal bursitis — 1 — A

IV. Muscle

    A. Basic Science* — 1 — B

    B. Clinical

TOPIC	SCORE	
	Knowledge	Instruction
1. Classification of Injury/Disease		
2. Evaluation**	1	B
3. Management***		
a. Non-Operative^A		
i. Tendinitis		
aa. Achilles	1	B
bb. Posterior tibial	1	B
cc. Peroneal	1	B
ii. Bursitis	1	B
aa. Retrocalcaneal bursitis	1	B
b. Operative^B		
i. Tendinitis		
aa. Achilles tendinitis/rupture	1	A
ii. Posterior tibial tendinitis/rupture	1	A
iii. Peroneal tendinitis/rupture	1	A
ii. Bursitis		
iv. Retrocalcaneal	1	A
V. Bone		
A. Basic Science*	1	B
B. Clinical		
1. Classification of Injury/Disease		
2. Evaluation**	1	B
3. Management***		
a. Non-Operative^A		
i. Osteochondritis dissecans of the talus	1	B
ii. Talar dome fractures	1	B
iii. Stress reactions - talus	1	B
iv. Fracture - talus	1	B
v. Fracture - malleoli	1	B
b. Operative^B		
i. Osteochondritis dissecans of the talus	2	A
ii. Talar dome fractures	2	A
iii. Fracture - talus	1	A
iv. Fracture - malleoli	1	A
VI. Nerve - Posterior MB, Saphenous, Peroneal tarsal tunnel		
VII. Vessel - Not applicable		

TOPIC	SCORE	
	Knowledge	**Instruction**
FOOT		
I. Ligament		
A. Basic Science*	1	B
B. Clinical		
1. Classification of Injury/Disease		
2. Evaluation**	1	B
3. Management***		
a. Non-Operative[A]		
i. Mid-foot - sprains and diastasis (Lisfranc injuries)	1	B
ii. Plantar fascia	1	B
b. Operative[B]		
i. Mid-foot - sprains and diastasis (Lisfranc injuries)	2	A
ii. Plantar fascia	2	A
II. Cartilage - Chondral injuries		
DJD - Hallux rigidus	2	B
III. Tendon - Ruptures		
Flexor tendons	2	B
Extensor tendon	2	B
IV. Muscle - Compartment syndrome	2	B
V. Bone		
A. Basic Science*	1	B
B. Clinical		
1. Classification of Injury/Disease		
2. Evaluation**	1	B
3. Management***		
a. Non-Operative[A]		
i. Toe injuries		
aa. Turf toe	1	B
bb. Hallux rigidus	1	B
cc. Sesamoid injuries	1	B
ii. Forefoot injuries		
aa. MTP joint injuries	1	B
bb. Bunions	1	B
cc. Metatarsal stress fracture	1	B
dd. Fractures	1	B
ee. Fractures at the base of the 5th metatarsal	1	B
ff. Osteonecrosis	1	B
gg. Tarsal coalition	2	B
iii. Midfoot injuries		
aa. Stress fractures	1	B
bb. Accessory navicular	1	B

TOPIC	Knowledge	Instruction
	SCORE	

TOPIC	Knowledge	Instruction
iv. Hindfoot injuries		
aa. Pes planus	1	B
bb. Tarsal bossing	1	B
cc. Calcaneal stress fracture	1	B
dd. Plantar fasciitis	1	B
b. Operative[B]		
i. Toe injuries		
aa. Hallus rigidus	2	C
bb. Sesamoid injuries	2	C
ii. Forefoot injuries		
aa. Bunions	2	C
bb. Metatarsal stress fractures	2	C
cc. Fractures	2	C
dd. Fractures at the base of the 5th metatarsal	2	A
ee. Osteonecrosis	2	C
iii. Midfoot injuries		
aa. Stress fractures	2	C
bb. Accessory navicular	2	C
iv. Hindfoot injuries		
aa. Pes planus	2	C
bb. Tarsal bossing	2	C
cc. Calcaneal stress fracture	2	C
dd. Plantar fasciitis	2	A
VI. Nerve		
A. Basic Science*	1	B
B. Clinical		
1. Classification - nerve entrapment syndromes	1	B
2. Evaluation**	1	B
3. Management***		
a. Non-Operative[A]		
i. Interdigital neuroma	1	B
ii. Tarsal tunnel syndrome	1	B
b. Operative[B]		
i. Tarsal tunnel syndrome	2	C
VII. Vessel - Not applicable		
VIII. Skin		
A. Basic Science*	1	B
B. Clinical		
1. Evaluation**	1	B
2. Management***		
a. Non-Operative[A]		
i. Blisters	1	B
ii. Hard corns	1	B
iii. Soft corns	1	B
iv. Tinea pedis	1	B
v. Plantar warts	1	B
vi. Ingrown toenails	1	B
b. Operative[B]		
i. Blisters	2	A
ii. Hard corns	2	A

TOPIC	SCORE Knowledge	Instruction

CERVICAL SPINE
I. Ligament

A. Basic Science*	1	B
B. Clinical		
1. Classification of Injury/Disease	1	B
2. Evaluation**	1	B
3. Management***		
a. Non-Operative[A]		
i. Neck sprains	1	B
ii. Facet subluxation/dislocation	1	B
iii. Dislocation	1	B
b. Operative[B]		
i. Facet subluxations/dislocations	2	C

II. Cartilage - Not applicable
III. Tendon - Not applicable
IV. Muscle - Not applicable
V. Bone

A. Basic Science*	1	B
B. Clinical		
1. Classification of Injury/Disease	1	B
2. Evaluation**	1	B
3. Management***		
a. Non-Operative[A]		
i. C-1 fractures	1	B
ii. Odontoid fractures	1	B
iii. Spinous process fractures	1	B
iv. Fractures & dislocations of the cervical spine	1	B
v. Spinal Stenosis	2	C
b. Operative[B]		
i. C-1 fractures	2	C
ii. Odontoid fractures	2	C
iii. Spinous process fractures	2	C
iv. Fractures & dislocations of the cervical spine	2	C
v. Spinal Stenosis	2	C

VI. Nerve

A. Basic Science*	1	B
B. Clinical		
1. Classification of Injury/Disease	1	B
2. Evaluation**	1	B
3. Management***		
a. Non-Operative[A]		
i. Brachial plexus injuries		
aa. Burners & stingers	1	B
bb. Traumatic avulsions	1	B
cc. Herniated Disk	1	B
ii. Spinal cord injury to include paralysis	1	B
b. Operative[B]		
i. Brachial plexus injuries	2	C
ii. Spinal cord injury to include paralysis	2	C
iii. Herniated Disk	2	C

VII. Vessel - Not applicable

TOPIC	SCORE	
	Knowledge	Instruction
SPINE		
I. Ligament		
A. Basic Science*	1	B
B. Clinical		
1. Classification of Injury/Disease	1	B
2. Evaluation**	1	B
3. Management***		
a. Non-Operative[A]		
i. Thoracolumbar sprains	1	B
ii. Lumbosacral sprains	1	B
II. Cartilage - Not applicable		
III. Tendon - Not applicable		
IV. Muscle		
A. Basic Science*	1	B
B. Clinical		
1. Classification of Injury/Disease	1	B
2. Evaluation**	1	B
3. Management***		
a. Non-Operative[A]		
i. Strains	1	B
ii. Contusions	1	B
V. Bone		
A. Basic Science*	1	B
B. Clinical		
1. Classification of Injury/Disease		
2. Evaluation**	1	B
3. Management***		
a. Non-Operative[A]		
i. Kyphosis	1	B
ii. Scoliosis	1	B
iii. Spinous process fracture	1	B
iv. Vertebral compression fractures of the thoracolumbar spine	1	B
v. Fracture/dislocations of the thoracolumbar spine	1	B
vi. Spondylolysis	1	B
vii. Spondylolisthesis	1	B
viii. Spondylitis and sacroilliatis	1	B
b. Operative[B]		
i. Spinous process fractures	2	C
ii. Vertebral compression fractures of the thoracolumbar spine	2	C
iii. Fracture/dislocation of the thoracolumbar spine	2	C
iv. Spondylolysis	2	C
v. Spondylolisthesis	2	C
VI. Nerve		
A. Basic Science*	1	B
B. Clinical		
1. Classification of Injury/Disease		
2. Evaluation**	1	B
3. Management***		
a. Non-Operative[A]		
i. Sciatica	1	B
ii. HNP	1	B
b. Operative[B]		
i. HNP	2	C
VII. Vessel - Not applicable		

Index

f indicates figure
t indicates table

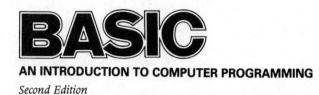

BASIC

AN INTRODUCTION TO COMPUTER PROGRAMMING

Second Edition

Brooks/Cole Series in Computer Science

Business BASIC
Robert J. Bent and George C. Sethares

BASIC: An Introduction to Computer Programming, Second Edition
Robert J. Bent and George C. Sethares

Beginning BASIC
D. K. Carver

Beginning Structured COBOL
D. K. Carver

FORTRAN with Problem Solving: A Structured Approach
Robert J. Bent and George C. Sethares